GRAINGER & ALLISON'S DIAGNOSTIC RADIOLOGY

Abdominal Imaging

SIXTH EDITION

GRAINGER & ALLISON'S DIAGNOSTIC RADIOLOGY

Abdominal Imaging

SIXTH EDITION

Michael M. Maher, MD, FRCSI, FRCR, FFR (RCSI)

Adrian K. Dixon, MD, MD(Hon caus), FRCP, FRCR, FRCS, FFRRCSI(Hon), FRANZCR(Hon), FACR(Hon), FMedSci

London   New York   Oxford   Philadelphia   St Louis   Sydney   Toronto

ELSEVIER

ISBN: 978-0-7020-6938-3

Executive Content Strategist: Michael Houston
Content Development Specialist: Louise Cook
Project Manager: Andrew Riley
Design: Christian Bilbow
Marketing Manager: Rachael Pignotti

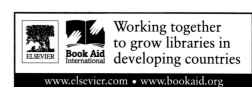

Working together
to grow libraries in
developing countries

www.elsevier.com • www.bookaid.org

Contents

PREFACE

The 20 chapters in this book have been selected from the contents of the Abdominal Imaging section in *Grainger & Allison's Diagnostic Radiology, Sixth Edition*. These chapters provide a succinct up-to-date overview of current imaging techniques and their clinical applications in daily practice and it is hoped that with this concise format the user will quickly grasp the fundamentals they need to know. Throughout these chapters, the relative merits of different imaging investigations are described, variations are discussed and recent imaging advances are detailed.

Grainger & Allison's Diagnostic Radiology has long been recognized as the standard general reference work in the field, and it is hoped that this book, utilizing the content from the latest sixth edition of this classic reference work, will provide radiology trainees and practitioners with ready access to the most current information, written by internationally recognized experts, on what is new and important in the radiological diagnosis of abdominal disorders.

LIST OF CONTRIBUTORS

Mohamed Abou El-Ghar, MD
Professor of Radiodiagnosis, Radiology Department, Urology and Nephrology Center, Mansoura University, Mansoura, Egypt

E. Jane Adam, MB, BS(Hons), MRCP, FRCR
Consultant Radiologist, St George's Healthcare NHS Trust, London, UK

Omar Agosto, MD
Clinical Assistant Professor, Diagnostic Radiology, Temple University School of Medicine; Director of Body MRI and Body CT, Diagnostic Radiology, Jeanes Hospital and Northeastern Ambulatory Care Center-Temple University Healthcare System, Philadelphia, PA, USA

Allan C. Andi, BSc(Hons), MRCS(Ed), FRCR
Consultant Radiologist, The Hillingdon Hospitals NHS Foundation Trust, London, UK

Susan M. Ascher, MD
Professor of Radiology, Georgetown University School of Medicine; Co-Director, Abdominal Imaging, Georgetown University Hospital, Washington, DC, USA

Jelle O. Barentsz, MD, PhD
Professor of Radiology, Department of Radiology, Prostate MR Reference Center, Radboud University Nijmegen Medical Center, Nijmegen, The Netherlands

Sue J. Barter, MBBS, MRCP, DMRD, FRCR, FRCP
Consultant Radiologist, Department of Radiology, Cambridge University Hospitals NHS Foundation Trust, Cambridge, UK

Lol Berman, FRCP, FRCR
Lecturer and Honorary Consultant, University Department of Radiology, Addenbrooke's Hospital, Cambridge, UK

Leonardo Kayat Bittencourt, MD
Radiologist, Department of Radiology, Federal University of Rio de Janeiro, Brazil

Joyce G.R. Bomers, MSc PhD
Candidate, Department of Radiology, Radboud University Nijmegen Medical Centre, Nijmegen, The Netherlands

Dina F. Caroline, MD, PhD
Professor of Radiology, Temple University Hospital, Philadelphia, PA, USA

Richard H. Cohan, BA, MD, FACR
Professor of Radiology, Department of Radiology, University of Michigan Hospital, Ann Arbor, MI, USA

Nigel C. Cowan, MA, MB, Bchir, FRCP, FRCR
Consultant Radiologist, The Manor Hospital, Oxford, UK

Maria Daskalogiannaki, MD, PhD
Consultant Radiologist, Radiology, University Hospital of Iraklion, Iraklion, Greece

Chandra Dass, MBBS, DMRD
Clinical Associate Professor, Department of Radiology, Temple University Hospital, Philadelphia, PA, USA

Tarek El-Diasty, MD
Professor of Radiology, Radiology Department, Urology and Nephrology Center, Mansoura University, Mansoura, Egypt

Alan H. Freeman, MBBS, FRCR
Consultant Radiologist, Department of Radiology, Addenbrooke's Hospital, Cambridge University Hospitals NHS Foundation Trust, Cambridge, UK

Susan Freeman, MRCP, FRCR
Consultant Radiologist, Department of Radiology, Cambridge University Hospitals NHS Foundation Trust, Cambridge, UK

Robert N. Gibson, MBBS, MD, FRANZCR, DDU
Professor, Department of Radiology, Royal Melbourne Hospital, Parkville, Victoria, Australia

Edmund M. Godfrey, MA, FRCR
Consultant Radiologist, Department of Radiology, Cambridge University Hospitals NHS Foundation Trust, Cambridge, UK

Nicholas Gourtsoyiannis, MD, PhD, FRCR(Hon), FRCSI(Hon)
Professor Emeritus, University of Crete, Medical School, Crete, Greece

Hedvig Hricak, MD, PhD, Dr(hc)
Chair, Department of Radiology, Memorial Sloan-
    Kettering Cancer Center, New York, NY, USA

Fleur Kilburn-Toppin, MA, MB, BChir, FRCR
Consultant Radiologist, West Suffolk Hospital,
    Bury St Edmunds, Suffolk, UK

David J. Lomas, MA, MB, BChir, FRCR, FRCP
Professor of Clinical MRI, University Radiology
    Department, Addenbrooke's Hospital, Cambridge,
    UK

Michael M. Maher, MD, FRCSI, FRCR, FFRRCSI
Professor of Radiology, University College Cork;
    Consultant Radiologist, Cork University Hospital
    and Mercy University Hospital, Cork, Ireland

Lorenzo Mannelli, MD, PhD
Radiologist, Department of Radiology, University of
    Washington, Seattle, WA, USA

**Patrick McLaughlin, MB BCh, BAO, BMedSc
FFRRCSI**
Lecturer in Radiology, Department of Radiology,
    University College Cork, Cork, Ireland

Lisa A. Miller, MD
Assistant Professor, Department of Diagnostic
    Radiology and Nuclear Medicine, University of
    Maryland Medical School, Baltimore, MD, USA

Stuart E. Mirvis, MD, FACR
Professor of Diagnostic Radiology; Director, Division
    of Emergency Radiology, Department of Radiology
    and Nuclear Medicine, University of Maryland
    School of Medicine, Baltimore, MD, USA

Robert A. Morgan, MB ChB, MRCP, FRCR, EBIR
Consultant Vascular and Interventional Radiologist,
    Radiology Department, St George's NHS Trust,
    London, UK

Iain D. Morrison, MBBS, MRCP, FRCR
Consultant Radiologist, Kent and Canterbury Hospital,
    East Kent Hospitals University NHS Foundation
    Trust, Canterbury, UK

**Owen J. O'Connor, MD, FFRRCSI, MB, BCh, BAO,
BMedSci**
Interventional Radiology Fellow, Radiology,
    Massachusetts General Hospital, Boston, MA, USA

Andrew Plumb, BMBCh, MRCP, FRCR
Research Fellow in Gastrointestinal Radiology,
    University College London Hospitals, London, UK

Panos Prassopoulos, MD, PhD
Professor of Radiology, Department of Radiology,
    University Hospital of Alexandroupoli, Democritous
    University of Thrace, Alexandroupoli, Greece

**Rodney H. Reznek, MA, FRANZCR(Hon),
FFRRCSI(Hon), FRCP, FRCR**
Emeritus Professor of Cancer Imaging, Cancer
    Institute, Queen Mary's University London,
    St Bartholomew's Hospital, West Smithfield,
    London, UK

Giles Rottenberg, MBBS, MRCP, FRCR
Consultant Radiologist, Department of Radiology,
    Guy's and St Thomas' NHS Foundation Trust,
    London, UK

Anju Sahdev, MBBS, MRCP, FRCR
Consultant Uro-Gynae Radiologist, Department of
    Imaging, St Bartholomew's Hospital, Barts Health,
    West Smithfield, London, UK

Evis Sala, MD, PhD, FRCR
University Lecturer and Honorary Consultant
    Radiologist, University Department of Radiology,
    Addenbrooke's Hospital, Cambridge, UK

Wolfgang Schima, MD, MSc
Professor, Department of Diagnostic and Interventional
    Radiology, KH Göttlicher Heiland Hospital; KH der
    Barmherzigen Schwestern Wien; Sankt Josef-
    Krankenhaus, Vienna, Austria

Nadeem Shaida, MRCP, FRCR, FHEA
Radiology Registrar, Department of Radiology,
    Cambridge University Hospitals NHS Foundation
    Trust, Cambridge, UK

Thomas Sutherland, MBBS, MMed, FRANZCR
Radiologist, Medical Imaging Department, St Vincent's
    Hospital, Melbourne, Victoria, Australia

Stuart A. Taylor, MBBS, BSc, MD, MRCP, FRCR
Professor of Medical Imaging, Centre for Medical
    Imaging, University College London, London, UK

Geert Villeirs, MD, PhD
Radiologist, Division of Genitourinary Radiology,
    Ghent University Hospital, Ghent, Belgium

Zaid Viney, MBBS, MRCP, FRCR
Consultant Radiologist, Department of Radiology,
    Guy's and St Thomas' NHS Foundation Trust,
    London, UK

Current Status of Imaging of the Gastrointestinal Tract: Imaging Techniques and Radiation Issues

Iain D. Morrison • Patrick McLaughlin • Michael M. Maher

CHAPTER OUTLINE

In this section on abdominal imaging, the imaging approach and appearances of lesions in the areas of the oesophagus, stomach, small bowel, large bowel, peritoneum, liver, biliary system and pancreas are covered in their respective chapters. In this chapter the relative merits of different imaging investigation are discussed, with most emphasis being placed on their utility in the acute abdominal pain setting. Issues regarding the radiation dose will be discussed. This becomes increasingly relevant now that computed tomography (CT) is frequently deployed early on in the management of patients with acute abdominal pain.

The plain abdominal radiograph (AXR) was for generations the staple investigation in the acute abdomen. Now there are many situations where CT or ultrasound (US) should be the first imaging investigation after clinical assessment of the patient. There are still scenarios where the AXR is very useful, and these will be discussed together with advice on interpretation, which can be difficult.

THE PLAIN ABDOMINAL RADIOGRAPH

For non-acute situations, the relatively small yield of information from a plain radiograph does not justify the radiation dose that it entails. There are exceptions, such as in the follow-up of renal calculi and in assessment of bowel transit times in constipation.

In the situation of the acute abdomen, a supine abdomen radiograph and an erect chest radiograph (CXR) can be regarded as the basic standard radiographs.

The erect CXR is invaluable in diagnosing visceral perforation since the X-ray beam is passing through any free gas under the diaphragm at an optimum angle, and at the correct exposure for visualisation. For this investigation the patient should ideally remain in the erect position for 10 min before radiography to allow time for any free gas to rise to the highest point, although this may not be achieved in practice. The supine radiograph should ideally be taken with an empty bladder, and should include the area from the diaphragm to the hernial orifices, which in practice means that the obturator foramina should be included.

Historically, an erect abdominal radiograph was performed additionally for the acute abdomen in order to assess the number and length of any fluid levels within bowel. This was thought to distinguish between obstruction and ileus. However, this distinction is highly unreliable, and evidence shows that the erect abdominal radiograph can be misleading.[1] The erect CXR appearances can be confusing when looking for free peritoneal gas, as discussed later in this chapter. Occasionally a left lateral decubitus radiograph can clarify, since small amounts of gas can be seen over the liver if there has been a perforation.

In the acute abdominal setting, plain radiography should only be requested in situations where it is likely to yield useful and not misleading information. Plain radiography is useful in diagnosing perforation of a viscus, and for assessing bowel dilatation (the main valid indications; see Table 1-1). Plain abdominal radiography is not helpful in diagnosing the common inflammatory conditions of the abdomen such as appendicitis,

TABLE 1-1 **Indications for Plain Radiographs in the Acute Abdomen**

Suspected viscus perforation
Bowel obstruction
Assessment of bowel wall pattern (e.g. ischaemia, colitis)
Intra-abdominal foreign body

TABLE 1-2 **Conditions That Can Simulate a Pneumoperitoneum**

Intestine between liver and diaphragm (Chilaiditi syndrome)
Subphrenic abscess
Curvilinear atelectasis in lung
Diaphragmatic irregularity/multiple humps
Subdiaphragmatic fat
Cysts in pneumatosis intestinalis

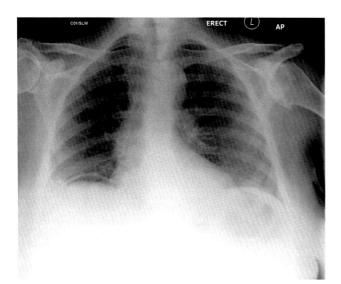

FIGURE 1-1 ■ Pneumoperitoneum. Erect chest radiograph. Free gas is seen between the liver and right hemidiaphragm.

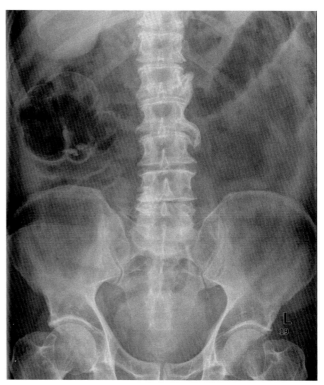

FIGURE 1-2 ■ Pneumoperitoneum in a patient with ulcerative colitis. Supine abdominal radiograph. Abnormal gas can be seen in the right upper quadrant (RUQ) over the liver. There is Rigler's sign with gas on both sides of the bowel wall in the RUQ.

diverticulitis, cholecystitis and pancreatitis. For this reason, plain radiography should be avoided in these situations unless there is the suspicion of perforation or bowel dilatation. Clinical assessment, US and CT all play a role in these inflammatory conditions.

ABNORMAL GAS DISTRIBUTION

Pneumoperitoneum

When analysing a plain radiograph of the abdomen, it is important to be able to attribute all the gas to normal anatomical structures, namely viscera. There are numerous causes for gas in abnormal places; the most frequent is pneumoperitoneum, but other causes include gas in the retroperitoneum, gall bladder, biliary tree, liver, kidneys, bladder and abscesses.

The presence of free intra-abdominal gas almost always indicates perforation of a viscus, for instance a peptic ulcer. Other causes include obstruction, inflammatory conditions, bowel ischaemia and colonoscopy. About 70% of perforated peptic ulcers will demonstrate free gas, a phenomenon rarely seen in the case of a perforated appendix. Small amounts of gas are detectable under the right hemidiaphragm on an erect CXR, outlining the smooth surface of the liver clearly (Fig. 1-1), but on the left it can be difficult to distinguish free gas from stomach and colonic gas. The diaphragm is seen as a relatively thin structure outlined by gas below, and lung above. The gas

under the right and left hemidiaphragms may join across the middle (cupola sign). There are many circumstances when interpretation of an erect CXR is difficult. Table 1-2 lists the most frequent situations when the radiologist or clinician may be fooled into thinking that there is a perforation (pseudo-pneumoperitoneum). A lateral decubitus radiograph can resolve the problem by demonstrating gas between the liver and the abdominal wall, but nowadays CT is usually requested when there is doubt. Since interpretation of the plain AXR can be unreliable, it is important to interpret the plain radiographic findings in the light of the clinical findings.

It is also important to be able to recognise the signs of pneumoperitoneum on supine AXRs, for example in patients being monitored for colitis. In many patients, particularly those who are unconscious, have suffered trauma, are old or are critically ill, perforation may be

TABLE 1-3 **Signs of Pneumoperitoneum on a Supine Radiograph**

Right upper quadrant gas
   Perihepatic
   Subhepatic
   Morrison's pouch
   Fissure for ligamentum teres
Rigler's (double wall) sign
Ligament visualisation
   Falciform (ligamentum teres)
   Medial umbilical (inverted V sign)
Triangular air

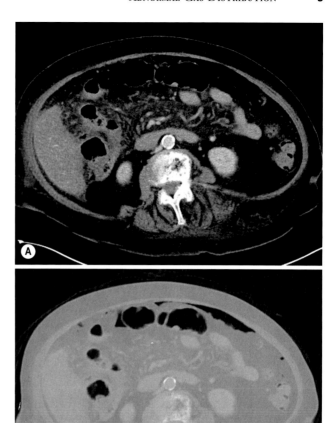

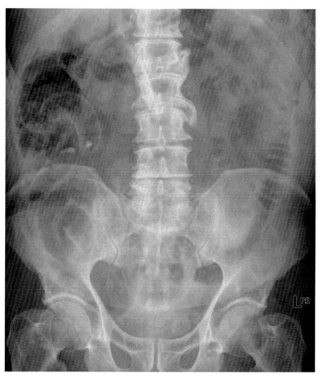

FIGURE 1-3 ■ **Pneumoperitoneum.** Supine abdominal radiograph. The falciform ligament is outlined by gas on both sides in the epigastric area to the right of the midline. There is also extraluminal gas and Rigler's sign in the right upper quadrant.

FIGURE 1-4 ■ **Free peritoneal gas due to perforated viscus.** (A) CT viewed on abdominal window settings. (B) The same image viewed on broad window settings. The free gas deep to the anterior abdominal wall is more conspicuous in (B).

clinically silent as it is overshadowed by other serious medical or surgical problems. In around half of patients with a pneumoperitoneum, gas may be detectable on the supine radiograph.[2] Almost half will have gas in the right upper quadrant adjacent to the liver, lying mainly in the subhepatic space and the hepatorenal fossa (Morrison's pouch). Visualisation of both the outer and inner walls of a bowel loop is known as Rigler's sign (Fig. 1-2). The bowel loops then take on a 'ghost-like' appearance. This sign can be difficult if several loops of bowel lie close together. The falciform or medial umbilical ligaments may be demonstrated by free gas lying on either side (Fig. 1-3). Air can be seen in the fissure for the ligamentum teres.[3] The signs are listed in Table 1-3.

CT is the most sensitive investigation for the detection of free peritoneal gas. Small volumes of free peritoneal gas can be seen over the liver and anteriorly in the central abdomen. Tiny pockets of free gas can also be seen in the peritoneal recesses. In order not to miss small amounts of free gas, the images should be reviewed on broad window settings (Fig. 1-4).

There are a number of causes of pneumoperitoneum without peritonitis. These are listed in Table 1-4.

Gas in Bowel Wall

If linear gas streaks are seen in the bowel wall, intestinal infarction should be suspected. Intestinal infarction is a most serious condition caused by thrombosis or embolism of the superior mesenteric artery. Other radiological signs are non-specific, consisting of slightly dilated loops of small bowel that may be gas-filled, or poorly seen when mainly fluid filled. The walls of the small-bowel loops may be thickened due to submucosal haemorrhage and oedema (Fig. 1-5). Free gas may be present if perforation has occurred. Intraluminal gas in the mesenteric veins or portal vein may be seen in advanced cases. These features can be readily demonstrated on CT.

TABLE 1-4 **Causes of Pneumoperitoneum without Peritonitis**

Silent perforation of viscus that has sealed itself in
  The aged
  Patients on steroids
  Unconscious patients
  The presence of other serious medical conditions
Postoperative (up to 7 days)
Peritoneal dialysis
Perforated cyst in pneumatosis intestinalis
Tracking down from pneumomediastinum
Stercoral ulceration
Vaginal-tubal entry of air

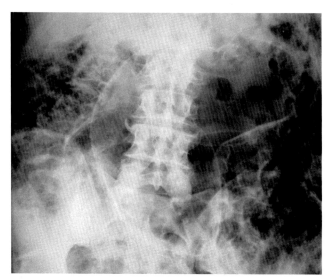

FIGURE 1-6 ■ **Pneumatosis coli.** Multiple small gas-filled cysts are seen in association with the colon. There is also free peritoneal gas.

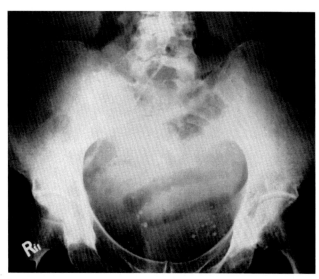

FIGURE 1-5 ■ **Mesenteric infarction.** Supine. Several gas-filled loops of small bowel lie in the pelvis. Note the abnormal irregular outline of the mucosa and the thickening of the bowel wall.

Pneumatosis cystoides intestinalis is an uncommon condition consisting of cyst-like collections of gas in the walls of hollow viscera. The aetiology is unknown, but there is an association with obstructive airways disease. The left hemicolon is the most common site, and the term pneumatosis coli is used to describe it. Most patients are past middle age; symptoms include vague abdominal pain, diarrhoea, constipation and mucus discharge. The cysts vary in size from 1 to 3 cm and lie both in the subserosa and submucosa. The plain radiographic appearances are characteristic, the gas-containing cysts giving rise to an appearance quite different from normal gas shadows (Fig. 1-6). Intermittently and subclinically these cysts rupture, producing a pneumoperitoneum without evidence of peritonitis. It is important to recognise pneumatosis as the cause of the pneumoperitoneum in such cases so as to avoid an unnecessary laparotomy.

Gas in Retroperitoneum

Gas can escape into the retroperitoneum, and the causes for this include perforation of a posterior peptic ulcer,

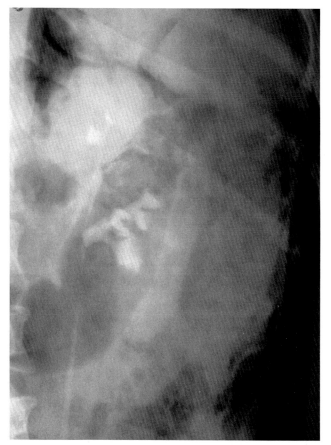

FIGURE 1-7 ■ **Retroperitoneal gas caused by perforated sigmoid diverticular disease.** Radiograph from an IVU series. There is gas between the layers of the abdominal wall and around the upper pole of the left kidney.

perforated sigmoid diverticular disease, colonoscopy and other iatrogenic causes. The gas may be best visible in the layers of the abdominal wall in the flanks, or around the kidneys (Fig. 1-7). Retroperitoneal gas can track superiorly into the mediastinum, and inferiorly into the

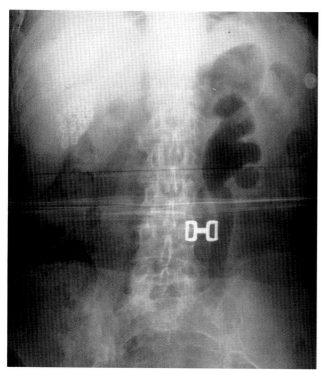

FIGURE 1-8 ■ **Emphysematous pyelonephritis.** Patient with diabetes mellitus and sepsis. The left renal collecting system and ureter are distended and gas-filled. There are also multiple dense gallstones in the gall bladder.

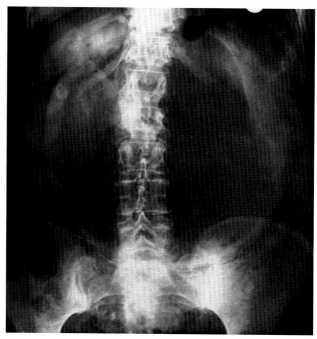

FIGURE 1-9 ■ **Gastric volvulus: supine.** Gas-filled, grossly dilated stomach, spherical in outline. Note also the linear gas within the wall of the stomach and visualisation of both sides of the stomach wall indicating free gas. At laparotomy a perforated gangrenous stomach had undergone volvulus around its transverse axis.

buttock and thigh. Gas in the soft tissues of the left thigh is a classical site for gas from a diverticular perforation.

Gas in Other Organs

Gas may also be identified in the biliary tree, portal veins, renal collecting systems (emphysematous pyelonephritis, Fig. 1-8), pancreas (infected necrosis or abscess), gall bladder wall and urinary bladder.

DILATATION OF BOWEL

Dilatation of the bowel occurs in mechanical intestinal obstruction, paralytic ileus and air swallowing. The radiological differentiation of these different causes depends mainly on the size and distribution of the loops of the bowel, and clinical correlation is essential.

Gastric Dilatation

Gastric dilatation can be caused by many conditions. Mechanical gastric obstruction may be benign, malignant or from extrinsic compression. It often leads to a huge fluid-filled stomach that retains its gastriform shape with little or no bowel gas beyond. This compares with the normal small gastric air bubble, usually just enough for the stomach to be identified. Paralytic ileus (often referred to as acute gastric dilatation) occurs mostly in elderly people, usually associated with considerable fluid and electrolyte disturbance.

Gastric volvulus is relatively rare and may result from twisting of the organ around its longitudinal or mesenteric axis. There is usually a collapsed small bowel, and virtually no gas is seen beyond the stomach. The stomach loses its gastriform shape and becomes spherical (Fig. 1-9). If oral contrast medium is given, there may be complete obstruction in the lower oesophagus, or if contrast medium does enter the stomach, it may not pass beyond the obstructed pylorus. After resuscitation and intubation, large amounts of gas can be seen in a dilated stomach. This sometimes occurs after air swallowing alone.

Distinction between Small- and Large-Bowel Dilatation

When a radiograph shows dilated bowel it is important to try to determine whether it is small or large bowel, or both. Useful differentiating features include the size and distribution of the loops. Dilated small-bowel loops are usually more numerous and arranged centrally in the abdomen. The loops show a small radius of curvature and rarely exceed 5 cm in diameter. The small-bowel folds (valvulae conniventes) form thin, frequent complete bands across the bowel gas shadow, prominent in the jejunum but becoming less marked in the ileum. The valvulae conniventes are much closer together than colonic haustra and become thinner when stretched, but still remain relatively close together as the calibre of the small bowel increases (Fig. 1-10). If the small-bowel blood supply is compromised, however, and the bowel

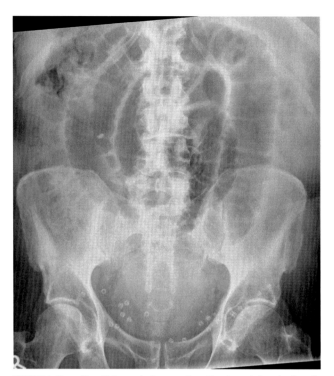

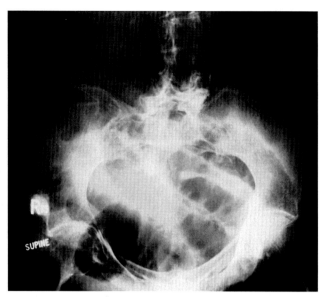

FIGURE 1-11 ■ **Small-bowel obstruction: strangulated right inguinal hernia, supine position.** Small-bowel dilatation with a grossly dilated loop passing down into the right inguinal region. Patient was an 80-year-old woman with abdominal pain and vomiting for 5 days.

FIGURE 1-10 ■ **Small-bowel obstruction.** Supine abdominal radiograph. There are distended loops of small bowel, identified by its central position, multiple loops and thin and frequent valvulae conniventes.

becomes oedematous or gangrenous, the valvulae conniventes may become thickened.

Problems in distinguishing the distal ileum from the sigmoid colon are relatively frequent as both may be smooth in outline and occupy a similar position, low in the central abdomen. Although haustra usually form thick incomplete bands across the colonic gas shadow, they sometimes form complete transverse bands, depending on the orientation of the loop. Haustra may be absent from the descending and sigmoid colon but can usually still be identified in other parts of the colon, even when it is massively distended.

Small-Bowel Dilatation

Small-bowel dilatation may be due to mechanical obstruction or paralytic ileus/pseudo-obstruction. In paralytic ileus there is no obstructing lesion. Small and large bowel may be dilated. Peritonitis and a postoperative abdomen are common causes, but there are many others including small-bowel ischaemia, metabolic disturbances, renal failure, drugs such as morphine and general debility. CT is valuable in determining whether there is an abrupt calibre change, which would point to a genuine small-bowel obstruction (SBO).

The causes of SBO are myriad, but can be largely divided into mural lesions (e.g. tumour, stricture due to Crohn's disease, irradiation), luminal (bezoar, gallstone, *Ascaris lumbricoides* bolus, intussusception) and extrinsic (adhesions, hernia, volvulus, abdominal malignancy). In the developed world the most common cause of SBO is

adhesions due to previous surgery, the obstruction being caused by a strangulated hernia in less than 10%.[4] In the undeveloped world, however, nearly three-quarters of cases are caused by a strangulated hernia. Mechanical obstruction of the small bowel normally causes small-bowel dilatation, with an accumulation of both gas and fluid, and a reduction in the calibre of the large bowel. On the plain radiograph it is important to look for a hernia, which may be identified as a gas-filled viscus below the level of the inguinal ligament (Fig. 1-11). Visualisation of a hernia does not always mean that it is the cause of the SBO.

Dilated loops of small bowel are readily identified if they are gas-filled on the supine radiograph. The string of beads sign, caused by a line of gas bubbles trapped between the valvulae conniventes, is seen only when very dilated small bowel is almost completely filled with fluid, and is virtually diagnostic of SBO. In a proportion of patients with SBO, the plain radiograph appears normal or only equivocally abnormal, since the dilated loops are mainly fluid-filled. Completely fluid-filled loops are not easily identified on plain radiographs, but are readily seen on CT (Fig. 1-12). The plain AXR has a sensitivity of around 66% for SBO.[5]

Where a gallstone is the cause of obstruction, this is known as gallstone 'ileus' (technically an obstruction, not an ileus). The gallstone passes into the duodenum by eroding the inflamed gall bladder wall. This condition is well known to clinicians, but relatively rare, accounting for about 2% of patients presenting with SBO. The diagnosis is frequently delayed or missed even though the characteristic radiological features of gallstone ileus are present in 38% of cases.[6] Over half the patients will have plain radiographic evidence of intestinal obstruction, and about one-third will have gas present in the biliary tree

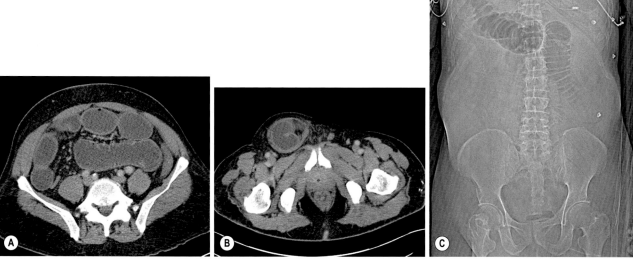

FIGURE 1-12 ■ **Small-bowel obstruction.** CT. (A) Multiple dilated small-bowel loops are filled with fluid. (B) The small-bowel obstruction is caused by strangulation of a right inguinal hernia. (C) CT scout image. Only a few of the distended loops are visible since most are filled with fluid.

(Fig. 1-13). Gas in the biliary tree can be recognised by its branching pattern, with gas being more prominent centrally. Gas in the portal vein, from which it must be distinguished, tends to be peripherally located in small veins around the edge of the liver. The obstructing gallstone, which is frequently located in the pelvic loops of ileum overlying the sacrum, can be identified in about one-third of patients on plain radiographs. Gas in the biliary tree is more commonly caused by previous sphincterotomy or biliary surgery, and may also be seen with perforation of a peptic ulcer into the common bile duct, and malignant fistula. Gas may rise into the biliary tree through a lax sphincter in the elderly.

Intussusception in adults nearly always develops as a result of a neoplasm of the bowel. Neoplasms arising in the submucosa such as lipoma, lymphoma and melanoma metastases show a propensity for intussusception. An intussusception may show on a plain radiograph as a soft-tissue mass, possibly part-outlined by gas (Fig. 1-14). If the intussusception is orientated end-on, a target sign may be seen. This consists of two concentric circles of fat density alternating with soft-tissue density.

In adults CT demonstrates the intussusception, a characteristic feature being the intussusceptum bringing mesenteric fat into the lumen of the intussuscipiens. The intussusception appears as a sausage-shaped mass or a target mass, depending on its orientation.[7] Multidetector CT and multiplanar imaging may help identify the features in an optimal plane. An underlying cause for the intussusception may also be apparent. Intussusception is occasionally diagnosed on CT during investigation of abdominal pain where the diagnosis has not been suspected (Fig. 1-15).

US can detect fluid-filled loops of small bowel, but US is not usually definitive in diagnosing the cause of the

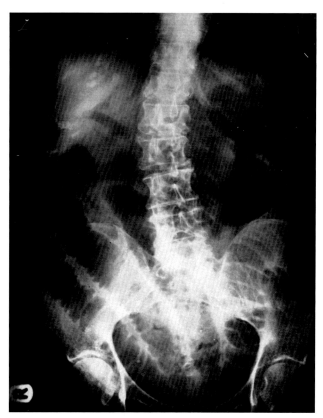

FIGURE 1-13 ■ **Gallstone ileus.** Supine radiograph showing evidence of small-bowel obstruction. In addition, gas can be identified within the right and left hepatic ducts and the common bile duct. The 79-year-old woman presented with a 5-day history of abdominal pain and vomiting.

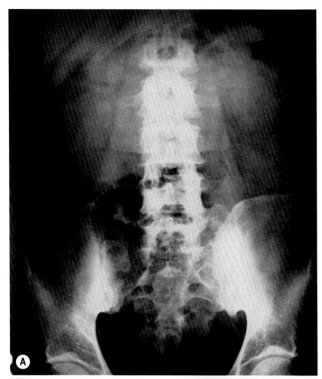

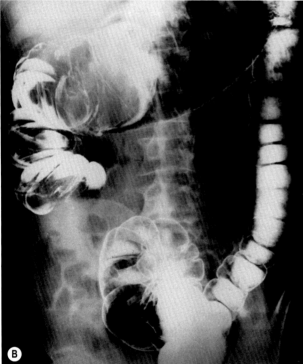

FIGURE 1-14 ■ **Intussusception.** (A) Supine. A soft-tissue mass is demonstrated extending across the upper abdomen and a crescent of gas is identified surrounding the head of the intussusception. (B) Barium enema. Huge intussusception identified in a 40-year-old man who had had abdominal pain for several months. A carcinoid tumour 10 mm in diameter was found to be responsible for the intussusception.

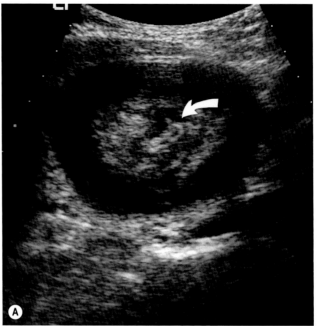

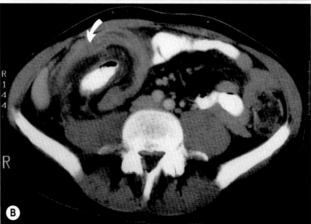

FIGURE 1-15 ■ **Ileocolic lymphoma leading to ileocolic intussusception.** (A) US image of the right iliac fossa showing the pseudotumour sign. The ileum can be seen centrally (arrow), surrounded by mesenteric fat that is hyperechoic, all within the thickened ascending colon. (B) CT showing oral contrast medium in the ileal lumen, the surrounding mesenteric fat accompanying the intussusceptum and the thickened ascending colon, which is the intussuscipiens (arrow).

obstruction, and it is not therefore usually recommended. If complete SBO has been diagnosed and the patient is to undergo surgery, further radiological examination is not strictly necessary, although most surgeons now find a preoperative diagnosis by CT very useful. If there is clinical doubt, partial obstruction, or when conservative management is planned, CT has a valuable role. CT will demonstrate dilated small-bowel loops, whether fluid- or gas-filled, and will add further information regarding the site and level of obstruction, and frequently the cause (Fig. 1-16).

Importantly, CT can add information on strangulation of a small-bowel loop, a sign that surgery is required. The mortality of SBO with strangulation rises from 5–8% to

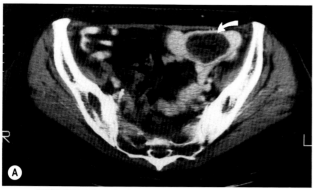

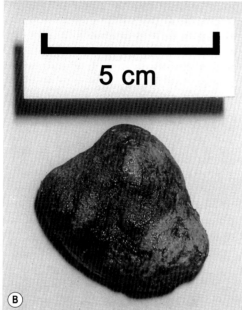

FIGURE 1-16 ■ **Small-bowel obstruction due to jejunal phyto-bezoar.** (A) CT through the upper pelvis demonstrating a filling defect within dilated jejunum (arrow). The bowel calibre was normal distal to this. (B) The phytobezoar after surgical removal.

20–37% compared to SBO without strangulation,[8] and mortality rises with treatment delay. CT signs of a closed loop include small-bowel dilatation, V-shaped or radial fluid-filled loops, mesenteric vessels converging towards the point of obstruction and a triangular loop with or without a whirl or beak. Where there is strangulation the bowel wall becomes thickened, and may be of high attenuation due to haemorrhage. Gas may be seen within the bowel wall and mesentery, and there may be congestion of the mesentery attached to the loop. There may be free peritoneal fluid whether strangulation is present or not.[9]

Where there is malignancy, additional staging information is gained by CT with the detection of lymphadenopathy, peritoneal deposits and other metastatic lesions. Adhesions are not visualised with certainty by any imaging technique, and are usually diagnosed on the basis of clinical history and exclusion. However, CT may demonstrate angulated and tethered loops which suggest the presence of adhesions. The CT sensitivity for adhesions is said to be around 73%.[8]

Large-Bowel Dilatation

There are numerous causes of large-bowel dilatation without obstruction, including paralytic ileus and pseudo-obstruction.

Pseudo-Obstruction

Pseudo-obstruction usually occurs in elderly patients. It mimics intestinal obstruction clinically and on the plain AXR. The plain radiographic appearances can be dramatic, showing a very dilated colon, and small-bowel distension as well. A contrast enema, CT or colonoscopy is required to exclude mechanical obstruction and to prevent an unnecessary laparotomy. The caecum may exceed the critical diameter of 9 cm when perforation is imminent, and a caecostomy or right-sided colostomy may even be required to prevent perforation.

Large-Bowel Obstruction

In the USA and Great Britain carcinoma of the colon is the commonest cause of large-bowel obstruction, about 60% of such carcinomas being situated in the sigmoid colon. Diverticulitis is the second most common cause of obstruction. In the USA, volvulus accounts for only 10% of cases of colonic obstruction, whereas for undeveloped countries a figure of 85% is quoted.[10] Adhesive obstruction of the large bowel is very unusual. Obstruction is much more common on the left side of the colon than the right. The plain radiographic findings depend on the site of obstruction and whether the ileocaecal valve is competent. In a minority of patients the ileocaecal valve remains competent and, despite increasing intracolonic pressure and marked distension of the caecum, the small bowel is not distended. More often, a closed ileocaecal valve also leads to small-bowel distension. In another group of patients, the ileocaecal valve is incompetent, the caecum and ascending colon are not unduly distended, while there is marked small-bowel distension. The obstructed colon almost invariably contains large amounts of air and can usually be identified by its haustral margin around the periphery of the abdomen (Fig. 1-17). When both small and large-bowel dilatation are present, the radiographic appearances may be identical to those seen in paralytic ileus.

The plain radiographic appearances of large-bowel obstruction are indistinguishable from pseudo-obstruction, and any patient with suspected large-bowel obstruction therefore requires another test to confirm the diagnosis. Traditionally this has been by way of an unprepared contrast enema, but now a CT is most frequently performed (Fig. 1-18).

There are some large-bowel obstruction syndromes leading to more specific radiological appearances on a plain radiograph. **Sigmoid volvulus** is the classical volvulus, occurring most frequently in old age or in patients with mental handicap or institutionalisation (Fig. 1-19). The usual mechanism is twisting of the sigmoid loop around the mesenteric axis. Although the classical radiographic changes may be present, in up to one-third of cases it is difficult to differentiate a twisted sigmoid from

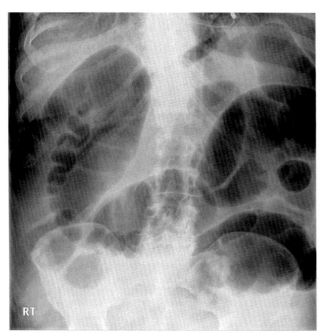

FIGURE 1-17 ■ **Large-bowel obstruction due to sigmoid carcinoma.** Supine abdominal radiograph. There are distended loops of colon due to obstruction.

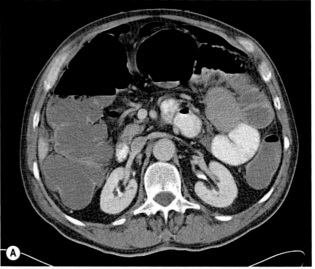

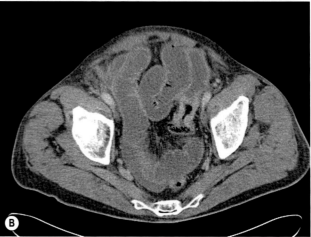

FIGURE 1-18 ■ **Large-bowel obstruction.** CT. (A) Multiple distended loops of colon. The dependent loops are fluid-filled. These are not visible on a plain radiograph. (B) The cause of the obstruction is demonstrated to be a stricture in the sigmoid colon, subsequently proven to be carcinoma.

a distended but non-rotated sigmoid, or from more proximal colonic distension.[11] When sigmoid volvulus occurs, the inverted U-shaped loop of sigmoid is usually massively distended and is commonly devoid of haustra, an important diagnostic point. The anhaustral margin can often be identified overlapping, respectively, the lower border of the liver shadow (the liver overlap sign), the haustrated, dilated descending colon (the left flank overlap sign) and the left side of the bony pelvis (the pelvic overlap sign). The top of the sigmoid volvulus usually lies very high in the abdomen (above the level of T10) with its apex on the left side.

If there is doubt about the diagnosis on the plain radiographs, however, a contrast enema should be performed. Features seen at the point of torsion include a smooth, curved tapering of the colonic lumen, like a hooked beak (the bird of prey sign); the mucosal folds often show a 'screw' pattern at the point of twist (Fig. 1-19).

Caecal volvulus can only occur when the caecum and ascending colon are on a mesentery. In comparison with sigmoid volvulus, it usually occurs in a younger age group, 30–60 years. In about half the patients, the caecum twists and inverts so that the pole of the caecum and the appendix occupy the left upper quadrant (Fig. 1-20). In other patients the twist occurs in an axial plane without inversion and the caecum still occupies the right half of the abdomen. The distended caecum can frequently be identified as a large viscus, which may be situated almost anywhere in the abdomen. The attached gas-filled appendix may be seen. There is often marked gaseous or fluid distension of the small bowel, which may sometimes obscure the caecal volvulus itself. The left side of the colon is usually collapsed.

ABNORMAL BOWEL WALL PATTERN

The gas within the bowel profiles the mucosa, allowing appreciation of the mucosal surface on plain radiographs. Adjacent bowel loops and peritoneal fat can delineate the outer extent of the bowel wall, and the wall thickness can therefore be judged.

Small-Bowel Ischaemia

Please see the above section on gas in the bowel wall. The small-bowel wall becomes thickened if there is acute ischaemia, as a result of haemorrhage and oedema (Fig. 1-5). Thickened bowel wall outlined by gas and adjacent fat may be evident on plain radiographs, but CT is far more sensitive; furthermore, small amounts of gas in the bowel wall are also better demonstrated. Gas in the bowel wall indicates infarction.

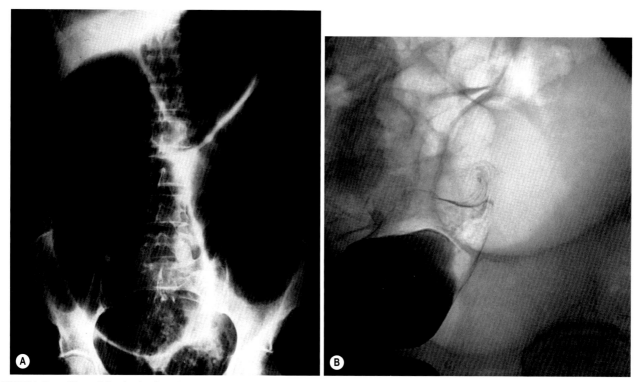

FIGURE 1-19 ■ Sigmoid volvulus in a 64-year-old woman. (A) Massively dilated distended gas-filled loop of sigmoid colon. (B) Contrast enema showing the twisted sigmoid colon (bird of prey sign).

Large-Bowel Ischaemia

Ischaemic colitis is characterised clinically by the sudden onset of abdominal pain, followed by bloody diarrhoea. The splenic flexure and proximal descending colon are most often involved, although other areas may be affected. The wall, particularly the submucosa of the colon, is thickened as a result of haemorrhage and oedema (Fig. 1-21). This can sometimes be detected on plain radiographs but in most cases a barium enema or CT is necessary. The term 'thumbprinting' has been used to describe the plain radiographic appearance of the submucosal thickening with its crescentic margins. The involved area of the colon acts as a functional obstruction so that the right side of the colon is frequently distended. In the long term, the affected area can fibrose to become a stricture.

Inflammatory Bowel Disease

The plain AXR can usually predict the extent of the mucosal lesions in acute inflammatory disease of the colon. An assessment of the extent of colitis, the state of the mucosa, the depth of ulceration and the presence or absence of toxic megacolon and/or perforation can be made. The extent of faecal residue is related to the extent of the colitis.[12] The disease is likely to be inactive where there are formed faeces, while a complete absence of faecal residue suggests extensive colitis. Intraluminal gas tends to accumulate as the colitis becomes more severe. Severe mucosal changes can be missed, however, if there is no intracolonic air to delineate the mucosal outline. A granular mucosa is shown as an even mucosal edge with blunting of the haustra, ulceration as an irregular mucosal edge with obliteration of the haustra and mucosal islands as large polypoid mucosal remnants separated by flat areas where large parts of the mucosa have been lost. When the bowel becomes dilated and the haustra disappear, the ulceration has penetrated the muscle layer and the patient moves into a high-risk group where urgent surgery must be considered. This is known as toxic megacolon (Fig. 1-22). In order to detect the development of this situation, daily plain AXR may be justified in order to monitor progress.

The reader is referred to Chapter 4 for information on small-bowel inflammatory disease.

Pseudomembranous Colitis

Pseudomembranous colitis may follow the administration of antibiotics, particularly the clindamycin and lincomycin groups. *Clostridium difficile* is frequently cultured in the stools. The plain radiograph is abnormal in around one-third of cases:[13] colonic dilatation (32%), thumbprinting, thickened haustra and abnormal mucosa (18%) may be identified (Fig. 1-23). The whole colon may be involved, but the transverse colon is the most frequently affected segment. The appearances may mimic acute inflammatory bowel disease, and other infective diarrhoeas, with or without immunosuppression, can look similar. CT is non-specific in the diagnosis of pseudomembranous colitis, and has been shown to be normal in 39% of cases, but CT can demonstrate markedly thickened mucosa, with oedema seen in the submocosa, and sometimes nodular mucosal thickening.[14] There may also be mild pericolonic inflammatory change in the fat.

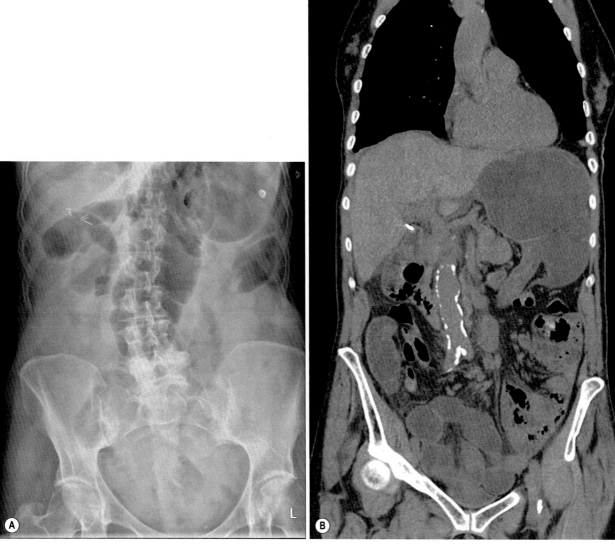

FIGURE 1-20 ▪ **Caecal volvulus.** (A) Supine abdominal radiograph. There is an inverted distended caecum extending up to the left upper quadrant. (B) Coronal CT reconstruction in the same patient. The terminal ileum can be seen entering the distended caecum in the left upper quadrant.

ACUTE ABDOMINAL INFLAMMATORY CONDITIONS

The plain AXR still has a role in the acute abdomen in the scenarios described above, but it offers very little information in the differential diagnosis of abdominal pain in the quadrants. Patients with suspected appendicitis, diverticulitis and cholecystitis should not receive a plain radiograph, since diagnostic signs are usually lacking, and the admitting team may misinterpret spurious findings.

Acute appendicitis is the commonest acute surgical condition in the developed world and carries an overall mortality rate of about 1%. When the clinical findings are typical, a prompt clinical diagnosis can be made, and radiological investigations are not indicated. However,

there is a long list of alternative diagnoses mimicking appendicitis (Table 1-5). Clinical diagnosis alone results in a normal appendix being found at appendicectomy in 10–15%, and in young women the negative appendicectomy rate is higher still.[15] Many argue that this rate of preventable operative intervention is unacceptable, and that either US or CT should be used more.

Plain radiographs of the abdomen are not indicated for suspected appendicitis. There are no specific plain radiographic signs of acute appendicitis but ileus can occur, and there may be obstruction as loops of small bowel become matted together or stuck to the inflamed appendix. There is a high positive correlation between the presence of an appendix faecolith and acute appendicitis (Fig. 1-24).

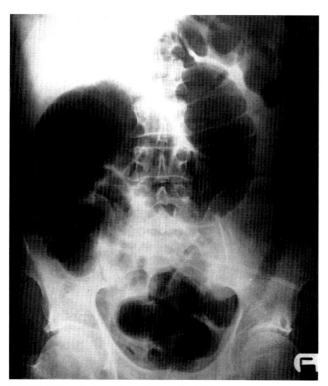

FIGURE 1-21 ■ **Ischaemic colitis.** A thick-walled oedematous descending colon outlined by gas. Slightly distended colon from caecum to splenic flexure, but with normal haustra and no evidence of abnormal mucosa.

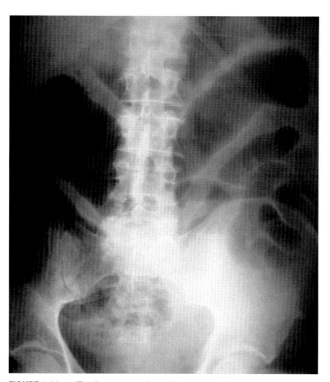

FIGURE 1-22 ■ **Toxic megacolon.** The ascending and transverse colon appears gas-filled and dilated with a thickened wall. There is an absence of haustral markings, indicating full-thickness mural inflammation.

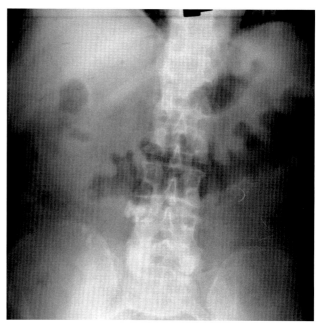

FIGURE 1-23 ■ **Pseudomembranous colitis.** There is gross mucosal oedema in the transverse colon. *Clostridium difficile* was grown.

TABLE 1-5   Diseases Mimicking Clinical Appendicitis Diagnosed at US

Ectopic pregnancy
Ovarian cyst ± torsion
Salpingitis
Endometriosis
Diverticulitis
Infectious ileocaecitis
Crohn's disease
Malignancy
Intussusception
Meckel's diverticulum
Cholecystitis
Urolithiasis
Mesenteric adenitis

Ultrasound in Appendicitis

Graded compression US is a well-documented technique for examining the appendix. The US probe is applied with gradually increased pressure over the right iliac fossa in order to displace bowel loops and examine the appendix.[16] US signs of acute appendicitis include visualisation of a blind-ending tubular structure, which is non-compressible, with a diameter of 7 mm or greater (Fig. 1-25). An appendicolith may be seen as a hyperechoic focus casting an acoustic shadow, and the surrounding inflammatory mass, which consists mainly of fat, is hyperechoic. An abscess or fluid around the appendix may be seen (Table 1-6). US of acute appendicitis has been reported to have a sensitivity of 78–98% and specificity of 85–98%.

There are interpretative pitfalls: false-negative results can arise in focal appendicitis of the appendiceal tip,

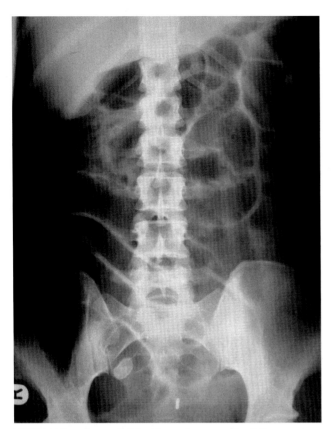

FIGURE 1-24 ■ Appendicitis. There is generalised ileus and an appendicolith in the right iliac fossa overlying the right side of the sacrum. At operation the appendix was gangrenous and perforated.

retrocaecal appendicitis, gangrenous or perforated appendicitis, a gas-filled appendix and a massively enlarged appendix, which is very unusual in the inflamed appendix. Pitfalls leading to a false-positive examination include a dilated fallopian tube, peri-appendicitis, inflammatory bowel disease and inspissated stool mimicking an appendicolith.[17] When the appendix has perforated it may be compressible at US. This phenomenon has been reported in 38% of paediatric perforations and 55% of adult perforations.[18] The main drawback of US is that in most instances, in most hands, a normal appendix is not visualised, and subsequently a negative US result, where the appendix is not seen, is of little value.[19] In a multicentre German study of 2280 patients with acute abdominal pain, US was not shown to lead to proven clinical benefit.[20] Similar results have been reported elsewhere. It is more useful in the clinically indeterminate group of patients, rather than when the diagnosis is considered very likely or very unlikely.

Nevertheless, US can diagnose a number of conditions that mimic appendicitis clinically (Table 1-5). When an experienced radiologist is available, US can be recommended in children where there is diagnostic doubt, in young women (due to the higher incidence of tubal disease) and in those patients who are pregnant.[21]

Computed Tomography in Appendicitis

A number of large prospective trials have demonstrated that CT is a highly accurate test for confirming or

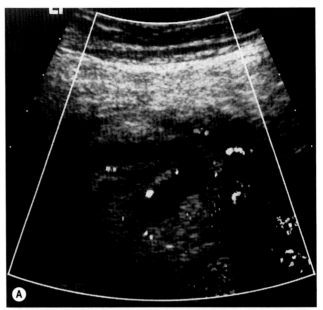

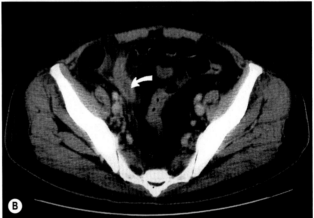

FIGURE 1-25 ■ Appendicitis. (A) US shows a thickened hypo-echoic tubular blind-ended structure in the right iliac fossa. The surrounding fat is hyperechoic. (B) CT shows the thickened inflamed appendix (arrow). (Courtesy of Dr A. McLean, St Bartholomew's Hospital, London.)

TABLE 1-6   Acute Appendicitis: US Signs

Blind-ending tubular structure
  Non-compressible
  Diameter 7 mm or greater
  No peristalsis
Appendicolith casting acoustic shadow
High echogenicity surrounding fat
Surrounding fluid or abscess
Oedema of caecal pole
Maximal tenderness over appendix

excluding appendicitis. CT signs of appendicitis include an appendix measuring greater than 6 mm in diameter, appendicolith and enhancement of its wall with intravenous contrast medium (Figs. 1-25B and 1-26). Surrounding inflammatory changes include increased fat attenuation, fluid, phlegmon, caecal thickening, abscess and extraluminal gas. Luminal contrast agent or air in the

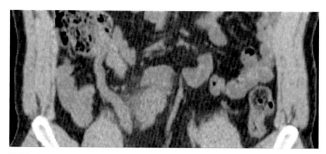

FIGURE 1-26 ■ **Appendicitis.** Coronal CT in a patient referred with renal colic. This unenhanced curved coronal CT along the length of the appendix shows the distended appendix along with subtle induration of the adjacent fat. The plain radiograph was normal.

caecum pointing towards the obstructed origin of the appendix has been called the arrowhead sign, and is present in 30% of cases of appendicitis.[22] Focal caecal thickening due to oedema at the origin of the appendix is referred to as a caecal bar.[23]

CT techniques for diagnosing appendicitis vary between authors. A focused technique examining the abdominopelvic junction exposes the patient to approximately one-third of the radiation dose of a full abdomen and pelvic examination (~3 vs 10 mSv).[24] However, this technique may not reveal other relevant diagnoses. Although authors debate the figures, a normal appendix is seen more frequently at CT than US; thus CT carries a better true negative rate. Much may depend on body habitus; US is well suited to thin patients and, especially, children.

Proponents for CT in acute appendicitis have achieved sensitivities and specificities of 100 and 95%, respectively, establishing an alternative diagnosis in 89%.[25] Several studies have reported overall accuracy of 93–98%.[24] Excellent results such as these come from radiologists specifically interested in CT of the acute abdomen, often examining patients where the diagnosis of acute appendicitis is deemed highly likely on clinical assessment. It does not follow that CT will perform as well in the hands of all radiologists in all centres, examining patients where the differential diagnosis is still broad. The high radiation dose from abdominal CT should be remembered. When recommending investigations in such patients it must be understood that they take varying amounts of additional time to organise and perform, and delay in treatment of appendicitis can be very detrimental to the clinical outcome. Imaging should not be a substitute for good clinical assessment.

Several studies have shown the negative appendicectomy rate to fall from over 20% to less than 9% with the liberal use of imaging.[26–29] In many institutions in the USA, CT is performed on all patients with acute right iliac fossa pain. Other studies have found that liberal use of CT and US does not reduce the negative appendicectomy rate.[30,31] A key strength of CT is its ability to make alternative diagnoses in right iliac fossa pain. These include mesenteric adenitis, terminal ileitis, Meckel's diverticulitis, typhlitis, appendagitis and omental infarction.[23]

Debate still continues over the use of CT and US in the setting of suspected acute appendicitis, and local practice will depend on the surgeons, radiologists, the age of the patient and the availability of imaging facilities/expertise at short notice.

Other Inflammatory Conditions

CT is the accepted best first investigation for suspected acute diverticulitis, on account of its ability to assess the extracolonic complications of the disease, namely inflammation, abscess, perforation and fistula formation. The degree of bowel obstruction, if present, can also be assessed. A CT also has the best chance of identifying alternative diagnoses in left iliac fossa pain. A barium study can only demonstrate the luminal component of the disease.

Ultrasound remains the first investigation of choice in suspected acute cholecystitis. For this condition the reader is referred to the chapter on the biliary system (see Chapter 8).

IMAGING THE ABDOMEN WITH CT: RADIATION ISSUES

When imaging acute abdominal conditions the choice of imaging investigation and technique is firstly guided by the clinical question at hand, secondly by availability of hardware and economic issues and thirdly by the local expertise of the radiographer and radiologist who acquire and interpret the study. Use of CT has increased exponentially in recent years; however, clinicians and their patients are becoming increasingly conscious of the exposure to ionising radiation associated with CT. This concern is motivated by recent coverage in the scientific literature and media which highlights the potentially increased cancer risk to patients as a result of the increasing use of CT in clinical medicine.[32]

Carcinogenesis is the primary concern and it is a proven stochastic effect of ionising radiation. A stochastic effect occurs randomly and no lower threshold of ionising radiation exposure exists where cancer induction does not occur. Carcinogenesis usually occurs many years remote from the exposure and is therefore of particular relevance in patients who are young and in patients who are subjected to repeated CT examinations over the course of their disease. Young cohorts who may be at particular risk of having a high cumulative effective dose include those with curable malignancies such as testicular cancer[33] and Hodgkin's lymphoma, those with inflammatory bowel disease particularly Crohns disease[34] or cystic fibrosis[35] and patients who repeatedly present with renal colic.[36]

Currently there is a considerable research and industry drive to reduce radiation exposure during CT while preserving image quality and diagnostic yield. One of the first technological steps towards CT dose reduction was to reduce inefficiencies of radiation delivery. Fixed tube kilovoltage and amperage settings were commonly used in older-generation CT systems. Using these fixed tube settings for CT of the abdomen and pelvis resulted in wider areas such as the mid-abdomen receiving the same exposure as narrower regions such as the pelvis. This inefficient method of dose delivery was the target of one of the most successful and now widely implemented dose reduction technologies, namely automatic tube current modulation.

AUTOMATIC TUBE CURRENT MODULATION

Automatic tube current modulation (ATCM) tailors the dose output of the CT tube to the patient size and shape based on the patient diameter and the X-ray attenuation of the tissues through which the fan beam is passing.[37] This automated process ensures that thicker regions of the body are imaged using higher tube currents than thinner, less attenuating areas. Initial trials examining the utility of ATCM found that diagnostic quality could be preserved while radiation exposure was significantly reduced. Early clinical trials demonstrated that dose reductions could be achieved in almost 90% of examinations and that the tube-current time product was reduced by on average 32% while using ATCM.[38] Further reductions in CT dose, beyond the elimination of inefficiencies in dose delivery, are inherently associated with an increase in image noise. Noise is the statistical variation in attenuation values of CT images which does not reflect anatomy and blurs image contrast. Increased image noise is particularly problematic when imaging pathological changes with a low lesion-background contrast. Accuracy in detecting small focal lesions of the liver, spleen and kidneys is negatively influenced by even a slight increase in image noise, whereas, when imaging the bowel and renal tract for potential urinary calculi, a higher amount of image noise is usually acceptable because of the higher lesion-background contrast.

Focused studies demonstrate preservation of diagnostic accuracy despite significant reductions in radiation dose and consequential increases in image noise in patient groups with Crohn's disease[39] and with urinary calculi[40] and also in cases of suspected appendicitis.[41]

Emerging CT noise reduction strategies have provided new strategies for reducing CT dose while maintaining image quality. These methods are already showing great promise in abdominopelvic CT and the widespread dissemination of technologies such as iterative reconstruction are likely to result in CT dose reductions on the order of 75% and greater in future years.

ITERATIVE RECONSTRUCTION ALGORITHMS

Iterative image reconstruction (IR) algorithms were used to generate images for the first commercial clinical CT systems but the limited processing abilities of computers in this generation forced manufacturers to use a more computationally efficient method of image reconstruction known as filtered back projection (FBP) at that time. The greater image noise associated with low-dose CT imaging is poorly handled by FBP alone and therefore IR is a more appropriate method for low-dose imaging reconstruction. Modern computers have allowed use of

this technology to enter the clinical domain where methods of iterative reconstruction currently represent the most exciting dose-optimising developments in CT.[42] Multiple generations of IR are being developed and tested by CT manufacturers. IR algorithms may operate on the image data or preferably on the raw projection data from the CT system itself but at least an IR algorithm operates on a combination of image and raw projection data. The images generated by algorithms such as ASIR have different qualities than those reconstructed with FBP. IR images were described as being 'waxy' or 'plastic' in appearance in the case of early algorithms but later generations of IR have yielded more acceptable images, which are mildly 'mottled', or 'pixelated'. Images generated by early IR algorithms such as ASIR are often blended with data reconstructed with traditional FBP to improve diagnostic acceptability and are therefore referred to as hybrid algorithms. Expert opinion in this area suggests that imagers tend to adapt to the new quality of these images in a relatively short period of time.[43]

Hybrid IR algorithms are typically noise-efficient, computationally fast and studies have indicated that images have good low-contrast detail and preserved image quality with radiation dose reductions of at least 30%.[42] Early investigations of the utility of ASIR,[44] IRIS[45] and SAFIRE[46] have shown that a diagnostically acceptable CT of the abdomen and pelvis can be acquired at approximately 50% less dose than was previously possible with FBP. By comparison pure iterative reconstruction algorithms result in diagnostically acceptable images de novo, which negates the requirement for blending with FBP data. Model-based iterative reconstruction (MBIR) is a commercially available form of pure IR developed by GE Healthcare. MBIR uses a model of the physical characteristics of the focal spot, the X-ray fan beam, the 3-dimensional interaction of the X-ray beam within the patient and the 2-dimensional interaction of the X-ray beam within the detector. Pure IR is computationally demanding and despite the use of parallel processing technology only 3 to 4 data sets can be reconstructed per hour at present. Early clinical trials suggest that low-dose abdominal CT reconstructed with pure IR is superior to hybrid IR such as ASIR and also outperforms FBP in both subjective image quality indices and objective image noise scores, facilitating dose reductions of approximately 80%[47] (Fig. 1-27).

CT DOSE REDUCTION IN CLINICAL PRACTICE

In practice, effective CT dose reduction is best achieved by careful patient selection, rigorous justification of CT examination and the application of suitable CT acquisition parameters. Monitoring and audit of one's own practice is recommended and may serve to identify aberrant trends in patient management or imaging which may result in an increase in patient cumulative effective dose. It is important that CT radiographers are involved in dose reduction strategies as this advances daily awareness and focus on the principles involved in

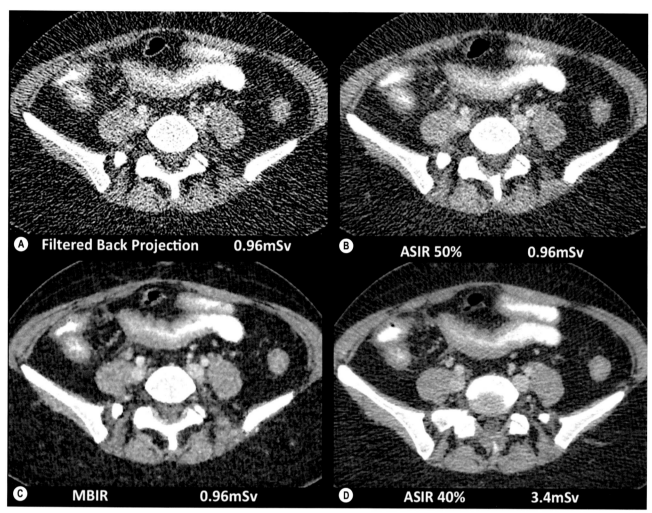

FIGURE 1-27 ■ **Low-dose CT with iterative reconstruction.** A 36-year-old female patient (BMI 23.6) with a known diagnosis of Crohn's disease. Axial contrast-enhanced images from low-dose CT abdomen and pelvis (0.96 mSv) reconstructed with (A) FBP, (B) 50% ASIR and (C) MBIR show a progressive reduction in image noise and increase in image quality with more advanced iterative reconstruction. (D) Corresponding image from the conventional dose CT abdomen and pelvis (3.4 mSv) reconstructed with 40% ASIR is provided for comparison with the low-dose images.

dose reduction and their appropriate application. Variations in CT dose between as well as within individual institutions serve to highlight the need for greater focus and consensus among those who are involved in the day-to-day acquisition and interpretation of CT. One recent study found a 32-fold variation in CT exposures among different centres, some even using the same CT machine.[48]

In conclusion radiation dose optimisation for abdominal CT is a progressive multidisciplinary process involving radiologists, CT radiographers, medical physicists and referring physicians. CT doses are trending in the right direction and continued multidisciplinary focus on CT dose reduction will result in a systematic reduction in cancer risk. Our responsibility is to first counsel patients accurately regarding the risks of ionising radiation exposure; secondly, to limit the use of those imaging investigations which involve ionising radiation to clinical situations where they are likely to change management; and thirdly, when an imaging investigation which results

in radiation exposure is deemed necessary, to ensure that a diagnostic quality imaging examination is acquired with lowest possible radiation exposure.

REFERENCES

1. Field S, Guy PJ, Upsdell SM, Scourfield AE. The erect abdominal radiograph in the acute abdomen: should its routine use be abandoned? Br Med J 1985;290:1934–6.
2. Menuck L, Siemers PT. Pneumoperitoneum importance of right upper quadrant features. Am J Roentgenol 1976;127:753–6.
3. Cho KC, Baker SR. Air in the fissure for the ligamentum teres: new sign of intraperitoneal air on plain radiographs. Radiology 1991;178:489–92.
4. Miller G, Baman J, Shrier I, Gordon PH. Etiology of small bowel obstruction. Am J Surg 2000;180(1):33–6.
5. Shrake PD, Rex DK, Lappas JC. Radiographic evaluation of suspected small-bowel obstruction. Am J Gastroenterol 1991;86:175–8.
6. Day EA, Marks C. Gallstone ileus. Am J Surg 1975;129:552–8.
7. Gayer G, Apter S, Hofmann C, et al. Intussusception in adults: CT diagnosis. Clin Radiol 1998;53:53–7.
8. Megibow AJ. Bowel obstruction: evaluation with CT. Radiol Clin North Am 1994;32:861–70.

9. Balthazar EJ, Birnbaum BA, Megibow AJ, et al. Closed-loop and strangulating intestinal obstruction: CT signs. Radiology 1992; 185:769–75.

10. Love L. Large bowel obstruction. Semin Roentgenol 1973;8: 299–322.

11. Young WS, Englebrecht HE, Stoker A. Plain film analysis of sigmoid volvulus. Clin Radiol 1978;29:553–60.

12. Bartram CI. Plain abdominal X-ray in acute colitis. Proc Roy Soc Med 1976;69:617–18.

13. Boland GW, Lee MJ, Cats A, Mueller PR. Pseudomembranous colitis: diagnostic sensitivity of the abdominal plain radiograph. Clin Radiol 1994;49:473–5.

14. Boland GW, Lee MJ, Cats AM, et al. Antibiotic-induced diarrhea: specificity of abdominal CT for the diagnosis of *Clostridium difficile* disease. Radiology 1994;191(1):103–6.

15. Birnbaum RA, Wilson SR. Appendicitis at the millennium. Radiology 2000;215:337–48.

16. Puylaert JBCM. Acute appendicitis: US evaluation using graded compression. Radiology 1986;158:355–60.

17. Jeffrey RB, Jain KA, Nghiem HV. Sonographic diagnosis of acute appendicitis: interpretive pitfalls. Am J Roentgenol 1994;162: 55–9.

18. Quillin SP, Siegel MJ, Coffin CM. Acute appendicitis in children: value of sonography in detecting perforation. Am J Roentgenol 1992;159:1265–8.

19. Roosevelt GE, Reynolds SL. Does the use of ultrasonography improve the outcome of children with appendicitis? Acad Emerg Med 1998;5:1071–4.

20. Franke C, Bohner H, Yang Q, et al. Ultrasonography for diagnosis of acute appendicitis: Results of a prospective multicenter trial. World J Surg 1999;23:141–6.

21. Birnbaum BA, Jeffrey RB. CT and sonographic evaluation of acute right lower quadrant abdominal pain. Am J Roentgenol 1998;170: 361–71.

22. Rao PM, Wittenberg J, McDowell RK, et al. Appendicitis: use of arrowhead sign for diagnosis. Am J Roentgenol 1997;202: 363–6.

23. Macari M, Balthazar EJ. The acute right lower quadrant: CT evaluation. Radiol Clin N Am 2003;41:1117–36.

24. Rao PM, Boland GWL. Imaging of acute right lower abdominal quadrant pain. Clin Radiol 1998;53:639–49.

25. Rao PM, Rhea JT, Novelline RA, et al. Helical CT technique for the diagnosis of appendicitis: prospective evaluation of a focused appendix CT examination. Radiology 1997;202:139–44.

26. Fuchs JR, Schlamberg JS, Shortsleeve MJ, Schuler JG. Impact of abdominal CT imaging on the management of appendicitis: an update. J Surg Res 2002;106:131–6.

27. Bendeck SE, Nino-Murcia M, Berry GJ, Jeffrey RB Jr. Imaging for suspected appendicitis: negative appendectomy and perforation rates. Radiology 2002;225:131–6.

28. Naoum JJ, Mileski WJ, Daller JA, et al. The use of abdominal computed tomography scan decreases the frequency of misdiagnosis in cases of suspected appendicitis. Am J Surg 2002;184:587–9; discussion 589–90.

29. Pena BM, Taylor GA, Fishman SJ, Mandl KD. The use of abdominal computed tomography scan decreases the frequency of misdiagnosis in cases of suspected appendicitis. Am J Surg 2002;184(6): 587–9; discussion 589–90.

30. Perez J, Barone JE, Wilbanks TO, et al. Liberal use of computed tomography scanning does not improve diagnostic accuracy in appendicitis. Am J Surg 2003;185:194–7.

31. McDonald GP, Pendarvis DP, Wilmoth R, Daley BJ. Influence of preoperative computed tomography on patients undergoing appendectomy. Am Surg 2001;67:1017–21.

32. Berrington de González A, Mahesh M, Kim K-P, et al. Projected cancer risks from computed tomographic scans performed in the United States in 2007. Arch Intern Med 2009;169(22):2071–7.

33. Joly F, Héron JF, Kalusinski L, et al. Quality of life in long-term survivors of testicular cancer: a population-based case-control study. J Clin Oncol 2002;20(1):73–80.

34. Desmond AN, O'Regan K, Curran C, et al. Crohn's disease: factors associated with exposure to high levels of diagnostic radiation. Gut 2008;57(11):1524–49.

35. O'Connell OJ, McWilliams S, McGarrigle A, et al. Radiologic imaging in cystic fibrosis: cumulative effective dose and changing trends over 2 decades. Chest 2012;141(6):1575–83.

36. Ferrandino MN, Bagrodia A, Pierre SA, et al. Radiation exposure in the acute and short-term management of urolithiasis at 2 academic centers. J Urol 2009;181(2):668–73.

37. Kalra MK, Maher MM, Toth TL, et al. Strategies for CT radiation dose optimization. Radiology 2004;230(3):619–28.

38. Kalra M, Maher M, Toth T, Kamath R. Comparison of z-axis automatic tube current modulation technique with fixed tube current CT scanning of abdomen and pelvis. Radiology 2004;232(2):347–53.

39. Kambadakone AR, Prakash P, Hahn PF, et al. Low-dose CT examinations in Crohn's disease: Impact on image quality, diagnostic performance, and radiation dose. Am J Roentgenol 2010;195(1): 78–88.

40. Ciaschini MW, Remer EM, Baker ME, et al. Urinary calculi: radiation dose reduction of 50% and 75% at CT—effect on sensitivity. Radiology 2009;251(1):105–11.

41. Kim K, Kim YH, Kim SY, et al. Low-dose abdominal CT for evaluating suspected appendicitis. N Engl J Med 2012;366(17): 1596–605.

42. Silva AC, Lawder HJ, Hara A, et al. Innovations in CT dose reduction strategy: application of the adaptive statistical iterative reconstruction algorithm. Am J Roentgenol 2010;194(1):191–9.

43. Nelson RC. New iterative reconstruction techniques for cardiovascular computed tomography: How do they work, and what are the advantages and disadvantages? J Cardiovasc Comput Tomogr 2011;5(5):286–92.

44. Singh S, Kalra MK, Hsieh J, et al. Abdominal CT: comparison of adaptive statistical iterative and filtered back projection reconstruction techniques. Radiology 2010;257(2):373–83.

45. May MS, Wüst W, Brand M, et al. Dose reduction in abdominal computed tomography: intraindividual comparison of image quality of full-dose standard and half-dose iterative reconstructions with dual-source computed tomography. Invest Radiol 2011;46(7): 465–70.

46. Winklehner A, Karlo C, Puippe G, et al. Raw data-based iterative reconstruction in body CTA: evaluation of radiation dose saving potential. Eur Radiol 2011;21(12):2521–6.

47. Singh S, Kalra MK, Do S, et al. Comparison of hybrid and pure iterative reconstruction techniques with conventional filtered back projection: dose reduction potential in the abdomen. J Comput Assist Tomogr 2012;36(3):347–53.

48. Dougeni E, Faulkner K, Panayiotakis G. A review of patient dose and optimisation methods in adult and paediatric CT scanning. Eur J Radiol 2012;81(4):e665–83.

CHAPTER 2

THE OESOPHAGUS

Edmund M. Godfrey • Alan H. Freeman

CHAPTER OUTLINE

ANATOMY AND FUNCTION

EXAMINATION

PATHOLOGICAL FEATURES

ANATOMY AND FUNCTION

Anatomy (Table 2-1)

The oesophagus is a fibromuscular tube that connects the pharynx in the neck to the stomach in the abdomen, traversing the thorax via the superior and posterior mediastinum. It begins below the cricopharyngeus muscle, at the lower edge of the cricoid cartilage and at the level of C6. In the neck, the oesophagus lies posterior to the trachea. As it descends through the mediastinum, it passes posterior to the aortic arch, the left main bronchus and the left atrium. At the diaphragm the oesophagus passes through the diaphragmatic hiatus at T10 accompanied by the vagus nerves, and ends at the gastric cardia at the level of T11. The abdominal oesophagus lies posterior to the left lobe of the liver. The oesophagus is therefore composed of a short cervical, a long thoracic, and short abdominal segments.[1]

In health, the oesophagus is lined by stratified, non-keratinising squamous epithelium. At the gastro-oesophageal junction there is an abrupt transition to columnar epithelium termed the 'Z-line' because of the irregular interdigitations between pale pink squamous and the darker columnar epithelia (Fig. 2-1). The gastro-oesophageal junction is usually found at a surprisingly constant 40 cm from the teeth.

The wall of the oesophagus is made up of five layers: the mucosa, the muscularis mucosa, the submucosa, the muscularis propria and adventitia.

Embryology

The stratified squamous epithelium of the oesophagus, together with its associated submucosal glands, is derived from the endoderm of the foregut. The striated muscle of the upper oesophagus is derived from branchial arches 4 and 6, whereas the smooth muscle of the lower oesophagus is derived from somite mesenchyme. The myenteric plexus is derived from neural crest cells.

Function

The oesophagus actively moves ingested material from the pharynx to the stomach, and to prevent reflux of stomach contents. Ingested material may also pass in the opposite direction during vomiting.

Passage of a food bolus is regulated by the upper and lower oesophageal sphincters. The upper oesophageal sphincter is a high-pressure zone at the pharyngo-oesophageal junction and comprises cricopharyngeus, thyropharyngeus and the superior part of the cervical oesophagus.[2] The lower oesophageal sphincter is a 2- to 3-cm high pressure zone at the gastro-oesophageal junction and is composed of the lower oesophageal muscle fibres and the diaphragmatic hiatus.[3] The gastro-oesophageal junction is anchored by the phreno-oesophageal, gastrosplenic, phrenicolienal and gastrophrenic ligaments. The important phreno-oesophageal ligament (or membrane) allows the oesophagus to slide longitudinally through the diaphragmatic hiatus whilst acting as a seal between the thoracic and abdominal cavities.[4]

Unlike the upper and lower oesophageal sphincters, the muscle of the interposed oesophageal 'body' is relaxed in the resting state. The swallowing reflex induces so-called primary peristaltic (or stripping) waves that travel at 3–4 cm/s. Secondary peristalsis occurs when oesophageal sensory receptors are activated by material persisting in the oesophagus after primary peristalsis. Tertiary contractions are non-propulsive and are seen in a variety of motility disorders[5] (Fig. 2-2). A further motility disturbance is the so-called feline oesophagus (Fig. 2-3). This takes the form of small horizontal transient contractions that are thought to arise from the muscularis mucosa. This finding, also known as the oesophageal shiver, is a normal feature of the cat's oesophagus, hence the term.

EXAMINATION

The oesophagus can be examined with any of the commonly used imaging techniques. The initial test of choice is usually endoscopy, with fluoroscopy reserved for frail patients, those with suspected motility disorders, or after surgery. Computed tomography (CT) is often the first-line test in the context of trauma.

Imaging is extensively used in the staging of oesophageal malignancy, particularly CT, positron emission

TABLE 2-1   **Anatomy of the Oesophagus**

	Muscle	Length (cm)	Innervation	Artery	Veins	Lymph
Cervical and upper thoracic	Striated	8	Sensory, motor and parasympathetic from vagus, some sensory from spinal nerves	Inferior thyroid	Inferior thyroid	Lower deep cervical nodes
Middle thoracic	Mixed	8	Vagus	Aortic branches	Azygos system	Mediastinal nodes
Lower thoracic and abdominal	Smooth	8	Vagus	Left gastric	Left gastric (NB varices)	Left gastric nodes

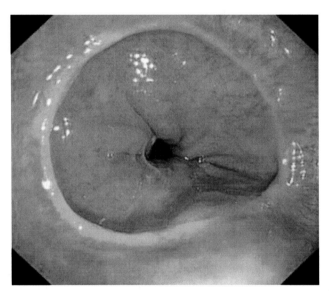

FIGURE 2-1 ■ **Endoscopic image demonstrating the normal Z-line.** (Image courtesy of Dr S Varghese, Cambridge University Hospitals.)

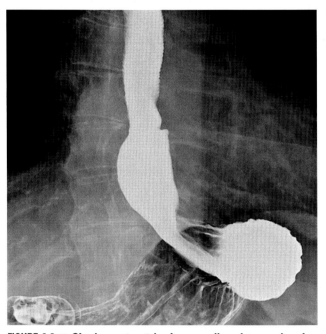

FIGURE 2-3 ■ **Single contrast barium swallow image showing feline oesophagus in a patient with a hiatal hernia.**

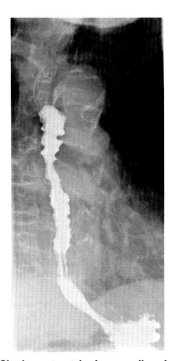

FIGURE 2-2 ■ **Single-contrast barium swallow image showing tertiary contractions of the oesophagus.**

tomography CT (PET-CT) and endoscopic ultrasound (EUS).

Plain Radiography

In most circumstances, plain radiographs reveal little useful information regarding the oesophagus, except in the context of foreign body ingestion.[6] Foreign bodies tend to lodge at one of the oesophageal constriction points:

- cricopharyngeus;
- aortic arch;
- left main bronchus; or
- diaphragmatic hiatus.

Otherwise a dilated, gas- or fluid-filled oesophagus (Fig. 2-4) may be identified incidentally during chest radiography for other indications.

Ultrasound

The majority of the oesophagus is inaccessible to conventional ultrasound examination. The short cervical and abdominal segments are amenable to imaging in this way, but this is rarely used in clinical practice.

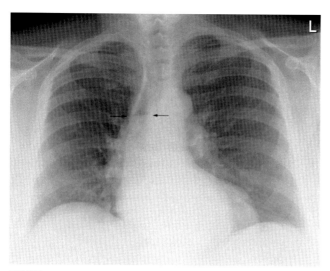

FIGURE 2-4 ■ A dilated, gas- and fluid-filled oesophagus is visible on the chest radiograph of this patient with achalasia (arrows indicate fluid level).

Fluoroscopy

Fluoroscopic examination of the oesophagus is frequently performed for a wide variety of indications. Barium suspensions are preferred for most indications; a density of 100% w/v is often used to provide a balance between good mucosal coating and not being too dense. If possible, double-contrast images should be obtained using an effervescent agent, usually in the erect position. These are complimentary to prone, single-contrast images.

Water-soluble contrast medium is used initially when a tear, perforation or anastomotic leak is suspected. Low osmolar agents such as Gastromiro (iopamidol) should always be used to prevent pulmonary oedema, which can occur following aspiration of high osmolar agents such as Gastrografin (meglumine diatrizoate).

In some institutions, when a leak is suspected, water-soluble contrast medium is followed with a barium suspension. Using barium in this way has been shown to be more sensitive for contained perforations, although it adds nothing in the detection of free leakage into the neck or mediastinum.[7]

Fluoroscopic examination of the oesophagus is tailored to the indication, but a suggested technique is as follows: control images should be obtained if the patient has had oesophageal or gastric surgery. In the erect position, double-contrast images are obtained in the lateral and PA projections of the cervical and upper oesophagus at 4 images per second. Right anterior oblique images of the mid and lower oesophagus are obtained at 2/s, also in double contrast. The patient is then moved to the prone position and images are obtained at 1/s during three separate, single bolus swallows to assess oesophageal motility and fully distend the gastro-oesophageal junction. The images obtained in the prone position are usually single contrast. Finally, a static image of the stomach to include the gastric fundus is obtained in the erect position.

The standard fluoroscopic examination may be augmented with additional procedures. As an example, where

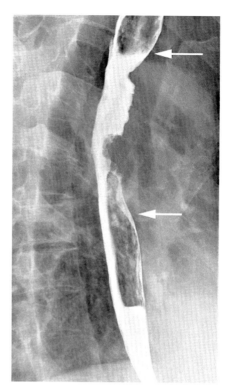

FIGURE 2-5 ■ Double-contrast barium swallow of a malignant stricture. Note the irregularity of the mucosa and shouldered, shelf-like margins (arrows indicate proximal and distal extent). Endoscopic biopsy confirmed a squamous cell carcinoma. (Image courtesy of Gillian Roe, St James's Hospital, Leeds.)

a patient describes a clear history of dysphagia but the images obtained appear normal, a swallow of biscuit dipped in barium or a barium tablet may uncover an occult stricture. If there are pharyngeal symptoms, images of the pharynx obtained during phonation are obtained.

Although no longer the first-line test for dysphagia, fluoroscopy remains an important test. It is well suited to evaluate motility disorders, the oesophagus following trauma or surgery, complex hiatal herniae and as a less invasive alternative to endoscopy in the frail, elderly patient (Fig. 2-5).

Endoscopy

Oesophagogastroduodenoscopy or 'endoscopy' is the initial investigation of choice for most oesophageal indications, particularly dysphagia. It permits the direct visualisation of the mucosa and, crucially, biopsies can be taken. In patients with high dysphagia, preliminary fluoroscopic assessment can be used to forewarn the endoscopist of a pharyngeal pouch, which hopefully reduces the risk of perforation.

For the procedure the patient is placed in the left lateral position. Increasingly, diagnostic endoscopy is performed without sedation, using pharyngeal local anaesthetic spray. Sedation with a short-acting benzodiazepine (e.g. midazolam) is an alternative for diagnostic procedures, and is preferred when intervention is planned.

In addition to a detailed diagnostic assessment of the mucosa, a wide variety of therapeutic manoeuvres may be

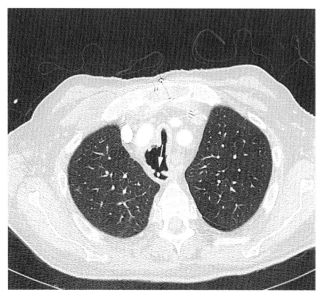

FIGURE 2-6 ■ CT image on lung window settings. There is a fistula (arrow) between the trachea and the oesophagus in this patient with metastatic squamous cell carcinoma. A nasogastric tube is present in the oesophagus.

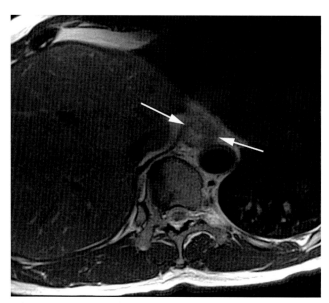

FIGURE 2-7 ■ Axial T2-weighted MR image of a distal oesophageal adenocarcinoma (arrows).

carried out endoscopically. The most common of these is the treatment of upper GI haemorrhage, which may be carried out using a variety of different techniques. Elective procedures include balloon dilatation and/or stenting of strictures, radiofrequency ablation (RFA) of dysplastic or malignant epithelium and injection of botulinum toxin for motility disorders. Endoscopic mucosal resection (EMR) deserves special note, as it is both therapeutic and the preferred method for staging early oesophageal tumours.[8]

CT

In the context of oesophageal disease, CT is most widely used in the staging of oesophageal cancer. A CT of the thorax, abdomen and pelvis should be acquired.[8] Good oesophageal and gastric distension is important: the patient should be given 1–1.5 L of water to drink as well as effervescent granules, and be imaged in the prone position. Intravenous contrast medium should be used whenever possible, with the upper abdomen imaged in both the arterial and portal venous phases.

For the investigation of patients with suspected oesophageal trauma (including Boerhaave's syndrome) and in the postoperative setting, positive oral contrast medium is required. As for fluoroscopic examinations, this should always be a low osmolar agent. For suspected tracheo-oesophageal fistula, an initial acquisition without the use of oral contrast medium is usually diagnostic (Fig. 2-6).

MRI

In current clinical practice, magnetic resonance imaging (MRI) is not used for imaging the oesophagus. Whether MRI may be useful for tumour or nodal staging in oesophageal cancer is an area of current research (Fig. 2-7).

Endoscopic Ultrasound

The highest spatial resolution imaging of the oesophagus is obtained using endoscopic ultrasound. This technique uses a high-frequency (7–12 MHz) ultrasound probe mounted at the end of an endoscope (an 'echoendoscope'). A radial echoendoscope produces ultrasound images that are perpendicular to the axis of the scope and is used for oesophageal cancer staging. A linear echoendoscope produces images parallel to its axis and it is this type of instrument that is used for EUS-guided fine needle aspiration (EUS-FNA).[9]

EUS is generally used to characterise abnormalities identified using other imaging techniques, in particular the staging of oesophageal cancer. Less frequently, EUS is used for the assessment of submucosal lesions of the oesophagus. The high frequency and close proximity of the ultrasound probe allow the delineation of five layers of the oesophageal wall: mucosa, muscularis mucosa, submucosa, muscularis propria and adventitia. The muscular layers are hypoechoic; hence, there is a five-layered alternating pattern. EUS-FNA allows sampling of structures deep to the oesophageal mucosa, particularly thoracic and upper abdominal lymph nodes. This can be particularly useful in the staging of oesophageal and lung malignancy, and in the diagnosis of tuberculosis.

Radionuclide Radiology Including PET-CT

For patients with oesophageal cancer, F18-fluorodeoxyglucose (FDG) PET-CT is now the standard of care if radical treatment is intended.[8] This is largely because of the high proportion of patients that have

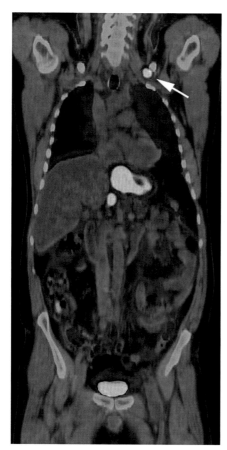

FIGURE 2-8 ■ Coronal PET-CT image of an FDG-avid left supra-clavicular lymph node (arrow) metastasis in a patient with a distal oesophageal adenocarcinoma.

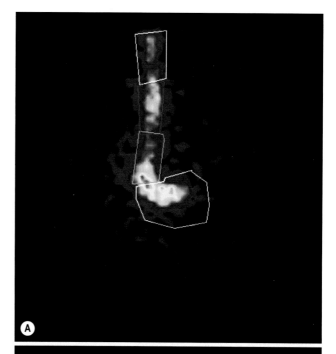

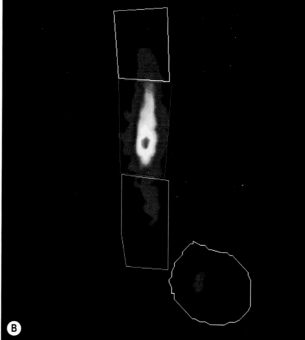

FIGURE 2-9 ■ Radioisotope imaging of the oesophagus. A normal examination is shown with isotope in the stomach (A), whereas in achalasia the isotope is retained in the oesophagus (B). (Images courtesy of Dr KK Balan, Addenbrooke's Hospital Cambridge.)

unsuspected metastatic disease at presentation (Fig. 2-8), and the superiority of PET-CT over other techniques for identifying it.[10] The improved anatomic localisation of integrated PET-CT means that it is preferable to separate PET and CT acquisitions.

Technetium-based radionuclide imaging of the oesophagus can be used for the identification of oesophageal motility disorders and gastro-oesophageal reflux disease (GORD). Patients can be imaged swallowing both liquid and solid material (usually ^{99m}Tc-labelled sulphur colloid and scrambled egg, respectively) (Fig. 2-9).

PATHOLOGICAL FEATURES

Oesophageal Cancer

Oesophageal cancer is the sixth most common cause of death from cancer in the UK. There are two major histological types: squamous cell carcinoma and adenocarcinoma. Although the squamous type has been more common historically (and still is worldwide), in the West it has been overtaken by adenocarcinoma due to the rise in obesity.[11]

Accurate preoperative staging of oesophageal cancer is difficult. The mobility of the oesophagus and its proximity to other organs make the assessment of local invasion problematic. Malignant lymph nodes are usually not enlarged,[12] and may first arise some distance from the tumour.[13] Furthermore, unsuspected metastases may be present in up to 30% of patients at diagnosis.[14] It is not surprising then that a variety of different tests are required for accurate staging. The patient with oesophageal cancer can face a whirlwind of tests, including endoscopy, CT,

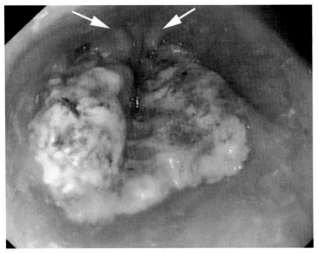

FIGURE 2-10 ■ **Endoscopic image of a distal oesophageal adeno-carcinoma.** Note the gastric folds (arrows) visible adjacent to the tumour, indicating the level of the gastro-oesophageal junction. (Image courtesy of Dr S Varghese, Cambridge University Hospitals.)

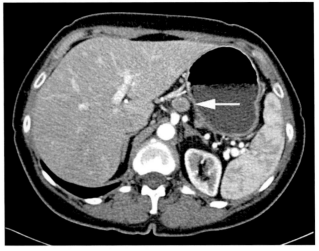

FIGURE 2-12 ■ **CT image of an enlarged coeliac lymph node (arrow) in a patient with a squamous cell carcinoma of the oesophagus.**

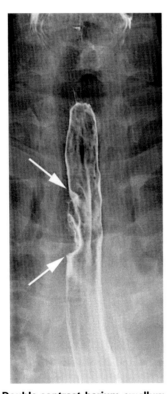

FIGURE 2-11 ■ **Double-contrast barium swallow image demonstrating a nodular mural lesion arising from the left side of the proximal oesophagus (arrows indicate proximal and distal extent).** This was confirmed as a squamous cell carcinoma on endoscopic biopsy.

EUS and PET-CT. This combination is crucial for determining appropriate therapy.

Initial diagnosis is usually with endoscopy as it permits histological confirmation with biopsy (Fig. 2-10). Despite this, a good-quality fluoroscopic examination can detect even early tumours (Fig. 2-11). If a stricture is identified using fluoroscopy and appears unequivocally benign, with symmetrical, smooth narrowing and a gradual tapering to normal calibre, malignancy can be confidently excluded.[15] The converse is also true: strictures with an ulcerated, irregular mucosa and shouldered, shelf-like margins can be considered malignant on imaging appearances alone.

The vast majority of patients will go on to CT as their initial staging investigation. Although less sensitive than EUS and PET-CT, it is relatively specific for identifying locally advanced or metastatic disease. Patients with these findings on CT are therefore spared further staging investigations. In the case of early tumours that appear to be T1 endoscopically, endoscopic mucosal resection (EMR) is the preferred initial staging technique.[8]

The introduction of the seventh edition of the TNM classification has resulted in a number of changes to oesophageal cancer staging:
1. Tumours of the gastro-oesophageal junction have been reclassified as lower oesophageal tumours if their epicentre is within 5 cm of the junction and they extend to involve the oesophagus.
2. T4 disease has been subdivided into resectable (T4a) and non-resectable (T4b) disease.
3. Positive nodal disease has been subdivided into N1, N2, and N3.
4. Coeliac axis (Fig. 2-12) and perioesophageal cervical lymph nodes (Fig. 2-13) have been reclassified as regional nodes rather than metastases.

CT for Oesophageal Cancer

The normal oesophagus should have a wall thickness of less than 5 mm on CT when adequately distended.[16] Tumours are usually seen as regions of wall thickening (Fig. 2-14). CT is rather limited in the local staging of oesophageal tumours because it is unable to delineate the layers of the oesophageal wall, and is therefore only useful for distinguishing between T1–3 and T4 (invasion of other structures). The sensitivity and specificity of CT

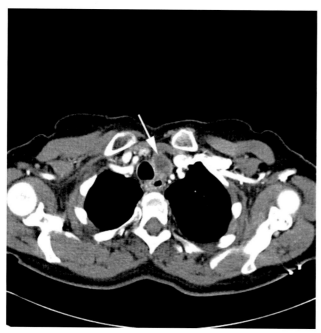

FIGURE 2-13 ■ **CT image of an enlarged left cervical perioesophageal lymph node (arrow) in a patient with squamous cell carcinoma of the oesophagus.**

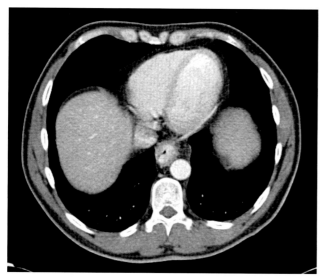

FIGURE 2-14 ■ **CT image of a lower oesophageal adenocarcinoma.** There are no features of invasion of adjacent organs such as the aorta. Statistically this tumour is most likely to be a T3 tumour, but a T2 could look identical; hence the requirement for EUS.

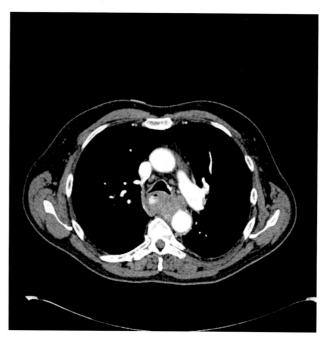

FIGURE 2-15 ■ **CT image of a lower oesophageal adenocarcinoma.** There is infilling of the triangle between the oesophagus, aorta and vertebral column. The tumour contacts the aorta for greater than 90°. The aortic contour is flattened adjacent to the tumour. These are all features of T4 invasion.

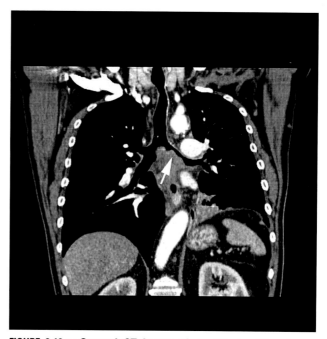

FIGURE 2-16 ■ **Coronal CT image of a patient with a lower oesophageal adenocarcinoma.** There is nodular protrusion of soft tissue from the tumour into the left main bronchus (arrow), in keeping with T4 invasion.

for T4 disease in a study of 94 patients with oesophageal squamous cell carcinoma were 66 and 84%, respectively.[17] Signs of T4 disease include tumour contact of more than 90° with the aorta (Fig. 2-15); loss of the triangle of fat between oesophagus, aorta and spinal column (Fig. 2-15); and nodular protrusion into the airways (Fig. 2-16).

For nodal staging of oesophageal cancer, CT is relatively insensitive, as the majority of malignant nodes are not enlarged.[12] In a recent meta-analysis the sensitivity and specificity for regional nodal disease were 50 and 83%, respectively.[18] In general, nodes with a short axis of greater than 1 cm should be considered malignant on CT. Common sites for nodal disease include perioesophageal, subcarinal, left gastric (Fig. 2-17) and coeliac territories.

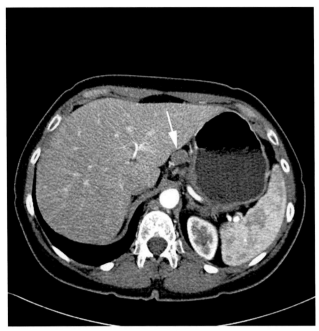

FIGURE 2-17 ■ CT image demonstrating an enlarged left gastric lymph node (arrow) in a patient with an oesophageal squamous cell carcinoma.

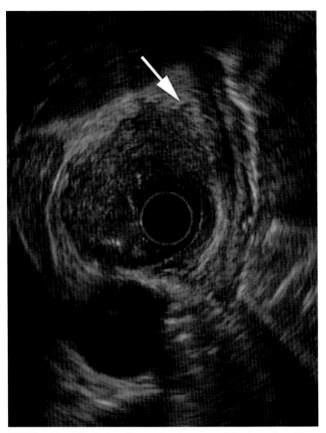

FIGURE 2-19 ■ **Radial endoscopic ultrasound image of a distal oesophageal adenocarcinoma.** The aorta is seen at 6 o'clock. The tumour is seen extending from 7 o'clock to 1 o'clock. There are pseudopodia (arrow) extending out from the tumour, indicating disruption of the muscularis propria and infiltration of the surrounding tissues, in keeping with T3 disease.

Visceral metastases are seen in the liver, the lungs, bones and the adrenal glands. In keeping with its performance for regional nodal involvement, CT is insensitive but relatively specific for metastatic disease, with a sensitivity in one meta-analysis of 52% and specificity of 91%.[18]

EUS for Oesophageal Cancer

EUS is superior to CT and PET-CT for T staging (Fig. 2-19). The sensitivity and specificity for identifying the various T stages of oesophageal cancer is high.[19] In some patients with advanced tumours, the stricture is too tight to prevent passage of the standard radial echoendoscope. An alternative oesophageal mini-probe (smaller because it lacks endoscopic video capability) can be used in some of these cases. If the tumour is not traversable with the standard echoendoscope, the T stage is almost always T3 or T4.

The number of lymph nodes involved seen on EUS correlates closely with patient survival. For nodal disease, EUS has a sensitivity higher than that of PET or CT but is less specific.[18]

Although metastatic disease can be identified with EUS on occasion (for example, in the left adrenal gland or liver) it does not provide the whole-body coverage necessary and so is always used in conjunction with cross-sectional imaging in practice.

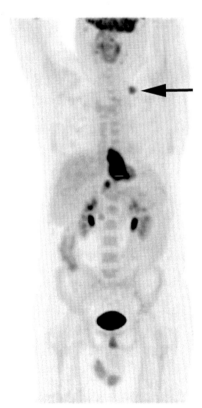

FIGURE 2-18 ■ Coronal PET MIP image demonstrating an FDG-avid left supraclavicular lymph node metastasis (arrow) in a patient with a distal oesophageal adenocarcinoma.

The most frequent sites for oesophageal cancer metastases are non-regional lymph nodes such as the supraclavicular and retroperitoneal abdominal lymph nodes. As is the case with gastric cancer, the left supraclavicular node is more frequently involved than the right (Fig. 2-18).

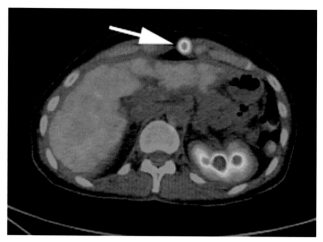

FIGURE 2-20 ■ **PET-CT image demonstrating a solitary region of abnormal FDG uptake in the anterior abdominal wall (arrow) of a patient with a distal oesophageal adenocarcinoma.** Ultrasound-guided fine needle aspiration of this lesion confirmed a metastasis.

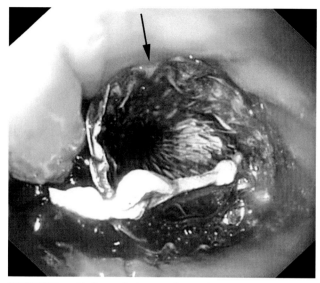

FIGURE 2-21 ■ **Endoscopic image of a patient with an oesophageal adenocarcinoma.** A self-expanding, covered metallic stent (arrow) has just been inserted. (Image courtesy of Dr S Varghese, Cambridge University Hospitals.)

EUS is particularly important for evaluating patients without nodal or metastatic disease on other techniques. This is because a fit patient with a T2 N0 M0 tumour will generally go straight to surgery, whereas a patient with a resectable but more advanced tumour will usually undergo neoadjuvant chemotherapy.

PET-CT for Oesophageal Cancer

In T1 tumours of the oesophagus, it is usually not possible to identify the tumour with PET, which should therefore be omitted if this stage is suspected endoscopically. If a tumour is not detectable by PET-CT, it will be T2 or less in 70% of cases.[20] PET-CT otherwise suffers the same limitations as CT in terms of mural invasion, and EUS is therefore the preferred technique for local staging.

Although the performance of PET for nodal staging has, to date, been variable,[10] the early results of combined PET-CT are more encouraging, probably because of improved anatomic localisation with fused images. In a study of 45 patients with squamous cell cancer the sensitivity and specificity were 93 and 92%, respectively. Whether these results can be replicated in oesophageal adenocarcinoma, which is generally less FDG avid, remains to be seen.

PET-CT is the technique of choice for identifying metastases to non-regional lymph nodes and other tissues such as the liver and skeletal muscle (Fig. 2-20). The ability of PET to correctly upstage up to 20% of patients means that it should be considered for all patients prior to radical treatment.[8] For single metastases, cytological or histological confirmation is recommended in view of the 4% false-positive rate.[21]

Treatment of Oesophageal Cancer

Treatment for oesophageal cancer covers a broad range of interventions that are dependent on the stage and type of the tumour, as well as the fitness of the patient and local availability.

For the earliest oesophageal tumours (T1a) that do not invade the submucosa, endoscopic mucosal resection is the preferred technique for removal. The EMR specimen is assessed histologically for deep invasion. If present, further treatment would be considered, including oesophagectomy.

At the other end of the staging spectrum, patients with invasion of major structures (T4b) or metastatic disease are offered palliative treatment. This includes a variety of manoeuvres for maintaining oesophageal patency, most commonly stenting (Figs. 2-21–2-23). Systemic treatment with palliative chemotherapy is used in patients with a good performance status. Radiotherapy has an important role, particularly for the more radiosensitive squamous cell carcinoma.

For patients with resectable disease, most will have nodal involvement, or a tumour extending through the muscularis propria (T3 disease). If this is the case, the patient will be offered neoadjuvant chemotherapy prior to surgery. Radical radiotherapy is an alternative treatment for squamous cell carcinoma. A variety of surgical approaches are used. The oesophagus is almost always substituted with a gastric conduit. Where this fails, a colonic interposition (Fig. 2-24) may be used, usually after an interval of several months.

Other Oesophageal Neoplasms

Other than adenocarcinoma and squamous cell carcinoma, true neoplasms of the oesophagus are uncommon. They can be categorised as benign or malignant, and according to whether they are mucosal or submucosal.

Benign Lesions

Glycogenic acanthosis, whilst not a neoplasm, requires mention as it is present in up to 30% of normal individuals. It manifests as mural nodules, usually measuring

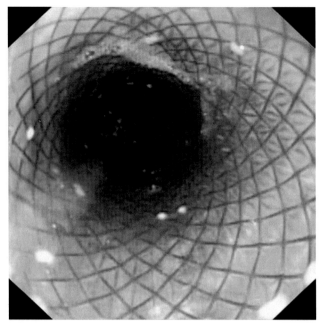

FIGURE 2-22 ■ **Endoscopic image of a patient with an oesophageal adenocarcinoma.** The oesophageal stent has now fully expanded, producing a viable lumen. (Image courtesy of Dr S Varghese, Cambridge University Hospitals.)

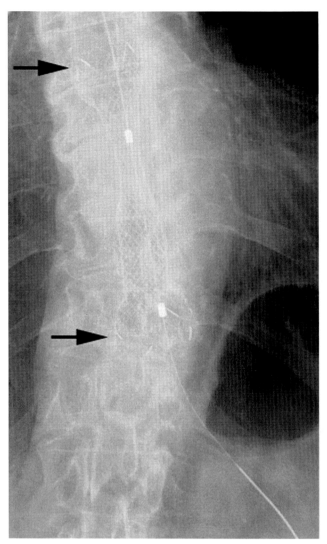

FIGURE 2-23 ■ **Fluoroscopic image of an oesophageal stent (arrows indicate proximal and distal extent of the stent) just after placement.** The guidewire and deployment device remain in situ.

2–5 mm, which are more easily seen as white/yellow plaques on endoscopy. These nodules/plaques are caused by the proliferation of glycogen-containing cells within the squamous epithelium. Glycogenic acanthosis is of no clinical consequence, although it may be associated with GORD, coeliac disease and rarely Cowden's syndrome. The multiplicity of lesions is usually helpful in making the diagnosis at fluoroscopy.

Papillomata are an uncommon benign tumour of the oesophagus, and comprise hyperplastic squamous epithelium. A papilloma usually appears as a solitary sessile polyp and will rarely measure more than 1 cm. In view of the non-specific appearance, biopsy is required to distinguish a papilloma from an early adenocarcinoma or squamous cell carcinoma.

The most common benign submucosal tumour of the oesophagus is the leiomyoma. This is in contrast to the rest of the gastrointestinal tract where gastrointestinal stromal tumours (GISTs) predominate. Endoscopically and on fluoroscopic studies, they appear as a smooth submucosal mass. On CT a homogeneous well-defined soft-tissue mass is the most common appearance, sometimes with a focus or two of punctate calcification. These findings are rather non-specific, so confirmation with EUS that the tumour arises from the muscularis mucosa, or less commonly the muscularis propria, is necessary.

Although not neoplastic, a congenital foregut duplication cyst (Fig. 2-25) may be identified as a submucosal mass on fluoroscopic or endoscopic examination of the oesophagus. These are very straightforward to characterise with MRI or endoscopic ultrasound; both techniques will demonstrate a simple cyst (Fig. 2-26).

Fibrovascular polyps are very rare pedunculated submucosal lesions that usually arise from the upper oesophagus (Fig. 2-27). As they tend to be rather soft, they can reach a considerable size before resulting in dysphagia. On CT they often have regions of both fat and soft-tissue attenuation (Fig. 2-28). They are notable for their potential for an unusual clinical presentation: regurgitation into the mouth, which can sometimes result in death by asphyxiation. Other submucosal lesions such as neurofibromata and lipomata are also rare.

Malignant Lesions

The vast majority of oesophageal malignant tumours are adenocarcinomas and squamous cell carcinomas. A number of rare malignancies are encountered, each representing around 1% of all oesophageal tumours. These include small cell carcinoma, gastrointestinal stromal tumours, melanoma, lymphoma and metastases.

Like small cell carcinoma of the lung, small cell carcinoma of the oesophagus is a highly aggressive primary

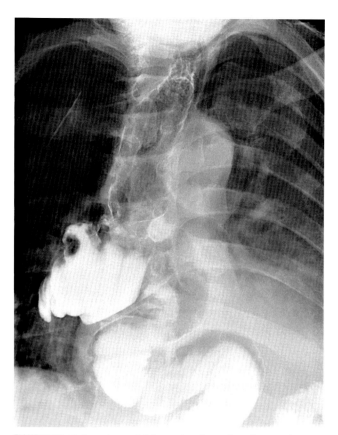

FIGURE 2-24 ■ **A water-soluble contrast swallow image demonstrating the normal appearance of a colonic interposition.** Note the normal haustral fold pattern of the colonic segment.

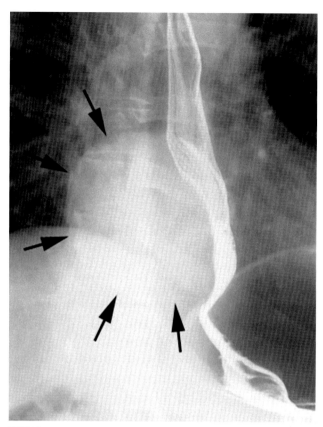

FIGURE 2-25 ■ **A barium swallow image demonstrating an extrinsic rounded lesion (arrows) causing compression of the distal oesophagus.**

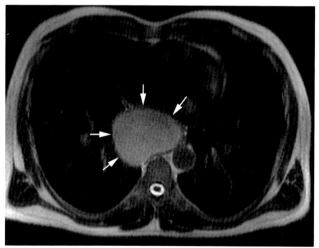

FIGURE 2-26 ■ **An MR study of the same patient as in Fig. 2-24 shows that the structure is of uniform high signal on T2-weighted MR imaging in keeping with a foregut duplication cyst (arrows).**

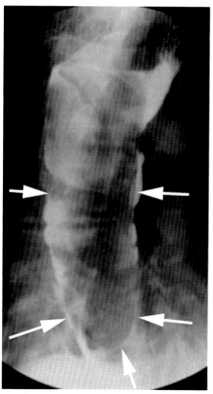

FIGURE 2-27 ■ **Barium swallow image demonstrating a grossly dilated oesophagus with a large filling defect (arrows) consistent with a fibrovascular polyp.** (Image courtesy of Dr DJM Tolan, Leeds Teaching Hospitals.)

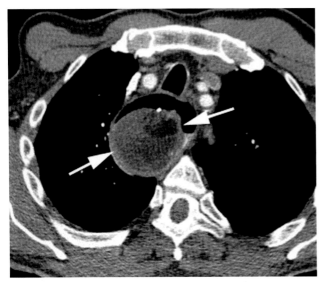

FIGURE 2-28 ■ **CT image of the same patient as in Fig. 2-26 demonstrating a grossly dilated oesophagus with a smooth intraluminal lesion (arrows) of mixed soft tissue and fat attenuation, confirmed as a fibrovascular polyp.** (Image courtesy of Dr DJM Tolan, Leeds Teaching Hospitals.)

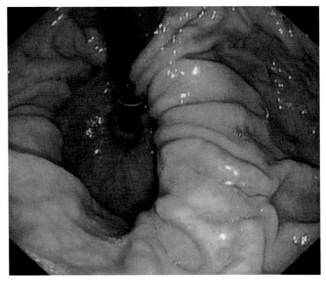

FIGURE 2-29 ■ **Endoscopic image during the 'J manoeuvre' with the endoscope retroflexed in the stomach.** The view is of the gastro-oesophageal junction from below, looking cranially. Gastric folds can be seen passing through the extrinsic narrowing of the diaphragmatic hiatus, diagnostic of a hiatal hernia. (Image courtesy of Dr S Varghese, Cambridge University Hospitals.)

malignancy. It tends to be advanced at diagnosis and to relapse quickly following treatment. Primary oesophageal malignant melanoma is similar to small cell carcinoma in that it confers a grave prognosis, is frequently advanced at presentation and behaves in a fashion similar to that of its better known extra-enteric counterpart. It should be considered as a diagnosis when endoscopic findings are of a pigmented lesion, although non-pigmented, amelanotic forms are also encountered.

GISTs are very rare in the oesophagus but much more common in the stomach and small bowel. They are of variable malignant potential. On EUS, oesophageal GISTs appear as submucosal lesions arising from the muscularis mucosa or the muscularis propria, and are therefore difficult to distinguish from a leiomyoma without tissue sampling.

Metastases to the oesophagus most commonly arise via direct extension, usually from carcinoma of the bronchus. Involved lymph nodes infiltrate the oesophagus, causing extrinsic compression and occasionally fistulae between the oesophageal lumen and the airways. Pancreatic cancer may also extend to directly involve the distal oesophagus and gastro-oesophageal junction. Lymphatogenous or haematogenous metastases result in a submucosal mass or masses, for example in breast cancer.

Hiatus Hernia

A hiatus hernia is when abdominal organs pass through the oesophageal hiatus into the chest. Usually the herniated organ is the abdominal segment of the oesophagus with part of the stomach, although greater omentum, colon, spleen, pancreas and small intestine are sometimes involved. Hiatal herniaes are divided into sliding and rolling varieties.

The majority of hiatal herniae are of the sliding type (approximately 90%). Weakening of the phreno-oesophageal membrane that usually anchors the distal oesophagus allows superior displacement of the gastro-oesophageal junction. The diaphragmatic hiatus is normally a muscular, slit-like opening in the right crus of the diaphragm passing anterior to posterior. In a well-established sliding hiatal hernia it becomes a more circular window, with atrophy of the surrounding muscular fibres. This change in configuration explains the main clinical consequence of sliding hiatal herniae: gastro-oesophageal reflux disease.

The diagnosis of a sliding hiatal hernia is made on fluoroscopy when gastric rugae are seen traversing the diaphragm, or when the oesophageal B-ring (variably present), representing the squamo-columnar junction, is seen 2 cm above the hiatus. Fluoroscopic and endoscopic assessment of small (less than 2 cm) sliding hiatal herniae is rather inaccurate and in the past has led to overdiagnosis. High-resolution manometry, although imperfect, is the current gold standard.[22] Both endoscopy (Fig. 2-29) and fluoroscopy are sufficient for diagnosing large sliding hiatal herniae.

The less common rolling hiatal hernia is caused by a focal defect in the phreno-oesophageal membrane, rather than generalised laxity. The gastric fundus herniates through the oesophageal hiatus, whereas the gastro-oesophageal junction remains below the diaphragm. In this context the chief concern is for progression to gastric volvulus with its concomitant risks of obstruction and infarction. As with sliding hiatal herniae, symptoms of gastro-oesophageal reflux may also be present. Rolling hiatal herniae are most easily diagnosed fluoroscopically, as are combined-type hiatal herniae (when the hernia consists of both rolling and sliding elements).

Gastro-Oesophageal Reflux Disease

The term gastro-oesophageal reflux disease (GORD) covers a spectrum of disorders including columnar-lined oesophagus, reflux oesophagitis and non-erosive reflux disease (where the patient has symptoms but the oesophagus is endoscopically normal). GORD is the commonest cause of oesophageal symptoms, and represents a major source of healthcare expenditure. A variety of causative factors, including dysfunction of the lower oesophageal sphincter, hiatus hernia, reduced resistance of the oesophageal mucosa to ulceration, reduced oesophageal and gastric emptying rates, and lifestyle choices such as smoking, have been identified.

Fluoroscopy has a limited role in the identification of gastro-oesophageal reflux. The gold standard test for establishing the presence of gastro-oesophageal reflux is 24-h pH monitoring, although in clinical practice a therapeutic trial of a proton pump inhibitor (PPI) is usually the initial step.

Endoscopy is the most accurate method for identifying the consequences of gastro-oesophageal reflux, as reflux oesophagitis and, particularly, columnar-lined oesophagus may be occult fluoroscopically.

Complications of GORD

Reflux Oesophagitis. Although best detected with endoscopy (Fig. 2-30), a nodular or granular appearance of the oesophageal mucosa on double-contrast fluoroscopic studies suggests early reflux oesophagitis (Fig. 2-31). When more advanced, ulcers or erosions may be seen.

If GORD is severe and untreated, a benign peptic stricture may form (Fig. 2-31). The typical fluoroscopic appearance of a smooth stricture, without shouldering, in the lower oesophagus enables the diagnosis of a peptic stricture to be made. If intramural pseudodiverticula or a stepladder appearance are present, these features lend

weight to the diagnosis. When fluoroscopic findings of a stricture are unequivocally benign, malignancy can be confidently excluded.[15]

Columnar-Lined Oesophagus. Columnar-lined oesophagus (also known as Barrett's oesophagus) is a condition where there is metaplasia of the distal oesophageal mucosa from the normal stratified squamous to columnar epithelium. It is essentially an endoscopic diagnosis, where there is replacement of the normal pale pink oesophageal mucosa with darker pink mucosa, macroscopically similar to that of the stomach, either circumferentially or in tongue-shaped areas extending up from the gastro-oesophageal junction (Fig. 2-32). A reticular pattern seen at double-contrast barium swallow is suggestive. The involved segment of oesophagus is often bell- or tent-shaped. When identified endoscopically, extensive biopsies are taken to assess for dysplasia, or even adenocarcinoma. If more than a 2-cm length of columnar-lined oesophagus is identified, the patient is offered surveillance endoscopy at 2-year intervals, and treated with a PPI. Columnar-lined oesophagus increases the risk of developing cancer by 30–60 times.[23]

Other Varieties of Oesophagitis

Eosinophilic oesophagitis is a recently described entity characterised in adults by dysphagia and food impaction.

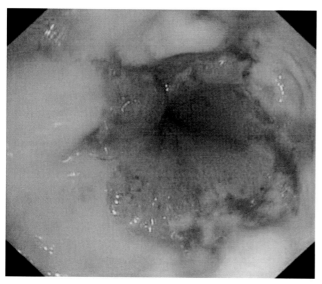

FIGURE 2-30 ▪ **Endoscopic image demonstrating erythema and ulceration of the distal oesophagus, diagnostic of oesophagitis.** (Image courtesy of Dr S Varghese, Cambridge University Hospitals.)

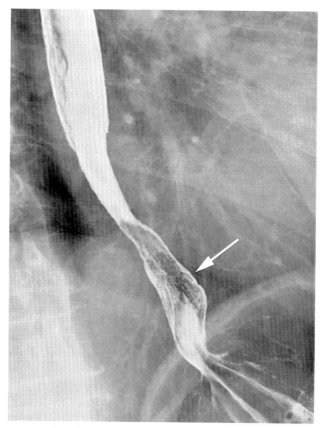

FIGURE 2-31 ▪ **Double-contrast barium swallow demonstrating a granular mucosa (arrow), indicating reflux oesophagitis below a benign stricture in the lower oesophagus.** (Image courtesy of Gillian Roe, St James's Hospital, Leeds.)

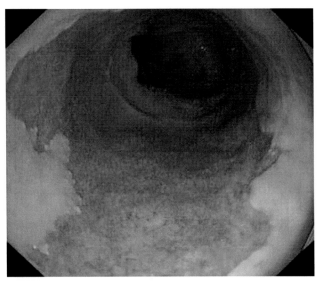

FIGURE 2-32 ■ **Endoscopic image demonstrating columnar-lined oesophagus.** Gastric folds are just visible in the distance, indicating the site of the gastro-oesophageal junction. Extending proximally from this region there is dark pink columnar mucosa. The pale pink mucosa is normal squamous oesophageal mucosa. (Image courtesy of Dr S Varghese, Cambridge University Hospitals.)

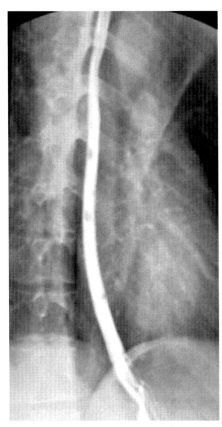

FIGURE 2-33 ■ **Single-contrast barium swallow image demonstrating a small-calibre oesophagus in a patient with eosinophilic oesophagitis.**

Endoscopic biopsies of the upper oesophageal squamous mucosa should demonstrate 15 or more eosinophils per high-powered field and other similar conditions (such as GORD) should be excluded prior to the diagnosis being made. The cause of eosinophilic oesophagitis remains unclear, although the finding that an exclusion diet can be effective supports an allergic aetiology. Fluoroscopic features may be seen at any segment of the thoracic oesophagus and include a small-calibre oesophagus, transient or fixed circular rings (Fig. 2-33) or a benign stricture.

Candida oesophagitis is the most common infectious cause of oesophagitis, and should be suspected when large or linear mural plaques are seen on fluoroscopy. It is more common in immunocompromised patients and those with oesophageal stasis, for example in achalasia. Other types of infectious oesophagitis including HIV and CMV oesophagitis usually manifest as one or more large ovoid or diamond-shaped ulcers.

Drug-induced oesophagitis has a variable appearance according to the culprit. Antibiotics such as tetracycline and doxycycline tend to cause small shallow ulcers. Potassium chloride and alendronate are more injurious and can lead to large ulcers and strictures. Radiation and caustic oesophagitis are usually suggested by the history. Both tend to produce long strictures, and predispose to squamous cell carcinoma.

Oesophageal Diverticula

In the upper and mid oesophagus, diverticula are thought to arise following scarring in mediastinal lymph nodes, for example secondary to tuberculosis. They are therefore termed traction diverticula. Pulsion diverticula, by comparison, are usually identified in the distal oesophagus, often associated with oesophageal dysmotility. Pseudodiverticula are tiny flask-shaped outpouchings within the mucosa (and hence not true diverticula) and are probably related to reflux oesophagitis (Fig. 2-34).

Motility Disorders

Fluoroscopic examination of the oesophagus is used in preference to endoscopy as the first-line test for suspected oesophageal motility disorders, but manometry is the gold standard. Gastro-oesophageal reflux disease is probably the commonest cause of disordered oesophageal motility. A number of distinct motility disorders including achalasia, diffuse oesophageal spasm and presby-oesophagus are recognised. In addition, systemic diseases such as scleroderma, diabetes or hypothyroidism may affect oesophageal motility. Finally, neuromuscular disorders such as stroke, Parkinson's disease, myotonic dystrophy and inclusion body myopathy may involve the oesophagus.

Achalasia

This motility disorder affects approximately 1 in 100,000 people. A history of dysphagia for solids and liquids, coupled with regurgitation and chest pain, are suggestive. Fluoroscopic examination classically reveals a grossly

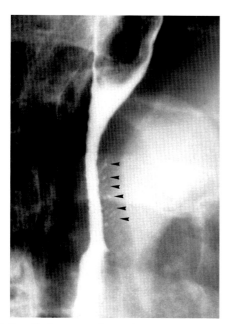

FIGURE 2-34 ■ Barium swallow demonstrating the typical appearances of oesophageal intramural pseudodiverticulosis. The small flask-shaped pits of contrast medium (arrowheads) represent dilated mucous glands and are associated with a benign stricture at the level of the aortic knuckle.

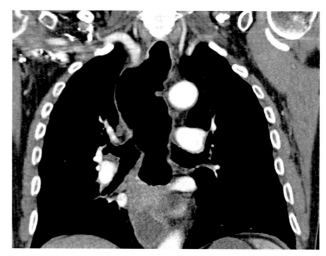

FIGURE 2-35 ■ Coronal CT image in a patient with a history of achalasia. A soft-tissue mass in the distal oesophagus was confirmed as a squamous cell carcinoma at endoscopic biopsy. Note the dilatation of the oesophagus, both proximal and distal to the tumour.

dilated oesophagus tapering down to a 'bird's beak' at the gastro-oesophageal junction. Earlier in the course of the disease, changes may be more subtle with a normal-calibre oesophagus and defective peristalsis distally. Barium retained in the oesophagus for longer than 5 min is a supportive finding.[24] When severe, the air–fluid level in the oesophagus may be visible on a chest radiograph. Immediate and pronounced relaxation of the gastro-oesophageal junction following a drink of hot water is evidence in favour of achalasia over a gastro-oesophageal cancer. Despite this, carcinoma is usually excluded with an endoscopy, and manometry may be arranged to confirm the diagnosis of achalasia. Patients with long-standing achalasia are at risk of aspiration pneumonia, and less commonly squamous cell carcinoma (Fig. 2-35).

Diffuse Oesophageal Spasm

This condition is five times less common than achalasia. Chest pain is usually a more prominent symptom than dysphagia. Like achalasia, characteristic findings may be seen at fluoroscopy, with a corkscrew appearance (Fig. 2-36). Endoscopic ultrasound may show thickening of the muscularis propria. The gold standard for diagnosis is manometry, where simultaneous, non-propulsive contractions of the lower oesophagus are interspersed with normal peristaltic waves.[25]

Presbyoesophagus

Motor disturbances of the oesophagus become more common with age. Often these cannot be attributed to a specific condition and the term presbyoesophagus is used. It is debatable as to whether it is a discrete entity, although

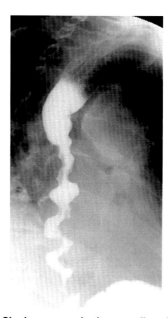

FIGURE 2-36 ■ Single-contrast barium swallow image demonstrating the classical corkscrew appearance of diffuse oesophageal spasm.

long-term GORD may be one of the major aetiological factors.[26]

Systemic Disorders

Scleroderma (progressive systemic sclerosis) preferentially involves the oesophagus over the rest of the gastrointestinal tract. The loss of smooth muscle from the muscularis propria results in fluoroscopic findings of reduced peristalsis, a patulous gastro-oesophageal junction and gastro-oesophageal reflux with its various complications. Manometry is the gold standard for diagnosis of oesophageal involvement, and endoscopy for assessing complications. In patients with lung disease related to scleroderma, a patulous oesophagus is seen in 80% of patients, often accompanied by enlarged mediastinal lymph nodes.[27] Although less common, similar oesophageal involvement may be seen with other connective tissue disorders.

Neuromuscular Disorders

A wide variety of neuromuscular disorders may result in dysphagia, including stroke, Parkinson's disease, myasthenia gravis, multiple sclerosis, motor neuron disease and inclusion body myositis. Although these disorders may involve the oesophagus, the dominant site of disease is usually oropharyngeal.

Inclusion body myositis is the most common myopathy presenting over the age of 40, with a prevalence similar to that of achalasia. It is underdiagnosed, maybe in part due to the variability in symptoms and signs at presentation. Given its propensity to affect skeletal muscle, it preferentially involves the upper oesophagus, as well as the pharynx and muscles of the limbs.[28]

Miscellaneous Conditions

Oesophageal Varices

The large majority of varices seen in the lower oesophagus and is of the uphill variety in the context of portal hypertension. They are termed uphill as blood flows in a superior direction from the left gastric veins of the portal system to systemic venous tributaries, usually of the azygos system. Less commonly, downhill varices may be seen in superior vena cava obstruction. Downhill varices are usually seen in the upper and mid-oesophagus. Both uphill and downhill varices are seen as serpentine filling defects at fluoroscopy, and may also be seen on CT.

Schatzki Ring

A Schatzki or B-ring is a circumferential ring of mucosa 2–3 mm in thickness at the Z-line (Fig. 2-37). If the luminal diameter of the ring is greater than 20 mm, it is very unlikely to cause dysphagia. Conversely if the luminal diameter is less than 13 mm, dysphagia is almost always present.[29]

Dysphagia Lusoria

The oesophagus may be compressed by a congenitally aberrant right subclavian artery. If this is symptomatic, a diagnosis of dysphagia lusoria is made. At CT the diagnosis is straightforward. Fluoroscopically an oblique tubular extrinsic impression is seen in the upper oesophagus (Fig. 2-38). Treatment is generally non-operative with PPIs unless symptoms are severe.[8]

Dysphagia Aortica

The acquired equivalent of dysphagia lusoria is compression of the posterior wall of the lower oesophagus by a tortuous or dilated aorta: hence the term dysphagia aortica. Older women of short stature are predisposed.

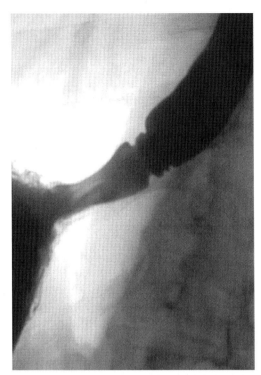

FIGURE 2-37 ■ An example of a fixed sliding hiatal hernia together with several 'B' or Schatzki rings.

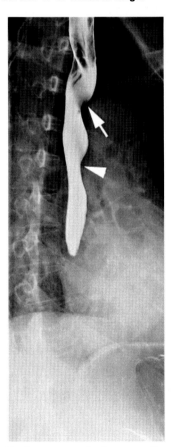

FIGURE 2-38 ■ Single-contrast barium swallow image of a patient with dysphagia lusoria. Note the normal impression made by the left main bronchus (arrowhead), and the deeper oblique impression superior to this (arrow) made by the aberrant right subclavian artery. (Image courtesy of Dr A Husainy, Leeds Teaching Hospitals.)

Trauma

The rib cage shields the oesophagus from blunt and penetrating injuries in most cases of external trauma. The commonest injury to the oesophagus is at endoscopy, with a perforation rate of between 0.008 and 0.018%.[30]

Vomiting can cause injuries of variable severity. A Mallory–Weiss tear is a minor injury consisting of a mucosal tear. Far more serious is the full-thickness injury in Boerhaave's syndrome. The classical clinical picture is of severe chest pain and surgical emphysema in the neck following vomiting, although these features may be absent in up to 50%. The technique of choice is usually CT, given its availability: a diagnosis should be reached as soon as possible given the grave consequences of delayed treatment and diagnosis.

REFERENCES

1. Oezcelik A, DeMeester SR. General anatomy of the oesophagus. Thorac Surg Clin 2011;21:289–97, x.
2. Sivarao DV, Goyal RK. Functional anatomy and physiology of the upper esophageal sphincter. Am J Med 2000;108(Suppl. 4a): 27S–37S.
3. Goyal RK, Chaudhury A. Physiology of normal esophageal motility. J Clin Gastroenterol 2008;42:610–19.
4. Kwok H, Marriz Y, Al-Ali S, Windsor JA. Phrenoesophageal ligament re-visited. Clin Anat 1999;12:164–70.
5. Patti MG, Gantert W, Way LW. Surgery of the oesophagus. Anatomy and physiology. Surg Clin North Am 1997;77: 959–70.
6. Young CA, Menias CO, Bhalla S, Prasad SR. CT features of esophageal emergencies. Radiographics 2008;28:1541–53.
7. Swanson JO, Levine MS, Redfern RO, Rubesin SE. Usefulness of high-density barium for detection of leaks after esophagogastrectomy, total gastrectomy, and total laryngectomy. Am J Roentgenol 2003;181:415–20.
8. Allum WH, Blazeby JM, Griffin SM, et al. Guidelines for the management of oesophageal and gastric cancer. Gut 2011;60: 1449–72.
9. Godfrey EM, Rushbrook SM, Carroll NR. Endoscopic ultrasound: a review of current diagnostic and therapeutic applications. Postgrad Med J 2010;86:346–53.
10. Chowdhury FU, Bradley KM, Gleeson FV. The role of 18F-FDG PET/CT in the evaluation of oesophageal carcinoma. Clin Radiol 2008;63:1297–309.
11. Chak A, Falk G, Grady WM, et al. Assessment of familiality, obesity, and other risk factors for early age of cancer diagnosis in adenocarcinomas of the oesophagus and gastroesophageal junction. Am J Gastroenterol 2009;104:1913–21.
12. Schroder W, Baldus SE, Monig SP, et al. Lymph node staging of esophageal squamous cell carcinoma in patients with and without neoadjuvant radiochemotherapy: histomorphologic analysis. World J Surg 2002;26:584–7.
13. Xu QR, Zhuge XP, Zhang HL, et al. The N-classification for esophageal cancer staging: should it be based on number, distance, or extent of the lymph node metastasis? World J Surg 2011;35: 1303–10.
14. Kato H, Miyazaki T, Nakajima M, et al. The incremental effect of positron emission tomography on diagnostic accuracy in the initial staging of esophageal carcinoma. Cancer 2005;103:148–56.
15. Gupta S, Levine MS, Rubesin SE, et al. Usefulness of barium studies for differentiating benign and malignant strictures of the oesophagus. Am J Roentgenol 2003;180:737–44.
16. Desai RK, Tagliabue JR, Wegryn SA, Einstein DM. CT evaluation of wall thickening in the alimentary tract. Radiographics 1991;11: 771–83; discussion 84.
17. Yamabe Y, Kuroki Y, Ishikawa T, et al. Tumor staging of advanced esophageal cancer: combination of double-contrast esophagography and contrast-enhanced CT. Am J Roentgenol 2008;191: 753–7.
18. van Vliet EP, Heijenbrok-Kal MH, Hunink MG, et al. Staging investigations for oesophageal cancer: a meta-analysis. Br J Cancer 2008;98:547–57.
19. Puli SR, Reddy JB, Bechtold ML, et al. Staging accuracy of esophageal cancer by endoscopic ultrasound: a meta-analysis and systematic review. World J Gastroenterol 2008;14:1479–90.
20. Walker AJ, Spier BJ, Perlman SB, et al. Integrated PET/CT fusion imaging and endoscopic ultrasound in the pre-operative staging and evaluation of esophageal cancer. Mol Imaging Biol 2011; 13:166–71.
21. Meyers BF, Downey RJ, Decker PA, et al. The utility of positron emission tomography in staging of potentially operable carcinoma of the thoracic oesophagus: results of the American College of Surgeons Oncology Group Z0060 trial. J Thorac Cardiovasc Surg 2007;133:738–45.
22. Kahrilas PJ, Kim HC, Pandolfino JE. Approaches to the diagnosis and grading of hiatal hernia. Best Pract Res Clin Gastroenterol 2008;22:601–16.
23. Cossentino MJ, Wong RK. Barrett's oesophagus and risk of esophageal adenocarcinoma. Semin Gastrointest Dis 2003;14:128–35.
24. Richter JE. The diagnosis and misdiagnosis of Achalasia: it does not have to be so difficult. Clin Gastroenterol Hepatol 2011;9: 1010–11.
25. Grubel C, Borovicka J, Schwizer W, et al. Diffuse esophageal spasm. Am J Gastroenterol 2008;103:450–7.
26. DeVault KR. Presbyesophagus: a reappraisal. Curr Gastroenterol Rep 2002;4:193–9.
27. Bhalla M, Silver RM, Shepard JA, McLoud TC. Chest CT in patients with scleroderma: prevalence of asymptomatic esophageal dilatation and mediastinal lymphadenopathy. Am J Roentgenol 1993;161:269–72.
28. Mastaglia FL. Sporadic inclusion body myositis: variability in prevalence and phenotype and influence of the MHC. Acta Myol 2009;28:66–71.
29. Schatzki R. The lower esophageal ring. Long term follow-up of symptomatic and asymptomatic rings. Am J Roentgenol Radium Ther Nucl Med 1963;90:805–10.
30. Newcomer MK, Brazer SR. Complications of upper gastrointestinal endoscopy and their management. Gastrointest Endosc Clin N Am 1994;4:551–70.

CHAPTER 3

THE STOMACH

Dina F. Caroline • Chandra Dass • Omar Agosto

ANATOMY

The oesophagus meets the stomach at the gastro-oesophageal (or oesophagogastric) junction (OGJ). The OGJ is formed by the lower oesophageal sphincter and the crural diaphragm, creating a barrier against acidic stomach contents. The stomach is divided into the cardia, fundus, body, antrum and pylorus. The medial and lateral curvatures of the stomach are known as the lesser and greater curvatures, respectively. The cardia connects the oesophagus to the stomach and lies close to the heart and left hemidiaphragm. The fundus is the rounded portion of the stomach that lies superior and posterior to the cardia. The body of the stomach lies distal to the cardia and comprises most of the organ. The body courses anteriorly and extends to the incisura angularis, which is an angle formed on the lesser curvature of the stomach. An imaginary line drawn from the incisura angularis perpendicular to the long axis of the stomach divides the body of the stomach from the distal third of the stomach or antrum. The pylorus with its short muscular cylindrical opening joins the stomach to the first part of the duodenum (Fig. 3-1). The antrum and pylorus course posteriorly to fix the second part of the duodenum retroperitoneally. Parietal cells, which produce hydrochloric acid, and chief cells, which produce pepsin precursors, are found in the fundus and body. Gastrin is produced in the antrum.

Histologically the stomach is composed of mucosa, submucosa, muscularis propria and serosa.[1] The mucosa is composed of an epithelial layer with innumerable invaginations (pits or fovea) where the gastric glands are found. Loose connective tissue, lamina propria, is found between the gastric pits. A thin band of smooth muscle, the muscularis mucosa, forms the deepest layer of the mucosa. The submucosa consists of loose connective tissue and contains vascular and lymphatic channels, lymphoid follicles and autonomic nerves. The muscularis propria forms the major muscular structure of the stomach and is composed of inner oblique, middle circular and outer longitudinal layers. The circular muscle is thickened at the pylorus to form the pyloric sphincter. The muscle acts as a valve, regulating the outflow of gastric contents into the duodenum.

The serosa is the outermost layer of the stomach and is continuous with the gastrocolic (greater omentum), gastrosplenic and gastrohepatic (lesser omentum) ligaments.

RADIOLOGICAL TECHNIQUES

FLUOROSCOPY

Though barium examinations still represent the main radiological investigations for examination of the stomach in most parts of the world, they have been increasingly replaced by endoscopy and cross-sectional imaging. There are four basic components or techniques which can be utilised during the performance of these examinations: (A) double-contrast, (B) compression, (C) mucosal relief and (D) barium filling.[2,3] Each has specific advantages as well as limitations in evaluating the stomach. Although it is rarely necessary to use all four of these components in a single examination, a thorough evaluation will typically utilise two or three of them.

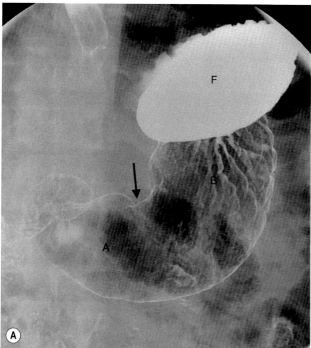

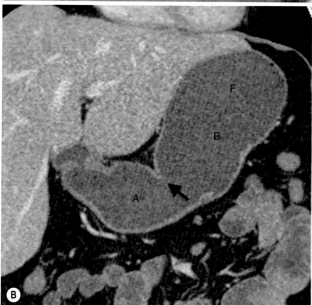

FIGURE 3-1 ▪ Normal stomach with patient lying supine. (A) Double-contrast fluoroscopic image of the stomach. Most of the barium collects in the fundus, which is a posterior structure. (B) Normal water-distended stomach on MDCT coronal image. Incisura angularis (arrow), fundus (F), antrum (A) and body (B) are seen.

The single-contrast upper gastrointestinal examination emphasises compression, barium filling and mucosal relief, whereas the double-contrast examination utilises these techniques to a limited degree.

The double-contrast examination remains invaluable in the evaluation of the mucosal details of the stomach. Antiperistaltic agents are sometimes used to prevent motion artefacts in morphological imaging. The double-contrast technique involves the ingestion of an effervescent, gas-producing agent. The gastric walls are then coated with 100–150 mL of ingested high-density barium suspension. The patient is rolled through at least 360° to coat the mucosa of the entire stomach. Spot radiographs are then obtained in multiple projections (Fig. 3-2).

A properly performed single-contrast examination will emphasise mucosal relief, compression and barium filling. Images may be obtained with the inpatient prone, supine and/or upright positions. Mucosal relief radiographs are particularly obtained at the onset of the examination in both the prone and supine positions, with the objective being demonstration of the gastric mucosal fold pattern. Compression technique is also utilised.

A complete examination of the stomach will include several of the described techniques and include views to show duodenum and duodenal sweep filling to the ligament of Treitz. In most cases, elements of both the double-contrast and single-contrast study will be utilised in a biphasic or multiphasic examination.

Water-soluble contrast for an upper GI examination is reserved for evaluation of a suspected perforation, usually due to peptic ulceration or to demonstrate postoperative anastomotic leaks. Barium may lead to granuloma formation and peritoneal fibrosis if it enters the peritoneal cavity and should be avoided in these circumstances. Water-soluble contrast is innocuous in this situation as the contrast medium will be absorbed by the peritoneum and excreted by the kidneys. If possible the patient should be examined in both prone and supine positions to exclude a leak from the anterior wall.

Gastric mucosa is characterised by two features, the areae gastricae, which form the mucosal surface pattern, and the gastric rugae, which form the gross or macromucosal pattern. The areae gastricae is composed of flat-polygonal tufts of mucosa separated by criss-crossing narrow grooves (sulci gastricae) which can be recognised in double-contrast studies as a reticular network of contrast filling the grooves between the mucosal tufts. The individual mucosal tufts normally have a diameter of 2–3 mm in the gastric antrum and 3–5 mm in the gastric body and fundus. Areae gastricae can be detected on double-contrast studies in nearly 70% of patients and are seen in greater frequency in the elderly.[4] Visualisation of the areae gastricae is considered an indicator of adequate coating of the stomach.

Gastric rugae are smooth folds that tend to parallel the long axis of the stomach and are about 3–5 mm thick on barium studies. These comprise mucosa and a portion of submucosa. Abnormal rugal folds become thicker than normal and may be nodular. Contractions of the muscularis mucosa (the deepest layer of the mucosa) in the antrum may be seen as fine transverse folds in up to 10% of the population[5] (Fig. 3-2C). In some cases these transverse folds, also known as gastric 'striae', may be seen in chronic antral gastrtis.

The fundus lies posteriorly in the left upper quadrant while the body and antrum course on a relatively horizontal plane to lie anteriorly and cross the midline. The distal antrum courses posteriorly to the right of the spine with the pylorus directed posteriorly. The greater curvature forms the anterior wall of the stomach and, similarly, the lesser curvature forms the posterior wall.[6] Variability in the length of the mesenteric attachments leads to a more horizontal orientation of the stomach in muscular and obese people, and a more vertical orientation in slender people and in the geriatric population.

CROSS-SECTIONAL IMAGING

Multidetector Computed Tomography (MDCT)

The role of CT for preoperative staging of gastric malignancy has been well established. Recent advances in MDCT with thin collimation offer the opportunity of near-isotropic imaging of the stomach in multiple planes, extending its role in the early detection of several gastric pathological processes. With proper distension of the stomach and optimally timed administration of intravenous contrast material, subtle luminal and mural lesions are evaluated with higher accuracy and a higher degree of confidence. Patient preparation includes no solid food for 6 h to empty the stomach. For dedicated CT evaluation of the stomach, stomach distension is achieved using negative contrast (6–8 g of effervescent gas-producing crystals with <10 cc water) or a neutral contrast (water, 750 mL approximately 15 min before imaging and an additional 250 mL table dose

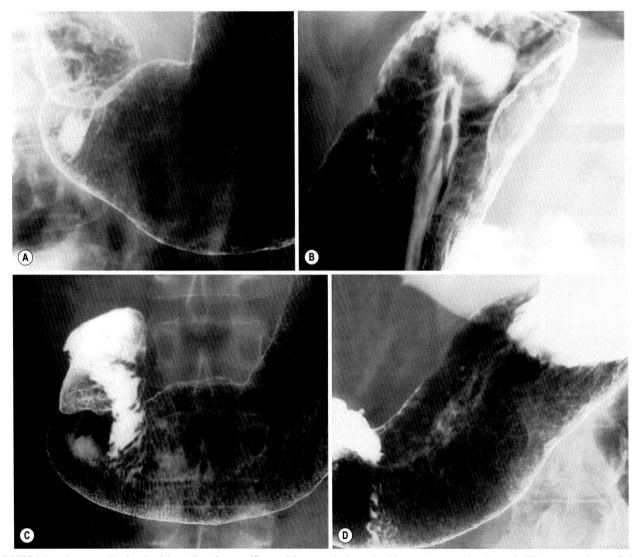

FIGURE 3-2 ■ Images obtained with patient in specific positions optimises double-contrast evaluation of different portions of the stomach. (A) Left proximal oblique (LPO) body and antrum. (Duodenal bulb also seen with double contrast.) (B) Right lateral. Fundus, cardia. This view is also used to evaluate the retrogastric region. Note: In this patient smooth, broad-based extrinsic impression from the spleen is present. (C) Supine body and antrum. In this case there is early filling of the duodenum. Note: Fine transverse antral folds. (D) Right proximal oblique (RPO) proximal body. If table is semi-upright the cardia and fundus will also be double contrast. Note: Areae gastricae, the polygonal lucencies demarcated by barium-filled grooves, which are normal mucosal features, are depicted in this image.

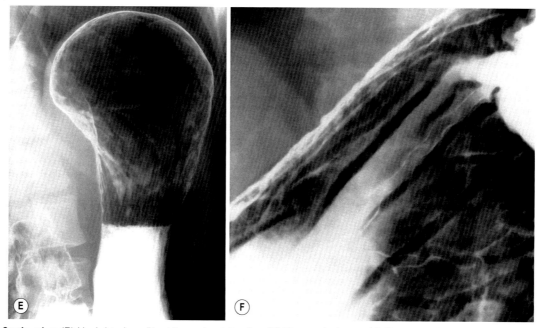

FIGURE 3-2, Continued ■ (E) Upright view. Double-contrast fundus. (F) Flow technique with fluoroscopic observation of thin coating of barium washing across the mucosal surface as the patient is turned from one side to the other. Optimal for demonstration of shallow depressions and protrusions of the mucosa of the dependent surface. Normal rugal folds on the non-dependent surface are 'etched in white', demarcated by a sharp thin line of barium. Normal folds on the dependent surface are seen as linear protrusions in the shallow barium pool.

immediately prior to the study). Antiperistaltic drugs may be used to to reduce motion artefacts. In order to optimise visualisation with water distension, the patients with suspected lesion in the upper one-third of the stomach (gastric cardia or fundus) may be imaged in the supine/left lateral decubitus position and lesions in the distal two-thirds in prone/30° RPO position; with gas contrast, the positions are reversed. Post-intravenous contrast images of the upper abdomen with an imaging delay of 40–45 s (late arterial phase to assess gastric wall enhancement) followed by images of the chest, abdomen and pelvis at 70 s (portal venous phase to identify liver and nodal metastases) are typically obtained. Images are commonly analysed in multiplanar reconstruction mode (MPR) (Figs. 3-3A,B). Additionally, in the case of air contrast, surface-shaded volume-rendered images (similar to images obtained on the single-contrast barium study) or endoluminal fly-through view (virtual gastroscopy), or a combination of both may be used[7,8] (Figs. 3-3C,D).

Based on its appearance in the arterial phase, the normal gastric wall is frequently described as single layered when only one high density layer is visualised or multilayered pattern, with a markedly enhanced inner mucosal layer, a middle hypoattenuating submucosal layer and an outer thin slightly higher attenuating muscular-serosal layer. Normal stomach wall thickness is a function of its degree of distension and normal values quoted in barium fluoroscopic literature are not applicable for CT gastrography. Optimal distension is critical for a successful CT gastrographic study.

Magnetic Resonance Imaging (MRI)

Dedicated MR imaging of stomach could be useful as an alternative for MDCT for locoregional staging of gastric malignancy. The patient preparation techniques are the same as for the CT and only water distension is used. Breath-hold fast T1W (2D fast gradient), T2W (2D fast spin echo) and post-gadolinium fat-suppressed T1W (3D fast gradient) images are routinely obtained. A trilaminar appearance of the normal gastric wall is well appreciated on T1W images, the middle layer representing submucosa with low T1 signal, compared to the inner wall (mucosa) and the outer wall (muscularis propria + serosa complex).[9] Image analysis techniques are the same as described for MDCT. The enhancement characteristics of most stomach pathology are similar to that seen in contrast-enhanced CT.

FDG-PET and FDG-PET-CT

The use of FDG-PET in the tumour (T) staging of gastric cancer and identifying primary gastric lymphoma is limited due to the variable and usually significant background physiological uptake of FDG by stomach. FDG-PET may have a role in staging due to its potential to identify extragastric involvement in both gastric carcinoma and lymphoma. The imaging protocol is similar to that used in other oncological applications of PET-CT. Qualitative visual approach with or without semiquantitative parameters (standard uptake value) is used for image interpretation. Strict adherence to a consistent protocol is of paramount importance when PET-CT is used for monitoring response to therapy.

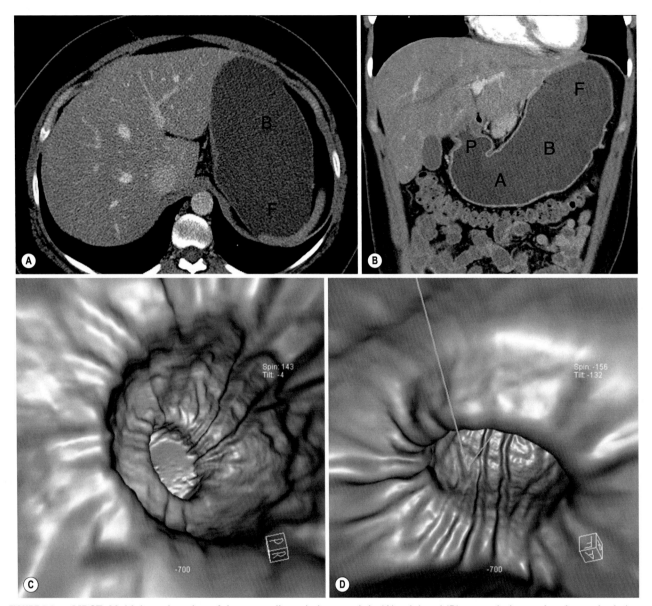

FIGURE 3-3 ■ **MDCT.** Multiplanar imaging of the water-distended stomach in (A) axial and (B) coronal planes showing a single layer of enhancing gastric wall. Fundus (F), antrum (A) and body (B) are seen. (C, D). Virtual endoscopy. (C) Normal appearance of gastric folds as seen on the virtual endoscopy. Images show a view from the fundus looking into the body of the stomach. (D) Normal appearance of the pylorus as seen on the virtual endoscope.

GASTRIC PATHOLOGY

INFLAMMATORY DISEASE AND INFILTRATIVE DISEASES

Helicobacter pylori and Diseases of the Stomach

Helicobacter pylori is a Gram-negative, flagellated, spiral bacterium that lives near the muscosal surface of the gastric mucosa. It is recognised as the strongest risk factor for the development of gastroduodenal ulcers.

Studies have shown *H. pylori* infection in 60–80% of gastric ulcers and 95% of duodenal ulcers.[10] Chronic active gastritis (superficial gastritis) is associated with *H. pylori* in close to 100% of cases. The organism was first isolated from gastric biopsies in the early 1980s by Marshall and Warren,[11] and by the early 1990s *H. pylori* was firmly established as the causative agent for PUD.[12] *Helicobacter pylori* is also considered by the World Health Organisation to be a dangerous carcinogen in the pathogenesis of gastric cancer[13] and has been associated with

MALT lymphoma (a low-grade B-cell lymphoma) of the stomach.[14] In particular, MALT lymphoma has been associated with the *H. pylori* strains expressing the Cag-a protein.[15]

Before the demonstration of *H. pylori* as the causative agent for PUD, the stomach was believed to be a sterile environment because of its acidity. *Helicobacter pylori* was found to produce the enzyme urease, and as a consequence creates an alkaline 'microenvironment' for the organism in the gastric mucus, thus allowing it to survive in the stomach.[16] Acute infection initially injures parietal cells, causing decreased gastric acid production. This is followed by the chronic stage of infestation, which is localised to the distal stomach and duodenum. Parietal cell function recovers, leading to abnormally high acid output. This causes antral gastritis and duodenitis, with approximately 1% of infected patients developing peptic ulcers every year.[17] Many factors appear to determine whether or not a person infected with *H. pylori* will develop ulcers or other diseases and in reality the majority of patients infected do not develop any associated diseases. The precise mechanism of ulcer formation is not known; however, eradication of the organism by combined antibiotic and antisecretory therapy increases the healing rate of ulcers and lowers the recurrence rate.[18]

Helicobacter pylori is found worldwide but is much more prevalent in developing countries. In developed countries the infection is more common in the lower socioeconomic groups, among ethnic and racial minorities, and in immigrants from less developed countries. It is more common in older patients from all the above groups. The precise mechanism of transmission is not known but it is likely to be oral–oral and/or faecal–oral.[19]

There is about 90% prevalence of *H. pylori* in adenocarcinoma arising in the body or antrum of the stomach. The risk of developing polyps and gastric cancer is six times higher in patients with *H. pylori* infection and gastric cancer is much more prevalent in countries where the rate of *H. pylori* infection is high. A large meta-analysis conducted by Fuccio et al. demonstrated that the eradication of *H. pylori* in high-risk populations decreases the risk of gastric cancer.[20] There is conflicting evidence regarding a possible association of *H. pylori* with non-ulcer dyspepsia[19] (Table 3-1).

Gastric Ulcer

Gastric ulcers penetrate the stomach wall through the mucosa into the submucosa and frequently the muscularis propria. Gastric ulcer is a common gastrointestinal disorder and is amenable to reliable radiographic detection. Almost all gastric ulcers (95%) are benign, with about 70% now shown to be caused by *H. pylori* infection and most of the remainder due to NSAIDs and alcohol abuse. Gastric ulcers are most prevalent in the distal stomach and along the lesser curvature. They are more common on the posterior wall of the stomach than the anterior wall and least common in the fundus.[21,22] Benign greater curvature ulcers found in the distal half of the stomach are most often associated with NSAID use. NSAID- and alcohol-related ulcers are most often seen on the greater curvature of the antrum, due at least in part to a direct toxic effect of the ingested material.[23] Benign ulcers are much less common in the fundus and along the proximal half of the greater curvature. These should always be considered suspicious for malignancy. Ulcers may be multiple, and in such cases each should be evaluated independently for criteria of benignancy.

In the elderly, ulcers are more evenly distributed throughout the stomach, particularly proximally along the lesser curvature.[24] Steroid use, hereditary factors, emotional stress and smoking are other factors that may play a contributory role in the development of gastric ulcers.

Radiographic fluoroscopic signs of gastric ulcers are described as to whether they are seen in profile or en-face (straight on). The location and size of the ulcer in the stomach and position of the patient during barium studies will determine which of the features will be shown in any specific case. Based on the radiographic features of an ulcer, a determination should be made as to whether it demonstrates benign, indeterminate or malignant characteristics. Ulcers with clear-cut benign features can be treated medically and followed to complete radiographic healing. Ulcers with indeterminate or malignant features must be evaluated endoscopically and biopsied. Most benign gastric ulcers detected on double-contrast barium studies are 5–10 mm in size. 'Giant' ulcers (>3 cm) are almost always benign but have a higher rate of complications of bleeding or perforation.

The en-face radiographic signs of gastric ulcers are best seen on double-contrast barium studies and to a lesser extent on compression views in the single-contrast examination. The primary sign of ulcer is a collection of barium in the ulcer crater along the dependent wall (Fig. 3-4A). Most benign ulcers are round or oval; some may have tear-drop or linear contour. If an ulcer is present on a non-dependent surface or is not filled with barium, it may be demonstrated as a 'ring' shadow, with barium coating the edge of the ulcer crater. If a ring shadow is seen with the patient in the supine position, and it is filled when the patient is turned prone, it is located on the anterior wall of the stomach. If the ulcer is on the posterior wall, it may be filled using the 'flow' technique—turning the patient with fluoroscopic guidance and observing while the barium bolus washes over the posterior wall.

En-face, a smooth mound of oedema is often seen surrounding the ulcer crater causing a circular filling defect. Radiating folds seen in healing ulcers should be

TABLE 3-1 **Prevalence of *Helicobacter pylori* Infection with Upper GI Disease**

Disease	Prevalence (%)
Active chronic gastritis	100
Duodenal ulcer	95
Gastric cancer (body or antrum)	80–95
MALT lymphoma	90
Gastric ulcer	60–80
Non-ulcer dyspepsia	35–60
Asymptomatic population	20–55

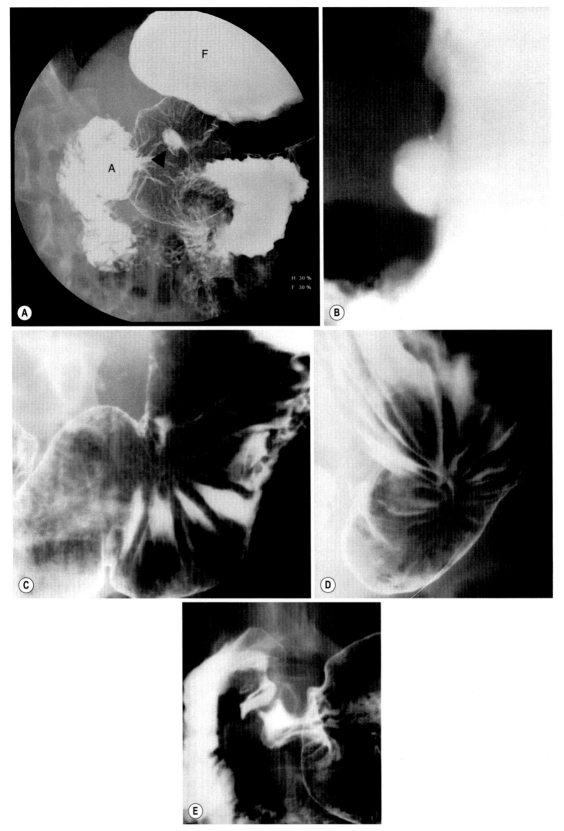

FIGURE 3-4 ■ **Gastric ulcer.** (A) Fluoroscopic image demonstrating a benign ulcer along the lesser curvature (arrowhead). Note: the stomach fundus (F) and the antrum (A). (B) Hampton's line, a thin line of radiolucency crossing the opening of an ulcer, a virtually infallible sign of a benign ulcer. (C) Focal retraction along the incisura angularis with small residual outpouching is present. Converging smooth folds no longer fill an ulcer crater. (D) Healing ulcer radiating folds converging to a linear scar. (E) Scarred antrum with constriction at site of previous ulcer causing narrowing and deformity.

TABLE 3-2 Ulcers

Findings	Benign	Malignant
Hampton's line	Present	Absent
Extends beyond gastric wall	Yes	No
Folds	Smooth, even	Irregular, nodular, may fuse
Associated mass	Absent	Present
Carman meniscus	Absent	Present
Ulcer shape	Round, oval, linear	Irregular
Healing	Heals completely	Rarely heals

smooth and symmetric and continue to the edge of the crater. The presence of normal areae gastricae extending to the ulcer crater is a sign of benignancy.

The classic description of a benign gastric ulcer refers to lesser curvature ulcers seen in profile. The ulcer, often referred to as the 'ulcer niche', projects beyond the lumen of the stomach.[25] Sometimes a pencil-thin line of lucency, 'Hampton's line', is present crossing the base of the ulcer[26] (Fig. 3-4B). This is believed to represent preserved gastric mucosa with undermining of the more vulnerable submucosa. This sign is not common, but is virtually diagnostic of a benign ulcer. More often there is a thicker (2–4 mm) smooth rim of lucency at the base of the ulcer termed the ulcer collar. This is also a sign of benignancy. When there is more visible oedema associated with an ulcer, it forms an ulcer mound. The ulcer mound should be a symmetrical gently sloping mass (Table 3-2).

Almost all (>95%) benign gastric ulcers heal in about 8 weeks when treated medically.[27] Benign ulcers may heal completely without any radiographic residua. As benign ulcers heal they may change shape from round or oval to linear crevices. There may be subtle retraction or stiffening of the affected wall (Fig. 3-4C). An easily recognisable radiographic sign of healed gastric ulcer is the presence of folds converging to the site of the healed ulcer. There may be a residual central pit or depression (Fig. 3-4D). The radiating folds should be uniform. Incomplete healing, irregularity of the folds, residual mass or loss of mucosal pattern all suggest the possibility of an underlying malignancy. The Carman meniscus sign is appreciated in the clinical setting of a large, flat ulcer with heaped-up edges. The edges of the ulcer trap a lenticular barium collection that is convex relative to the lumen when the edges are folded upon themselves during compression. These findings are indicative of a malignant gastric ulcer. Occasionally benign ulcers may heal with significant scarring. Severe retraction of the greater curvature from healed ulceration of the lesser curvature may cause narrowing of the mid-body of the stomach. Healing of antral ulcers may form prominent transverse folds or significant antral narrowing and deformity (Fig. 3-4E). Such scarring may lead to significant obstruction, an important complication of peptic ulcer disease (PUD).

The use of CT in the evaluation of gastric ulcers has been studied by several authors in recent years. Evaluation of the stomach by MDCT has been found to be useful in the detection and characterisation of benign and

malignant gastric ulcers. The differences between malignant and benign ulcers are important in treatment planning and follow-up of patients with gastric ulcers. Evaluation by virtual gastroscopy (VG) and/or MPR has been studied and certain advantages and disadvantages have been elucidated.[28]

The benefits of VG include the ability to evaluate for mucosal changes which include morphological changes that are similar to conventional gastroscopy. Another benefit is that since optical endoscopic criteria have been well established for benign and malignant ulcers, then similar criteria can be applied to VG. Characteristics of malignant ulcers on VG include: 'irregular or angulated shape; uneven base; asymmetric edge; bulbous enlargement; fusion or disruption of gastric folds reaching the crater edge'.[28] Benign ulcer criteria by VG include: 'smooth, regular, round or oval shape; even base; sharply demarcated or round edges; converging gastric folds with smooth tapering and radiation'.[28]

The use of MPR images allows for better visualisation of ulcers in multiple planes, facilitating better detection and characterisation of the ulcers. MPR also provides mural and extramural information, including, but not limited to, enhancement patterns of the gastric wall, lymphadenopathy and evaluation of adjacent organs. Characteristics of malignant ulcers on MPR images include: 'strong enhancement of the wall at the site of ulcer greater than adjacent wall; marked periulcer wall thickening with loss of normal wall stratification; perigastric fat infiltration, lymphadenopathy or metastatic disease'.[28] Characteristics of benign ulcers include: 'no excessive enhancement when compared to adjacent gastric wall; mild periulcer wall thickening with preservation of wall stratification'[28] (Fig. 3-5A). It is, however, important to understand that some of the features for benign and malignant lesions may overlap and differentiation of benign from malignant ulcers may not be determined by CT alone. MDCT evaluation remains complementary to conventional endoscopy (gastroscopy).[29] Surgical complications like penetration and perforation are easily identified on MDCT using water-soluble contrast medium (Fig. 3-5B).

Gastric Erosions

Gastric erosions or aphthous ulcers are superficial ulcerations that do not penetrate the muscularis mucosa. They usually appear as small, shallow collections of barium 1–2 mm in diameter surrounded by a radiolucent rim of oedema. These are called 'complete' or 'varioliform' erosions (Fig. 3-6A). When the halo of oedema is lacking, the erosions are called 'incomplete' (Fig. 3-6B). These appear as short linear or serpentine lines or dots of barium. Gastric erosions are most easily detected radiographically when they are multiple and complete. They are most often detected on double-contrast barium studies but may also be seen with compression technique.[30] Single or incomplete erosions are commonly detected endoscopically but are infrequently identified radiographically.[31] Erosions heal without scarring. Gastric erosions are most often causally related to *H. pylori* infection.[32] Other causes include alcohol, NSAID ingestion

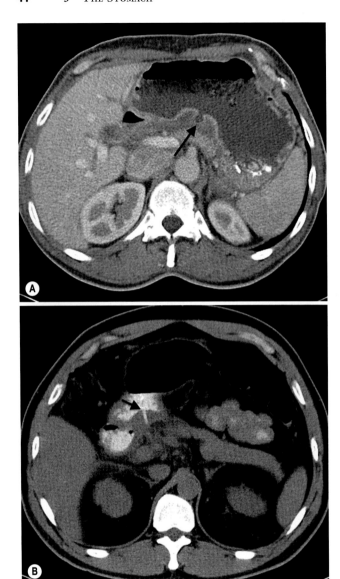

FIGURE 3-5 ▪ **Gastric ulcer on CT.** (A) Axial CT image showing benign ulcer (arrow) along the lesser curvature with a crater and surrounding smooth mound. (B) Axial CT shows perforated gastric ulcer in the posterior gastric antrum with leaking contrast (arrow), focal wall thickening and adjacent fat stranding.

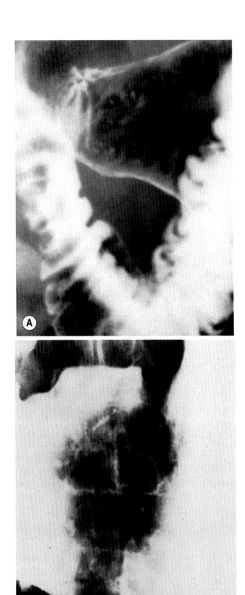

FIGURE 3-6 ▪ **Gastric erosions.** (A) Complete or 'varioliform' erosions in antrum seen on double-contrast views. (B) Incomplete erosions in antrum on compression view. The erosions do not have a rim of oedema.

and Crohn's disease. They may also be seen as a response to stress: for example, in patients with severe trauma.

Gastritis

Gastritis is a descriptive term with sometimes conflicting pathological, endoscopic and radiographic definitions. It is now better understood that many causes of gastritis, including *H. pylori*, alcohol and NSAID gastritis, lead to similar morphological changes.[30] The most common findings are thick (>5 mm) folds with or without nodularity (Fig. 3-7). Erosions, while less commonly seen, are a frequent sign of *H. pylori* gastritis. Other signs of gastritis include antral narrowing, inflammatory polyps and prominent areae gastricae. The radiological findings are similar to endoscopic findings.

It is important to note that there is considerable overlap of findings between patients who are biopsy positive or negative for *H. pylori*. Therefore it is often not possible at this time to distinguish between ulcers and gastritis caused by *H. pylori* or those caused by chemical irritants (alcohol, NSAIDs and other aetiologies of gastritis).[33] Owing to the prevalence of *H. pylori*, its association with many gastric diseases and effective treatment options, it is important for the radiologist to recognise findings that suggest the presence of the infection. It has been shown that thickened gastric folds, although nonspecific, is still the single most useful radiographic sign for the diagnosis of *H. pylori* gastritis and that the combination of thick folds and enlarged areae gastricae may be the most specific findings.[34]

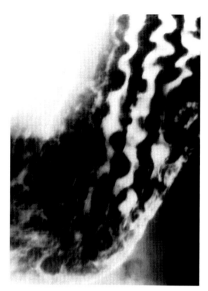

FIGURE 3-7 ■ **Diffuse erosive gastritis with thick nodular folds.** Erosions are scattered along the folds.

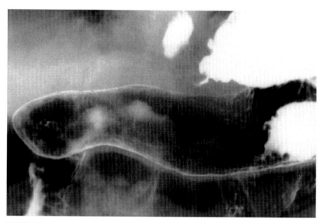

FIGURE 3-8 ■ **Atrophic gastritis.** Diffuse atrophy of the muscosal folds in a narrowed featureless stomach.

Atrophic Gastritis

Atrophic gastritis is a combination of atrophy of the gastric glands with histological inflammatory changes. Atrophic gastritis is found in more than 90% of patients with pernicious anaemia and is characterised by loss of parietal and chief cells, leading to achlorhydria, and atrophy of the mucosa and mucosal glands.[35] Atrophic gastritis causes a decrease in the production of intrinsic factor, which in turn causes malabsorption of vitamin B_{12}.

Radiographic findings of atrophic gastritis include loss of rugal folds and a tubular, featureless narrowed stomach (Fig. 3-8). Areae gastricae may be absent. The radiographic features are non-specific, but because of the important prognostic implications of atrophic gastritis, an appearance suggesting this diagnosis should trigger an appropriate clinical work-up.

There is an association with gastric polyps and carcinoma[36] and ulcers, both benign and malignant, may occur. Intestinal metaplasia, which may be seen histologically in atrophic gastritis, is considered a premalignant condition. The diagnosis of intestinal metaplasia may be suggested by areas of focal enlargement of the areae gastricae.[37]

Infectious Gastritis

Helicobacter pylori gastritis is by far the most common infection affecting the stomach. Tuberculosis, histoplasmosis and syphilis are usually lumped together with other granulomatous processes causing gastritis. Ulceration, thick folds and mucosal nodularity are common features, with antral narrowing being a late feature of these diseases. *Monilia* (*Candida*) may involve the stomach. This almost always occurs in the presence of severe oesophageal disease. Prominent aphthous ulceration may be seen in such cases.[38]

In immunocompromised patients, cytomegalovirus, crytosporidiosis and toxoplasmosis may occur. Radiographic findings are non-specific but there are some suggestive signs. Deep ulceration, and even fistulisation to adjacent structures may be seen with cytomegalovirus.[39] *Cryptosporidium* primarily affects the small bowel, causing severe diarrhoea and thick, small bowel folds. It rarely involves the stomach but has been shown to cause deep ulcers, antral narrowing and rigidity.[40,41] *Strongyloides* is a parasitic infection with a worldwide distribution affecting the stomach, duodenum and proximal small bowel evidenced by thickened, effaced folds and narrowing. In advanced cases, the stomach may be narrowed and have thickened folds.

Crohn's and Other Granulomatous Diseases

Granulomatous conditions of the stomach include Crohn's disease, sarcoidosis, tuberculosis, syphilis and fungal diseases. Crohn's disease is a chronic inflammatory bowel disease primarily affecting the ileum and colon. Gastroduodenal involvement occurs in up to 20% of cases, most often in the presence of ileocolitis.[42] When the upper gastrointestinal tract is affected by Crohn's disease, both the stomach and duodenum are commonly affected. However, involvement of the duodenum alone is more common than the stomach alone.[43] A wide range of symptoms may be seen in patients with gastroduodenal Crohn's disease; some are asymptomatic, others have symptoms more typical of PUD or with symptoms related to antral narrowing or gastric outlet obstruction. Diarrhoea caused by associated ileocolic disease is common. Gastrocolic fistula is an unusual complication. When it occurs, disease of the transverse colon extending to the stomach is most often the cause.[44] Radiographic findings of gastric Crohn's disease almost always demonstrate involvement of the antrum alone or antrum and body of the stomach.[45] With early disease, findings include aphthous ulcers, larger discrete ulcers, thickened and distorted folds and sometimes a nodular ('cobblestone') mucosa (Fig. 3-9). These are indistinguishable from aphthous ulcers or erosions due to other causes. These findings represent the non-stenotic phase of Crohn's disease. Stenotic disease caused by scarring and fibrosis can result in narrowing of the gastric antrum and pylorus into a funnel or 'rams-horn' shape, sometimes leading to

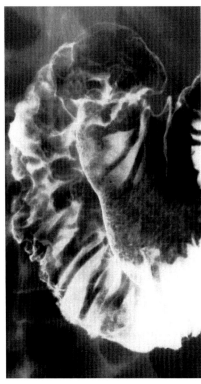

FIGURE 3-9 ■ **Crohn's disease.** Multiple aphthous (superficial) erosions are present on the antrum. Duodenal folds are thick and nodular (cobblestone mucosa).

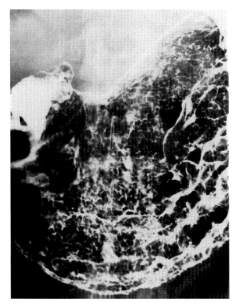

FIGURE 3-10 ■ **Hypertrophic gastritis.** Image from a patient with a recently healed lesser curvature ulcer. This characteristic enlargement and prominence of the areae gastricae can be correlated with an increased incidence of gastric hypersecretion and PUD.

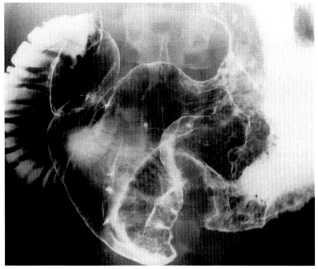

FIGURE 3-11 ■ **Ménétrier's disease.** Classic appearance with massively enlarged folds in the body without abnormality in the antrum.

foreshortening of the stomach which can be so severe that it simulates a partial gastrectomy. This scarred, funnel-shaped antroduodenal region may also be seen in other granulomatous diseases, including tuberculosis, syphilis, sarcoidosis and eosinophilic gastroenteritis. Antral narrowing may also mimic scirrhous gastric carcinoma.[46]

Hypertrophic Gastritis

Hypertrophic gastritis is characterised radiographically by thickened folds, often greater than 10 mm in width, predominantly in the fundus and body, which are the acid-producing regions of the stomach. While the term is often used descriptively, the entity of hypertrophic gastritis is associated with glandular hyperplasia and increased acid secretion.[47,48] Histologically, inflammation is not a prominent feature; thus, 'gastritis' is somewhat a misnomer. The areae gastricae pattern will become more prominent[49] (Fig. 3-10). There is a high prevalence of duodenal and gastric ulcers in these patients. Many cases that had been previously classified as hypertrophic gastritis may in fact have been due to *H. pylori* infection. The differential diagnosis is primarily Ménétrier's disease and lymphoma.

Ménétrier's Disease

Ménétrier's disease is a rare entity well known in the radiology literature because of its dramatic and characteristic appearance. This condition is characterised by

hypertrophy of gastric glands, achlorhydria and hypoproteinaemia. Loss of protein from the hyperplastic mucosa into the gastric lumen results in a protein-losing enteropathy, and may produce disabling symptoms. The disease is characterised by markedly enlarged, often bizarre gastric folds most prominent in the proximal stomach and along the greater curvature.[50] Radiographically, upper gastrointestinal or CT show massively thickened often lobular folds (Fig. 3-11). The folds remain pliable, which helps to differentiate it from carcinoma, where the stomach becomes rigid and aperistaltic. While in the classic description of Ménétrier's disease the antrum is spared, it has been found to be involved in up to 50% of cases[51] causing diffuse involvement of the stomach. Another feature of Ménétrier's disease is the finding of increased fluid in the small bowel, which in turn may prevent optimal mucosal coating with barium.

Zollinger–Ellison Syndrome

Patients with Zollinger–Ellison syndrome may have thickened gastric folds and increased gastric secretions. This syndrome is caused by gastrinomas, which are non-beta islet cell tumours that secrete gastrin, stimulating acid secretion in the stomach. Seventy-five per cent of the tumours are found in the pancreas and 15% in the duodenum. A small number are extraintestinal. The tumours may be malignant and metastases, primarily to the liver, are present in up to half of the cases. Zollinger–Ellison is one of the manifestations of multiple endocrine neoplasia (MEN) type I (also called Wermer syndrome), which includes parathyroid, pituitary and adrenal tumours. In some cases MEN type I may be associated with carcinoid tumours.

Eosinophilic Gastroenteritis

Eosinophilic gastroenteritis is characterised by focal or diffuse infiltration of the gastrointestinal tract by eosinophils. The clinical presentation includes crampy abdominal pain, diarrhoea, distension and vomiting, often in an atopic or asthmatic patient.[52] Peripheral eosinophilia is a frequent accompaniment. Any segment of the gastrointestinal tract may be affected but it most often involves the stomach, especially the antrum and the proximal small bowel.

The clinical and imaging features depend on which layers of the GI tract wall are involved.[53] Involvement may be predominantly mucosal, muscular or subserosal.[54] Many cases are panmural and eosinophilic ascites is often seen in such cases.[55–57] Radiographically, eosinophilic gastritis is characterised by fold thickening of the stomach and small bowel. Antral narrowing and rigidity with mucosal nodularity are frequently seen[58] (Fig. 3-12).

Corrosive Ingestion

Ingestion of caustic chemicals may cause severe injury to the stomach, sometimes leading to gastric necrosis, perforation and death. Acids are more injurious to the stomach and duodenum. Since the stomach secretes hydrochloric acid, it has the ability to neutralise alkaline agents. However, the already acidic gastric contents have no ability to neutralise strong ingested acids such as sodium hypochlorite (household bleach).

The consequences of ingesting a corrosive agent follow a distinct course. First, there is necrosis, with sloughing of the mucosal and submucosal layers. In severe cases, full-thickness necrosis of the gastric wall may lead to perforation. In less severe cases, the denuded gastric wall develops a granulating surface and the formation of collagen then leads to fibrosis and stricture. The final result is a deformed, contracted and occasionally

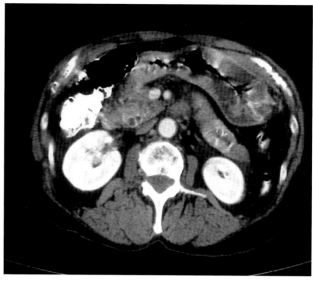

FIGURE 3-12 ■ **Eosinophilic gastroenteritis.** CT shows diffuse thickening of the gastric wall in a patient proven to have eosinophilic gastroenteritis. No ascites was present. Symptoms resolved with steroid therapy.

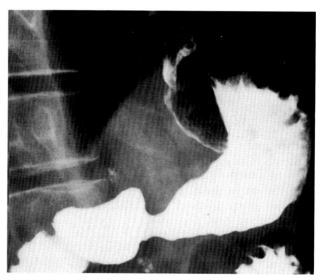

FIGURE 3-13 ■ **Corrosive gastritis following the ingestion of household bleach.** The distal stomach has undergone considerable scarring and contraction in a manner similar to syphilitic gastritis or linitis plastica.

obstructed stomach which often necessitates total gastrectomy.

The radiographic findings in corrosive gastritis depend on the severity of the chemical insult and the time that has elapsed since injury. Initially, swelling and irregularity of the gastric mucosa are seen, occasionally with visible blebs. As the mucosa sloughs, barium flows beneath it and the mucosa may then be seen as a thin radiolucent line paralleling the outline of the stomach. After a week or two, fibrotic contraction of the stomach becomes evident (Fig. 3-13). In severe cases, the lumen of the stomach may be no larger than that of the duodenal bulb.

Amyloidosis

Amyloidosis is a rare condition that may cause gastric fold and/or wall thickening and rigidity. Luminal narrowing may mimic infiltrative tumour (linitis plastica). The condition is caused by the deposition of amyloid, a protein–saccharide complex in the stomach.[59] Findings are non-specific and the diagnosis is confirmed by biopsy.

NEOPLASTIC DISEASES

Mucosal Polyps

Gastric epithelial polyps are typically asymptomatic and found incidentally in upper endoscopic or radiological studies. Approximately 1–4% of patients who undergo gastric biopsy have gastric polyps in the Western world, with much higher rates reported from the East. The prevalence and the type of the polyps encountered depend on the population being studied; hyperplastic and adenomatous polyps are highest in an *H. pylori*-infected population and fundic gland polyps are related to increased proton pump inhibitor (PPI) usage. Larger polyps can be symptomatic from bleeding or distal prolapse producing gastric outlet obstruction. Polyps are important because of their variable intrinsic malignant potential and their occurrence in patients who have other risk factors for developing gastric malignancy. For these reasons most polyps are biopsied or resected if possible, along with multiple topographic biopsies of the rest of the gastric mucosa. Surveillance is indicated in patients with higher risk for gastric cancer.[60]

Hyperplastic polyps are the most common type seen in association with insulted gastric mucosa (*H. Pylori* gastritis, atrophic gastritis, pernicious anemia, ulcers and erosions, gastric surgical sites and bile reflux gastritis). They are randomly distributed throughout the stomach, usually multiple, uniform and of an average size of 1 cm, but may reach much larger dimensions (Fig. 3-14). Though they have low malignant potential, the risk increases in polyps more than 2 cm in size; therefore larger polyps are completely excised.

Fundic gland polyps appear to be on the rise due to increased use of PPI therapy and are currently the commonest type found in upper endoscopy in the United States.[61] They are traditionally considered a variant of hamartomatous polyps, and distributed exclusively in the gastric fundus and proximal body (Fig. 3-15). They are small (usually <0.5 cm), multiple and sessile. They may occur sporadically, or in association with familial adenomatous polyposis (FAP) or, more commonly, in response to chronic PPI therapy. Polyps associated with PPI use have virtually no malignant potential.

Adenomatous polyps or adenomas are microscopically similar to colonic adenoma. They are usually solitary, sessile or pedunculated, and often seen in the antrum in association with atrophic gastritis. They are also seen in polyposis syndromes (FAP, Gardner's syndrome, Turcot syndrome). They are premalignant with high-grade dysplastic changes and are currently redefined as non-invasive intraepithelial neoplasia (NiN) in keeping with their biological profile.[62] The presence of invasive

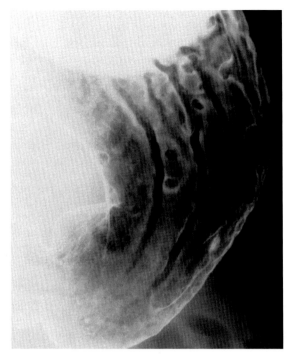

FIGURE 3-14 ■ Hyperplastic polyps in the body of the stomach in a double-contrast study—multiple, small, sessile and uniform in size.

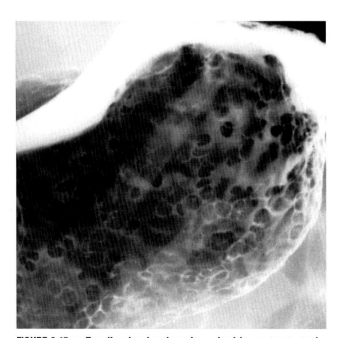

FIGURE 3-15 ■ Fundic gland polyps in a double-contrast study, morphologically identical to hyperplastic polyps, but seen in the fundus and proximal body of the stomach in this patient with familial adenomatous polyposis (FAP).

carcinoma in an adenoma correlates with increasing size, villous histology and higher grades of dysplasia.

Hamartomatous polyps occur sporadically or in polyposis syndromes (Peutz–Jeghers, juvenile polyposis, Cronkhite–Canada and Cowden). These are the least common types, with no specific endoscopic or radiographic findings. Though the term hamartoma implies a non-neoplastic tumour, they may coexist with adenomatous polyps.[63]

The different subtypes of polyps are radiographically indistinguishable. Smaller mucosal polyps are well circumscribed with smooth, nodular or lobulated surface on barium double-contrast studies. They are sessile or pedunculated and when viewed in profile form acute angles with adjacent gastric wall. Larger polyps have a lobulated surface and areas of erosion or ulceration mimicking malignant growth.[64]

Mesenchymal Tumours

Benign mesenchymal tumours arising in the submucosa constitute the second most common type of benign lesion in the stomach after mucosal polyps. Gastrointestinal stromal tumour (GIST) is the most common mesenchymal tumour of the GI tract, with two-thirds of them occurring in the stomach and the remainder in the small bowel. GIST is much less common compared to tumours of gastric epithelial and lymphomatous origin. Adults older than 50 years are usually affected. GIST is thought to arise from the stem cells in muscularis propia, (interstitial cell of Cajal, the gut pacemaker). Most GISTs (95%) are characterised by the expression of *Kit* receptor (CD117), with resultant increase in tyrosine kinase activity leading to cell hyperproliferation. In the past GIST was misdiagnosed as a smooth muscle tumour because under light microscopy both share many features. Clinical presentation depends on the site and the size of the tumour; GI bleeding is more common than obstruction as a presenting symptom. Primary treatment is complete surgical resection of the mass. Approximately 20–25% of gastric GISTs are clinically malignant. Tumour size and mitotic activity are the best predictors of clinical malignancy. Gastric GISTs are less aggressive than enteric GISTs. Metastases commonly develop in the abdominal cavity and the liver. Lymphatic involvement and lung metastases are extremely rare. First-line treatment for metastatic disease is the selective tyrosine kinase inhibitor, imatinib mesylate. Most tumours are sporadic; however, a small percentage (5%) of the GISTs are associated with 1 of 3 tumour syndromes: neurofibromatosis type 1 (NF1), Carney triad and familial GIST syndrome, in order of decreasing frequency.[65]

Smaller tumours are discovered incidentally during radiological study, endoscopy or even surgery. They often form solid subserosal, intramural or less commonly polypoid intraluminal masses with intact mucosa (Fig. 3-16A). Post-contrast CT and MR show more homogeneous enhancement of the mass. Common radiological presentation of a larger lesion is that of a heterogeneously enhancing, exophytic mass (Fig. 3-16B). The heterogeneity is due to cyst formation, necrosis, haemorrhage, ulceration and cavitary changes. Pooling of air and oral contrast may be seen within the mass if the luminal margin is ulcerated. Liver metastases are usually hypervascular. Pre-contrast MR imaging findings of liver metastases are non-specific with low T1 and high T2 signal. Intense late arterial phase enhancement and almost complete portal venous phase washout are seen both on CT and MRI.[66]

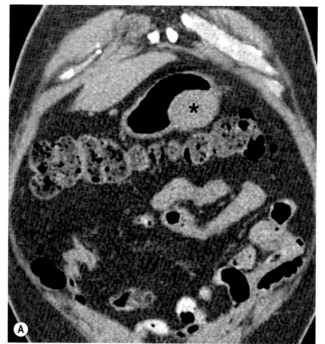

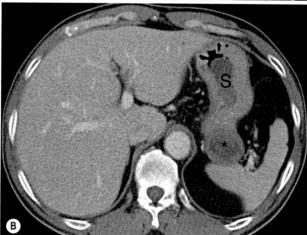

FIGURE 3-16 ■ **Gastric GIST.** (A) Coronal CT image showing a small GIST (*) with both intraluminal and exophytic component. (B) Different patient with a necrotic fundal mass (*), which is totally exophytic, a feature that is diagnostic of GIST. S = stomach.

Non-stromal mesenchymal tumours like neuroma, leiomyoma and glomus tumours are uncommon with non-specific radiographic findings. A definite diagnosis of gastric lipoma can be made both on CT and MRI due to the characteristic appearance of fat (Fig. 3-17).

Gastric Carcinoma

Approximately 90 to 95% of all malignant gastric tumours are adenocarcinomas; the remainder include lymphoma, stromal tumour and neuroendocrine tumours. Carcinoma of the stomach is considerably more prevalent in Eastern Asia (Japan, Korea, China). Much of the early diagnostic techniques and management guidelines have been developed in Japan. In the West, most gastric

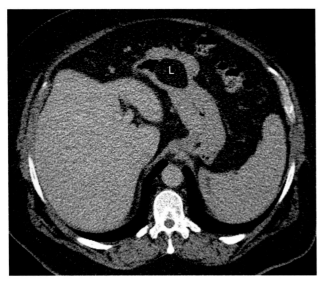

FIGURE 3-17 ■ **Gastric lipoma.** Fat density luminal mass (L) with a thin capsule in the gastric antrum, the most common site.

cancers are detected at an advanced stage, possibly due to non-availablity of mass screening programmes and the non-specific symptoms of the early disease. Peak age incidence is between 50 and 70 years. A third of the lesions occur each in the antrum, body and the fundus-cardiac region of the stomach; the remaining 10% are diffusely infiltrative. The overall declining incidence of gastric carcinoma in the distal stomach is related to aggressive treatment of *H. pylori* infection; but an increasing incidence of proximal gastric cancer has been recently observed amoung young adults in the United States. Chronic atrophic gastritis, *H. pylori* infection and some polyposis syndromes are considered definite risk factors for gastric cancer. Multiple dietary factors and autoimmune gastritis are also implicated. Photofluorography has been the dominant method recommended for mass screening in Japanese national guidelines. However, other screening methods (endoscopy, *H. pylori* antibody and serum pepsinogen testing) are also used with variable success rates in different parts of the world.[67]

Early Gastric Cancer

The concept of early gastric cancer (EGC) originated in Japan and refers to a lesion confined to the gastric mucosa and submucosa, irrespective of lymph nodal metastases (T1, any N). Patients may be asymptomatic or present with non-specific symptoms. The Japanese system classifies the EGC into three types (type I polypoid >5 mm, protruding into the lumen; type II superficial, which is further subtyped as IIa elevated <5 mm, IIb flat, IIc depressed; type III excavated).[68] Limited recent literature is available about the role of double-contrast upper gastrointestinal examination for EGC.[69,70] With the widespread use of endoscopy, multiple endoscopic biopsies of suspicious lesions are considered the diagnostic procedure of choice for early gastric cancer. Endoscopic resection for EGC is also shown to improve the quality of life.[71] Recent advances in MDCT techniques like

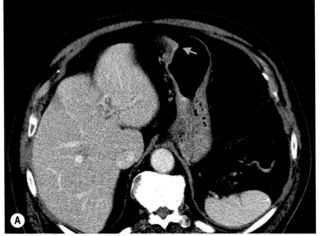

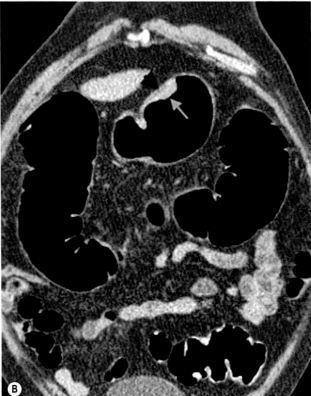

FIGURE 3-18 ■ **Early gastric cancer (EGC) type I, confined to mucosa (T1 lesion).** (A) Axial and (B) coronal MPR CT images show a type 1 polypoid lesion (arrow) in the lesser curvature of the stomach. These post-contrast images show abnormal focal mucosal hyperenhancement with preservation of the outer hypodense stripe (arrowhead), which represents submucosa.

multiplanar reformatting (MPR), surface shading, virtual gastroscopy, and post-contrast dynamic imaging have significantly improved the detection rate of type 1 EGC. The common CT appearance of the T1 lesion is focal thickening of the inner layer, nearly well enhanced with visible low-attenuation outer layer and clear perigastric fat plane (Fig. 3-18). T1 lesions without gastric wall thickening or hyperenhancement are extremely difficult to positively identify on MDCT. Some mucosal changes associated with EGC, which are not detected on the

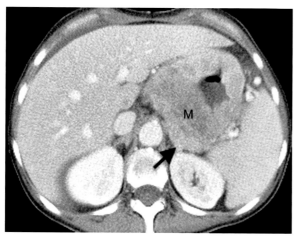

FIGURE 3-19 ■ **Advanced gastric cancer (T4B lesion).** Large heterogeneously enhancing mass (M) with poorly defined margin in the body of the stomach. There is loss of posterior perigastric fat plane and direct invasion of the left adrenal gland, which shows nodular enlargement (arrow).

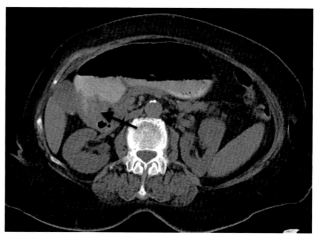

FIGURE 3-20 ■ **Gastric outlet obstruction.** Distended stomach containing air and barium caused by antral invasion by adenocarcinoma (arrow).

standard MPR images, may be demonstrated with surface-shaded images or virtual gastroscopy.[72]

Advanced Gastric Cancer

Advanced gastric cancer (AGC) invades the muscularis propria and further spreads outward. This is the most common form diagnosed in Western countries. The gross radiographic morphology of advanced lesions is classically described as polypoid, infiltrative or ulcerative, with considerable overlap among them. Tumours most frequently present as large, irregular polypoid masses that may or may not be ulcerated. The margins may exhibit a shelf, and form an acute angle with the gastric wall indicating the mucosal origin of the tumour. This may become less obvious as the tumour enlarges (Fig. 3-19). Although most large mucosal masses in the stomach will prove to be gastric carcinomas, there are a number of other benign and malignant conditions that may have a similar radiographic appearance and biopsy confirmation is always required. A tumour originating in the antrum may cause severe narrowing and gastric outlet obstruction (Fig. 3-20).

The term 'malignant ulcer' is used to indicate an ulcer within a gastric mass, usually a carcinoma and less often a lymphoma. Even though the fluoroscopic and CT features of benign and malignant ulcers have been described, endoscopic biopsy confirmation is routinely obtained in current clinical practice.

Infiltrative cancers can have non-scirrhous or scirrhous (desmoplastic) histology. Non-scirrhous tumours manifest as stomach wall thickening and rugal fold thickening. Scirrhous lesions are aggressive and exhibit wall thickening with loss of mucosal folds. Linitis plastica is a descriptive term for diffuse scirrhous tumour, where the stomach appears as a narrowed, rigid structure (leather bottle stomach) and is better appreciated in fluoroscopic imaging compared to endoscopy[64] (Fig. 3-21).

Post-surgical cancer is discussed under postoperative complications.

Staging of Gastric Cancer

TNM staging by the AJCC/UICC is commonly used for gastric cancer and two key changes are included in their 7th edition *Tumour Staging Manual*. Tumours arising at the gastro-oesophageal junction or arising in the stomach 5 cm or less from the oesophagogastric junction and crossing the oesophagogastric junction, are staged using the TNM system for oesophageal cancer. Secondly, the stomach T categories (Table 3-3)[73] have been harmonised with the T categories of the rest of the tubular gastrointestinal tract, from oesophagus to colorectum.[74] Surgical resection of the primary tumour and regional lymph nodes is the most definite therapy. The important prognostic factors influencing survival in resectable gastric cancer are depth of invasion and the presence or absence of nodal metastases. Investigational CT criteria for T staging have been established and also recently revised to reflect the 7th edition TNM staging.[73] Limited experience is available using MRI for staging gastric cancer. T1W images show intermediate signal intensity in regions affected by carcinoma compared to the surrounding normal mucosa and muscularis propria. Low signal intensity on T2W images and high signal intensity on opposed phase images are also noted.[75,76] Abnormal focal thickening (6 mm or greater), loss of the trilaminar appearance and differential enhancement compared to the surrounding normal wall (usually hyperenhancement due to neovascularity, but sometimes iso- or hypoenhancement), are common findings in affected areas similar to MDCT.

Certain limitations of both MDCT and MRI still exist in T staging for AGC. Massive submucosal infiltration makes T1 and T2 differentiation difficult. Differentiation between T2 and T3 is hindered by the non-visiblity of subserosa and serosa as separate entities.[9,76] In practice, for AGC, the differentiation between serosal (T4A) versus the adjacent organ invasion (T4B) is more

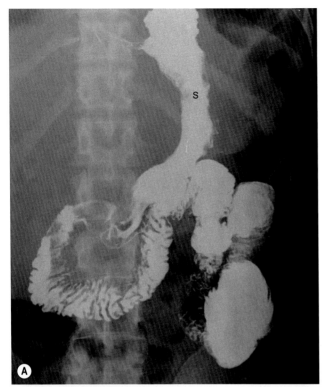

TABLE 3-3   **T-Category Definitions, Gastric Cancer**

TX	Primary tumour cannot be assessed
T0	No evidence of primary tumour
Tis	Carcinoma in situ: intraepithelial tumour without invasion of the lamina propria
T1	Tumour invades lamina propria, muscularis mucosae or submucosa
T1a	Tumour invades lamina propria or muscularis mucosae
T1b	Tumour invades submucosa
T2	Tumour invades muscularis propria
T3	Tumour penetrates subserosal connective tissue without invasion of visceral peritoneum or adjacent structures. T3 tumours also include those extending into the gastrocolic or gastrohepatic ligaments, or into the greater or lesser omentum, without perforation of the visceral peritoneum covering these structures
T4	Tumour invades serosa (visceral peritoneum) or adjacent structures
T4a	Tumour invades serosa (visceral peritoneum)
T4b	Tumour invades adjacent structures such as spleen, transverse colon, liver, diaphragm, pancreas, abdominal wall, adrenal gland, kidney, small intestine and retroperitoneum

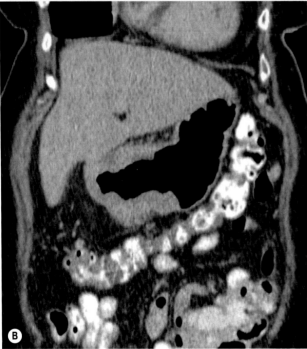

FIGURE 3-21 ■ **Linitis plastica.** (A) Single-contrast fluoroscopic image shows luminal narrowing from infiltrative carcinoma of nearly the entire stomach, resulting in a 'tubular stomach' (S). (B) Unenhanced coronal CT in a different patient shows infiltrative cancer involving the distal body and the antrum with luminal narrowing.

meaningful to surgeons for treatment planning. Cachexia and distended stomach frequently efface fat planes in patients with advanced cancer, hindering proper differentiation of T3 and T4. Also, obliteration of the fat planes by inflammatory or desmoplastic reactions results

in overstaging. Therefore, focal change in the CT attenuation or MR signal intensity within the adjacent organs is required to make a diagnosis of adjacent organ invasion (T4b), not simply loss of intervening fat plane. The pancreas, left lobe of the liver, spleen and transverse colon may all be involved by direct extension of tumour. Early or miliary peritoneal carcinomatosis without ascites or tumour invasion of mesocolon are difficult to detect preoperatively on both MDCT and MR imaging.

The N category is defined in the TNM staging system on the basis of the number of metastatic nodes involved, whereas the anatomical nodal stations are used in the Japanese system (JCGC 13th edn). A wide range of accuracy for N staging has been reported with CT and MRI, depending on the threshold size criteria (usually > 6–8 mm in short axis) considered to identify nodal metastases. Also the metastatic nodal margin, architecture and the enhancement pattern can be different. Nevertheless, CT (or MRI) evaluation of N staging is still challenging. In the preoperative evaluation, it is reasonable to use more sensitive criteria at the expense of specificity to allow detection of potentially pathological nodes. It is recommended to indicate all visible lymph nodes regardless of their size and leave it to histology for accurate N staging. The common nodal groups involved are perigastric, celiac axis, para-aortic and portahepatis nodes. Recent literature suggests that the accuracy of MDCT is comparable to EUS for both T and N staging.[77] Both EUS and MDCT are now considered complimentary techniques for locoregional staging of gastric cancer.[78]

CT and MRI are the techniques of choice for M staging (liver, peritoneum, lung, pancreas, retroperitoneum, adrenal, ovary (Krukenberg tumour) and diaphragm) of the gastric cancer. With the higher sensitivity of CT and the high specificity of FDG-PET, fusion of these imaging techniques (PET-CT) will be more useful than either alone for peritoneal metastases. Diagnostic laparoscopy is highly sensitive for identifying peritoneal metastases.[79]

The detection of gastric carcinoma by FDG-PET is limited by (1) some histological subtypes (mucinous, signet ring and poorly differentiated adenocarcinoma) are not FDG-avid, (2) highly variable and sometimes intense focal physiological uptake within the normal gastric wall, (3) spatial resolution limits the ability to distinguish primary mass and the immediate perigastric nodal metastases and (4) the lack of unified criteria in how to interpret imaging findings.[80] FDG-PET has a better positive predictive value for lymph nodal metastases when compared to CT, especially for N3 metastases, which is important in the management of gastric cancer as treatment strategy may change from curative surgery to palliative measures. Metabolic response in FDG-avid tumours helps to identify therapy responders from non-responders earlier than morphological imaging techniques (Fig. 3-22).

Gastric Lymphoma

The gastrointestinal tract is the commonest site of extra-nodal lymphoma and the stomach is the most frequent

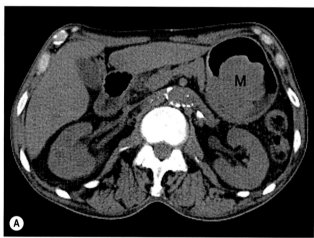

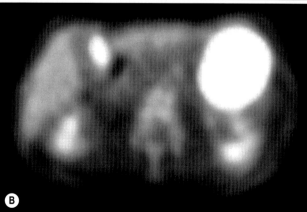

FIGURE 3-22 ■ **PET-CT in advanced gastric cancer.** (A) Un-enhanced axial CT image shows a large polypoid mass (M) in the posterior body of the stomach. The perigastric fat planes are preserved. (B) FDG-PET image at the same level shows intense uptake in this moderately differentiated adenocarcinoma.

site of gastrointestinal lymphoma. Gastric involvement may be primary, i.e confined to the stomach and the regional lymph nodes, or secondary, as part of generalised disease. Primary gastric lymphomas are almost exclusively of non-Hodgkin's type (NHL), mostly of large B-cell type. Lymphoma of mucosa-associated lymphoid tissue (MALToma) is an indolent subtype of marginal cell type NHL, which is closely linked with chronic *H. pylori* infection, in particular strains expressing the Cag-a protein.[15] Normally, there is no lymphoid tissue in the gastric mucosa. It is postulated that *H. pylori* infection may trigger the acquisition of MALT and subsequent inflammatory response may be a prerequisite for the development of MALToma, which may transform to intermediate or high-grade B-cell NHL. However, high-grade NHL may also arise de novo. Inflammatory bowel disease, coeliac disease, HIV infection and immunosuppression after solid organ transplant are other risk factors for gastric lymphoma.[81]

Lymphoma may involve any portion of the stomach in a diffuse or focal pattern. Though early lymphoma is confined to the mucosa and submucosa, gastric lymphomas are usually advanced at presentation. Primary gastric lymphoma has no typical radiographic appearance, and may mimic any of the appearances of gastric carcinoma. Radiographic findings of lymphoma, in both double-contrast barium and CT studies, parallel their gross morphological subtypes. The most common appearance is that of an infiltrating lesion extending over a large area of the stomach with diffuse mural and fold thickening (Fig. 3-23A). Ulcerations may or may not be present. Other presentations are those of a bulky, polypoid mass, multiple submucosal nodules or single or multiple ulcers.[8] CT may be helpful in differentiating gastric lymphoma from carcinoma. Preservation of perigastric fat planes at CT is more likely to be seen in lymphoma than in carcinoma, particularly in the presence of bulky tumour. In addition, the stomach remains pliable even with extensive lymphomatous infiltration, and the lumen is preserved, making gastric outlet obstruction an uncommon feature. However, NHL should be recognised as another cause of linitis plastica, an appearance that results from dense infiltration of lymphomatous tissue in the gastric wall without associated fibrosis. Adenopathy is seen both with carcinoma and lymphoma, but if it extends below the renal hila or if the lymph nodes are bulky, lymphoma is more likely.[82]

While FDG-PET has a well-established role generally in lymphoma, evaluation of primary gastric lymphoma is challenging due to unpredictable physiological FDG uptake in the stomach and variability in the degree of uptake in different histological subtypes (Fig. 3-23B).[83] PET-CT helps to detect extragastric involvement in diffuse large B-cell subtype. Also FDG-PET has proven to be helpful in evaluating the response to treatment.

Carcinoid

Though the stomach is the least common site of gastrointestinal carcinoids, they are clinically significant due to the associated endocrinopathies that involve the stomach itself. Gastric carcinoids are well-differentiated endocrine

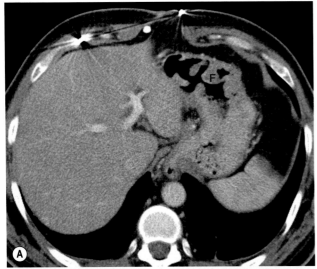

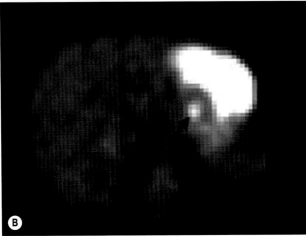

FIGURE 3-23 ■ **Primary gastric lymphoma, Large B-cell NHL.**
(A) CT shows diffuse wall thickening in the body of the stomach
with giant folds (F). (B) The corresponding FDG-PET image
shows intense tracer uptake in the involved area. Also seen is
a hypermetabolic lymphomatous perigastric node (arrow).

neoplasms that arise in the mucosa and/or submucosa.
Three clinicopathological types are described.[84] Type I
is most commonly associated with enterochromaffin-like
cell hyperplasia, hypergastrinaemia and chronic atrophic
gastritis, with or without pernicious anemia. Type II is
the least common, seen in the hypergastrinaemic state
of Zollinger–Ellision syndrome as part of multiple
endocrine neoplasia (MEN 1). The association between
hypergastrinaemia-induced   gastric   enterochromaffin-
like (ECL) cell hyperplasia/dysplasia and subsequent
neoplasia has been demonstrated in both human and
animal models.[85] Both types present as small multiple
nodules with or without central ulceration in the setting
of diffuse gastric wall thickening. Type III are sporadic
tumours and not associated with hypergastrinaemic state.
Unlike types I and II tumours, type III tumours are large
solitary ulcerative lesions. They are aggressive and are
more likely to be locally invasive with nodal and hepatic
metastases. Carcinoid syndrome may be seen in patients
with liver metastases.

Metastatic Disease

Metastatic tumours to the stomach are uncommon and
occur late in the course of the disease. The most common
primary tumours that metastasise to the stomach are
breast, malignant melanoma and lung. Blood-borne
metastases to the stomach initially appear radiographically as small intramural masses, usually multiple, that are
indistinguishable from benign disease. As the disease
progresses, they may assume similar morphology to
primary gastric tumours. These may contain central
ulcerations, having a bull's-eye appearance. This is most
frequently seen in metastatic melanoma, lymphoma and
Kaposi's sarcoma. Breast carcinoma may produce a linitis
plastica-type appearance, indistinguishable from primary
gastric carcinoma.

MISCELLANEOUS CONDITIONS

Positional Abnormalities

The stomach is attached to several peritoneal reflections,
permitting its relative mobility. These include the gastrohepatic ligament (lesser omentum), the gastrosplenic
ligament and the gastrocolic ligament, which is part of
the greater omentum. The oesophagogastric junction
passing through the oesophageal hiatus of the diaphragm
normally fixes the proximal stomach while the distal
stomach is anchored at the pyloroduodenal junction.

Hiatus Hernia

Hiatal hernias are the most common positional abnormality in which the stomach herniates into the chest
through the diaphragmatic hiatus when there is widening
of the opening between the diaphragmatic crura. The
prevalence of hiatal hernia increases with age and is
present in over 50% of the aged population. Most hiatal
hernias are small, involving a protrusion of a part of the
gastric fundus at least 1.5–2 cm above the diaphragm. At
the opposite extreme the entire stomach may be intrathoracic. Hiatal hernias may be divided into four types.
Sliding hiatal hernias are the most common type of hiatal
hernia (type 1) (Fig. 3-24A). In this type of hernia the
gastro-oesophageal junction slides proximally through
the diaphragmatic hiatus to assume an intrathoracic location. Small or moderate-sized hiatal hernias are often
reducible, changing in size and configuration during
barium evaluation. They are best demonstrated with the
patient recumbent in the right anterior oblique position.
Sliding hiatal hernias are often accompanied by gastro-
oesophageal reflux and reflux oesophagitis.

In comparison to sliding hiatal hernias, in paraoesopha-
geal hernias (type 2) the gastro-oesophageal junction is
in its normal position below the diaphragm. The proximal stomach herniates through the oesophageal hiatus
usually to the left of the distal oesophagus in the posterior
mediastinum. This type of hernia is important because it
is more prone to incarceration and obstruction than a
sliding hernia.

Mixed hiatal hernia (type 3) is a combination of both
types 1 and 2 together, with the gastro-oesophageal

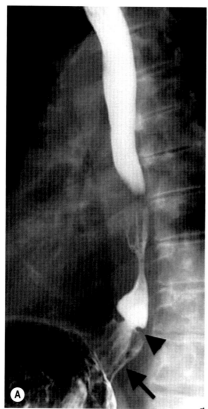

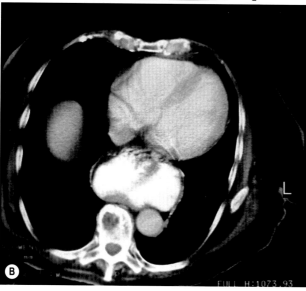

FIGURE 3-24 ■ **Hiatal hernia.** (A) Fluoroscopic image demonstrates type 1 hiatal hernia with gastric folds in the herniating portion of the stomach cardia (arrow) above the diaphragm with an incidental Schatzki ring (arrowhead). (B) MDCT shows barium-filled stomach in the chest (type 3).

junction above the hiatus (Fig. 3-24B). Type 4 hiatal hernia is composed of an intrathoracic stomach which may demonstrate organoaxial rotation.[86]

Traumatic diaphragmatic hernias result from a tear in the diaphragm either from a direct penetrating injury or from a sudden increase in intra-abdominal pressure during blunt trauma. These hernias are almost always on

the left side. Herniation may occur immediately after trauma or may be delayed by many years. Diagnosis is often difficult both due to lack of specificity of symptoms and because it is often confused with simple elevation of the hemidiaphragm. On barium studies the recognition of the gastric hernia lateral to the normal oesophageal hiatus is crucial. CT is also often helpful in diagnosis.

Gastric Volvulus

Gastric volvulus occurs when the stomach twists on itself between the points of its normal anatomical fixation. It is clinically important as it may cause gastric outlet obstruction or vascular compromise resulting in a surgical emergency. Classically, it presents with violent retching with minimal amount of vomitus, severe epigastric pain and difficulty in passing a nasogastric tube. Gastric volvulus is most common in the elderly but may occur at any age. Most of the time gastric volvulus involves a stomach that is partially or totally intrathoracic and that rotates between the normally positioned gastric ligaments. Other predisposing factors include phrenic nerve palsy, eventration of the diaphragm, traumatic diaphragmatic hernia, gastric distension and abnormalities of the spleen.[87]

Gastric volvulus is often divided into two types depending on the plane of torsion. In organoaxial volvulus the stomach rotates along its long axis, which is a line drawn between the cardia and the pylorus. Rotation may be to the right or left. The configuration of the torsed stomach depends on the original shape and position of the stomach (horizontal or vertical). If the normal stomach was in a horizontal position, volvulus flips the stomach upward so that the greater curvature is superior to the lesser curvature (Fig. 3-25). If the stomach was originally vertically orientated, volvulus causes a right–left twist.

Mesenteroaxial volvulus is less common but more likely to have significant clinical consequences. In this type of volvulus the stomach rotates on an axis perpendicular to the long axis of the stomach along a line joining the middle of the lesser curvature to the greater curvature. This corresponds to the axis of the mesenteric attachments of the greater and lesser omentum.[88] The characteristic appearance is an 'upside-down stomach' with the distal antrum and pylorus assuming a position cranial to the fundus and proximal stomach. This type of volvulus is often associated with traumatic diaphragmatic ruptures.

Radiographic signs of gastric volvulus include an air–fluid level of the stomach in the mediastinum and upper abdomen on upright plain radiography. On barium studies and on CT, the stomach may be inverted with the greater curvature above the lesser curvature, or the pylorus above the cardia and the torsed area identified as the source of the obstruction.[89]

Gastric Pneumatosis

Disruption of the gastric mucosa permits air to enter the gastric wall. When this occurs without an underlying infection it is called gastric emphysema[90] (Fig. 3-26A). Causes include corrosive ingestion, gastric ulcer, gastric

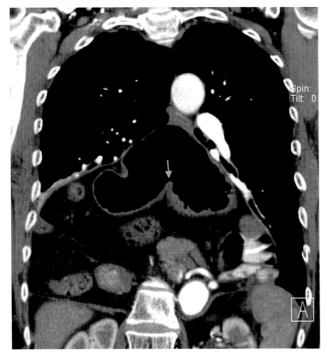

FIGURE 3-25 ■ **Gastric volvulus, organoaxial type.** MDCT coronal image shows an inverted stomach with the greater curvature above the lesser curvature (arrow).

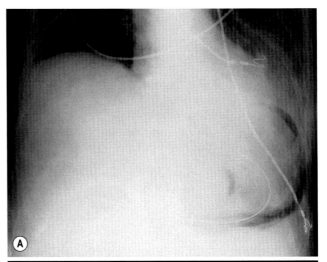

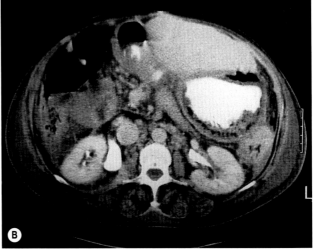

FIGURE 3-26 ■ **Gastric emphysema.** (A) Abdominal radiograph in a patient with ischaemic gastritis after extensive abdominal surgery showing curvilinear lucency outlining the stomach wall. (B) CT of a patient with infectious emphysematous gastritis.

outlet obstruction, chronic obstructive pulmonary disease (COPD), ischaemia and trauma.

Air in the gastric wall caused by an acute infection with a gas-forming organism is called emphysematous gastritis (Fig. 3-26B). *Escherichia coli* and *Clostridium welchii* are the usual causative agents. Acute panmural infectious gastritis by non-gas-forming organisms may also occur and is referred to as phlegmonous gastritis. Causative infectious agents include alpha-haemolytic streptococcus, *Staphylococcus aureus*, *E. coli*, *C. welchii* and *Streptococcus pneumoniae*. Infectious gastritis with any organism is unusual but is always a fulminant process associated with a high morbidity.

The radiological findings in both emphysematous gastritis and gastric emphysema include thin, curvilinear lines of radiolucent gas paralleling the gastric wall. CT is highly sensitive in detecting gastric wall gas.

Prepyloric Web (Antral Mucosal Diaphragm)

Prepyloric web, believed to be a congenital lesion, occurs as a diaphragm-like, exaggerated fold of gastric mucosa[91] oriented perpendicular to the long axis of the stomach. The thin web demarcates the distal antrum into a third small chamber between the proximal antrum and duodenal bulb. It appears as a thin persistent circumferential smooth band within 3–4 cm of the pylorus. The antral chamber produced by the web may mimic a second duodenal bulb. While usually asymptomatic, it may present with symptoms of gastric outlet obstruction.

Diverticula

Gastric diverticula are most common in the posterior aspect of the fundus,[92] below the oesophagogastric junction and near the lesser curvature,[93] or rarely in the antrum (Fig. 3-27A). These are true diverticula, i.e. containing muscularis propria, and thus are capable of peristalsis. They may be several centimetres in size and readily fill with barium. They rarely present a diagnostic dilemma but may mimic a submucosal mass if they fail to fill with barium. They may be mistaken for a gastric ulcer. In certain cases the CT appearance may be less specific if there is no luminal contrast medium or air.

Intramural or partial gastric diverticula describes a rare anomaly in which there is invagination of gastric mucosa into the gastric wall. These diverticula are usually smaller than 1 cm in size and have a lenticular shape in profile with a small opening into the gastric lumen.[94,95] (Fig. 3-27B). They are typically located on the greater curvature of the distal antrum and are generally considered to be asymptomatic. Radiologically they may present

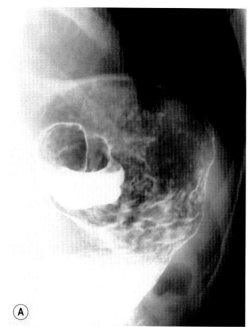

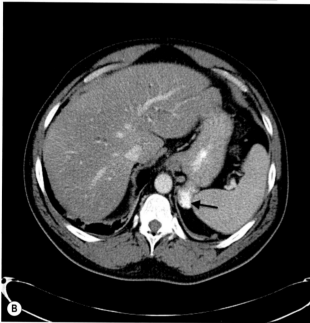

FIGURE 3-27 ■ **Gastric diverticulum.** (A) The patient is upright and a barium/air level is present in the fundal diverticulum. (B) MDCT in a different patient with fundal diverticulum (arrow).

a problem as they can be mistaken for ulcers, or for aberrant (ectopic) pancreatic rests, which typically occur in the same region.

Hypertrophic Pyloric Stenosis

Hypertrophic pyloric stenosis (HPS) is a relatively frequent congenital disorder diagnosed in infancy. Presentation in adults occasionally occurs. The morphological features are due to hypertrophy and hyperplasia of the circular muscle with some contribution by the longitudinal muscle. The hypertrophied muscle lengthens and

narrows the pyloric channel. Radiographically, there is lengthening of the pyloric channel (2–4 cm long) with smooth symmetrical narrowing. The hypertrophied muscle bulges retrogradely into the antrum, creating a 'shoulder'. In infants, HPS ultrasound is the technique of choice in the diagnosis of HPS.

A similar appearance may be seen with acquired hypertrophy of the distal antrum and pylorus. This is usually a sequela of peptic or other inflammatory disease.[92] This form of pyloric stenosis typically lacks the retrograde bulge of muscle.

Varices

Gastric varices are seen in most patients who have portal hypertension and oesophageal varices. Gastric veins provide one of the collateral pathways when there is obstruction of the portal vein. The presence of gastric varices in the absence of oesophageal varices is a sign of splenic vein thrombosis most often associated with pancreatitis or pancreatic carcinoma.[96]

Varices are most often seen in the fundus around the oesophagogastric junction sometimes involving the proximal body. They appear as widened, effaceable polypoid folds. They may be nodular-appearing, 'grape-like' or appear mass-like, in which case they may mimic gastric cancer.[97-99] Rarely they occur in the antrum without fundal involvement.[100] Transabdominal and endoscopic US are important techniques for definitive diagnosis of gastric varices. Varices are also well demonstrated on constrast-enhanced MDCT and MRI. Differential diagnosis for thick polypoid gastric folds includes hypertrophic gastritis, Ménétrier's disease and lymphoma (Fig. 3-28).

Gastric Distention

Gastric distension may be obstructive or non-obstructive. PUD and gastric cancer account for more than 90% of cases of gastric outlet obstruction. PUD is the most common cause of gastric outlet obstruction in adults. Duodenal and pyloric channel and distal antral ulcers are the usual culprits. Obstruction is caused by one or more factors including spasm, scarring, acute inflammation and muscle hypertrophy. Carcinoma of the distal antrum or pylorus is the second most common cause of gastric outlet obstruction. Infrequent causes include Crohn's disease, sarcoidosis, tuberculosis, syphilis (granulomatous diseases) and pancreatitis or pancreatic cancer.

Abdominal radiographs show the outline of the dilated air-filled stomach or downward displacement of the transverse colon by a fluid or an air-filled stomach. Barium studies are less than ideal for the delineation of the obstruction. CT is superior in depicting a mass or abnormal gastric wall when gastric malignancy is the cause of obstruction (Fig. 3-20).

Non-obstructive gastric dilatation may be acute or chronic. Rapid sudden gastric distension or gastric ileus occurs most often as a complication of abdominal surgery or acute trauma. Chronic gastric dilatation is common in diabetics, where gastroparesis, i.e. delayed gastric emptying, due to decreased or absent gastric peristalsis, occurs

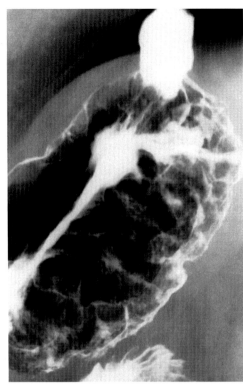

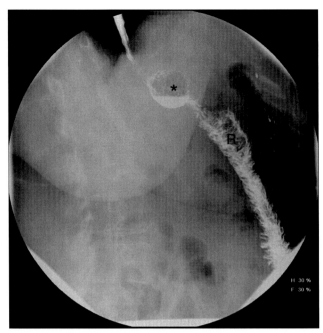

FIGURE 3-29 ■ **Normal gastric bypass study.** Single-contrast upper GI barium study shows the small gastric pouch (*) with free flow of barium into the Roux limb (R).

FIGURE 3-28 ■ **Gastric varices.** Multiple nodular and serpigenous submucosal masses in the fundus suggesting gastric varices.

in 20–30% of patients. These are most often poorly controlled diabetics.[101] Delayed gastric emptying can also be encountered after pancreaticoduodenectomy (Whipple's procedure) for pancreatic cancer or other pathological processes in the periampullary region. Nuclear medicine gastric emptying studies are commonly used to evaluate gastric motility disorders.

Ectopic Pancreas

Ectopic pancreas (pancreatic rest, aberrant pancreas) is the presence of pancreatic tissue in the submucosa of the luminal gastrointestinal tract. On imaging studies it is most commonly visible along the greater curvature of the antrum. The ectopic pancreatic tissues are usually solitary deposits that appear as sharply defined submucosal nodules usually <2 cm. A central depression that collects barium, thought to represent a rudimentary duct, is present in about 50% of cases. When this is present, the appearance is pathognomonic. If there is no central depression, the appearance is indistinguishable from other small submucosal lesions. If the central barium collection is prominent, ulceration is also a diagnostic consideration.

THE POSTOPERATIVE STOMACH

Gastric surgery is performed most commonly because of neoplasms, as an antireflux procedure, to bypass obstruction and for weight reduction. Complications of bariatric

surgery are an important source of morbidity and mortality, although the complication rate has vastly improved over the years since this has become an important way of treating morbid obesity. Imaging plays an important role in bariatric surgery, predominantly in the postoperative period, and it is important for the radiologist to be familiar with common postoperative appearances.

Bariatric Surgery for Obesity

Obesity is defined by having a body mass index of 30 kg/m² or greater in adults. According to the Centers for Disease Control and Prevention (CDC) website (as of July 2011), the United States has had a dramatic increase in obesity in the past 20 years. More than one-third of US adults are obese (35.7%). In England approximately a quarter of adults (26%) are classified as obese.[102] Conditions related to obesity include stroke, heart disease, sleep apnoea, type 2 diabetes and its related complications, among others. Surgical treatment for morbid obesity has burgeoned over the past years. The Roux-en-Y gastric bypass and gastric banding procedures are both increasingly performed laparoscopically for weight reduction. The laparoscopic Roux-en-Y gastric bypass is the most popular bariatric surgery in the United States although laparoscopic gastric banding is becoming increasingly popular.[103]

The laparoscopic Roux-en-Y gastric bypass (LRYGB) surgery consists of creating a gastric pouch measuring 10–30 mL, which is separated from the distally excluded gastric remnant. A portion of the jejunum (Roux limb) is mobilised and anastomosed end-to-side with the newly created small gastric pouch. The Roux limb is then anastomosed side-to-side with the biliopancreatic limb (proximal jejunum) (Fig. 3-29). The Roux limb may course retrocolic (through a newly created transverse mesocolon defect) or antecolic as well as antegastric or retrogastric.[103]

The laparoscopic adjustable gastric band procedure consists of placing a silicon band around the fundus of the stomach, just about 3 cm from the OE junction and therefore creating a small gastric pouch. Unlike in LRYGB, there is still a connection to the rest of the stomach through a stoma. The size of the stoma and pouch can be adjusted by accessing the attached port, which is usually placed anterior to the left rectus sheath.[103]

Sleeve gastrectomy, in which a large portion of the greater curvature is removed, creating a tubular-shaped stomach, is another procedure gaining popularity. It has lower morbity than Roux-en-Y procedures and shows promising long-term results.

Other Surgeries

In the past, partial gastrectomy was often performed for PUD. This consists of antrectomy, vagotomy and creation of either a gastroduodenostomy (Billroth I) (Fig. 3-30) or a gastrojejunostomy (Billroth II). This treatment approach has decreased significantly with medical anti *H. pylori* treatment and it is currently reserved for refractory cases.

Pyloroplasty may be used to treat ulcer disease, and consists of widening of the lumen of the pylorus to facilitate gastric emptying. This is frequently combined with a vagotomy. In the postoperative state, the normal pyloric contours are lost, and a pouch-like deformity may be observed.

Fundoplication procedures are performed to prevent gastro-oesophageal reflux and produce a characteristic deformity of the gastric cardia. The Nissen, Toupe and Dor fundoplications are the three commonly performed. The Nissen consists of 360° wrap, while the Toupe and Dor fundoplications have a 270° posterior wrap and a 180° anterior wrap, respectively.[104] These procedures are now most often performed laparoscopically.

Partial gastrectomy and gastroenterostomy are also performed, along with cholecysto- or choledochojejunostomy as part of Whipple's procedure.

Complications of Gastric Surgery

During the early postoperative period several complications may be observed. Submucosal haemorrhage may lead to outlet obstruction, which is usually self-limited and subsides within 10 days.[105] Leakage from the duodenal stump or anastomosis after gastrojejunostomy is the most common cause of death during the postoperative period.[106,107] The incidence of this complication is 1–5%, with a mortality rate of 40–50%.[106] Stump leakage usually occurs during the first 2 weeks after surgery. Ischaemia of the stomach, leading to necrosis and fistula formation, is another serious postoperative complication, associated with a significant morality rate.[107] Fortunately, this is rare. Leakage can usually be diagnosed after ingestion of water-soluble contrast material. Persistent severe diarrhoea caused by inadvertent gastroileostomy instead of gastrojejunostomy also is best diagnosed by upper gastrointestinal examination.[108]

Complications from LRYGB and gastric banding procedures are well known and are frequently detected by fluoroscopy and/or MDCT. Gastric bypass complications include but are not limited to: leaks (from any of the anastomosis sites), anastomotic narrowing (early due to oedema or early stricture), patulous anastomosis, gastrogastric fistula, ulcer, small bowel obstruction (internal hernias or less likely postoperative adhesions), haemorrhage and abscess formation.[109,110] In particular, an internal hernia may be caused by herniation of the Roux limb and other loops of small bowel through the surgically created defect in the transverse mesocolon in the setting of a retrocolic approach (Fig. 3-31). Other possible sites for internal hernias include defect at the meseteric site of the enteroenterostomy, and posterior to the Roux limb (Peterson hernia). A study by Lockhart et al.[111] showed that mesenteric swirl sign is the best CT indicator of internal hernias after laparoscopic Roux-en-Y gastric bypass.

Complications from gastric banding procedures may be divided into early complications and late complications. Early complications include misplacement of the band, perforation, and early slippage. Late complications may include pouch dilatation, band herniation, spontaneous variation in volume, erosion through the gastric wall and migration/slippage of the band.[112] Slippage is herniation of the stomach through the band upward, and

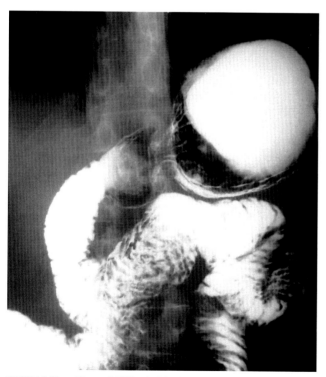

FIGURE 3-30 ■ **Normal Billroth I barium study.** The stomach is foreshortended by antrectomy and gastroduodenostomy.

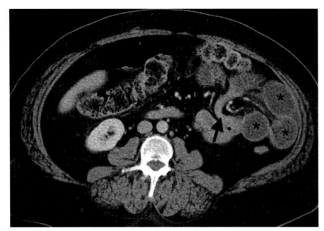

FIGURE 3-31 ▪ **Roux-en-Y gastric bypass, retrocolic.** Dilated small bowel loops (*) caused by internal hernia through the transverse mesocolon defect (arrow).

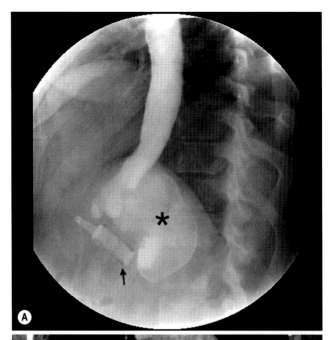

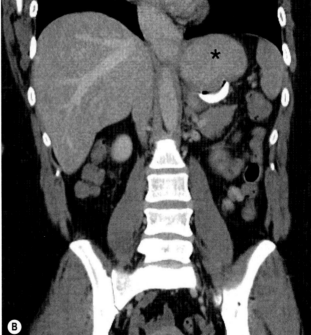

FIGURE 3-32 ▪ **Gastric band slippage.** (A) Fluoroscopic lateral image demonstrates posterior band slippage with protusion of the fundus and proximal body (*) above the gastric band (arrow). (B) MDCT coronal image of the same patient showing stomach fundus and proximal body (*) above the gastric band.

therefore causing eccentric gastric pouch enlargement. Slippage may be anterior or posterior, based on which portion of the stomach herniates upward through the band. The enlarged eccentric gastric pouch is posterior and inferior in posterior slippage and anterior and superior in anterior slippage.[113] Fluoroscopy and MDCT may be used to detect band slippage (Fig. 3-32). Band slippage may be caused by faulty surgical technique or recurrent vomiting, among other causes.[113]

Marginal ulcerations occur in 3–10% of patients who have been operated on for PUD.[108,114] They occur within the first 2 cm of anastomosis on the jejunal side and are usually caused by inadequate vagotomy.

Afferent loop obstruction may be acute or chronic. This is usually caused by herniation of the afferent loop through a surgically created mesocolon defect behind the gastroenteric anastomosis.[106] Chronic afferent loop obstruction occurs because of preferential gastric emptying into the afferent loop.[106,108] Patients present with intermittent bilious vomiting, weight loss, malabsorptions and steatorrhoea. The symptoms are secondary to stasis with accumulation of secretions in the afferent loop. Preferential filling of the afferent loop is seen on upper gastrointestinal examination. Barium is retained within the afferent loop on delayed films, and regurgitation of contrast material into the stomach from the afferent loop may be recognised. This syndrome may be associated with a very long afferent loop.

Efferent loop obstruction is usually caused by spasm and inflammation. It is manifested between the fifth and tenth postoperative days,[106,108] usually after removal of the nasogastric tube, and is usually a self-limiting phenomenon not requiring specific treatment. Upper gastrointestinal examination reveals delayed transit in the efferent loop.

Prolapse and intussusception may occur at the anastomosis postoperatively. Jejunogastric intussusception is the most common abnormality of this type. Either the afferent or the efferent loop may be involved, although the efferent loop is involved in 75% of cases.[115]

Bezoars are well-recognised complications after Billroth I and II procedures, especially when these are accompanied by vagotomies. Gastric bezoars are more common after the Billroth I procedure,[116] and bezoars in the small bowel after Billroth II anastomoses. They have also been reported after Roux-en-Y bypass. These are usually phytobezoars related to an improper diet postoperatively[117] and may be recognised radiographically as

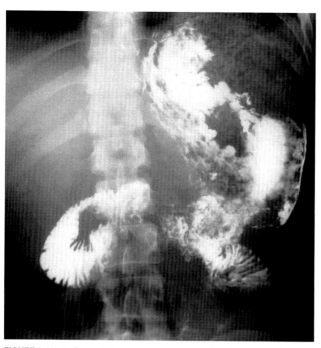

FIGURE 3-33 ■ **Gastric bezoar.** Large mass in stomach solidified retained ingested fibrous material mixed with air in the patient after a Billroth II anastomosis.

irregularly coated masses in either the stomach or the small bowel that tend to move freely within the lumen (Fig. 3-33). Those in the small intestine may produce obstruction.

Primary gastric carcinoma occasionally develops in the gastric remnant, with reports being somewhat more frequent in Europe than in the United States. Reports of the incidence of this complication range from 0.3 to 11%.[118] These tumours represent approximately 1% of all gastric cancers. It is reported that the patients have a relatively high incidence of atrophic gastritis.[119] On upper gastrointestinal examination, these tumours may demonstrate a lack of distensibility of the gastric remnant. Obstruction, either at the stoma or at the gastro-oesophageal junction, may be seen. A pattern of enlarged rugae with intraluminal masses or gastric ulcer formation may also be seen.

ADVANCES IN GASTRIC IMAGING

Recent technical developments in high-resolution multi-planar MDCT and image analysis have sparked renewed interest in using CT to evaluate gastric disease. Multiple studies from countries with high incidence of gastric cancer suggest significantly improved accuracy of non-invasive evaluation of stomach pathology, now comparable to upper endoscopy. Large-scale prospective studies are needed to identify the role of non-invasive imaging in the detection of early cancers. Consistent criteria for a reproducible PET-CT reporting system for staging, and evaluation of response to therapy need to be established. Increasing awareness about the risks of radiation coupled with recent advances in fast imaging techniques will increase the role of MR imaging as a safe and reliable alternative in the near future.

REFERENCES

1. Gore RM, Lichtenstein JE. The gastrointestinal tract: anatomic-pathologic basis of radiologic findings. In: Traveras JM, Ferrucci JT, editors. Radiology. 4th ed. Philadelphia: Lippincott-Raven; 1998. Chapter 4.
2. Kawai K, Tanaka H. The fundamentals of an X-ray diagnosis. In: Differential Diagnosis of Gastric Diseases. Chicago: Year Book; 1974. pp. 11–53.
3. Gelfand DW. Gastrointestinal Radiology. New York: Churchill Livingstone; 1984. pp. 29–46; 55–66.
4. Rubesin SE, Levine MS, Laufer I. Double-contrast upper gastrointestinal radiography: a pattern approach for diseases of the stomach. Radiology 2008;246:33–48.
5. Cho KC, Gold BM, Printz DA. Multiple transverse folds in the gastric antrum. Radiology 1987;164:339–41.
6. Meyers MA. Dynamic Radiology of the Abdomen. 4th ed. New York: Springer-Verlag; 1994.
7. Chen CY, Hsu JS, Wu DC, et al. Gastric cancer: prospective local staging with 3D multi-detector row CT—correlation with surgical and histipathological results. Radiology 2007;242:472–82.
8. Ba-Ssalamah A, Prokap M, Uffmann M, et al. Dedicated multi-detector CT of the stomach: spectrum of diseases. Radiographics 2003;23:625–44.
9. Kim I, Kim SW, Shin HC, et al. MRI of gastric carcinoma: Results of T and N staging in an in vitro study. World J Gastroenterol 2009;15:3992–8.
10. Amieva MR, EL-Omar EM. Host-bacterial interactions of *Helicobacter pylori* infection. Gastroenterology 2008;134(1):306–23.
11. Marshall BJ, Warren JR. Unidentified curved bacilli in the stomach of patients with gastritis and peptic ulceration. Lancet i:1311–15. 1984.
12. NIH Consensus Conference. *Helicobacter pylori* in peptic ulcer disease: NIH Consensus Development Panel on *Helicobacter pylori* in peptic ulcer disease. JAMA 1994;272:65–9.
13. IARC monographs on the evaluation of carcinogenic risks to humans: schistosomes, liver flukes and *Helicobacter pylori*. Lyon: International Agency for Research on Cancer; 1994. pp. 177–240.
14. Wotherspoon AC, Ortiz-Hidalgo C, Falzon MR, et al. *Helicobacter pylori*-associated gastritis and primary B-cell gastric lymphoma. Lancet 1991;338:1175–6.
15. Lin WC, Tsai HF, Kuo SH, et al. Translocation of *Helicobacter pylori* CagA into Human B lymphocytes, the origin of mucosa-associated tissue lymphoma. Cancer Res 2010;70(14):5470–8.
16. Marshall BJ, Barrett L, Prakash C, et al. Urea protects *Helicobacter (Campylobacter) pylori* from the bactericidal effect of acid. Gastroenterology 1990;99:697–702.
17. Cullen DJ, Collins BJ, Christiansen KJ, et al. When is *Helicobacter pylori* infection acquired? Gut 1993;34:1681–2.
18. Graham DY, Lew GH, Klein PD, et al. Effect of treatment of *Helicobacter pylori* infection on long term recurrence of gastric or duodenal ulcer. Ann Intern Med 1992;116:707–8.
19. Pattison PC, Combs M, Marshall BJ. *Helicobacter pylori* and peptic ulcer disease: evolution to revolution to resolution. Am J Roentgenol 1997;168:1415–20.

20. Fuccio L, Zagari RM, Eusebi LH, et al. Meta-analysis: can *Helicobacter pylori* eradication treatment reduce the risk for gastric cancer? Ann Intern Med 2009;151(2):121–8.

21. Gelfand DW, Dale WJ, Ott DJ. The location and size of gastric ulcer: radiologic and endoscopic evaluation. Am J Roentgenol 1994;143:755–8.

22. Thompson G, Stevenson GW, Somers S. Distribution of gastric ulcers by double-contrast barium meal with endoscopic correlation. J Can Assoc Radiol 1983;34:296–7.

23. Kottler RE, Tuft RJ. Benign greater curve gastric ulcer: the 'sump-ulcer'. Br J Radiol 1981;54:651–4.

24. Amberg JR, Zboralske FF. Gastric ulcers after 70. Am J Roentgenol 1966;96:393–9.

25. Haudek M. Zur rontgenologischen Diagnose der Ulcerationen in der pars media des magnes. Munchen Med Wschr 1910;57: 1587–91.

26. Schumacher EC, Hampton AO. Radiographic differentiation of benign and malignant ulcers. Ciba Clin Symp 1956;8:161–71.

27. Levine MS, Creteur V, Kressel HY, et al. Benign gastric ulcers: diagnosis and follow-up with double-contrast radiography. Radiology 1987;164:9–13.

28. Chen C-Y, Jaw T-S, Kuo Y-T, et al. Differentiation of gastric ulcers with MDCT. Abdom Imaging 2007;32:688–93.

29. Gossios K, Tsianos E. CT evaluation of benign gastric lesions. Ann Gastroenterol 2004;17(1):31–6.

30. Laufer I, Hamilton J, Mullens JE. Demonstration of superficial gastric erosions by double-contrast radiography. Gastroenterology 1975;68:387–91.

31. Ott DJ, Gelfand EW, Wu SC, Kerr RM. Sensitivity of single- vs double-contrast radiology in erosive gastritis. Am J Roentgenol 1982;138:263–6.

32. Graham DY, Go MF. *Helicobacter pylori*: current status. Gastroenterology 1993;105:279–82.

33. Gelfand DW, Ott DJ. *Helicobacter pylori* and gastroduodenal diseases: a minor revolution for radiologists. Am J Roentgenol 1997;168:1421–2.

34. Sohn J, Levine MS, Furth EE, et al. *Helicobacter pylori* gastritis: radiographic findings. Radiology 1995;195:763–7.

35. Joske RA, Finckh ES, Wood IJ. Gastric biopsy: a study of 1000 consecutive successful gastric biopsies. Q J Med 1955;24: 269–94.

36. Elsborg L, Mosbech J. Pernicious anaemia as a risk factor in gastric cancer. Acta Med Scand 1979;206:315–18.

37. Levine MS. Inflammatory conditions of the stomach and duodenum. In: Gore RM, Levine MS, editors. Textbook of Gastrointestinal Radiology. 3rd ed. Philadelphia: Saunders Elsevier; 2008. Chapter 34.

38. Cronan J, Burrell M, Trepeta R. Aphthoid ulcerations in gastric candidiasis. Radiology 1980;134:607–11.

39. Agel NM, Tanner P, Drury A, et al. Cytomegalovirus gastritis with perforation and gastrocolic fistula formation. Histopathology 1991;18:165–8.

40. Megibow AJ, Balthazar EJ, Hulnick DH. Radiology of nonneoplastic gastrointestinal disorders in acquired immune deficiency syndrome. Semin Roentgenol 1987;22:31–41.

41. Falcone S, Murphy BJ, Weinfeld A. Gastric manifestations of AIDS: radiographic findings on upper gastrointestinal examination. Gastrointest Radiol 1991;16:95–8.

42. Levine MS. Crohn's disease of the upper gastrointestinal tract. Radiol Clin North Am 1987;225:79–91.

43. Legge DA, Carlson HC, Judd ES. Roentgenologic features of regional enteritis of the upper gastrointestinal tract. Am J Roentgenol 1970;110:355–60.

44. Laufer I, Joffe N, Stolberg H. Unusual causes of gastrocolic fistula. Gastrointest Radiol 1977;2:21–5.

45. Cohen WN. Gastric involvement in Crohn's disease. Am J Roentgenol 1967;101:425–30.

46. Marshak RH, Maklansky D, Kurzban JD, et al. Crohn's disease of the stomach and duodenum. Am J Gastroenterol 1982;77: 340–3.

47. Stempien SJ, Dagradi AE, Reingold IM, et al. Hypertrophic hypersecretory gastropathy. Am J Dig Dis 1964;9:471–93.

48. Tan D T D, Stempien SJ, Dagradi AE. The clinical spectrum of hypertrophic hypersecretory gastropathy. Gastrointest Endosc 1971;18:69–73.

49. Rose C, Stevenson GW. Correlation between visualization and size of the areae gastricae and duodenal ulcer. Radiology 1981; 139:371–4.

50. Reese DF, Hodgson JR, Dockerty MB. Giant hypertrophy of the gastric mucosa (Ménétrier's disease): a correlation of the roentgenographic, pathologic, and clinical findings. Am J Roentgenol 1962;88:619–26.

51. Olmsted WW, Cooper PH, Madewell JE. Involvement of the gastric antrum in Ménétrier's disease. Am J Roentgenol 1976; 126:524–9.

52. Schulman A, Morton PCG, Dietrich BE. Eosinophilic gastroenteritis. Clin Radiol 1980;31:101–4.

53. Lee CM, Changchien CS, Chen PC, et al. Eosinophilic gastroenteritis: 10 years experience. Am J Gastroenterol 1993;88:70–4.

54. Klein NC, Hargrove RL, Sleisenger MH, et al. Eosinophilic gastroenteritis. Medicine 1970;49:299–319.

55. Goldberg HI, O'Kieffe D, Jenis EH, et al. Diffuse eosinophilic gastroenteritis. Am J Roentgenol 1973;119:342–51.

56. Balfe DM. Eosinophilic gastritis. Am J Roentgenol 1989;152: 1322.

57. Wehunt WD, Olmsted WW, Neiman HL, et al. Eosinophilic gastritis. Radiology 1976;120:85–9.

58. MacCarthy RL, Talley NJ. Barium studies in diffuse eosinophilic gastroenteritis. Gastrointest Radiol 1990;15:183–7.

59. Carlson HC, Breen JF. Amyloidosis and plasma cell dyscrasias: gastrointestinal involvement. Semin Roentgenol 1986;21: 128–38.

60. Carmack SW, Genta RM, Graham DY, et al. Management of gastric polyps: a pathology based guide for gastroenterologists. Nat Rev Gastroenterol Hepatol 2009;(6):331–41.

61. Park YD, Lauwers GY. Gastric polyps: classification and management. Arch Pathol Lab Med 2008;132(4):633–40.

62. Rugge M, Nitti D, Farinati F, et al. Non-invasive neoplasia of the stomach. Eur J Gastroenterol Hepatol 2005;17:1191–6.

63. Calva D, Howe JR. Hamartomatous polyposis syndromes. Surg Clin North Am 2008;88(4):779–817.

64. Rubesin SE, Levine MS, Laufer I. Double-contrast upper gastrointestinal radiography: a pattern approach for disease of the stomach. Radiology 2008;246:33–48.

65. Miettinen M, Lasota J. Gastrointestinal stromal tumors. Review on morphology, molecular pathology, prognosis, and differential diagnosis. Arch Pathol Lab Med 2006;130:1466–78.

66. Sandrasegaran K, Rajesh A, Rydberg J, et al. Gastrointestinal stromal tumors: clinical, radiologic and pathologic features. Am J Roentgenol 2005;184 (3):803–11.

67. Hamashima C, Shibuya D, Yamazaki H, et al. The Japanese guidelines for gastric cancer screening. Jpn J Clin Oncol 2008; 38:259.

68. Japanese Gastric Cancer Association. Japanese classification of gastric carcinoma—2nd English edition. Gastric Cancer 1998; 10–24.

69. Low VH, Levine MS, Rubesin SE, et al. Diagnosis of gastric carcinoma: sensitivity of double-contrast barium studies. Am J Roentgenol 1994;162:329–34.

70. Levine MS, Rubesin SE, Laufer I. Barium studies in modern radiology: do they have a role? Radiology 2009;250:18–22.

71. Gotoda T. Endoscopic resection of early gastric cancer: The Japanese perspective. Curr Opin Gastroenterol 2006;22:561.

72. Lee IJ, Lee JM, Kim SH, et al. Diagnostic performance of 64-channel MDCT in the evaluation of gastric cancer: differentiation of mucosal cancer (T1a) from submucosal involvement (T1b and T2). Radiology 2010;(255):805–14.

73. Furukawa K, Miyahara R, Itoh A, et al. Diagnosis of the invasion depth of the gastric cancer using MDCT with virtual gastroscopy: comparison with staging with endoscopic ultrasound. Am J Roentgenol 2011;197:867–75.

74. Washington K. Editorial: 7th edition of the AJCC Cancer Staging Manual: Stomach. Ann Surg Oncol 2010;17:3077–9.

75. Palmowski M, Grenacher L, Kuntz C, et al. Magnetic resonance imaging for local staging of gastric carcinoma: results of an in vitro study. J Comput Assist Tomogr 2006;30:896–902.

76. Kim II Young. MR imaging of gastric carcinoma. In: Ismaili N, editor. Management of Gastric Cancer. InTech; 2011. pp. 19–36.

77. Kwee RM, Kwee TC. Imaging in local staging of gastric cancer: a systematic review. J Clin Oncol 2007;25:2107–16.

78. Hwang SW, Lee DH, Lee SH, et al. Preoperative staging of gastric cancer by endoscopic ultrasonography and multidetector-row computed tomography. J Gastroenterol Hepatol 2010;25: 512–18.

79. Lim JS, Kim MJ, Yun MJ, et al. Comparison of CT and 18F FDG-PET for detecting peritoneal metastases on the preoperative evaluation of gastric carcinoma. Korean J Radiol 2006;7: 249–56.

80. Hopkins S, Yang G. FDG PET imaging in the staging and management of gastric cancer. J Gastrointest Oncol 2011;2(1): 39–44.

81. Parsonnet J, Hansen S, Rodriguez L, et al. Recent developments in our understanding of gastric lymphoma. Am J Surg Pathol 1996;20 (suppl I):S1–7.

82. Ghai S, Pattison J, Ghai S, et al. Primary gastrointestinal lymphoma: spectrum of imaging findings with pathological correlation. Radiographics 2007;27(5):1371–88.

83. Radan L, Fischer D, Bar-shalom R, et al. FDG avidity and PET/CT patterns in primary gastric lymphoma. Eur J Nucl Med Mol Imaging 2008;35:1428–4330.

84. Binstock A, Johnson CD, Stephens DH, et al. Carcinoid tumors of the stomach: a clinical and radiographic study. Am J Roentgenol 2001;176:947–51.

85. Modlin IM, Lye KD, Kidd M. A 5-decade analysis of 13,715 carcinoid tumors. Cancer 2003;97(4):934–59.

86. Canon CL. Gastrointestinal tract. In: Lee JKT, Sagel SS, Stanley RJ, Heiken JP, editors. Computed Body Tomography with MRI Correlation. 4th ed. Philadelphia: Lippincott Williams & Wilkins; 2006. Chapter 11.

87. Balthazar EJ. Positional abnormalities of the stomach. In: Taveras JM, Ferrucci JT, editors. Radiology Diagnosis-Imaging-Intervention. 4th ed. Philadelphia: Lippincott-Raven; 1998. Chapter 20.

88. Gerson DE, Lewicki AM. Intrathoracic stomach: when does it obstruct? Radiology 1976;119:257–64.

89. Menuck L. Plain film findings of gastric volvulus herniating into the chest. Am J Roentgenol 1976;126:1169–74.

90. Kussin SZ, Henry C, Navarro C, et al. Gas within the wall of the stomach: report of a case and review of the literature. Dig Dis Sci 1982;27:949.

91. Felson B, Berkman YM, Hoyumpa AM. Gastric mucosal diaphragm. Radiology 1969;92:513–17.

92. Eisenberg RL, Levine MS. Miscellaneous abnormalities. In: Gore RN, Levine MS, editors. Textbook of Gastrointestinal Radiology, vol. 1. 3rd ed. Philadelphia: Saunders Elsevier; 2008. Chapter 38.

93. Palmer ED. Collective review: gastric diverticula. Int Abstr Surg 1951;92:417–28.

94. Rabushka SE, Melamed M, Melamed JL. Unusual gastric diverticula. Radiology 1968;90:1006–8.

95. Treichel J, Gerstenberg E, Palme G, et al. Diagnosis of partial gastric diverticula. Radiology 1976;119:13–18.

96. Muhletaler C, Gerlock J, Goncharenko V, et al. Gastric varices secondary to splenic vein occlusion: radiographic diagnosis and clinical significance. Radiology 1979;132:593–8.

97. Swischuk LE. Gastric varices presenting as 'pseudotumors' of the cardia. Am J Dig Dis 1967;12:839.

98. Belgrard R, Carlson HC, Payne WS, Cain JC. Pseudotumoral gastric varices. Am J Roentgenol 1964;91:751–6.

99. Carucci LR, Levine MS, Rubesin SE. Tumorous gastric varices: radiographic findings in 10 patients. Radiology 1999;212: 861–5.

100. Csos T, Meyers MA, Baltaxe HA. Nonfundic gastric varices. Radiology 1972;105:579–80.

101. Gramm HF, Reuter K, Costello P. The radiologic manifestations of diabetic gastric neuropathy and its differential diagnosis. Gastrointest Radiol 1978;3:151–5.

102. NHS Information Centre. Statistics on Obesity, Physical Activity and Diet: England, 2012. Available at: http://www.ic.nhs.uk/statistics-and-data-collections/health-and-lifestyles/obesity/statistics-on-obesity-physical-activity-and-diet-england-2012. Accessibility verified 19 March 2012.

103. Gore RM, Smith CH. Postoperative stomach and duodenum. In: Gore RN, Levine MS, editors. Textbook of Gastrointestinal Radiology, vol. 1. 3rd ed. Philadelphia: Saunders Elsevier; 2008. pp. 707–25.

104. Canon CL, Morgan DE, Einstein DM. Surgical approach to gastroesophageal reflux disease: what the radiologist needs to know. Radiographics 2005;25:1485–99.

105. Burhenne HJ. Postoperative defects of the stomach. Semin Roentgenol 1971;6:182–92.

106. Burrell M, Curtis AM. Sequelae of stomach surgery. CRC Crit Rev Diagn Imag 1977;10:17–97.

107. Hardy JH. Problems associated with gastric surgery. Am J Surg 1964;108:699–716.

108. Jay BS, Burrell M. Iatrogenic problems following gastric surgery. Gastrointest Radiol 1977;2:239–57.

109. Scheirey CD, Scholz FJ, Shah PC, et al. Radiology of the laparoscopic Roux-en-Y gastric bypass procedure: conceptualization and precise interpretation of results. Radiographics 2006;26: 1355–71.

110. Yu J, Turner MA, Cho S-R, et al. Normal anatomy and complications after gastric bypass surgery: helical CT findings. Radiology 2004;231:753–60.

111. Lockhart ME, Tessler FN, Canon CL. Internal hernia after gastric bypass: sensitivity and specificity of seven CT signs with surgical correlation and controls. Am J Roentgenol 2007;188:745–50.

112. Mehanna MJ, Birjawi G, Moukaddam HA, et al. Complications of adjustable gastric banding, a radiological pictorial review. Am J Roentgenol 2006;186(2):522–34.

113. Blachar A, Blank A, Gavert N. Laparoscopic adjustable gastric banding surgery for morbid obesity: imaging of normal anatomic features and postoperative gastrointestinal complications. Am J Roentgenol 2007;188(2):472–9.

114. Burhenne HJ. The retained gastric antrum: preoperative roentgenologic diagnosis of an iatrogenic syndrome. Am J Roentgenol 1967;101:549–97.

115. Poppel MH. Gastric intussusceptions. Radiology 1962;78: 602–8.

116. Szemes GC, Amberg JR. Gastric bezoars after partial gastrectomy: report of five cases. Radiology 1968;90:765–8.

117. Moskowitz H. Phytobezoars of the small bowel following gastric surgery. Radiology 1974;13:23–6.

118. Feldman F, Seaman WB. Primary gastric stump cancer. Am J Roentgenol 1972;115:257–67.

119. Kobayashi S, Prolla JC, Kirsner JB. Late gastric carcinoma developing after surgery for benign conditions. Am J Dig Dis 1970;15:905–12.

CHAPTER 4

The Duodenum and Small Intestine

Nicholas Gourtsoyiannis • Panos Prassopoulos • Maria Daskalogiannaki •
Patrick McLaughlin • Michael M. Maher

THE DUODENUM

ANATOMY AND NORMAL APPEARANCES

The duodenum measures 20–30 cm in length. It forms an incomplete circle surrounding the head of the pancreas and is described as having first, second, third and fourth parts.

The first (superior) part contains the duodenal cap or bulb and passes superiorly, posteriorly and to the right before turning down to become the second part. Posteriorly it is devoid of peritoneum. The second (descending) portion passes down anterior to the right kidney and posterior to the transverse colon. Above and below the transverse colon it is covered with peritoneum. The duodenum turns to the left and passes horizontally in front of the spine as the third (horizontal) part before it ascends in front and to the left of the aorta as the fourth

(ascending) part to end at the duodenojejunal flexure (ligament of Treitz).

At barium examination, parallel, or nearly parallel, folds are seen passing upwards from the base of the duodenal cap. They are effaced when the hypotonic duodenum is distended by gas at double-contrast barium examination. The mucosa of the remainder of the duodenum is thrown into numerous folds that disappear on distension. The circular folds, termed valvulae conniventes, are permanent; they begin in the second part of the duodenum and extend throughout the small intestine.

The ampulla of Vater can be seen in 65% of patients during routine double-contrast barium examination and the accessory papilla of Santorini's duct (also known as the minor duodenal papilla) in 25%. The ampulla of Vater is recognised by its fold pattern: a hooded fold and a distal longitudinal fold are usual, and oblique folds are frequently present. The accessory papilla is sited about 10 mm proximal to the ampulla. On a prone view the ampulla lies on the medial wall and the accessory papilla on the anterior wall.

RADIOLOGICAL INVESTIGATION

Barium Studies

The barium examination is the principal radiological technique for examining the duodenal lumen, although the technique has largely been replaced by endoscopy. It is easier to detect abnormalities if the duodenum is relaxed. Hypotonia is produced by IV injection of 20 mg of hyoscine butylbromide (Buscopan) or 0.2 mg of glucagon. With the table horizontal, the patient is first turned onto their right side so that barium fills the duodenum. The patient is next rotated onto their left side and gas passes rapidly from the stomach into the duodenum. Then, with the patient in the right anterior oblique position, a number of double-contrast views of the duodenal cap and duodenal loop (Fig. 4-1) are taken. Water-soluble contrast medium should be used in patients with suspected perforation of the stomach or duodenum. The examination is best performed under fluoroscopic control; alternatively, a right decubitus radiograph is taken after a short interval. Hypotonic duodenography is performed by placing a duodenal catheter in the lower part of the descending duodenum and injecting about 40 mL of barium suspension. The smooth muscle relaxant is then injected intravenously and air is injected through the catheter to distend the duodenum and radiographs of the duodenal loop are taken.

Other Imaging Techniques

Angiography can be invaluable in the diagnosis of acute duodenal haemorrhage, when endoscopy has failed to locate the bleeding site. Ultrasound (US) and computed tomography (CT) are used to evaluate secondary involvement of the duodenum by malignant disease and CT may also be helpful in assessing the extent of duodenal neoplasms.

PEPTIC ULCERATION

On double-contrast barium examination, duodenal ulcer craters are shown as sharply defined, constant collections of barium (Fig. 4-2), sometimes with a surrounding zone of oedema or radiating folds. Anterior wall ulcers are normally shown best on the prone view.

Postbulbar Ulceration

Postbulbar ulcers are occasionally seen, mostly on the concave border of the second part or in the immediate postbulbar area. The ulcer is shown as a typical crater, frequently with spasm of the opposite wall. There may be narrowing of the lumen and thickening of the mucosal folds. In some cases scar formation may obscure the ulcer crater. Postbulbar ulcers usually fail to heal on medical treatment.

Complications of Peptic Ulceration

The principal complications of duodenal ulceration are perforation, bleeding, stenosis and penetration of adjacent organs. Free perforation is usually diagnosed on the

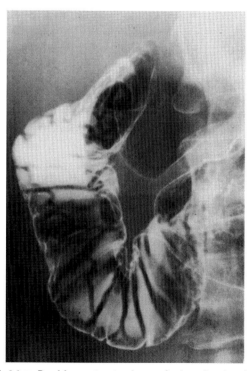

FIGURE 4-1 ■ **Double-contrast view of the duodenal loop.** The normal duodenal cap is also seen.

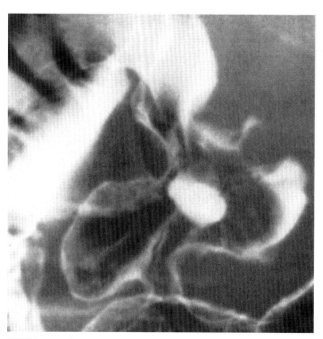

FIGURE 4-2 ■ **Duodenal ulceration.** The duodenal cap is deformed and a moderate-sized ulcer crater is outlined with barium.

clinical and plain radiographic findings. Occasionally, a water-soluble contrast examination may be necessary to confirm the diagnosis. The perforation is sometimes localised or 'walled-off' with marked deformity of the duodenum due to the adjacent inflammatory reaction. Bleeding caused by duodenal ulceration is diagnosed by endoscopy and/or angiography. Duodenal stenosis may become quite marked and result in obstruction. Barium examination in this situation will show an excessive amount of fluid in a dilated stomach with considerable delay in emptying.

GASTRIC HETEROTOPIA

Gastric heterotopia is present in a small percentage of normal people. Irregular filling defects, varying in size from 1 to 6 mm, are seen in the duodenal cap extending from the pylorus distally (Fig. 4-3). Gastric heterotopia should be differentiated from lymphoid hyperplasia of the duodenal bulb, which usually requires endoscopy.

DIVERTICULA

Duodenal diverticula are present in 2–5% of barium studies; most are an incidental finding. They are usually in the descending part of the duodenum, with 85% arising from the medial surface (Fig. 4-4). Frequently they are in contact with the pancreas and may be embedded in its surface. Occasionally, a diverticulum contains aberrant pancreatic, gastric, or other functioning tissue and is the site of ulceration, perforation, or gangrene. Symptoms may also develop due to the retention of food or a foreign body. Cholangitis or pancreatitis may result from the aberrant insertion of the common bile duct or pancreatic duct into an intraluminal diverticulum.

NEOPLASMS

Benign Neoplasms

Benign neoplasms of the duodenum are uncommon and often symptomless. Brunner's gland hyperplasia is seen as single or multiple polypoid lesions in the first part of the duodenum (Fig. 4-5), often with a characteristic cobblestone appearance. Patients usually present with typical symptoms of peptic ulceration. A single Brunner's gland adenoma is occasionally seen. Adenomatous polyps feature as solitary, mostly sessile, polypoid, intraluminal filling defects on barium studies, or as soft-tissue masses on CT. Villous adenomas exhibit a characteristic 'cauliflower' or 'soap bubble' appearance on barium studies, caused by the trapping of barium in the crevices between the multiple frond-like projections of the tumour. Benign lymphoid hyperplasia is an occasional finding shown as multiple small rounded filling defects of uniform size (Fig. 4-6). Other benign neoplasms of the duodenum include periampullary adenomas (Fig. 4-7), gastrointestinal stromal tumours (GISTs), lipomas (Fig. 4-8) and neurogenic tumours or hamartomas exhibiting the same features as in the small intestine.

Malignant Neoplasms

Primary Carcinoma

Carcinoma of the papilla of Vater (also known as the ampulla of Vater) is the type most frequently encountered, usually presenting with jaundice. Barium studies

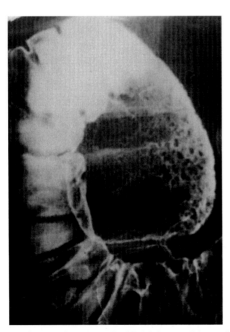

FIGURE 4-3 ■ **Gastric heterotopia.** Multiple small irregular filling defects of varying size are seen in the duodenal cap. (Courtesy of Dr J. Virjee.)

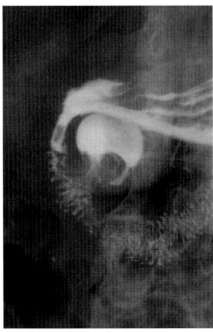

FIGURE 4-4 ■ **Duodenography.** A large diverticulum is demonstrated arising from the medial surface of the descending duodenum. The filling defect corresponds to the ampulla of Vater.

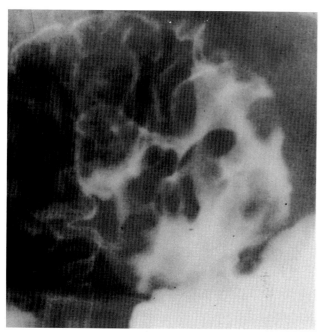

FIGURE 4-5 ▪ **Brunner's gland hyperplasia.** Multiple filling defects are seen in the duodenal cap. Biopsies obtained at endoscopy showed Brunner's gland hyperplasia.

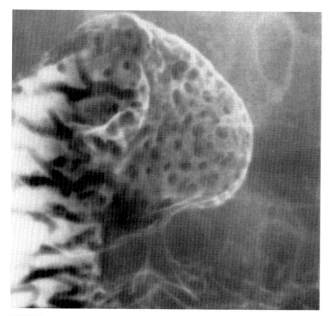

FIGURE 4-6 ▪ **Lymphoid hyperplasia.** Multiple small filling defects characteristic of lymphoid hyperplasia are shown on a double-contrast view of the duodenal cap. (Reproduced from Darrah, E. R. Nolan, D, J. 1999. Hosp Med 60:10–18, with permission.)

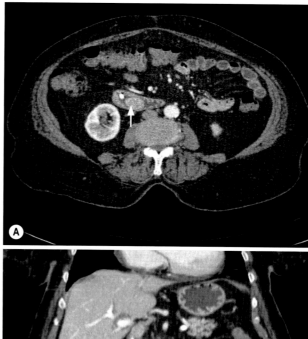

FIGURE 4-7 ▪ **Periampullary adenoma.** (A) Axial image and (B) coronal reconstruction. Enhanced CT with water used as oral contrast shows a sharply defined mass (arrows) within the lumen of the second duodenal part extending to the infrapapillary area. A biliary stent is also seen.

show an enlarged papilla of Vater with irregular borders, sometimes with spiculation and ulceration. Non-papillary carcinomas of the duodenum are adenocarcinomas and usually present clinically as duodenal obstruction. Barium examination shows the neoplasm as an ulcerative, polypoid or annular lesion. On CT, primary carcinomas are seen mostly as focal masses with asymmetric mural thickening with varying degrees of luminal narrowing (Fig. 4-9). Coincident adenopathy or hepatic metastases may be present. Other malignant primary neoplasms occasionally encountered in the duodenum include GISTs and lymphomas.

Secondary Involvement

The duodenum may be invaded by malignant neoplasms from adjacent organs or be the site of metastases. Carcinoma and lymphoma of the stomach can spread directly across the pylorus to involve the duodenum. This is reported to occur in up to 40% of lymphomas and 25% of adenocarcinomas of the gastric antrum.[1]

Carcinoma of the head of the pancreas frequently causes changes in the duodenal loop. There may be widening of the duodenal loop, a double contour, irregularity of the inner border and stricturing or distortion of the valvulae conniventes. Carcinoma of the tail of the pancreas may compress or invade the duodenum, resulting in mucosal destruction, which may ultimately result in bleeding or obstruction clinically.

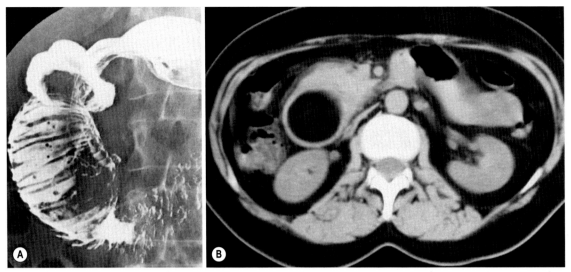

FIGURE 4-8 ■ **Lipoma.** (A) A large intraluminal filling defect is seen occupying and distending the second part of the duodenum on a barium examination. (B) CT shows the lesion to be a well-defined, round mass with low attenuation values, characteristic of fat.

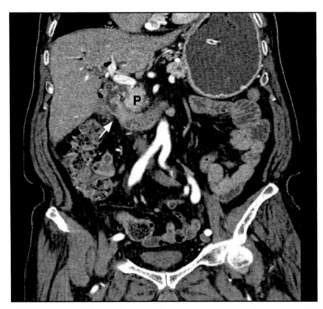

FIGURE 4-9 ■ **Primary duodenal adenocarcinoma.** Enhanced CT with water used as oral contrast agent shows asymmetric mural thickening and encroachment of the lumen at the second portion of the duodenum (arrow). Dilatation of the common bile duct is also seen. The head of the pancreas (P) appears normal.

OTHER CONDITIONS

Pancreatitis

Duodenal ileus may be seen on plain radiographs in acute pancreatitis. Mucosal oedema, enlargement of the duodenal loop and enlargement of the papilla of Vater are characteristic findings on barium studies.

Crohn's Disease

The duodenum is affected in about 4% of patients with Crohn's disease. The radiological appearances are similar

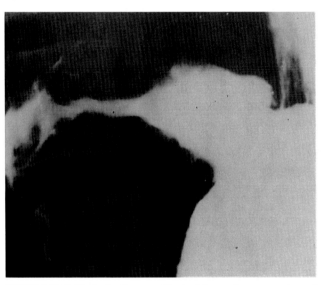

FIGURE 4-10 ■ **Crohn's disease.** Marked irregular narrowing of the antrum and first portion of the duodenum, giving the 'pseudo post-Billroth I' appearance.

to those in the more distal parts of the small intestine. The valvulae conniventes are frequently thickened. At a more advanced stage of the disease, there may be strictures with eccentric or concentric narrowing. Cobblestoning, asymmetry and skip lesions may be seen but fissure ulcers, sinuses and fistulae are uncommon in the duodenum. The disease may cause tubular narrowing of the antrum and proximal duodenum in continuity (Fig. 4-10), resulting in the 'pseudo post-Billroth I' appearance.

Tuberculosis

Tuberculosis of the duodenum is rare. Barium studies show narrowing of the lumen, sometimes with destruction of the mucosa and ulceration, mostly involving the descending duodenum. Tuberculous mesenteric lymphadenitis, in the absence of intrinsic duodenal tuberculosis, may produce extrinsic pressure on the duodenum and cause obstruction.

Progressive Systemic Sclerosis

In patients with neuromuscular disorders, particularly progressive systemic sclerosis and visceral myopathy, the duodenum is frequently involved. There may be dilatation, which is often more pronounced in the second, third and fourth parts. The dilated duodenum may be slow to empty and the grossly dilated, atonic organ may produce a sump effect.

Intramural Haematoma

The most common cause of intramural haematoma is blunt abdominal trauma. Intramural haematoma is usually seen on barium studies as a concentric obstructive lesion in the duodenum. Infiltration of blood and oedema may result in thickening of the valvulae conniventes. CT shows the extent of the haematoma, seen as a large mixed-attenuation mass, surrounding the duodenum (Fig. 4-11).

Traumatic Rupture

The most frequent site of rupture is at the junction of the second and third parts of the duodenum. CT is the primary imaging technique for assessment. Imaging findings include retroperitoneal air adjacent to the duodenum, extravasation of oral contrast in the retroperitoneum, oedema in the duodenal wall and stranding in the peripancreatic fat.[1]

Vascular Conditions

Abdominal aortic aneurysms may compress the third part of the duodenum and they occasionally cause obstruction. The duodenum, when faintly opacified with oral contrast medium and stretched around an aneurysm, may be misinterpreted as a contained leak or as a patch of

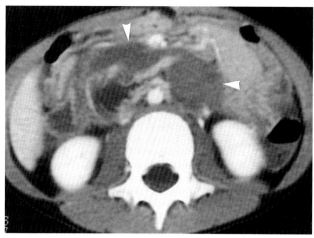

FIGURE 4-11 ■ **Intramural haematoma.** CT shows a mass of mixed attenuation, characteristic of haematoma, surrounding the third portion of the duodenum (arrowheads).

perianeurysmal inflammation. Aortoenteric fistulae most often involve the duodenum, particularly the third part of the duodenum. An aortoenteric fistula should always be suspected in patients who have undergone aortic graft surgery and present with gastrointestinal haemorrhage. The superior mesenteric artery compression syndrome is a rare form of high intestinal obstruction, which is believed to be caused by narrowing of the normal angle between the aorta and superior mesenteric artery. Strong to-and-fro peristalsis and duodenal dilatation may be seen during a symptomatic episode on barium meal examination. Superior mesenteric artery compression is seen as a sharp cut-off in the right anterior oblique position, with the compression and proximal dilatation persisting in the prone position. MDCT is useful to define the distance between aorta and superior mesenteric artery.

Duodenal varices are encountered occasionally in the duodenal cap and loop. They occur mainly in patients with extrahepatic portal hypertension, but may occur in portal hypertension without evidence of extrahepatic obstruction.

THE SMALL INTESTINE

ANATOMY AND NORMAL APPEARANCES

The small intestine measures approximately 5 m in length and extends from the duodenojejunal flexure to the ileocaecal valve. It is attached by its mesentery to the posterior abdominal wall and this allows it to be mobile. The proximal two-fifths constitute the jejunum and the distal three-fifths the ileum. The jejunum lies mainly in the left upper and lower quadrants and the ileum in the lower abdomen and the right iliac fossa. The jejunal and ileal branches of the superior mesenteric artery provide the blood supply.

Normally the small intestine is in a collapsed or partially collapsed state. Its calibre diminishes as it passes distally. During peristalsis the maximum diameter of the jejunal loops is 4 cm and of the ileal loops 3 cm. The valvulae conniventes have a circular configuration and are about 2 mm thick in the distended jejunum, becoming more spiral shaped and about 1 mm thick in the ileum. They may be absent in the distended terminal ileum, resulting in a rather featureless outline.

RADIOLOGICAL INVESTIGATION

Compared to the upper gastrointestinal tract and large bowel, the small intestine is much less amenable to examination with endoscopy, and as a result, radiological investigations play a pivotal role in the diagnosis of small intestinal disease. CT, MRI, barium and US examinations all have a role in the assessment and diagnosis of small intestinal pathology. In many circumstances each of the aforementioned modalities may be used in a complementary fashion. The choice of initial examination will depend on the clinical issue in question. Plain abdominal radiography often has a limited role. Angiography and nuclear medicine studies can be of value in selected cases.

Plain Radiographs

Patients who present acutely with suspected perforation or obstruction of the small intestine are investigated initially with plain abdominal radiographs.

Barium Studies

The barium follow-through is performed following a barium meal examination of the oesophagus, stomach and duodenum. The small bowel meal is a modification of the follow-through, which specifically focuses on the small intestine. Five hundred millilitres of a 30–40% weight/volume suspension of barium sulphate is given to the patient, who is encouraged to drink it as fast as possible. Cold water is used in the preparation of the suspension to stimulate gastric emptying and reduce transit time. Full-length prone radiographs are exposed at 10, 30 and 60 min. All segments of the small intestine are examined fluoroscopically and compression is applied.

Enteroclysis

Barium introduced directly into the small intestine gives excellent visualisation by challenging the distensibility of intestinal loops, thereby making it easier to identify the presence of morphological abnormalities. The technique the current authors use is similar to Sellink's method.[2] A 10 French (10Fr) radio-opaque Nolan tube (William Cook Europe A/S) is passed via the nasogastric route to the duodenum so that its tip lies at or just distal to the duodenojejunal flexure, or preferably 5–10 cm into the jejunum. A total of 800–1200 mL of barium suspension diluted to 20% weight/volume is infused, using a pump, at about 75 mL min^{-1}. Radiographs of the barium-filled jejunum and ileum are then taken (Fig. 4-12). Double-contrast methods have been employed successfully, including the air-contrast method and by using barium suspension followed by an aqueous suspension of methylcellulose. Detailed mucosal changes, particularly small ulcers, are well shown by the air-contrast method. However, as air does not distend the intestine as well as dilute barium, sinuses and fistulae are often not demonstrated and stenoses may be overlooked.

Computed Tomography

CT is becoming increasingly important in evaluating mural and extramural lesions and in assessing mesenteric involvement and ancillary intra-abdominal findings associated with inflammatory or neoplastic small intestinal diseases. Careful choice of CT imaging and

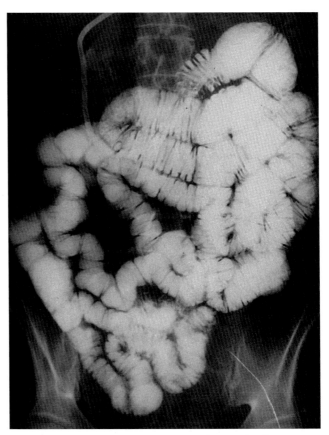

FIGURE 4-12 ■ Normal enteroclysis examination.

reconstruction technique is vital to the identification and characterisation of small intestinal abnormalities. Maximising the spatial and contrast resolution by acquiring isotropic multiplanar data sets with appropriate delivery of oral and intravenous contrast agents results in significantly improved diagnostic performance.

Intravenous contrast administration is essential for a comprehensive CT examination of the small intestine. Peak enhancement of the small intestinal mucosa, known as the enteric phase, occurs approximately 50 s after intravenous injection or 14 s after peak aortic enhancement.[3] Multiphase CT protocols, employing combinations of unenhanced, arterial, enteric and delayed phases, may be helpful in certain clinical situations such as the evaluation of intestinal bleeding.[4]

For routine CT imaging, opacification of the intestinal lumen is achieved using orally administered positive contrast material such as iodinated or dilute barium solutions, starting approximately 1 h prior to the examination. CT enterography involves the use of larger volumes of neutral Hounsfield unit (0–30 HU) oral contrast agents, ingested orally at a faster rate to distend the small intestine. Many neutral Hounsfield unit oral contrast agents have been described in the literature ranging from commercial products such as polyethylene glycol-based bowel preparation medications and VoLumen (Bracco Diagnostics, Princeton, NJ, USA), a low density (0.1%) barium sulphate solution to simpler solutions such as water or milk with or without the addition of bulking agents such as methylcellulose, locust bean gum and

Mucofalk (Dr F. Pharma, Freiburg, Germany), a plant husk extract. Neutral oral contrast agents are gaining widespread acceptance and are more frequently used when a detailed CT study of the small bowel wall or mesenteric vessels is required. Although the site and severity of mucosal disease and mural enhancement patterns of the small intestine are much better assessed with neutral or negative oral contrast agents,[5-7] positive enteric contrast agents remain valuable in patients with suspected perforation, abscess or extramural complications of Crohn's disease and some authors also maintain that positive enteric contrast agents may also increase the conspicuity of cystic and subtle soft-tissue disease of the mesentery and peritoneum.

Adequate distension of the small bowel improves the diagnostic accuracy of CT when neutral oral contrast agents are employed.[7] CT enterography typically results in greater distension than routine oral preparation techniques but studies comparing CT enterography with CT enteroclysis demonstrate that absolute bowel distension is better when enteroclysis is performed.[8-11] CT enteroclysis is performed by administering contrast medium directly into the small intestine through a nasojejunal tube (Fig. 4-13). Water or methylcellulose solution is typically used as a neutral luminal contrast agent but iodinated water-soluble contrast medium or a dilute barium solution can be used to provide positive luminal contrast. Although there are few comparative studies, diagnostic accuracy rates do not seem significantly different between CT enterography and CT enteroclysis, but a majority of studies report greater patient tolerance with CT enterography.[8-11]

Ultrasound

Ultrasound does not employ ionising radiation and therefore is particularly useful when imaging young patients with Crohn's disease who often require repetitive imaging procedures during the variable clinical course of this disease.[12] Ultrasound of the small intestine requires high-frequency (5–17 MHz) linear array probes, which provide increased spatial resolution of the intestinal wall.[13] Colour or power Doppler imaging and contrast-enhanced US (CEUS) provide more detailed

information on mural and extraintestinal vascularity, which may reflect inflammatory disease activity.[14] High-resolution ultrasonography is quick and non-invasive but diagnostic accuracy is dependent on operator experience. In clinical practice, US plays a rather limited role in the diagnosis and management of other small intestinal disorders but small intestinal obstruction can also be recognised and primary intestinal neoplasms may be identified using a dedicated US technique.

Magnetic Resonance Imaging

MR imaging (MRI) provides excellent soft-tissue contrast and three-dimensional imaging capabilities, which are of importance when studying the small intestine. Prerequisites for a state-of-the-art MRI examination of the small intestine include adequate bowel distension, homogeneous intraluminal contrast and dynamic multiphase intravenous contrast enhancement. Imaging sequences should have a high temporal resolution to reduce bowel motion artefacts and, if required, cine sequences to facilitate the dynamic assessment of intestinal motility. Good spatial resolution is fundamental and allows adequate depiction of the bowel wall and perienteric soft tissues. These prerequisites can be provided by a comprehensive MR enteroclysis (MRE) examination protocol, which includes small bowel intubation, administration of a biphasic contrast agent, heavily T2-weighted (T2W) single-shot turbo spin-echo (SSTSE) images for MR fluoroscopy and for monitoring the infusion process, T2W imaging employing half-Fourier acquisition single-shot turbo spin-echo (HASTE) and true FISP sequences (Fig. 4-14), and dynamic T1-weighted (T1W) imaging using a post-gadolinium FLASH sequence with fat suppression (Fig. 4-15). This protocol can provide anatomic demonstration of the

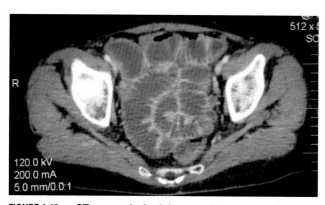

FIGURE 4-13 ■ **CT enteroclysis.** Adequate distension of the small bowel (SB) loops with clear delineation of the SB wall and valvulae conniventes.

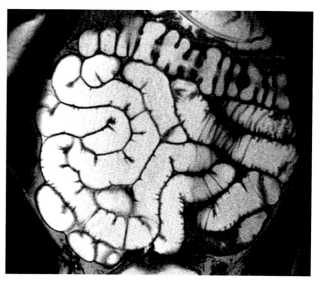

FIGURE 4-14 ■ **Coronal true FISP MR image demonstrating small bowel at its entire length.** The use of an iso-osmotic water solution as an intraluminal contrast agent results in homogeneous opacification of the bowel lumen. Note the increased conspicuity of the normal bowel wall due to the high-resolution capability and total absence of motion.

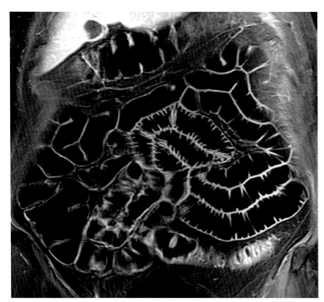

FIGURE 4-15 ■ **Two-dimensional FLASH coronal MR image with fat saturation, after IV administration of gadolinium and glucagon.** Normal small bowel wall and valvulae conniventes are demonstrated with excellent conspicuity.

acute active bleeding angiography is successful when the rate of blood loss exceeds 0.5 mL min^{-1}. Acute lower gastrointestinal bleeding is, however, frequently intermittent rather than continuous, resulting in a high rate of negative angiographic examinations. In the clinical context of acute active bleeding, it is important to avoid barium or other fluoroscopic studies using oral contrast agents before angiographic studies, as oral contrast will significantly impact the quality of the angiographic study.

Nuclear Medicine Studies

Nuclear medicine studies are useful alternative and adjunctive methods in the investigation of small bowel pathology. Leucocyte scintigraphy and FDG-PET are helpful in the diagnosis of suspected inflammatory bowel disease and/or the assessment of current disease activity. Older techniques, like pertechnetate scintigraphy for the detection of a Meckel's diverticulum, have yet to be surpassed by more modern imaging methods. Scintigraphy with labelled red cells remains a useful examination for localisation of intestinal bleeding. Carcinoid tumours of the small bowel may be elegantly demonstrated by scintigraphy and PET techniques are already proving useful in small bowel oncology.

Radionuclide Imaging of Meckel's Diverticulum

Radionuclide scintigraphy, using ^{99m}Tc-pertechnetate, is a well-established non-invasive technique for identifying a Meckel's diverticulum that contains gastric mucosa, as this agent is concentrated in the mucus-secreting cells and the parietal cells of the gastric mucosa in both the stomach and the diverticulum. The technique is more accurate in the paediatric age group than in adults.

normal intestinal wall, identification of wall thickening and neoplasms, lesion characterisation and/or evaluation of disease activity, assessment of the extent of exoenteric/mesenteric disease and information concerning intestinal motility.

Angiography

Selective visceral angiography of the small intestine can detect the site of obscure bleeding when extensive barium studies and endoscopy are negative. It is also used to determine the bleeding site in patients who present with massive acute bleeding from the small intestine. In

THE ABNORMAL SMALL INTESTINE

CROHN'S DISEASE

Crohn's disease (CD) is a chronic relapsing immune-mediated inflammatory disorder that results from a dysregulated immune response to luminal antigens including normal intestinal bacterial flora in genetically susceptible individuals.[15,16] A decrease in common intestinal infections in Westernised countries is accompanied by an increase in non-infectious inflammatory bowel diseases and the prevalence of CD in the USA has dramatically increased since the 1980s.[17] There is a bimodal distribution of patient age at disease onset, with a large peak at 20 years and smaller peak at 50 years.[18,19] CD often manifests with non-specific symptoms such as diarrhoea, weight loss and abdominal pain but specific clinical evidence of inflammatory bowel disease may be present in up to one-third of patients including signs of perianal fistulae, tags or fissures and aphthous ulceration.[20]

Abdominal pain and diarrhoea, often accompanied by weight loss, are the most frequent presenting symptoms.

Patients may present with an 'acute abdomen', indistinguishable from acute appendicitis. Other presenting symptoms are anaemia, retardation of growth, anorexia and weight loss. Acute intestinal obstruction due to stenosis is occasionally the presenting symptom, as are fistulae, particularly fistula in ano.

This chronic, progressive, transmural disease may affect any part of the gastrointestinal tract, but mostly involves the small intestine. The extent of involvement varies considerably but the terminal ileum is almost always affected. Approximately 15% of CD patients initially present with features of colitis alone and 35–45% of patients may develop perinanal complications over the course of their disease.[17,19] Less commonly, CD patients may present with isolated gastroduodenal and jejunal disease and this pattern is more common in CD patients who present within the paediatric age range.[21] In patients with previous right hemicolectomy for Crohn's disease, the site of anastomosis in the small bowel represents the most common site of recurrence.

Radiological Appearances

The most characteristic feature of Crohn's disease of the small intestine is the variety of its radiological appearances and the multiplicity of imaging features often seen in the majority of patients (Table 4-1).

Aphthoid ulcers, which are a characteristic feature, are usually visualised as small collections of barium with surrounding radiolucent margins due to oedema. Fissure ulcers are seen in profile, may penetrate deep into the thickened intestinal wall and may lead to abscess formation at their base and/or to the development of sinuses and fistulae. Fistulae pass to adjacent loops of ileum, the caecum, the sigmoid colon or the urinary bladder and occasionally to the skin or the vagina. Longitudinal ulcers (Fig. 4-16) running along the mesenteric border of the ileum are a characteristic but infrequent sign of the disease process. Cobblestoning (Fig. 4-17) is fairly common and is caused by a combination of longitudinal and transverse ulceration, separating intact portions of mucosa.

Narrowing of the intestinal lumen is frequent, as are strictures, which may be short, long, single or multiple, the latter being virtually diagnostic of Crohn's disease. Solitary strictures (Fig. 4-18) are a common finding; they may be accompanied by proximal dilation and, in the absence of additional evidence of Crohn's disease, have to be differentiated from other causes of stricture formation (Table 4-2). Discontinuous involvement of the intestinal wall is shown either as skip lesions or asymmetry. Asymmetrical involvement of the intestinal wall produces characteristic 'pseudodiverticula', which represent small patches of normal intestine in an otherwise severely involved segment. Inflammatory polyps (pseudopolyps) are seen in Crohn's disease as small, discrete round filling defects, but are not a frequent finding. A smooth, featureless outline replacing the normal mucosal pattern, without any significant changes in the calibre of the lumen, may occasionally be seen. Thickening of the wall of the diseased bowel is shown radiologically as displacement of the adjacent barium-filled loops. Mesenteric inflammation and fibrofatty proliferation of the peritoneal fat also contributes to displacement of the bowel loops. The

TABLE 4-1 Radiological Signs of Crohn's Disease

Ulceration
Discrete ulcers
Fissure ulcers
Longitudinal ulcers
Cobblestoning
Thickening of the valvulae conniventes
Stenosis
Dilatation proximal to stenosis
Asymmetrical involvement
Skip lesions
Inflammatory polyps (pseudopolyps)
Featureless outline
Thickened wall
Enlarged ileocaecal valve
Gross distortion
Adhesions

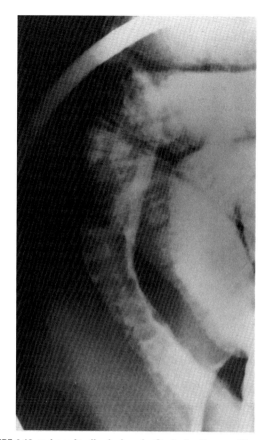

FIGURE 4-16 ■ **Longitudinal ulcer in Crohn's disease.** There is a long, longitudinal ulcer involving the mesenteric border of the terminal ileum.

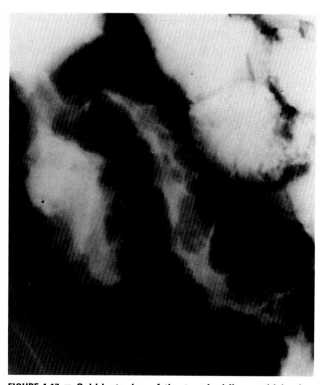

FIGURE 4-17 ■ **Cobblestoning of the terminal ileum, thickening of the wall of the terminal ileum, and an enlarged ileocaecal valve in Crohn's disease.**

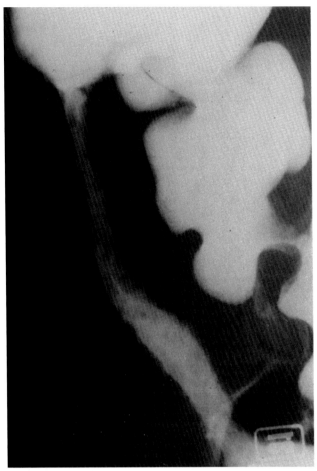

FIGURE 4-18 ■ **Long stricture in Crohn's disease.** A long segment of narrowing is seen in the ileum just proximal to the site of an ileocolic anastomosis in a patient who had undergone a previous resection for Crohn's disease.

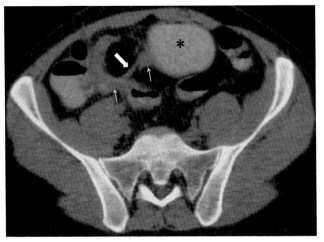

FIGURE 4-19 ■ **Crohn's disease.** Enteroenteric fistula (thick arrow) between two involved small bowel loops. Bowel wall thickening (thin arrows) and prestenotic dilatation is also seen (asterisk).

TABLE 4-2 Strictures of the Small Intestine

Crohn's disease
Tumours
Primary carcinoma
Carcinoid
Lymphoma (including malignant histiocytosis)
Invasion from other organs
Metastases
Tuberculosis
Actinomycosis
South American blastomycosis
Strongyloidiasis
Anisakiasis
Radiation damage
Ischaemia
Intramural haemorrhage
Diverticular mass
Appendix mass
Endometriosis
Eosinophilic gastroenteritis
Idiopathic ulcerative enteritis
Behçet's disease
Non-steroidal anti-inflammatory drugs

valvulae conniventes are blunted, flattened, thickened and distorted or straightened in approximately 50% of patients with Crohn's disease. These early changes are due to hyperplasia of the lymphoid tissue causing obstructive lymphoedema.

Cross-sectional imaging is increasingly important in the initial diagnosis and follow-up of patients with Crohn's disease, because of its ability to directly image the intestinal wall, assess for mucosal inflammation and also because it facilitates the accurate diagnosis of extramural disease such as sinuses, fistulae, phlegmon and abscess formation (Fig. 4-19). Identification of interloop, pelvic and abdominal wall abscesses is essential for appropriate patient management as their presence often contraindicates the use of advanced immunosuppressive medications such as the anti-TNF agent infliximab.

On CT, the thickened bowel wall may enhance homogeneously or may demonstrate a stratified 'target' appearance (Fig. 4-20). Mural stratification is often seen in active lesions after IV contrast administration. Multisegmental discontinuous small intestine disease, known as 'skip lesions', is highly suggestive of Crohn's disease,[22,23] particularly when the bowel wall thickening is asymmetric or ulceration is seen (Fig. 4-21). Perienteric changes that occur in mesentery and peritoneum include mesenteric hypervascularity, fat stranding and fibrofatty proliferation which is caused by an accumulation of mesenteric fat related to the chronic inflammatory process.[24]

MR enteroclysis (MRE) is a robust, but technically challenging, technique for the evaluation of small bowel in patients with Crohn's disease.[25] Characteristic lesions such as bowel wall thickening (Fig. 4-22), linear and fissure ulcers (Fig. 4-23) and cobblestoning are accurately depicted on T2-weighted MR sequences.[26] Fat-suppressed, T2-weighted sequences are required to identify submucosal oedema and T1-weighted post-contrast sequences are required to identify mucosal hyperenhancement. MRE is comparable with conventional enteroclysis in assessing the number and extent of

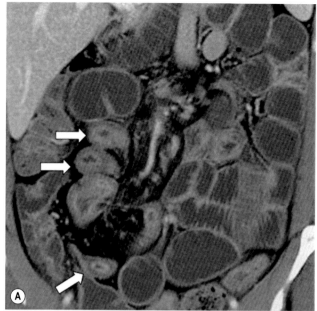

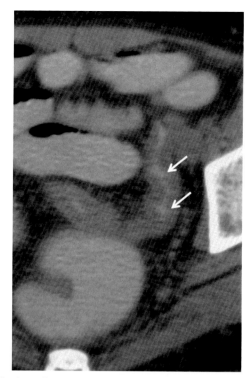

FIGURE 4-21 ■ **Crohn's disease.** Involved small bowel segment with intestinal wall thickening and ill-defined deep ulcers (arrows) on CT.

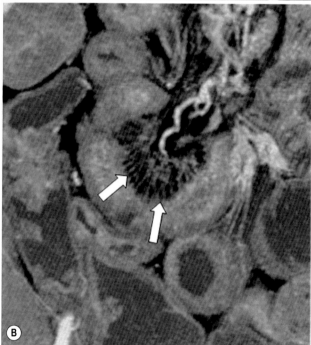

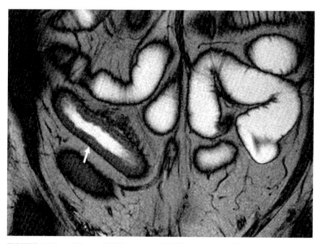

FIGURE 4-20 ■ **Crohn's disease.** (A) Coronal reconstruction image of CT enterography shows thickened distal ileal loops and mural stratification resulting in a 'target' appearance (arrows). Prestenotic dilatation is also seen. (B) A coronal, three-dimensional projection of the same patient showing the vascular engorgement (arrows) of an involved ileal loop (comb sign).

FIGURE 4-22 ■ **True FISP coronal MR image of a patient with Crohn's disease of the terminal ileum.** Moderate luminal narrowing and mural thickening is shown. Black boundary artefact (arrow) can be easily differentiated from the thickened bowel wall, exhibiting moderate signal intensity.

involved small bowel segments and in demonstrating luminal narrowing and/or prestenotic dilatation. MRE has a clear advantage over conventional enteroclysis in demonstrating extramural manifestations and/or complications of Crohn's disease, including abscesses. Sinuses and fistulous tracts manifest as high signal tracts on T2-weighted, fat-saturated MR images with avid enhancement following gadolinium-based contrast material administration.

Evaluation of all imaging studies in patients with Crohn's disease should always include a search for the extraintestinal manifestations of Crohn's disease, which include renal calculi, erosive sacroiliitis and for evidence of sclerosing cholangitis.[27] Complications of Crohn's disease related to the disease process include both gastrointestinal adenocarcinomas and carcinoid tumours[28] but the radiologist should also be aware of emerging reports of an increased risk of lymphoma in Crohn's

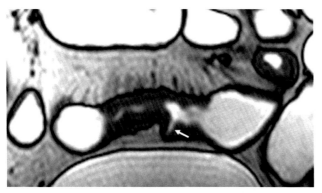

FIGURE 4-23 ■ **A 34-year-old male patient with active Crohn's disease (Crohn's Disease Activity Index (CDAI) = 244).** Coronal true FISP spot MR view demonstrates luminal narrowing and wall thickening in a segment of distal ileum. A fissure ulcer (arrow) penetrating the thickened wall and increased mesenteric vascularity are also disclosed. (With permission from Gourtsoyiannis, N. C., Papanikolaou, N., Karantanas, A. 2006. Magnetic resonance imaging evaluation of small intestinal Crohn's disease. Best Pract Res Clin Gastroenterol 20:137–156.)

patients receiving long-term immunosuppressive medications such as azathioprine or anti-TNF agents.[29–32]

COELIAC DISEASE

Coeliac disease is a gluten-related immune-mediated enteropathy in genetically susceptible individuals. The prevalence of coeliac disease has increased dramatically over the past 50 years largely due to improvements in serological analysis.[33] Patients usually present with clinical symptoms of malabsorption, such as diarrhoea, weight loss, steatorrhoea, malnutrition, anaemia and abdominal pain. Patients with coeliac disease are at greater risk of developing malignant neoplasms of the small intestine, including lymphoma and adenocarcinoma. Enteropathy associated T-cell lymphoma should be suspected when there is a history of abdominal pain or systemic B-symptoms such as weight loss, night sweats and fever.

The diagnosis of coeliac disease is established by demonstrating the abnormal villous pattern on specimens obtained at peroral jejunal biopsy. Radiological examination should be reserved for patients with normal jejunal biopsy, those with a suspected complication such as lymphoma, or those whose symptoms fail to respond to a gluten-free diet.

Radiological appearances on barium studies include dilatation of bowel loops, increased intestinal fluid, straightened and thickened valvulae conniventes in the jejunum and presence of numerous mucosal folds in the ileum (jejunisation). Transient non-obstructive intussusception may be also seen. CT is especially useful in clinically unsuspected adult patients, in whom it may demonstrate bowel dilatation and fluid excess, bowel wall thickening, a jejunoileal fold pattern reversal, transient small bowel intussusception, extraintestinal findings like benign mesenteric lymphadenopathy of low attenuation and complications of coeliac disease such as lymphoma.

Rarer complications in patients with coeliac disease include cavitary mesenteric lymph node syndrome, which results in enlarged, fluid-attenuation mesenteric lymph nodes with thin, peripherally enhancing rims[34] and ulcerative jejunoileitis. Ulcerative jejunoileitis results in diffuse mucosal ulceration predominantly in the jejunum. Appearance of ulcerative jejunoileitis on MDCT enteroclysis is best described by Boudiaf et al., who found, in an analysis of three cases, circumferential mural thickening with a bilaminar 'double halo' configuration resulting from a high-attenuation 'inner halo' of mucosal hyperenhancement and an 'outer halo' of mural thickening with soft-tissue attenuation.[35] Ulcerative jejunoileitis is reported to simulate Crohn's disease on imaging and also on capsule endoscopy examinations.[36]

MRI may be useful in coeliac disease, especially in paediatric patients in whom avoidance of exposure to ionising radiation is particularly important. Like CT, it can identify jejunisation of the ileum, jejunoileal fold pattern reversal, mural thickening due to submucosal oedema and varying degrees of inflammation, transient intussusception, benign mesenteric lymphadenopathy, small-volume ascites and vascular engorgement.

NEOPLASMS

Primary neoplasms of the small intestine account for only 3–6% of gastrointestinal neoplasms. The clinical presentation is often non-specific, making their detection particularly challenging. The reported mean time period between the onset of symptoms and diagnosis is approximately 3 years for benign tumours and almost 2 years for malignant neoplasms.[37] The radiological features of these tumours, as shown by enteroclysis and CT, correlate very well with the morphological changes seen in the gross pathology specimens.[38]

Specific subtypes of small intestinal neoplasms have a predilection for different regions along the small intestine.[39] Adenocarcinoma is usually proximal and it is the most common primary small intestinal malignancy of the duodenum and jejunum.[40] Carcinoid tumours are most commonly seen in the ileum and small intestinal lymphoma has a relatively homogeneous distribution along the small intestine but shows a minor predilection for the distal ileum.[41,42]

Malignant Neoplasms

The epidemiology of primary small intestine malignancies is changing. In 1987, the small intestinal malignancies were adenocarcinoma (45%), carcinoid (29%), lymphoma (16%) and sarcomas (10%).[39] By the year 2000, the incidence of carcinoid tumours had exceeded adenocarcinoma, rising to represent 44% of all small intestinal (SI) neoplasms in 2005. Carcinoid tumours are now the most common small intestinal malignant neoplasms in the USA.[43] Similar changes in the incidence of carcinoid tumours have been identified in epidemiological studies from Sweden and the United Kingdom but changes in the pathological classification of these tumours, as well as improvements in endoscopy and imaging techniques, appear to be at least partly responsible.[44,45] Despite the many improvements in imaging, which improve diagnostic capability, and improvements in the medical and surgical management of small intestinal neoplasms over the last 20 years, the reported 5-year survival remains unaltered for all histologic subtypes.[43] Careful and specific imaging technique is fundamental to the evaluation of small intestinal neoplasms. Accurate identification of early-stage tumours may allow for complete surgical resection, which is associated with much improved survival.

Carcinoid Tumour

Carcinoid tumours of the small intestine are regarded as low-grade malignant neoplasms. Almost 90% of them are located distally and they may be multiple in approximately one-third of cases. Carcinoid tumours arise within the basal portion of the mucosa and often extend into the submucosa, infiltrating the intestinal wall and serosa. Less frequently, intraluminal growth results in a polypoid lesion. Invasion of the muscular layers of the intestinal wall may lead to fibrosis of the surrounding submucosa, the mesentery and mesenteric vessels.

The primary tumour rarely produces symptoms, largely because of its small size and its deep mucosal location. Abdominal pain, diarrhoea or an abdominal mass may be encountered, but gastrointestinal haemorrhage is extremely rare.

The radiological features of carcinoid tumour on barium examinations are non-specific and reflect the stage of evolution of the pathological process at the time of examination. These features may be those of: (A) the primary lesion, appearing as solitary or multiple, round, smoothly outlined intraluminal filling defects (Fig. 4-24); (B) those of a secondary mesenteric mass, causing stretching, rigidity and fixation of ileal loops; (C) those due to interference with the ileal blood supply, resulting in thickening of valvulae conniventes and chronic ischaemic intestinal changes; or (D) those of fibrosis associated with tumour spread, presenting as sharp angulation of a loop or a stellate, spoke-like arrangement of adjacent loops.

Similar to barium examinations, the primary tumour may be difficult to identify on cross-sectional imaging. CT or MR may reveal a mucosal or submucosal nodule, which typically enhances avidly on arterial phase images. Carcinoid tumours are best recognised on the basis of secondary changes which occur in the mesentery. Carcinoid tumours produce serotonin and other vasoactive substances such as histamine, dopamine and kallikrein, which induce a strong desmoplastic reaction which results in local fat stranding and spiculated or stellate soft-tissue thickening on CT. There may be kinking of the adjacent bowel loops, sometimes resulting in intestinal obstruction, and there may be vascular encasement, resulting in segmental bowel wall thickening and oedema secondary to ischaemia. Since 30% of small bowel carcinoid tumours are multicentric, the entire bowel should be examined carefully for additional tumour locations (Fig. 4-25). CT enterography/enteroclysis may improve the detection rate of even small carcinoid deposits in the small bowel.

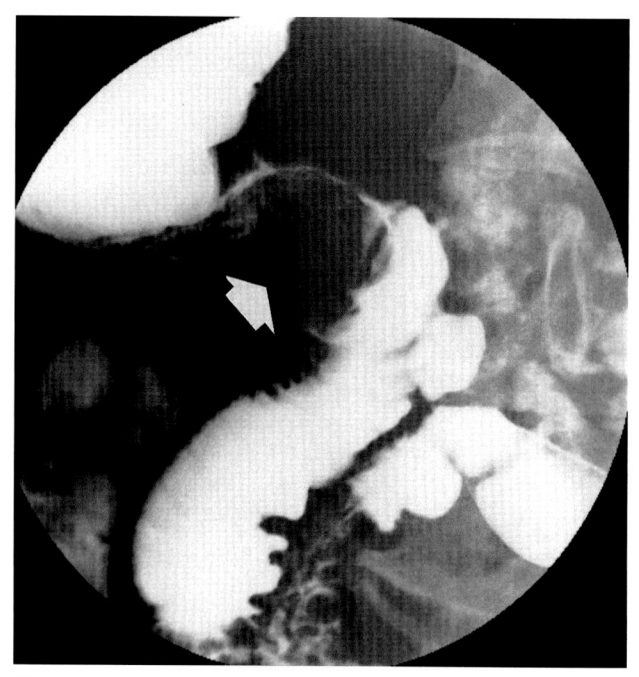

FIGURE 4-24 ■ **Carcinoid tumour.** A round, well-defined, intraluminal filling defect (arrow) is seen in the distal ileum of a patient who presented with symptoms of intermittent obstruction but without any manifestations of the carcinoid syndrome.

Hepatic metastases are seen slightly more frequently with carcinoid tumours than other primary SI neoplasms[40] and may result in 'carcinoid syndrome', which is characterised by flushing, diarrhoea, palpitations and wheezing. Dystrophic calcification in metastatic nodes, liver metastases or in the mesenteric mass may be encountered in up to 70% of cases.[46]

Adenocarcinoma

Primary adenocarcinoma of the small intestine is a chemoresistant tumour with an aggressive clinical nature.[47] It is usually a solitary lesion mostly located in the proximal small intestine; they are classically short and often present symptomatically with signs of partial or complete small bowel obstruction due to their predominantly radial growth pattern. Its appearance on enteroclysis includes an annular constricting lesion, a filling defect, a polypoid and/or ulcerated mass, or a combination of the above. Infiltrative adenocarcinoma, featuring as circumferential narrowing with mucosal destruction and shouldering of the margins (Fig. 4-26), is the most common type. On cross-sectional imaging, adenocarcinoma typically appears as a focal region of wall thickening, not exceeding 1.5 cm, compromising the lumen either concentrically or asymmetrically. The tumour mass is usually irregular and shows mild to moderate contrast enhancement. Infiltration of the mesentery is seen with advanced disease and associated lymphadenopathy is found in almost 50% of patients. An increased risk of small intestinal adenocarcinoma is seen in coeliac disease, Crohn's disease and in a number of familial cancer syndromes including Peutz–Jehgers syndrome and familial adenomatous polyposis (FAP). Importantly, hereditary non-polyposis colon

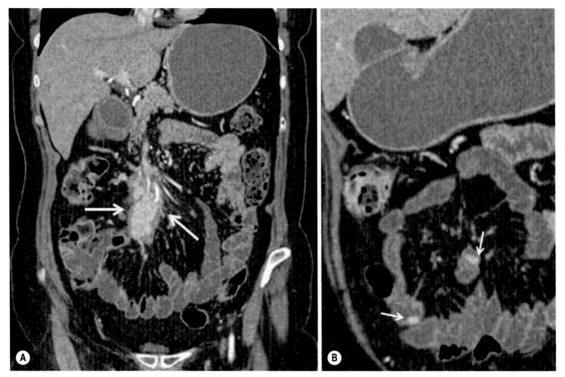

FIGURE 4-25 ■ **Multicentric carcinoid tumour.** (A) Coronal reformatted CT enterographic image shows a hypervascular mesenteric carcinoid tumour (arrows) encasing mesenteric vessels. (B) Enhancing mural nodules in ileum (small arrows) represent two additional tumour deposits.

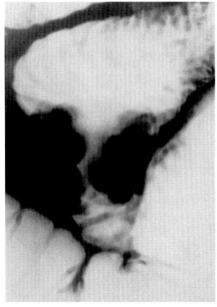

FIGURE 4-26 ■ **Carcinoma.** A spot compression view of a segment of jejunum shows a tight constricting lesion with mucosal destruction and shouldered margins.

cancer (HNPCC) is thought to be responsible for 5–10% of all small intestine adenocarcinomas.[48]

Lymphoma

Lymphoma represents 20% of primary small intestinal malignancies. The clinical presentation depends on whether bowel involvement is primary or secondary, and on the features of any associated disorders, such as adult coeliac disease, immunoproliferative disease or immunodeficiency syndromes. The distal or terminal ileum is most commonly involved. Mediterranean-type lymphoma, complicating immunoproliferative small intestinal (alpha-chain) disease, is an exception, as it affects the duodenum and proximal jejunum. The diagnosis of primary small intestinal lymphoma requires that there is no peripheral or mediastinal lymphadenopathy, no evidence of hepatic or splenic involvement, a normal white blood cell differential and tumour involvement must be predominantly in the GI tract.[49] Secondary GI involvement is comparatively frequent, occurring in approximately 10% of patients with limited-stage non-Hodgkin's lymphoma (NHL) at the time of diagnosis, and up to 60% of those dying from advanced NHL.[50]

Characteristic radiological signs include luminal narrowing with mucosal destruction, occasional shouldering of the margins and stricture formation, broad-based ulceration, cavitation (Fig. 4-27), thickening of the valvulae conniventes, discrete intraluminal filling defects and an extraluminal mass. Small nodules or polyps may be seen throughout the small intestine. Focal 'aneurysmal' dilatation, caused by extensive lymphomatous invasion of the muscle layers and neural plexuses, is characteristic but only occasionally seen. Ileoileal fistula formation may result from a cavitating mass invading adjacent ileal loops.

Small intestinal lymphomas usually have a more homogeneous attenuation on CT and typically show less contrast enhancement than other SI neoplasms[35]

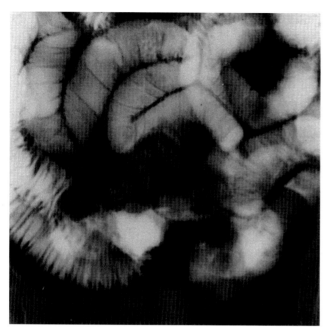

FIGURE 4-27 ■ **Lymphoma.** A large mass is seen infiltrating and compressing the pelvic loops of ileum. There is also a large cavitating ulcer that has eroded a number of loops of intestine, producing an ileoileal fistula. The patient presented with abdominal pain, weight loss, anaemia and a palpable mass.

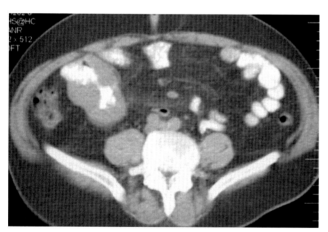

FIGURE 4-28 ■ **Lymphoma shown by CT.** Involved ileal loop exhibiting extensive mural thickening, luminal narrowing and ulcerations seen as broad-based extraluminal contrast medium projections to the thickened bowel wall.

(Fig. 4-28). Mesenteric adenopathy, when present, is typically bulky, sometime progressing to a characteristic 'sandwich-like' mass of confluent mesenteric lymphomatous tissue encasing the mesenteric vasculature and bowel loops.

Gastrointestinal Stromal Tumours

Gastrointestinal stromal tumours are rare mesenchymal neoplasms which arise from the interstitial cells of Cajal in the subepithelial bowel wall. GISTs represent less than 10% of all primary SI neoplasms.[51] and may arise in any segment of the alimentary tract but also may occasionally arise from peritoneal structures such as the omentum or small intestinal mesentery. GISTs exhibit a wide spectrum

of clinical behaviour from benign, small, incidentally depicted nodules to frank malignant lesions. The pathologically defining feature of GISTs is their expression of KIT (CD 117), a tyrosine kinase growth factor receptor. Immunoreactivity for KIT distinguishes GISTs from other mesenchymal tumours, like leiomyomas, leiomyosarcomas, schwannomas and neurofibromas and determines the appropriateness of KIT inhibitor therapy.[52] GISTs display highly variable clinical behaviour and typically grow in an exoenteric direction, sometimes extending to the mucosal surface, resulting in focal ulceration. Exoenteric GISTs are typically larger than other SI neoplasms at the time of diagnosis, sometimes growing to more than 30 cm,[40] and they often demonstrate internal degenerative changes, such as necrosis, haemorrhage, calcification, fistula or secondary infection.

The characteristic finding on barium examinations is a large, inhomogeneous extrinsic mass, displacing or distorting adjacent loops of intestine. There may be associated mucosal ulceration, cavitation or fistula formation. CT or MR usually demonstrate a classically smooth, lobulated mass but this appearance does not exclude malignant change. Large GISTs that display signs of direct extension into adjacent organs and vessels are more likely to metastasise[53] to the liver or peritoneum.

Secondary Neoplasms

In day-to-day practice the radiologist will more frequently encounter secondary rather than primary SI neoplasms; transcoelomic spread is typical of ovarian, gastric or colonic primaries,[54] whereas hematogenous spread is more commonly recognised from primary lesions such as melanoma, lung, breast, cervix and squamous carcinomas of the head and neck.[55] Lymphatic spread plays a minor role in the spread of neoplasms to the small intestine; spread of caecal carcinoma to the terminal ileum is a classic example.

Transcoelomic spread usually results in segmental rather than focal small intestinal changes. Tethering of the mucosal folds may be a conspicuous feature on barium examinations. Intraperitoneal seeding of abdominal neoplasms frequently localises in the right lower quadrant at the distal mesentery (Fig. 4-29). Stasis in the lower recess of the small intestinal mesentery results in the deposition and growth of secondary deposits. As a result the ileal loops in the right lower quadrant become separated with angled tethering of the mucosal folds, and the narrowed loops may align in a parallel configuration described as 'palisading'.

Haematogenous metastases to the small intestine may result in small, focal, nodular or more diffusely infiltrating obstructive lesions. Metastatic melanomas often appear as multiple submucosal polypoid lesions with central ulceration or cavitation, giving a 'bull's eye' or 'target' appearance, on barium studies.

Benign Neoplasms

Benign small intestinal neoplasms account for approximately 0.5–2% of all gastrointestinal tract neoplasms.

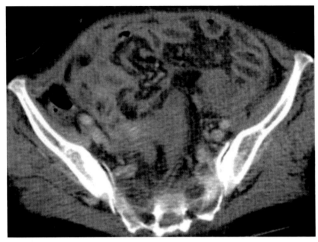

FIGURE 4-29 ■ Peritoneal carcinomatosis involving the small bowel wall. CT enteroclysis demonstrates irregular thickening of the small bowel wall—more pronounced at the right lower abdomen—confluent and adhered intestinal loops and lumen narrowing or lack of distensibility due to numerous, small, malignant peritoneal implants from ovarian carcinoma, 'covering' the surface of the small bowel wall. Mesenteric infiltration is also present.

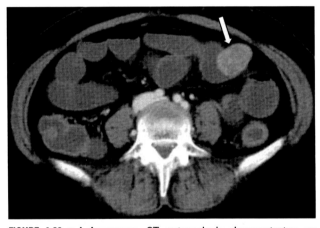

FIGURE 4-30 ■ Leiomyoma. CT enteroclysis demonstrates an oval clearly defined and homogeneously enhancing mass with intra- and extraluminal extension (arrow).

There are more than 12 histopathological types, amongst which adenoma and leiomyoma are the most common and the only two with definite malignant predisposition. Lipomas, vascular and neurogenic tumours, hamartomas and heterotopias are less frequently encountered.

Leiomyoma is the most common symptomatic benign neoplasm. Patients usually present with acute bleeding. In cases of intraluminal tumours a broad-based, smooth, round or semilunar filling defect is usually seen, whereas with extraluminal masses there is displacement and distortion of neighbouring bowel loops. Bidirectional or dumb-bell tumours combine features of both (Fig. 4-30). Tenting deformity of the intestinal wall, ulceration and signs of intussusception may also be encountered.

Ancillary CT findings include a round or semilunar, homogeneous soft-tissue mass associated with the intestinal wall, showing marked homogeneous or rim contrast enhancement and absence of mesenteric changes or metastasis. A peripheral crescent-shaped necrosis of the mass, shown on contrast-enhanced CT, US or MRI is additionally suggestive of the diagnosis. On angiography, leiomyoma appears as a well-defined, round or lobulated hypervascular mass.

Adenomatous polyps and **villous adenomas** are two terms widely used to designate the growth pattern and gross morphology of adenomas. Adenomatous polyps are often symptomless. On barium studies they appear as small, smooth, round or oval intraluminal filling defects, and are often solitary and sessile. When multiple, they usually affect a single segment, are of different sizes and may be pedunculated. Villous adenomas are usually >3 cm in size, are invariably broad based and present radiographically as lobulated cauliflower-like filling defects, exhibiting multiple radiolucent striations, interspersed with frond-like projections.

Hamartomatous polyps are a developmental anomaly and may be present in large numbers in the small intestine of patients with the Peutz–Jeghers syndrome. Recurrent abdominal pain caused by intussusception is the most common clinical presentation. The polyps are shown on barium studies as multiple round or lobulated filling defects and are often pedunculated; intussusception is frequently demonstrated (Fig. 4-31) but this may also be seen with adenomatous polyps (Fig. 4-32).

Lipoma is the third most common benign neoplasm. On barium studies, lipomas appear as sharply marginated, solitary, sessile, intraluminal filling defects, averaging 3–4 cm in size. They are easily deformed by peristalsis or compression during fluoroscopy. On CT, they feature as smooth ovoid masses, exhibiting attenuation values of fat.

INFECTIONS AND INFESTATIONS

Imaging is not routinely indicated in cases of acute infectious enteritis. A history of acute rather than chronic diarrhoea is typical and stool culture remains the best diagnostic approach. Nevertheless, the imaging manifestations of infectious enteritis may be encountered by the radiologist when other pathologies such as acute appendicitis or Crohn's disease are clinically suspected and imaging is requested. Infectious enteritis may result from a wide range of viral, bacterial, parasitic or antibiotic-associated pathogens.

Mesenteric Adenitis

Infectious enteritis as well as bacterial or viral pharyngitis may precipitate a syndrome known as mesenteric adenitis. Mesenteric adenitis is a common cause of right lower quadrant pain in children and has been found in one study to be the final diagnosis in approximately 16% of patients presenting with symptoms of acute appendicitis.[56] Mesenteric lymph nodes measuring greater than 5 mm in their shortest axis are present in almost two-thirds of asymptomatic children; therefore judicious clinical correlation and a short-axis size threshold of 10 mm

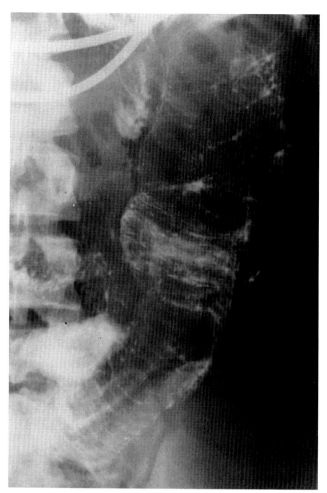

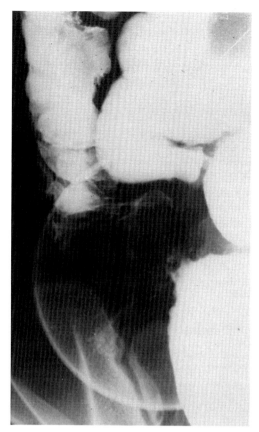

FIGURE 4-33 ■ **Tuberculosis.** A short, irregular stricture, about 4 cm long, is shown to involve the terminal ileum and ileocaecal valve. The narrowing caused considerable delay in the passage of barium, and dilatation of the ileum proximal to the stricture can be seen. The patient presented with intestinal obstruction.

FIGURE 4-31 ■ **Peutz–Jeghers syndrome.** Jejunal intussusception is seen resulting from the presence of multiple hamartomatous polyps in a patient with Peutz–Jeghers syndrome.

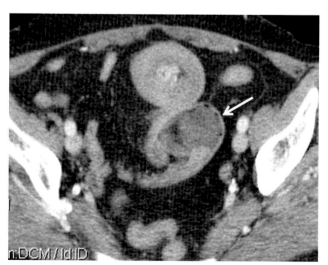

FIGURE 4-32 ■ **Polyp associated with jejunoileal intussusception.** Contrast-enhanced CT demonstrates invaginated mesenteric fat and vessels, as well as bowel wall thickening of the intussusceptum and intussuscipiens. A round hypodense soft-tissue mass corresponding to the polyp is seen (arrow) and serves as the 'lead point'.

is recommended in the literature.[57] Cross-sectional imaging reveals mesenteric lymph nodes measuring greater than 10 mm in short axis, which may occasionally be accompanied by thickening of the ileal wall.[58]

Tuberculosis

Intestinal tuberculosis is rare in Europe. Patients usually present with abdominal pain, fever, weight loss, diarrhoea, intestinal obstruction and, rarely, with bowel perforation. Lesions are often multiple and usually involve more than one site. The ileum is most commonly affected, particularly the terminal ileum and the ileocaecal junction (Fig. 4-33). Discrete ulcers, usually transverse and circumferential, mucosal fold thickening and stricture formation are the main radiological features.

In ileocaecal tuberculosis, the terminal ileum is narrowed and thickened, the ileocaecal valve becomes rigid, irregular, gaping and incompetent and the caecum is usually involved, classically resulting in a conical shape to the caecum on barium examination.[59] CT shows bowel wall thickening with homogeneous attenuation and lack of mural stratification. Occasionally there may be stenotic and transmural fistulating disease which can be almost indistinguishable from Crohn's disease. The presence of enlarged, low-attenuation, mesenteric nodes with enhancing peripheral rings and imaging signs of tuberculous peritonitis, such as diffuse omental and mesenteric infiltration, nodules, peritoneal thickening and ascites, are important clues in differentiating between abdominal tuberculosis and CD.[60]

Yersiniosis

The term yersiniosis refers to infections caused by the Gram-negative bacilli *Yersinia enterocolitica* and *Yersinia pseudotuberculosis*. Acute inflammation of the terminal ileum occurs and the clinical presentation is often indistinguishable from acute appendicitis, with right iliac fossa pain and tenderness, fever, diarrhoea and, occasionally, vomiting. The radiological changes of yersiniosis are limited to the distal 20 cm of ileum. The mucosal folds are tortuous, increased in number and thickened with the typical small, discrete nodular filling defects of lymphoid hyperplasia. Some thickening of the wall of the terminal ileum may be present.

Actinomycosis

Abdominal actinomycosis is a rare condition caused by *Actinomyces israelii*, a common saprophyte in the mouth, throat and gastrointestinal tract. Predisposing factors include overt gastrointestinal perforation, previous surgery, neoplasms, diabetes mellitus, steroid therapy and poor dental hygiene. The appendix is the site most commonly affected in the abdominal cavity and the clinical presentation often suggests an appendiceal abscess. Barium studies and/or CT may show a mass causing ileocaecal compression. Sinus tracts and enteroenteric, enterocolic, enterocutaneous and enterovesical fistulae may also be demonstrated.

CHRONIC RADIATION ENTERITIS

Radiation enteritis is a form of intestinal ischaemia resulting from damage to vascular endothelial cells that leads to endarteritis obliterans. High radiation doses or radiation treatment over a short time or large treatment volumes result in a higher incidence of chronic radiation enteritis. The distal ileum, particularly the pelvic loops, is the most frequent site of intestinal damage. The time interval between the radiation therapy and the development of symptoms varies considerably and may be as long as 25 years. The typical clinical presentation of patients with chronic radiation enteritis is colicky abdominal pain, diarrhoea, malabsorption and intermittent small intestinal obstruction.

Radiological features include thickening of the valvulae conniventes, mural thickening, effacement of the mucosal pattern, ulceration and fixation and angulation of small intestinal loops. 'Mucosal tacking', seen as spiking and distortion of the mucosal folds on the antimesenteric border of the intestine caused by adhesions to the inflamed and thickened mesentery, is rather characteristic. Luminal narrowing and stenosis, single or multiple, are frequent findings (Fig. 4-34), sometimes leading to obstruction. Sinuses and fistulae are

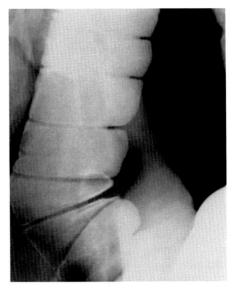

FIGURE 4-34 ■ **Radiation stricture.** This spot view of a barium infusion examination shows a short, tight stricture of the terminal ileum in a patient who 4 years earlier had undergone radiotherapy for carcinoma of the uterus.

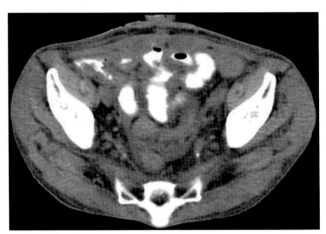

FIGURE 4-35 ■ **Radiation enteritis.** CT shows mural thickening, fixation and angulation of intestinal loops and segmental lumen narrowing.

uncommon findings. Mural thickening is best assessed on CT. It is demonstrated as a target configuration representing a combination of submucosal oedema and mucosal hyperenhancement secondary to acute inflammation. Homogeneous mural thickening is more characteristic of the chronic, healing fibrotic phase (Fig. 4-35).

MECHANICAL SMALL INTESTINAL OBSTRUCTION

The most common causes of small intestinal obstruction are adhesions, external or internal hernias, primary or secondary neoplasms and Crohn's disease.

Abdominal CT has contributed greatly to the management of patients with acute small intestinal obstruction by accurately demonstrating the level and sometimes the

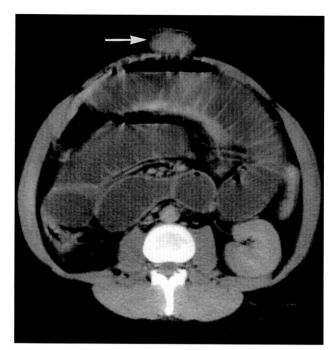

FIGURE 4-36 ■ **CT—small intestinal obstruction.** A section through the mid-abdomen shows dilated, mainly fluid-filled, small intestinal loops. The stretched valvulae conniventes can clearly be identified in some segments. The obstruction was due to an incarcerated paraumbilical hernia, the edge of which can be identified (arrow).

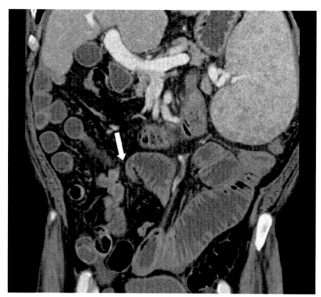

FIGURE 4-37 ■ **Small bowel obstruction secondary to an adhesive band.** Enhanced CT, coronal reformation image of a patient with splenic lymphoma shows the transition zone (arrow) between the dilated, fluid-filled jejunal loops proximal to the site of obstruction and the collapsed loops distally. No mass or mural thickening is seen at the transition zone. Note the micronodular lymphomatous splenic involvement.

cause of obstruction and also by demonstrating important signs of threatened bowel viability. CT's ability to exclude other causes of an acute abdomen makes it particularly valuable in the acute clinical setting. It is especially beneficial in high-grade obstruction and in patients with a history of a previous abdominal malignancy, hernias (Fig. 4-36), inflammatory bowel disease, a palpable abdominal mass or sepsis. The identification of a definite point of obstruction, the 'transition zone', with dilated small bowel loops proximal to the site of obstruction and collapsed loops distally, is the most reliable CT criterion for diagnosing small bowel obstruction (Figs. 4-37 and 4-38). Small bowel 'faeces sign' may be a useful CT sign that facilitates identification of the 'transition zone'. It is defined as the presence of faeces-like material mixed with gas bubbles within dilated small bowel loops proximal to the site of obstruction resulting from stasis and water absorption (Fig. 4-39). The differentiation of simple obstruction from closed-loop and strangulated obstruction is a crucial issue. Characteristic CT appearances in closed-loop obstruction include U- or C-shaped configuration of dilated loops and a fixed radial distribution of several dilated loops with prominent stretched mesenteric vessels converging towards the point of torsion. CT findings suggestive of strangulation include wall thickening with increased attenuation, poor or no contrast enhancement of the bowel wall, engorgement of mesenteric vasculature, mesenteric haziness and intestinal pneumatosis. Detection of ischaemic changes in the bowel wall and/or attached mesentery implies strangulation, necessitating emergency laparotomy. MRI is an alternative to CT in

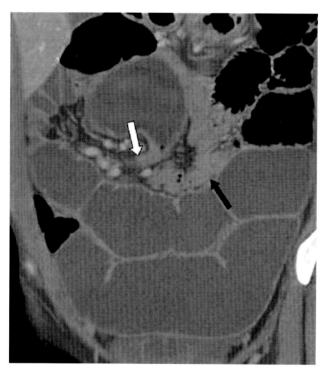

FIGURE 4-38 ■ **Adhesive small bowel obstruction.** Enhanced CT, coronal reformation image shows the transition zone (white arrow), distended, fluid-filled proximal jejunal loops and collapsed distal loops (black arrow). No mass is seen.

the diagnosis of intestinal obstruction in cases where radiation to the patient is to be avoided (Fig. 4-40).

CT enterography and CT enteroclysis can combine the advantages of volume challenge in detecting and grading partial obstruction with the ability of CT to

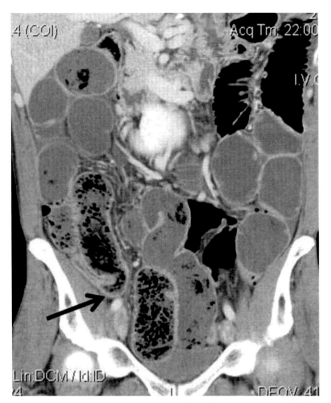

FIGURE 4-39 ■ **Small bowel obstruction.** Contrast-enhanced CT, coronal reformation image demonstrates the small bowel 'faeces sign' proximal to the transition zone (arrow).

demonstrate the cause and any pertinent extraintestinal manifestations, including vascular impairment.

ACUTE MESENTERIC ISCHAEMIA

Acute mesenteric ischaemia can be the result of arterial embolism or thrombosis, venous occlusion or low-flow states. Patients usually present with severe abdominal pain. The early diagnosis of bowel ischaemia is difficult both clinically and radiologically. MDCT has greatly improved the diagnosis of acute mesenteric ischaemia but careful attention to CT technique is required. The use of water as oral contrast medium allows better assessment of the bowel wall. A rapidly administered IV bolus of contrast medium and dual-phase imaging are required for accurate mesenteric vessel evaluation. With regard to diagnostic accuracy, a meta-analysis conducted in 2010 found that MDCT has a high sensitivity and specificity (93 and 96%, respectively) for the detection of acute mesenteric ischaemia.[61]

The imaging manifestations of SI ischaemia are protean and vary according to the nature and severity of vascular insufficiency.[62] Acute transmural SI infarction typically results in mural thinning and small intestinal dilatation with reduced or absent mural enhancement.[62] In contrast, non-occlusive mesenteric ischaemia typically results in mural thickening and mucosal hyperenhancement and ischaemia related to mesenteric venous thrombosis results in marked mural thickening, mucosal

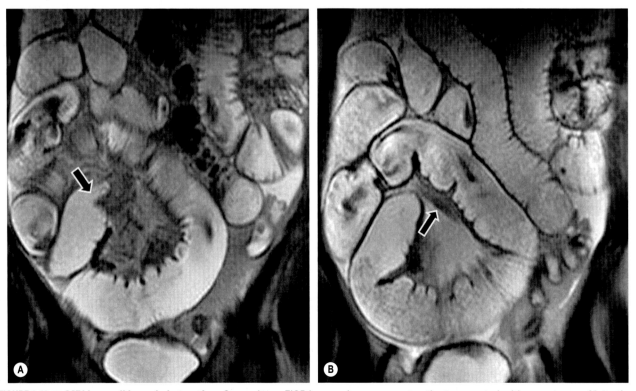

FIGURE 4-40 ■ **MRI in small bowel obstruction.** Coronal true FISP images in a pregnant patient presented with symptoms of intestinal obstruction. (A) Dilatation of small bowel loops and identification of the 'transition zone' (arrow). (B) Demonstration of an adhesion (arrow) responsible for the intestinal obstruction.

hyperenhancement, mesenteric stranding and vascular engorgement.[62] Ascites is present in approximately two-thirds of patients with acute intestinal ischaemia but is a more prominent feature in cases of mesenteric venous thrombosis.[62]

The presence of solid visceral infarcts should also prompt suspicion for a cardioembolic cause of intestinal ischaemia. Knowledge of the patient's cardiac rhythm is important, as there is a wide spectrum of CT findings in mesenteric ischaemia related to atrial fibrillation. These signs are dependent on the size and location of the embolus but include segmental bowel dilatation, wall thickening, altered mural enhancement, mesenteric stranding and ascites.[63]

The presence of pneumatosis intestinalis and superior mesenteric/portal venous gas were once considered ominous signs in cases of acute intestinal ischaemia; however, a wide range of non-ischaemic causes are now known, including infection, inflammation, neoplastic and even respiratory causes such as asthma.[62,64]

VASCULITIS

Systemic vasculitis should be suspected when there are imaging signs of intestinal ischaemia involving young patients or atypical sites such as the stomach, duodenum or rectum.[62] Vasculitis should also be suspected when there is recurrent involvement in different small bowel segments with or without improvement and also when there are solid visceral infarcts.[65] The mesenteric and renal vessels should be scrutinised for aneurysms which are most commonly seen in polyarteritis nodosa but may also be found in systemic lupus erythematosus, Wegener's granulomatosis, rheumatoid vasculitis and Churg–Strauss syndrome. Systemic lupus erythematosus may result in serositis causing ascites, lymphadenopathy and more diffuse bowel wall thickening.

OCCULT GASTROINTESTINAL BLEEDING

Multidetector CT angiography has an undisputed role in the diagnosis of acute gastrointestinal bleeding and, importantly, also successfully guides interventional management by facilitating selective catheterisation and embolisation of bleeding vessels.[66,67] Emerging evidence now also defines a role for CT in the evaluation of occult or low-grade gastrointestinal bleeding. Multiphasic concontrast-enhanced CT protocols with neutral 'enterographic contrast' appear more sensitive and may reveal focal masses, angiodysplasia or may reveal discrete foci of enhancement which persist on the delayed phases consistent with active extravasation. One recent but small study comparing multiphasic contrast-enhanced CT enterography with wireless capsule endoscopy found significantly greater sensitivity with CT enterography than capsule endoscopy (88 vs 38%) in identifying a source of occult gastrointestinal bleeding.[4] The primary benefit of CT enterography over capsule endoscopy in this study was its superior ability in identifying focal small intestinal tumours but in clinical practice CT enterography and capsule endoscopy are complementary, particularly in the investigation of benign causes of blood loss such as angiodysplasia and mucosal inflammation.

DIVERTICULA AND BLIND LOOPS

Jejunal Diverticula

Jejunal diverticula are uncommon. They result from mucosal herniation along the mesenteric border. Symptomatic patients present with abdominal pain, distension, weight loss and megaloblastic anemia—the 'blind loop' syndrome. Symptoms develop as a result of bacterial overgrowth and can be effectively treated with antibiotics and replacement therapy. Less common complications include acute diverticulitis with or without perforation or mesenteric abscesses, bleeding and small bowel obstruction.

On barium examination jejunal diverticula are usually multiple and are seen as fairly large outpouchings with a relatively narrow neck. In cases with jejunal diverticulitis, CT can assess the extent of the inflammatory process and suggest the correct diagnosis.

Meckel's Diverticulum

Meckel's diverticulum results from failure of the yolk sac to close during fetal life and is present in 0.5–3% of the population. It is located on the antimesenteric border of the ileum, 30–90 cm from the ileocaecal valve, and ranges in size from 0.5 to 13 cm. It is estimated that approximately 20–40% of Meckel's diverticula cause symptoms. Complications associated with the abnormality include ulceration, bleeding, perforation, inflammation, intussusception, internal hernia, volvulus and adhesions. Ectopic gastric mucosa is present in the diverticulum in 20% of adults and 95% of children who present with bleeding.

The preoperative diagnosis of Meckel's diverticulum may be difficult. Radionuclide imaging with ^{99m}technetium pertechnetate (^{99m}Tc-pertechnetate) is more accurate in the paediatric age group than in adults. On enteroclysis, it is seen as a blind-ending sac arising from the antimesenteric border of the ileum (Fig. 4-41). A triradiate pattern of mucosal folds or a triangular plateau is sometimes present at the base of the diverticulum. The diverticulum may become inverted and give the appearance of a polypoid filling defect, often presenting with intussusception.

The demonstration of a persistent vitelline artery is a hallmark for the angiographic diagnosis of Meckel's diverticulum in patients who present with chronic gastrointestinal bleeding.

Blind Loops

Other causes of 'blind loop' syndrome include strictures of the small intestine and surgically produced blind loops. Blind pouches are a complication of side-to-side intestinal anastomosis. A blind pouch is invariably a short length of proximal bowel that lies beyond the stoma. It can become quite large, and patients may develop abdominal

pain, distension, steatorrhoea, weight loss and megaloblastic anaemia.

Ileal Diverticula

Acquired diverticula of the ileum are rare. They are
usually small, few in number and are located on the
mesenteric border of the terminal ileum. Complications
are extremely rare but perforation, diverticulitis, fistula
formation and bleeding have been reported.

NEUROMUSCULAR DISORDERS

Progressive systemic sclerosis, visceral myopathies and
visceral neuropathies can produce diffuse disorders of

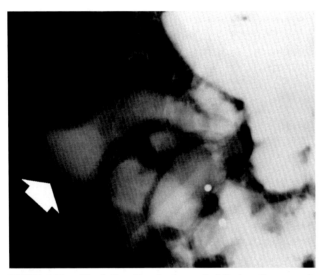

FIGURE 4-41 ■ Meckel's diverticulum. A blind-ending sac is
shown arising from the antimesenteric border of the distal
ileum (arrow).

gastrointestinal motility and patients may present with
recurring symptoms and signs of intestinal obstruction in
the absence of true mechanical obstruction.

In progressive systemic sclerosis barium examination
shows dilatation of the duodenum and jejunum, diminished peristalsis, decreased motility and delayed transit.
Sacculations, also known as pseudodiverticula, are seen
frequently as large, broad-based outpouchings with a
somewhat squared contour (Fig. 4-42A). Similar appearances, with the exception of pseudodiverticula, may be
seen in visceral myopathy. A characteristic sign of progressive systemic sclerosis is an increased number of
mucosal folds—the 'wire spring or 'hidebound' appearance (Fig. 4-42B).

NODULAR LYMPHOID HYPERPLASIA AND IMMUNOGLOBULIN DEFICIENCY

Nodular lymphoid hyperplasia is frequently seen in the
terminal ileum and colon of children and young adults
and is considered to be a normal finding. In older people,
nodular lymphoid hyperplasia is commonly associated
with immunoglobulin deficiency and, in particular, with
the late-onset type of variable hypogammaglobulinaemia.
The lymphoid nodules are multiple, small, discrete,
round in shape and measure 1–3 mm. The nodules are
seen throughout the small intestine in most patients with
immunoglobulin deficiency, increasing in number from
the proximal to the distal end. The colon is frequently
involved throughout its length.

WHIPPLE'S DISEASE

Whipple's disease is a rare condition related to a Gram-
positive bacillus, *Tropheryma whippelii*. Presenting symptoms include abdominal pain, diarrhoea, malabsorption,

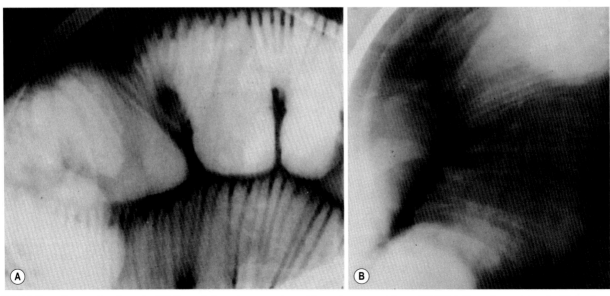

FIGURE 4-42 ■ Systemic sclerosis. (A) Sacculation shown as broad-based outpouchings. (B) Dilatation of a segment of intestine with
the 'hidebound' appearance of the valvulae conniventes seen on a spot compression view.

lymphadenopathy and polyarthritis. The characteristic radiological change is thickening of the valvulae conniventes, often with a nodular appearance in the proximal small intestine. CT findings include non-specific bowel wall thickening and low-density retroperitoneal and mesenteric lymphadenopathy, due to increased amount of fat and fatty acids.

INTESTINAL LYMPHANGIECTASIA

Intestinal lymphangiectasia may be primary, part of a generalised hypoplasia of the lymphatic channels, seen in children or young adults, or secondary to lymph flow obstruction by retroperitoneal fibrosis or malignant infiltration of the mesenteric or retroperitoneal lymph nodes. The diagnosis of the primary form can be made by demonstrating dilated submucosal lymphatics on histology, following peroral jejunal biopsy.

Enteroclysis shows non-specific uniformly thickened, closely set and parallel valvulae conniventes and/or a micronodular mucosal surface pattern. CT will demonstrate mural thickening or alternative causes of secondary lymphangiectasia.

EOSINOPHILIC GASTROENTERITIS

Eosinophilic gastroenteritis is characterised by eosinophilic infiltration of the walls of the stomach and small intestine. It is a rare disease, which may affect all age groups but typically presents in the third to fifth decades with a male predominance.[68,69] The aetiological role of ingested food allergens is substantiated by patient response to dietary modification (± corticosteroids) and the fact that more than 50% of cases occur in patients with a history of atopy.[70] Any portion of the gastrointestinal tract may be involved, but the SI and the stomach are the most common sites of disease.[16] Gastric involvement is seen radiologically as nodularity and narrowing of the pyloric antrum. The imaging manifestations of eosinophilic enteritis involving the small intestine vary depending on which layer (mucosa, muscle, serosa) of the intestinal wall is involved.[71] Mucosal eosinophilic enteritis results in fold thickening, polyps and mucosal ulcers that are visible on both CT and barium examinations. Disease of the muscularis propria results in small intestinal thickening with stricture formation and serosal disease results in ascites, lymphadenopathy, omental thickening and aggregation of small intestinal loops.[16] Initial treatment response to oral corticosteroids is often dramatic but approximately 50% of patients develop chronic disease.[70,72] Eosinophilic gastroenteritis should be suspected in any patient with small intestinal imaging changes accompanied by peripheral eosinophilia.[72]

MASTOCYTOSIS

Mast cell disease or mastocytosis is a condition in which mast cell infiltration of the skin and other tissues has occurred. It is nearly always characterised by a typical skin rash, known as urticaria pigmentosa. Involvement of the small intestine is frequent and is shown radiologically as thickening of the valvulae conniventes with associated nodular mucosal defects, 2–5 mm in diameter. The mucosal nodules are usually seen in short segments of jejunum but can occur in the ileum.

ANGIO-OEDEMA

Angio-oedema may present with acute abdominal pain and infrequently the segmental SI involvement may mimic the skip lesions more commonly seen in Crohn's disease.[6] Angio-oedema is caused by abnormal leakage of serum into the extravascular spaces and results in long segment or diffuse small intestinal imaging changes. These changes include small intestinal thickening with submucosal oedema and mucosal hyperenhancement creating the 'target sign' often with prominent mesenteric vessels and associated ascites.[73] SI angio-oedema may be idiopathic or hereditary but it also is recognised, with similar imaging features, in patients receiving ACE inhibitor therapy.[74]

AMYLOIDOSIS

Infiltration of the gastrointestinal tract with amyloid occurs in the majority of patients with primary amyloidosis. The radiological appearances vary from symmetrical thickening to effacement of the valvulae conniventes. The degree of thickening of the valvulae is related to the amount of vascular amyloid infiltration. Large deposits of amyloid may form intraluminal masses in the barium-filled small intestine. Diminished motility and atrophy of the valvulae may result from amyloid deposited throughout the layers of the intestinal wall and the lumen of the intestine may become dilated. CT findings are non-specific but typically include symmetric wall thickening of the affected small bowel.

ACQUIRED IMMUNE DEFICIENCY SYNDROME

With the advent of highly active antiretroviral therapy, the prevalence of opportunistic small intestinal infections in HIV patients has dramatically declined worldwide.[75] When small intestinal infection is suspected in HIV patients, a diverse range of pathogens such as *Mycobacterium avium-intracellulare* (MAI), *Cryptosporidium*, *Cryptococcus*, cytomegalovirus (CMV) and the HIV virus itself should be considered.[75,76] Cryptosporidiosis is the most common cause of enteritis in the HIV patient and results in mild thickening of the bowel wall with a moderate amount of fluid within the lumen. The proximal small intestine is the most common site for MAI infection, which typically results in wall thickening and mesenteric lymphadenopathy.[77] CMV more commonly involves the caecum but may also result in a terminal ileitis.[77] Kaposi's sarcoma and AIDS-related lymphomas may also involve the small intestine in AIDS patients, producing bulky retroperitoneal and mesenteric nodal masses that may be indistinguishable from opportunistic MAI infection.

BEHÇET'S DISEASE

Occasionally the small intestine, particularly the ileocaecal region, is involved in Behçet's disease. The appearances usually resemble ileocaecal tuberculosis or Crohn's disease.

GRAFT-VERSUS-HOST DISEASE

Intestinal graft versus host disease (GVHD) may involve any portion of the gastrointestinal tract, from the oesophagus to the rectum. Signs and symptoms include a maculopapular skin rash, nausea, vomiting, abdominal pain, tenderness and secretory diarrhoea. The risk of developing GVHD depends on the graft type, degree of human leucocyte antigen matching and donor and recipient characteristics such as age, sex and parity. Acute GVHD is said to occur within 100 days of the transplant and the small intestine is involved in GVHD in 75–100% of cases. Typical imaging findings include moderate mural thickening, mild bowel dilation and mural stratification resulting from a combination of submucosal oedema and mucosal hyperenhancement, which is a hallmark of this condition.[78] Apart from key features in the clinical history, intestinal GVHD differs from other pathologies such as Crohn's disease due to the diffuse, long length of bowel typically extending from duodenum to rectum and bowel wall thickening is typically mild. Infective differentials are more difficult to exclude, particularly when patients are immunocompromised. Stool cultures should be performed to evaluate for *Clostridium difficile* but rectal biopsy is often required to differentiate from infection with viral pathogens such as CMV.

NON-STEROIDAL ANTI-INFLAMMATORY DRUG ENTERITIS

Non-specific ulceration of the small intestine, with blood and protein loss, may develop in patients on long-term treatment with non-steroidal anti-inflammatory drugs (NSAIDs). Characteristic pathological findings include concentric, circumferential diaphragm-like narrowings, resulting from submucosal fibrosis secondary to focal ulceration. These diaphragm-like narrowings, which can progress to strictures, can be depicted clearly on enteroclysis.

REFERENCES

1. Cho KC, Baker SR, Alterman DD, et al. Transpyloric spread of gastric tumors: comparison of adenocarcinoma and lymphoma. Am J Roentgenol 1996;167:467–9.
2. Gourtsoyiannis NC, Grammatikakis J, Papamastorakis G, et al. Imaging of small intestinal Crohn's disease: comparison between MR enteroclysis and conventional enteroclysis. Eur Radiol 2006;16:1915–25.
3. Schindera ST, Nelson RC, DeLong DM, et al. Multi-detector row CT of the small bowel: peak enhancement temporal window—initial experience. Radiology 2007;243:438–44.
4. Huprich JE, Fletcher JG, Fidler JL, et al. Prospective blinded comparison of wireless capsule endoscopy and multiphase CT enterography in obscure gastrointestinal bleeding. Radiology 2011;260:744–51.
5. Aiyappan SK, Kalra N, Sandhu MS, et al. Comparison of neutral and positive enteral contrast media for MDCT enteroclysis. Eur J Radiol 2012;81:406–10.
6. Macari M, Megibow AJ, Balthazar EJ. A pattern approach to the abnormal small bowel: observations at MDCT and CT enterography. Am J Roentgenol 2007;188:1344–55.
7. Megibow AJ, Babb JS, Hecht EM, et al. Evaluation of bowel distention and bowel wall appearance by using neutral oral contrast agent for multi-detector row CT. Radiology 2006;238:87–95.
8. Minordi LM, Vecchioli A, Mirk P, Bonomo L. CT enterography with polyethylene glycol solution vs CT enteroclysis in small bowel disease. Br J Radiol 2011;84:112–19.
9. Negaard A, Paulsen V, Sandvik L, et al. A prospective randomized comparison between two MRI studies of the small bowel in Crohn's disease, the oral contrast method and MR enteroclysis. Eur Radiol 2007;17:2294–301.
10. Negaard A, Sandvik L, Berstad AE, et al. MRI of the small bowel with oral contrast or nasojejunal intubation in Crohn's disease: Randomized comparison of patient acceptance. Scand J Gastroenterol 2008;43:44–51.
11. Lawrance IC, Welman CJ, Shipman P, Murray K. Small bowel MRI enteroclysis or follow through: which is optimal? World J Gastroenterol 2009;15:5300–6.
12. Desmond AN, O'Regan K, Curran C, et al. Crohn's disease: factors associated with exposure to high levels of diagnostic radiation. Gut 2008;57:1524–9.
13. Strobel D, Goertz RS, Bernatik T. Diagnostics in inflammatory bowel disease: ultrasound. World J Gastroenterol 2011;17:3192–7.
14. Migaleddu V, Quaia E, Scanu D, et al. Inflammatory activity in Crohn's disease: CE-US. Abdom Imaging 2011;36:142–8.
15. Podolsky DK. Inflammatory bowel disease. N Engl J Med 2002;347:417–29.
16. Shanbhogue AKP, Prasad SR, Jagirdar J, et al. Comprehensive update on select immune-mediated gastroenterocolitis syndromes: implications for diagnosis and management. Radiographics 2010;30:1465–87.
17. Loftus EV. Clinical epidemiology of inflammatory bowel disease: Incidence, prevalence, and environmental influences. Gastroenterology 2004;126:1504–17.
18. Fleischer DE, Grimm IS, Friedman LS. Inflammatory bowel disease in older patients. Med Clin North Am 1994;78:1303–19.
19. Polito JM, Childs B, Mellits ED, et al. Crohn's disease: influence of age at diagnosis on site and clinical type of disease. Gastroenterology 1996;111:580–6.
20. Lewis RT, Maron DJ. Anorectal Crohn's disease. Surg Clin North Am 2010;90:83–97.
21. Sinha R, Verma R, Verma S, Rajesh A. MR enterography of Crohn disease: part 1, rationale, technique, and pitfalls. Am J Roentgenol 2011;197:76–9.
22. Choi D, Jin Lee S, Ah Cho Y, et al. Bowel wall thickening in patients with Crohn's disease: CT patterns and correlation with inflammatory activity. Clin Radiol 2003;58:68–74.
23. Tolan DJM, Greenhalgh R, Zealley IA, et al. MR enterographic manifestations of small bowel Crohn disease. Radiographics 2010;30:367–84.
24. Herlinger H, Furth EE, Rubesin SE. Fibrofatty proliferation of the mesentery in Crohn disease. Abdom Imaging 1998;23:446–8.
25. Prassopoulos P, Papanikolaou N, Grammatikakis J, et al. MR enteroclysis imaging of Crohn disease. Radiographics 2001;21 Spec No:S161–72.
26. Sinha R, Verma R, Verma S, Rajesh A. MR enterography of Crohn disease: part 2, imaging and pathologic findings. Am J Roentgenol 2011;197:80–5.
27. Pariente B, Cosnes J, Danese S, et al. Development of the Crohn's disease digestive damage score, the Lémann score. Inflamm Bowel Dis 2011;17:1415–22.
28. Boltin D, Levi Z, Halpern M, Fraser GM. Concurrent small bowel adenocarcinoma and carcinoid tumor in Crohn's disease—case report and literature review. J Crohn's Colitis 2011;5:461–4.

29. Kandiel A, Fraser AG, Korelitz BI, et al. Increased risk of lymphoma among inflammatory bowel disease patients treated with azathioprine and 6-mercaptopurine. Gut 2005;54:1121–5.

30. O'Donnell S, Murphy S, Anwar MM, et al. Safety of infliximab in 10 years of clinical practice. Eur J Gastroenterol Hepatol 2011; 23:603–6.

31. Parakkal D, Sifuentes H, Semer R, Ehrenpreis ED. Hepatosplenic T-cell lymphoma in patients receiving TNF-α inhibitor therapy: expanding the groups at risk. Eur J Gastroenterol Hepatol 2011; 23:1150–6.

32. Brown SL, Greene MH, Gershon SK, et al. Tumor necrosis factor antagonist therapy and lymphoma development: twenty-six cases reported to the Food and Drug Administration. Arthritis Rheum 2002;46:3151–8.

33. Rubio Tapia A, Kyle RA, Kaplan EL, et al. Increased prevalence and mortality in undiagnosed celiac disease. Gastroenterology 2009;137:88–93.

34. Huppert BJ, Farrell MA. Case 60: Cavitating mesenteric lymph node syndrome. Radiology 2003;228:180–4.

35. Boudiaf M, Jaff A, Soyer P, et al. Small-bowel diseases: prospective evaluation of multi-detector row helical CT enteroclysis in 107 consecutive patients. Radiology 2004;233:338–44.

36. LePane CA, Barkin JS, Parra J, Simon T. Ulcerative jejunoileitis: a complication of celiac sprue simulating Crohn's disease diagnosed with capsule endoscopy (PillCam). Dig Dis Sci 2007;52:698–701.

37. Maglinte DD, O'Connor K, Bessette J, et al. The role of the physician in the late diagnosis of primary malignant tumors of the small intestine. Am J Gastroenterol 1991;86:304–8.

38. Gourtsoyiannis N, Makó E. Imaging of primary small intestinal tumours by enteroclysis and CT with pathological correlation. Eur Radiol 1997;7:625–42.

39. Weiss NS, Yang CP. Incidence of histologic types of cancer of the small intestine. J Natl Cancer Inst 1987;78:653–6.

40. Bilimoria KY, Bentrem DJ, Wayne JD, et al. Small bowel cancer in the United States. Ann Surg 2009;249:63–71.

41. Kim SJ, Choi CW, Mun YC, et al. Multicenter retrospective analysis of 581 patients with primary intestinal non-Hodgkin lymphoma from the Consortium for Improving Survival of Lymphoma (CISL). BMC Cancer 2011;11:321.

42. Nakamura S, Matsumoto T, Iida M, et al. Primary gastrointestinal lymphoma in Japan. Cancer 2003;97:2462–73.

43. Bilimoria KY, Bentrem DJ, Wayne JD, et al. Small bowel cancer in the United States: changes in epidemiology, treatment, and survival over the last 20 years. Ann Surg 2009;249:63–71.

44. Hemminki K, Li X. Incidence trends and risk factors of carcinoid tumors: a nationwide epidemiologic study from Sweden. Cancer 2001;92:2204–10.

45. Ellis L, Shale MJ, Coleman MP. Carcinoid tumors of the gastrointestinal tract: trends in incidence in England since 1971. Am J Gastroenterol 2010;105:2563–9.

46. Gore RM, Mehta UK, Berlin JW, et al. Diagnosis and staging of small bowel tumours. Cancer Imaging 2006;6:209–12.

47. Nicholl MB, Ahuja V, Conway WC, et al. Small bowel adenocarcinoma: understaged and undertreated? Ann Surg Oncol 2010;17: 2728–32.

48. Rodriguez-Bigas MA, Vasen HF, Lynch HT, et al. Characteristics of small bowel carcinoma in hereditary nonpolyposis colorectal carcinoma. International Collaborative Group on HNPCC. Cancer 1998;83:240–4.

49. Dawson IM, Cornes JS, Morson BC. Primary malignant lymphoid tumours of the intestinal tract. Report of 37 cases with a study of factors influencing prognosis. Br J Surg 1961;49:80–9.

50. Paryani S, Hoppe RT, Burke JS, et al. Extralymphatic involvement in diffuse non-Hodgkin's lymphoma. J Clin Oncol 1983;1:682–8.

51. Howe JR, Karnell LH, Scott-Conner C. Small bowel sarcoma: analysis of survival from the National Cancer Data Base. Ann Surg Oncol 2001;8:496–508.

52. Gustafsson BI, Siddique L, Chan A, et al. Uncommon cancers of the small intestine, appendix and colon: an analysis of SEER 1973–2004, and current diagnosis and therapy. Int J Oncol 2008;33: 1121–31.

53. Hong X, Choi H, Loyer EM, et al. Gastrointestinal stromal tumor: role of CT in diagnosis and in response evaluation and surveillance after treatment with imatinib. Radiographics 2006;26:481–95.

54. Buckley JA, Fishman EK. CT evaluation of small bowel neoplasms: spectrum of disease. Radiographics 1998;18:379–92.

55. Richie RE, Reynolds VH, Sawyers JL. Tumor metastases to the small bowel from extra-abdominal sites. South Med J 1973;66: 1383–7.

56. Vignault F, Filiatrault D, Brandt M, Garel L. Acute appendicitis in children: evaluation with US. Radiology 1990;176:501–4.

57. Simanovsky N. Importance of sonographic detection of enlarged abdominal lymph nodes in children. J Ultrasound Med 2007;26: 581–4.

58. Macari M, Hines J, Balthazar E, Megibow A. Mesenteric adenitis: CT diagnosis of primary versus secondary causes, incidence, and clinical significance in pediatric and adult patients. Am J Roentgenol 2002;178:853–8.

59. Boudiaf M, Zidi SH, Soyer P, et al. Tuberculous colitis mimicking Crohn's disease: utility of computed tomography in the differentiation. Eur Radiol 1998;8:1221–3.

60. Makanjuola D. Is it Crohn's disease or intestinal tuberculosis? CT analysis. Eur J Radiol 1998;28:55–61.

61. Menke J. Diagnostic accuracy of multidetector CT in acute mesenteric ischaemia: systematic review and meta-analysis. Radiology 2010;256:93–101.

62. Wiesner W, Khurana B, Ji H, Ros PR. CT of acute bowel ischaemia. Radiology 2003;226:635–50.

63. Barajas RF, Yeh BM, Webb EM, et al. Spectrum of CT findings in patients with atrial fibrillation and nontraumatic acute abdomen. Am J Roentgenol 2009;193:485–92.

64. Segatto E, Mortelé KJ, Ji H, et al. Acute small bowel ischaemia: CT imaging findings. Semin Ultrasound CT MR 2003;24: 364–76.

65. Ha HK, Lee SH, Rha SE, et al. Radiologic features of vasculitis involving the gastrointestinal tract. Radiographics 2000;20(2000): 779–94.

66. Geffroy Y, Rodallec MH, Boulay-Coletta I, et al. Multidetector CT angiography in acute gastrointestinal bleeding: why, when, and how. Radiographics 2011;31:E35–46.

67. Graça BM, Freire PA, Brito JB, et al. Gastroenterologic and radiologic approach to obscure gastrointestinal bleeding: how, why, and when? Radiographics 2010;30:235–52.

68. Tien F-M, Wu J-F, Jeng Y-M, et al. Clinical features and treatment responses of children with eosinophilic gastroenteritis. Pediatr Neonatol 2011;52:272–8.

69. Talley NJ, Shorter RG, Phillips SF, Zinsmeister AR. Eosinophilic gastroenteritis: a clinicopathological study of patients with disease of the mucosa, muscle layer, and subserosal tissues. Gut 1990; 31:54–8.

70. Zhang L, Duan L, Ding S, et al. Eosinophilic gastroenteritis: clinical manifestations and morphological characteristics, a retrospective study of 42 patients. Scand J Gastroenterol 2011;46: 1074–80.

71. Khan S. Eosinophilic gastroenteritis. Best Pract Res Clin Gastroenterol 2005;19:177–98.

72. de Chambrun GP, Gonzalez F, Canva J-Y, et al. Natural history of eosinophilic gastroenteritis. Clin Gastroenterol Hepatol 2011;9: 950–6.

73. De Backer AI, De Schepper AM, Vandevenne JE, et al. CT of angioedema of the small bowel. Am J Roentgenol 2001;176: 649–52.

74. Scheirey CD, Scholz FJ, Shortsleeve MJ, Katz DS. Angiotensin-converting enzyme inhibitor-induced small-bowel angioedema: clinical and imaging findings in 20 patients. Am J Roentgenol 2011;197:393–8.

75. Huppmann AR, Orenstein JM. Opportunistic disorders of the gastrointestinal tract in the age of highly active antiretroviral therapy. Hum Pathol 2010;41:1777–87.

76. Tzimas D, Wan D. Small bowel perforation in a patient with AIDS. Diagnosis: small bowel infection with *Cryptococcus neoformans*. Gastroenterology 2011;140:1882, 2150.

77. Koh D, Langroudi B, Padley SPG. Abdominal CT in patients with AIDS. Imaging 2002;14:246–9.

78. Mahgerefteh SY, Sosna J, Bogot N, et al. Radiologic imaging and intervention for gastrointestinal and hepatic complications of hematopoietic stem cell transplantation. Radiology 2011;258: 660–71.

THE LARGE BOWEL

Stuart A. Taylor • Andrew Plumb

ANATOMY

The large bowel comprises the colon, rectum and anus. Knowledge of cross-sectional radiological anatomy of the colon is of increasing importance given the requirement for accurate pre-treatment staging of malignancy. The caecum, ascending colon and descending colon are covered anteriorly by visceral peritoneum and approximately 50% of the posterior aspect of these segments is retroperitoneal. The retroperitoneal colon has an adventitial layer, separating muscle from peritoneal fat. The anterior peritoneum runs medially onto the rudimentary mesocolon and laterally onto the abdominal wall as parietal peritoneum.[1] The transverse and sigmoid colon have a mesentery formed from a double layer of visceral peritoneum sandwiching connective and adipose tissue with vessels, nerves and lymphatics. The outer muscularis propria of the colon has two layers, an inner circular and an outer longitudinal, with the myenteric (Auerbach's) nerve plexus in between. The outer layer is thin, except where it is condensed into three narrow bands called the taeniae coli that contain more collagen and elastic tissue than muscle. Three rows of haustral sacculations arise between the taeniae, with haustral clefts between the sacculations. In the distal colon, haustra form only when the taeniae contract. The intraperitoneal colon is covered by mesenteric serosa. Subserosal fat in the caecum and sigmoid accumulates in small peritoneal pouches to form the epiploic appendages that may encase diverticula in the sigmoid. The superior mesenteric artery supplies the colon proximal to the splenic flexure via the ileocolic, right and mid-colic branches. The colon distally is supplied by the left colic, sigmoid and superior rectal artery branches of the inferior mesenteric artery. The marginal artery is a vascular arcade in the mesenteric border giving off short branches, the vasa recta, which penetrate the muscle layer close to the taenia mesocolica, and long branches entering between the taenia omentalis and libra.

The veins and lymphatics follow the course of the arteries, draining up into the portal vein and celiac nodes, respectively. The mid-rectal veins drain into the internal iliac vein and so into the systemic circulation via the inferior vena cava. In the rectum, lymph drains superiorly via superior rectal artery nodes to the inferior mesenteric chain, posteriorly by nodes around the median sacral artery, and laterally around the middle rectal artery to the internal iliac chain.

The rectum is defined as beginning at the third sacral level, although the sacral promontory is often taken surgically as the reference point. Others define it as the distal 15 cm of large bowel before the anus. Anteriorly the rectum is covered by peritoneum to the level of the junction of the upper two-thirds and lower one-third. The lateral and posterior aspects of the upper rectum and all the lower one-third are surrounded by the mesorectum, which is composed of loose adipose connective tissue containing the small perirectal lymph nodes and the superior rectal vessels. The mesorectum itself is enclosed by the mesorectal fascia (Fig. 5-1).[2] Posteriorly the mesorectal fascia is separated from the presacral fascia by the thin retrorectal space; anteriorly it blends with the urogenital septum (Denonvillier's fascia/rectovaginal septum), superiorly it is contiguous with the sigmoid mesentery, and inferiorly it terminates close to the anus in the parietal fascia covering the levator ani. There is no haustration in the rectum, but the valves of Houston create folds in the rectum. The presacral space is normally less than 1 cm at the fourth sacral segment, as measured from a lateral pelvic view during double-contrast examination, but may be up to 2 cm in the elderly and obese. The anus has a complex sphincter arrangement with an internal sphincter of smooth muscle (a continuation of the circular muscle coat of the distal rectum) and an external sphincter of striated muscle. Between these, the longitudinal layer, comprising striated and smooth muscle with extensive fibroelastic tissue,

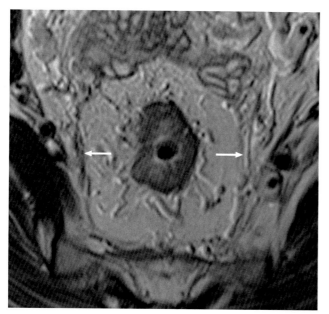

FIGURE 5-1 ■ Axial T2-weighted MRI depicts the mesorectal fascia (arrows) as a low signal layer enveloping the mesorectal fat.

TABLE 5-1   Contrast Enhancement Pattern and Differential Diagnosis

Pattern	Main Differential Diagnosis
Avid	Ischaemia
	Acute inflammatory bowel disease
	Malignancy
	Acute infection
Moderately	Malignancy
homogeneous	Lymphoma
	Chronic inflammatory bowel disease or chronic ischaemia
Heterogeneous	Malignancy
	Lymphoma (especially after treatment)
	Infiltration, e.g. endometriosis
Layered	Inflammatory bowel disease
enhancement	Infection
(target sign)	Ischaemia
	Vasculitis
	Graft versus host disease
	Radiation colitis
Reduced	Ischaemia

anchors the anus in position. The vascular subepithelial tissues seal the canal to maintain continence. The pelvic floor is an anatomical and functional unit and consists of muscles and connective tissue in three contiguous supporting layers. From cranial to caudal, these include the fascial layer or endopelvic fascia, the intermediate pelvic diaphragm and the urogenital diaphragm. The muscular pelvic diaphragm consists mainly of the levator ani complex.

The colonic mucosa is columnar in type with goblet and some enterochromaffin cells arranged in crypts (of Lieberkühn). The surface pattern consists of fine parallel grooves running transversely with short intercommunicating branches, and is called the innominate groove pattern. The lamina propria contains lymphoid follicles, the submucosa, adipose tissue with neural elements (Meissner plexus), blood vessels and lymphatics.

RADIOLOGICAL INVESTIGATION

The mainstays of colonic radiological investigation are intraluminal contrast examinations and cross-sectional techniques. Although cross-sectional imaging is largely replacing contrast studies, the latter still have a role in specific clinical situations.

A water-soluble contrast enema (Gastrografin diluted 3 : 1 with water or Urografin 150; Schering AG, Berlin, Germany) allows real-time evaluation of colonic anatomy and is most commonly used to test the integrity of surgical anastomoses, define colonic calibre, for example in suspected megacolon, delineate colonic fistulae and exclude mechanical obstruction. These agents are hypertonic and produce diarrhoea. Proximal to colonic strictures, water shifts will distend the colon and perforation resulting from this has been reported; care must be taken

not to overfill the bowel proximal to a stricture. Isotonic contrast agents produce less fluid shifts and are increasingly used.

A double-contrast barium enema (DCBE) involves full bowel preparation, an IV smooth muscle relaxant, partial filling of the colon with a barium suspension and insufflation of air or carbon dioxide to distend the colon. The objective is to acquire a series of images so that the entire colon is seen in double contrast, with no segment obscured by a barium pool or coated poorly.

CT can be performed either with (CT colonography) or without gaseous distension of the colon – in general, gaseous distension improves diagnostic accuracy for colonic abnormality, although it is more invasive and not always appropriate in acute situations. Standard abdominal CT protocols may include colonic opacification using orally administered contrast (2% barium or Gastrografin suspension), typically commencing the day before the examination, together with IV contrast medium administration. Rectal contrast agents may be used, for example in suspected perforation or appendicitis. The colonic wall should be not more than 3 mm thick. The pericolic fat should be homogeneous with only a few vascular channels. The normal colonic mucosa enhances after intravenous contrast administration, but the pattern of mural enhancement in abnormal colon may provide clues as to the underlying diagnosis (Table 5-1).

CT colonography (CTC) describes CT of the gas-distended colon. The use of oral contrast agents to tag residual colonic contents as higher attenuation is becoming mainstream, and can be combined with full or reduced laxative preparation, or without any additional laxative ('prepless CTC'). High osmolar contrast agents such as Gastrografin have a laxative effect and can be used as a single colonic preparatory agent. Distension of the colon is preferably performed using carbon dioxide and automated insufflation devices give superior distension to manual techniques.[3] Distension is improved with IV hyoscine butylbromide (Buscopan, Boehringer,

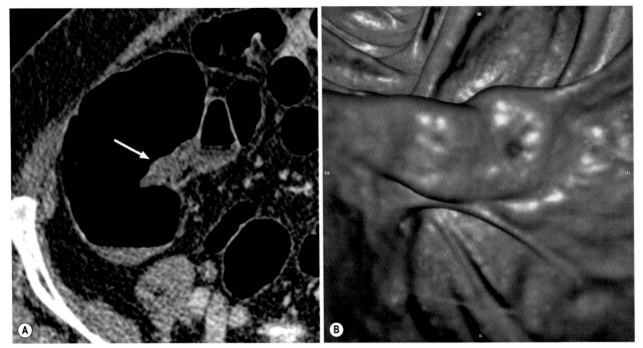

FIGURE 5-2 ■ (A) 2D CT colonogram of the normal ileocaecal valve (arrow). (B) The 3D endoluminal reconstruction shows the bicuspid, lobulated contour.

Ingelheim, Germany).[4] Supine and prone acquisitions (or decubitus views, if prone positioning is not possible) are essentially mandatory to ensure full mucosal visualisation. Review is performed using a combination of two-dimensional (2D) axial and multiplanar reconstructions, together with three-dimensional (3D) endoluminal reconstructions. Cross-correlation between 2D and 3D images is required to differentiate normal colonic structures such as the ileocaecal valve (Fig. 5-2), haustral folds and faecal residue from pathological entities. Collimation with multidetector CT is typically 1–2.5 mm. Intravenous contrast administration is not required for colonic evaluation.

MR colonography (MRC) follows similar principles to CTC, and is most commonly performed after bowel purgation, although non-laxative approaches are possible. Colonic distension is achieved with 1.5–2 L warm water or gas (carbon dioxide or air). Bright lumen MRC uses a gadolinium-spiked water enema and typically a 3D T1-weighted spoiled GRE sequence is used. Dark lumen MRC uses air, carbon dioxide or water and is more widely performed, although it requires the administration of intravenous gadolinium.[5]

Evacuation proctography (EP) is a study of the dynamics of rectal evacuation. Conventionally the procedure has been performed using X-ray fluoroscopy, but MRI proctography is gaining increasing acceptance. The rectum is distended using thick barium paste (fluoroscopy) or air/ultrasound jelly (MRI). During the fluoroscopic procedure, a video recording is made of the voluntary evacuation of the paste. The small bowel should be opacified with a dilute barium suspension to show any enterocele, and some advocate contrast filling of the bladder and vagina. No such extracolonic organ opacification is required for MRI proctography and evacuation

is captured using a rapid dynamic sequence such as true fast imaging with steady-state precession. Proctography may be viewed in three stages: rest, evacuation and recovery. At rest, the anorectal junction is normally just above the plane of the ischial tuberosities. Evacuation is initiated by 3 cm descent of the pelvic floor, widening of the anorectal angle, and relaxation of the anal sphincters. The rectum distal to the main fold is squeezed by raised intra-abdominal pressure against the levator ani to form a 'zone of evacuation' that empties in less than 30 s. On MRI proctography, organ prolapse is conventionally measured with respect to the pubococcygeal line.[6]

Abdominal ultrasonography requires a graded compression technique for good views of the colon. Gas distension often prevents visualisation of both walls, but the haustral pattern of the anterior wall should still be seen. Usually only the low reflective muscularis propria and reflective submucosa are identified. The bowel wall thickness may be measured, Doppler flow assessed and the pericolic tissues interrogated. Endosonography allows higher frequency probes to be used (10–20 MHz range) to show the wall layers in detail. The sonographic pattern is created by a mixture of interface reflections between, and reflections from, the thin layers. A four-layer pattern is seen in the anal canal (Fig. 5-3), with a five-layer pattern in the rectum (see Fig. 5-4).

TUMOURS

Polyps

A polyp is an elevated mucosal lesion (Table 5-2). The majority occur sporadically in the general population, although there are many rare polyposis syndromes. The

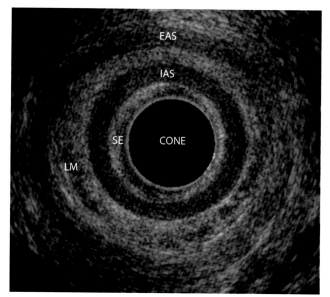

FIGURE 5-3 ■ **Normal male endosonographic mid anal canal anatomy.** The internal anal sphincter (IAS) is a hyporeflective structure. The external anal sphincter (EAS) is commonly hyporeflective in comparison to the surrounding fat. Women tend to have a more echogenic EAS. The longitudinal muscle (LM) can also be seen in the intersphincteric plane. The subepithelium (SE) is of quite variable thickness and is generally echogenic.

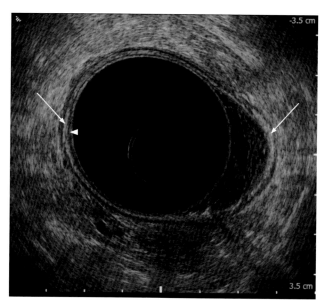

FIGURE 5-4 ■ **Endorectal ultrasound of an early rectal cancer.** The normal layered rectal wall architecture is shown on the left of the image, with (from superficial to deep) the echogenic superficial mucosa, hypoechoic deep mucosa (arrowhead), echogenic submucosa (arrow) and hypoechoic muscularis propria. The tumour is confined by submucosa (right arrow) and does not reach the muscularis propria (T1 stage).

TABLE 5-2   Classification of Polyps and Polyposis Syndrome

Histological Type	Single or Few in Number	Polyposis
Epithelial	Adenoma—tubular, villous, tubulovillous Adenocarcinoma	Familial adenomatous polyposis, Turcot's syndrome Cowden's disease
Hamartomatous	Juvenile Metaplastic	Juvenile polyposis Peutz–Jeghers syndrome Metaplastic polyposis
Inflammatory	Post-inflammatory polyp	Post-inflammatory polyposis
Nonepithelial	Lipoma, carcinoid, GIST, benign lymphoid, neurofibroma	Lymphomatous polyposis, Metastatic, neurofibromatosis
Miscellaneous	Endometriosis	Cronkhite–Canada syndrome

GIST = gastrointestinal stromal tumour.

most clinically significant polyps are adenomas. By definition, adenomas contain dysplasia i.e. intra-epithelial neoplasia. Colorectal cancer (CRC) represents extension of this neoplasia beyond the muscularis mucosae into the submucosa. Perhaps two-thirds of CRC originates via an adenomatous precursor (the adenoma-carcinoma sequence).[7] Detection of polyps is therefore clinically important, particularly as their removal substantially reduces subsequent carcinoma risk.

Adenoma prevalence depends largely on age, gender and family history. They are rare under the age of 30, but are seen in around 30% of individuals over 50 years. They are commoner in men than women and a first-degree relative with colorectal cancer confers about 50% additional risk. Around 50% occur in the rectosigmoid, 25% in the descending colon, 10% in the transverse and 15% in the caecum and ascending. Right-sided adenomas increase in older subjects.[8]

Certain factors increase the chance of invasive malignancy in an adenoma. Size is most important; the risk of invasion in a series of over 11,000 adenomas was negligible for <5 mm polyps, 2% for polyps between 0.6 and 1.5 cm in diameter, 19% for 1.6–2.5 cm polyps, 43% for 2.6–3.5 cm polyps and 76% for polyps of >3.5 cm.[9] Morphology is also important. Pedunculated polyps, which have a stalk separating the dysplastic epithelium from the deeper submucosa are often considered cured once resected, if the neoplasia is confined to the polyp's stalk (Haggitt levels 1, 2 or 3). Sessile polyps have a similar diameter at their base and near the top—they are roughly hemispheric. These have an intermediate risk of invasive malignancy for a given size. So-called 'flat polyps' are not truly polypoid and hence are probably better termed 'flat lesions'. A flat lesion is defined as being less than 2.5 mm in height above the colonic mucosal surface at endoscopy, or 3 mm on radiology.[10] Flat lesions may be depressed rather than elevated relative to the colonic mucosa. Such flat depressed lesions carry a higher risk of invasive cancer for a given size, whereas other subtypes of flat lesions are generally less aggressive. They can be very challenging to detect, both at endoscopy and on imaging. Pathological subtype is a third key factor. Villous adenomas are higher risk than tubular or tubulovillous lesions. Barium enema may suggest a villous histology when the surface is lacelike or granular due to the trapping of barium in the villous interstices. Similar trapping of oral contrast may occur on CT, although imaging features in general are non-specific.

Non-adenomatous polyps were once felt of lesser clinical importance due to a lower risk of malignancy, although this perspective is evolving. Traditionally, polyps were divided into adenomas, hyperplastic polyps and others (including juvenile, inflammatory, lymphoid and other rare polyps). Some polyps which were historically classified as hyperplastic have microscopic architectural distortion and are now termed sessile serrated adenomas. Their genes can show errors in sequences of repeated DNA, termed microsatellite instability (MSI) and/or gene hypermethylation (CpG island methylator phenotype, CIMP). They feed into a second major pathway of colorectal carcinogenesis termed the 'serrated pathway' which is hypothesised to account for up to 35% of CRC.[11] This implies polyps other than conventional adenomas may have clinical significance. Furthermore, even true hyperplastic polyps may harbour some genetic alterations also seen in CRC and share many risk factors with adenomas and CRC. They may represent a marker that an individual is at higher risk of subsequent CRC or genuinely represent precursor lesions.

Polyposis Syndromes

Familial Adenomatous Polyposis. Familial adenomatous polyposis (FAP) is caused by a mutation of the APC tumour suppressor gene on chromosome 5q21, and accounts for about 1% of CRC. Inheritance is autosomal dominant. APC is generally the first gene mutated in the sporadic adenoma-carcinoma sequence: individuals with FAP are therefore already one step along the pathway of tumourigenesis. More than 100 adenomas have to be present for the diagnosis; typically several hundred polyps are present. These may cause rectal bleeding, diarrhoea and mucus discharge. All affected patients eventually develop CRC. Preventative proctocolectomy is therefore recommended.

Extracolonic polyps also occur. Gastric adenomas and hamartomas are present and almost 100% of FAP patients have duodenal adenomas clustered around the ampulla (possibly due to the co-carcinogenic effect of bile). There is a 5% risk of periampullary duodenal carcinoma, a major cause of death in those who have had proctocolectomy. Extraintestinal manifestations include multiple osteomas of the skull and mandible, epidermal cysts (often facial), congenital hypertrophy of retinal pigment epithelium, abnormal dentition and desmoid tumours. Gardner's syndrome is a variant of FAP with prominent skeletal and skin manifestations. Desmoid formation is often precipitated by trauma or surgery. These benign

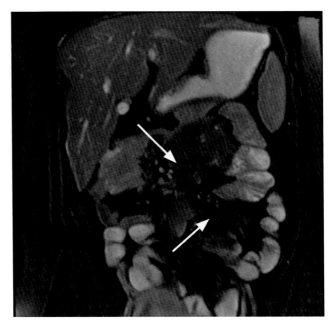

FIGURE 5-5 ■ Coronal fat-suppressed T2-weighted MRI in this patient with FAP shows abnormal infiltrative low signal (arrows) invading the small-bowel mesentery in keeping with desmoid disease. (Image courtesy of Dr Arun Gupta, St Mark's Hospital.)

fibromatous tumours are locally invasive and involve the abdominal wall, small-bowel mesentery or retroperitoneum. Previously, desmoid disease was a major cause of morbidity and mortality, although this has improved with advances in surgical expertise. In the early stages CT and MRI show ill-defined mesenteric infiltration with small-bowel tethering (Fig. 5-5), before mass development (which may be huge). Imaging often underestimates the extent of disease at surgical resection.

Hereditary Non-polyposis Colorectal Cancer (Lynch Syndrome). Hereditary non-polyposis colorectal cancer (HNPCC) is an autosomal dominant condition caused by faults in DNA mismatch repair (MMR) genes and probably accounts for 5% of all CRC. The lifetime risk of CRC in HNPCC is 70–85%. Genetically, these tumours exhibit high levels of microsatellite instability (MSI). Other tumours are also increased, notably of the endometrium, small bowel and renal pelvis/ureter. Clinical criteria for this condition follow the '3-2-1 rule': (A) three or more relatives with a HNPCC-associated cancer, (B) two or more successive generations affected, (C) one or more tumours diagnosed before the age of 50 years, (D) one should be a first-degree relative of the other two. Cancers occur at an earlier age in HNPCC (mean 45 years); about 70% are in the proximal colon and multiple tumours are common. Small polyps at an early age may be present.

Peutz–Jeghers Syndrome. This autosomal dominant condition is characterised by mucocutaneous pigmentation and intestinal hamartomas, mainly in the stomach and small bowel. Large-bowel polyps are fewer, but are larger, often pedunculated, and may bleed. There is an increased risk of gastrointestinal tract cancer, including

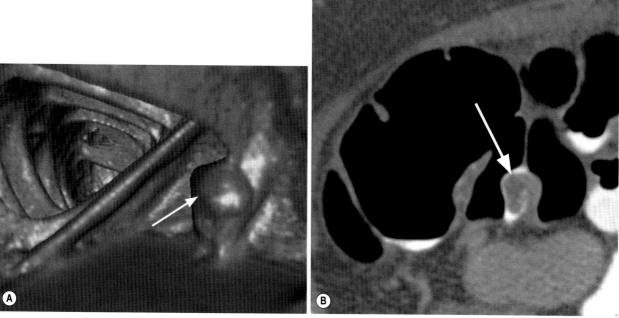

FIGURE 5-6 ■ (A) Endoluminal CTC image depicts a polyp (arrow) growing on a haustral fold just above residual colonic fluid. (B) The corresponding 2D image shows a stalked lesion (arrow) coated by a thin rim of tagged fluid.

CRC. Extraintestinal cancers are also increased, particularly of the ovary, cervix, thyroid, testis, pancreas and breast.

Rare Polyposes. There are a number of other rare polyposes. Turcot's syndrome is an association between colorectal adenomas/carcinomas and primary brain tumours. It can arise via a HNPCC-type defect in mismatch-repair genes or FAP-type defect in the APC gene. Sebaceous gland tumours occurring with HNPCC-type tumours is called Muir–Torre syndrome. Cowden's syndrome is an autosomal dominant trait with hamartomatous intestinal polyposis and lesions of the skin, mucous membranes, breast, thyroid and dysplastic cerebellar gangliocytoma. Juvenile polyposis is also autosomal dominant and presents in infancy with multiple juvenile hamartomatous polyps in the stomach, small bowel and colon. CRC risk is increased. Cronkhite–Canada syndrome is a diffuse intestinal polyposis that is associated with alopecia, hyperpigmentation of the skin and nail atrophy secondary to gross malabsorption. Serrated polyposis (previously known as hyperplastic or metaplastic polyposis) is a very rare condition with increased CRC risk and is diagnosed when there are multiple or large, proximally located, serrated colonic polyps.

Radiographic Features of Polyps

CT Colonography. CTC is the most accurate radiological technique for polyp detection, surpassing double-contrast barium enema (DCBE)[12] and approaching that of colonoscopy for larger polyps.[13] The entire colonic surface must be visualised using either a primary 2D approach with 3D problem-solving or a primary 3D

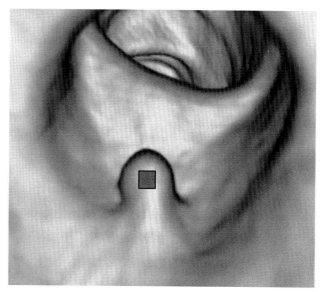

FIGURE 5-7 ■ **CTC endoluminal view shows an 8-mm polyp.** A small square has been overlaid on the polyp surface by the CAD software to aid detection.

endoluminal fly-through with 2D problem-solving (Fig. 5-6). The exact analysis method used is less important than the training and experience of the reporting individual.[14] Computer-aided detection (CAD) increases sensitivity with only a small reduction in specificity and should be used as a second reader to maximise its benefit (Fig. 5-7).[15] Once a polyp candidate is detected, it must be interrogated further to confirm its nature. Faecal residue may mimic a polyp; variable attenuation due to internal gas content is a distinguishing feature from the

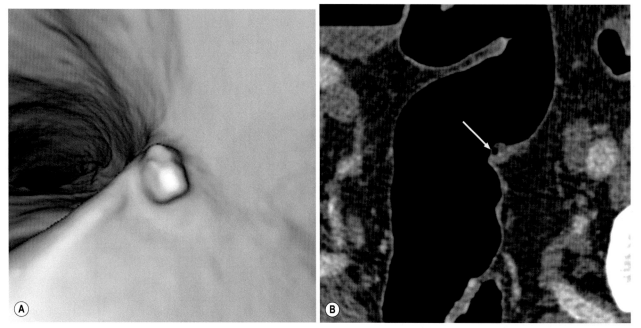

FIGURE 5-8 ■ (A) 3D view from CT colonogram shows a polypoid lesion that might be mistaken for a sessile polyp. However, the 2D view (B) shows a tiny locule of gas (arrow), demonstrating that this is, in fact, retained faecal residue.

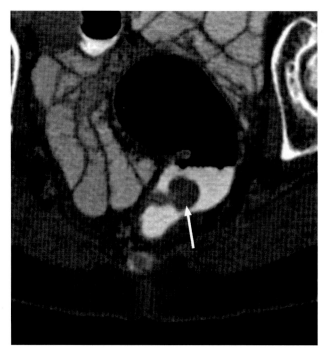

FIGURE 5-9 ■ 2D axial CT colonogram image shows a peduncu-lated rectal polyp (arrow) bathed by tagged fluid.

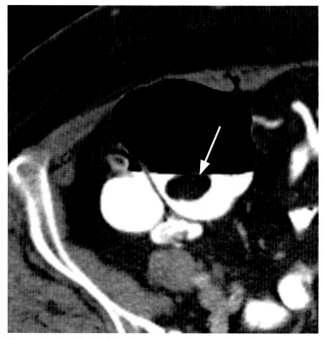

FIGURE 5-10 ■ Axial CT colonogram image with faecal tagging shows a smooth, lobulated fat-density polypoid lesion (arrow), diagnostic of a lipoma.

usual homogeneous soft-tissue attenuation of a polyp (Fig. 5-8). Faecal tagging (use of oral contrast to label or 'tag' residual colonic contents) improves both sensitivity and specificity; lesions which might be obscured by retained liquid residue can be seen within the higher-density fluid (Fig. 5-9) and tagged stool will not be mistaken for a polyp due to its high attenuation. Stool often moves between the prone and supine acquisitions. The

mesenteric colon may be mobile and changes in colonic position between the supine and prone acquisition may suggest 'movement' of a polyp; use of fixed landmarks such as diverticula or haustral folds may be helpful. Lipomas may be polypoid on 3D but the fat density on 2D is diagnostic (Fig. 5-10). Diverticula are seen as extra-luminal pockets of gas. An inverted diverticulum may simulate a polyp on 3D, but on 2D the gas content

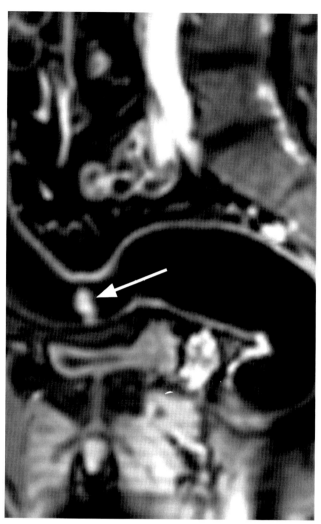

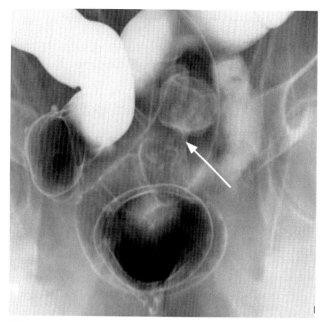

FIGURE 5-12 ■ **Prone-angled view of the rectum at double-contrast barium enema shows a large, pedunculated polyp (the arrow shows the stalk).** (Image courtesy of Professor Steve Halligan, University College London Hospital.)

FIGURE 5-11 ■ **Sagittal image from post-contrast fat-suppressed T1-weighted MR colonogram showing an enhancing sigmoid polyp (arrow).** (Image courtesy of Dr Anno Graser, University of Munich.)

indicates its true nature. Flat lesions can be very hard to detect and may only manifest as subtle wall thickening on 2D images (often best appreciated on an abdominal window setting) or minor protuberance or irregularity on 3D images. CAD can help detect flat lesions[16] and newer CAD algorithms will improve performance further.

MR Colonography. Dark-lumen sequences depict polyps as enhancing protrusions from the normal mucosa (Fig. 5-11). Endoluminal projections are feasible but may appear pixelated due to the current lower spatial resolution of MR.

Double-Contrast Barium Enema. As CTC rises in popularity, so DCBE declines. However, substantial numbers are still performed and interpretation skills will be needed for the foreseeable future. Polyps *en face* create a ring shadow with a sharp inner border and a fading outer margin. Viewed obliquely, a protruding polyp creates the 'bowler hat sign', which points towards the colonic lumen. The stalk and target signs are features of

pedunculation. The stalk is outlined by two parallel lines of barium that run obliquely to the axis of the lumen, distinguishing it from a haustral fold (Fig. 5-12). The 'target sign' is created when the head and stalk are superimposed. A polyp may create a filling defect in the barium pool, assuming it is not too deep.

Colorectal Cancer

Primary CRC is the third commonest cancer in the UK with around 40,000 new cases a year (2008 figures). It is the second commonest cause of cancer death. The lifetime risk is 1 in 15 for men and 1 in 19 for women. The risk increases with age, with almost three-quarters of cases seen in people aged 65 or more. Family history is a factor in around 20% of cases of CRC. Other risk factors include obesity, cigarette smoking and chronic inflammatory bowel disease. Anti-inflammatory medications such as aspirin and NSAIDs may be protective, as may diets low in red meat and high in fibre.

Just over half of all CRCs arise in the rectum or sigmoid; the rectum alone accounts for one-third of cases. Overall 5-year survival is about 50%. Major prognostic factors include local tumour stage, vascular or lymphatic invasion, preoperative elevation of carcinoembryonic antigen (CEA) and tumour differentiation (grade).

Colon cancer and rectal cancer are currently treated slightly differently. The mainstay of therapy for both is surgical excision, but in the rectum it is more difficult to achieve adequate clearance margins to prevent local recurrence whilst avoiding significant complications. The static nature and pelvic position of the rectum, however, make it amenable to chemoradiotherapy, which has been shown to decrease local recurrence in later-stage disease.

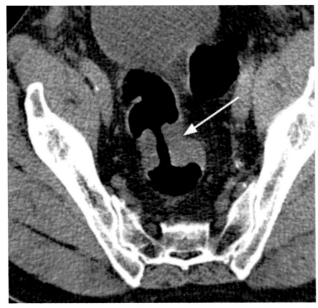

FIGURE 5-13 ■ **2D axial CT colonogram image demonstrating a circumferential tumour (arrow).**

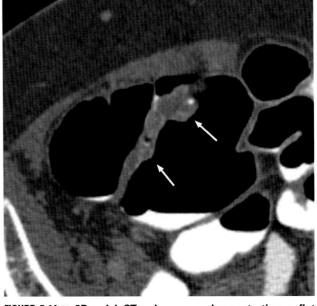

FIGURE 5-14 ■ **2D axial CT colonogram demonstrating a flat cancer manifesting as lobulated fold thickening (arrows).**

UICC/TNM	Tumour Extent	Dukes'	5-year Survival
Stage I	Invasion submucosa T1 Invasion muscularis propria T2 No nodal involvement, no distant metastasis	A	85–95%
Stage II	Invasion outside muscularis propria T3 Invasion visceral peritoneum T4a Invasion other organs T4b No nodal involvement, no distant metastasis	B	60–80%
Stage III	1–3 lymph nodes involved N1 >3 N2	C	30–60%
Stage IV	Distant metastasis in one organ M1a Distant metastasis in >1 organ or peritoneum M1b	D	<10%

TABLE 5-3   Colorectal Cancer Staging (TNM 7th edition)

UICC, Union for International Cancer Control (formerly International Union Against Cancer).

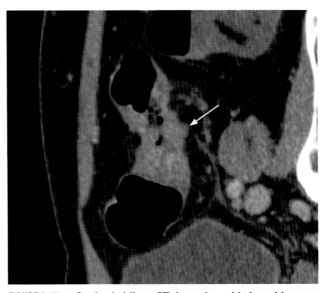

FIGURE 5-15 ■ **Sagittal oblique CT through a mid-sigmoid cancer shows an irregular outer margin (arrow) with soft tissue extending into the pericolic fat, indicating T3 disease.**

Local staging is therefore particularly important in rectal cancer. Both colon and rectal cancers can be staged according to the Dukes' and TNM systems (Table 5-3).

Colon Cancer

CTC has equivalent sensitivity to colonoscopy for detecting colorectal cancer,[17] although one advantage of colonoscopy is the ability to obtain biopsy confirmation of malignancy. CTC depicts annular or semi-annular lesions with shouldered ends and luminal narrowing (Fig. 5-13). Flat or plaque-like cancers show wall thickening and irregularity (Fig. 5-14). At conventional CT, malignancy is usually seen as an area of focal wall thickening (>3 mm), often with extension into the pericolic fat and local nodal enlargement (Fig. 5-15). Tumours are usually homogeneous but may be heterogeneous in the context of large adenocarcinomas or mucinous tumours or when associated with abscess formation. Mucinous tumours, both primary and metastatic, also have a propensity to calcify.

CT can estimate the T stage, with accuracy for identification of disease extension beyond the bowel wall of around 86%.[18] Colonic segments with a mesentery are

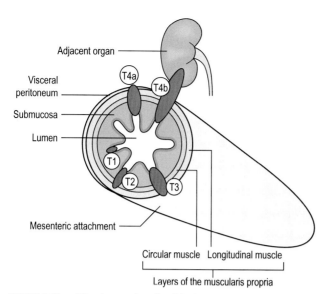

FIGURE 5-16 ■ **The layers involved in T1–T4 colorectal cancers according to the TNM, 7th edition.** Note how the mesenteric attachments determine the likelihood of T3 versus T4a disease status.

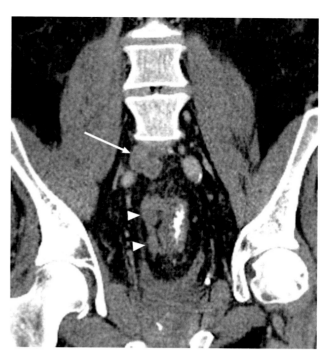

FIGURE 5-17 ■ **Coronal CT in this patient with a low rectal cancer demonstrates undulating expansion of a draining rectal vein (arrowheads), which is filled by abnormal soft tissue, typical of EMVI.** There are abnormal lymph nodes (arrow) just below the aortic bifurcation.

fully enveloped by visceral peritoneum and hence tumours here are more likely to achieve T4a status (Fig. 5-16). In the retroperitoneal colon, there may be direct retroperitoneal invasion which may compromise the retroperitoneal surgical margin, a risk factor for local recurrence. Generally, CT is better suited to broad categorisation of tumours into good-prognosis and poor-prognosis groups. Such classification predicts outcome almost as well as histopathological analysis.[19] This allows targeting of poor-prognosis patients for neoadjuvant chemotherapy, a topic under evaluation in clinical trials. Adverse prognostic features are unequivocal T3 tumours, T4 tumours and tumours with extramural vascular invasion (EMVI).[20] T3 disease should be suspected when there is extension of a discrete mass through the muscle coat into pericolic fat. EMVI is recognised by nodular or undulating expansion of colic veins (Fig. 5-17).

CT performs poorly for nodal staging, as size thresholds are neither sensitive nor specific. Abnormal clustering of normal-sized nodes has been used as an alternative criterion but does not substantially improve performance. Ascites and omental or peritoneal nodularity indicate disseminated intraperitoneal disease.

Barium enema is useful for cancer detection but provides limited information about the tumour stage. Randomized trial data show that, in symptomatic adults, barium enema misses twice as many cancers as CTC.[12] Annular lesions are generally easier to detect than plaque-like growths (Fig. 5-18).

Rectal Cancer

Treatment of rectal cancer involves *en bloc* resection of the tumour, rectum and mesorectum (total mesorectal excision, TME) to minimise the risk of local recurrence. The dissection plane extends along the mesorectal fascia, constituting the circumferential resection margin (CRM).

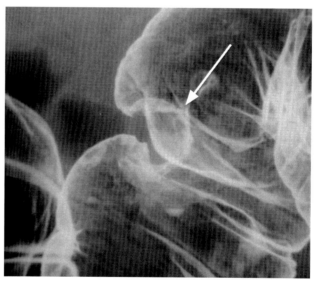

FIGURE 5-18 ■ **Double-contrast barium enema shows a distal transverse cancer (arrow) which has shortened and distorted the colonic contour.** (Image courtesy of Professor Steve Halligan, University College London Hospital.)

MRI is the imaging investigation of choice for local staging of rectal cancer. In particular, thin section (3-mm) T2-weighted (T2W) fast spin-echo (SE) sequences at right angles to the cancer provide information on local stage and relationship to the mesorectal fascia. Preoperative MRI stratifies tumours into three main groups: those highly likely to have an involved CRM after surgery; intermediate-risk tumours that do not threaten the

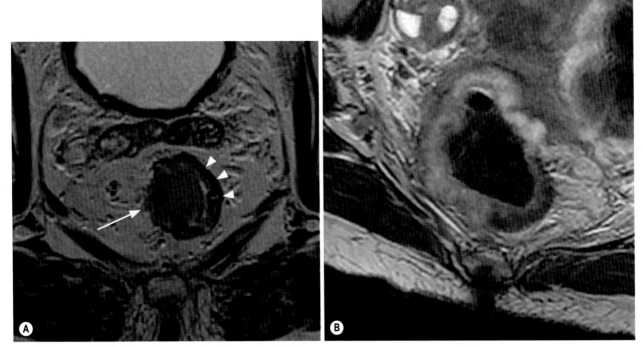

FIGURE 5-19 ■ **Axial T2-weighted MR through a mid-rectal cancer.** The normal low-signal muscularis propria (arrowheads) is intact on the left but breached by intermediate signal tumour (arrow) between 8 and 9 o'clock, indicating T3 disease. The tumour is well away from the circumferential resection margin (A). Conversely, (B) shows a different patient, with tumour abutting the resection margin. Surgery will almost certainly leave a positive margin, and hence increase the risk of local recurrence.

CRM; and low-risk tumours. The first group require pre-operative downsizing and/or downstaging with chemoradiotherapy to allow an attempt at curative surgery by TME; in the second group, operative therapy may be supplemented by pre-operative radiotherapy which reduces local recurrence rates; and the third group can undergo primary surgery with good local control rates without the toxicity of radiotherapy. CRM involvement is likely if MRI shows tumour within 1 mm of the mesorectal fascia (Fig. 5-19). Low rectal tumours that extend into the intersphincteric plane are also very high risk.[21]

Some early tumours (T1 and T2) can be treated by local resection alone. Transanal endoscopic microsurgery (TEM) removes the cancer without the need for a full TME. Endorectal ultrasound (ERUS) is not able to resolve the mesorectal fascia, but has better differentiation of the wall layers than MRI and higher accuracy for early stage (T1 or T2) disease. ERUS should therefore be performed to confirm local resectability (see Fig. 5-4).

Nodal staging is challenging on MRI, but important, as nodes outside the CRM will not be resected routinely. Morphological features are more useful than size criteria. Irregular outline and heterogeneous internal signal are suspicious. Diffusion-weighted imaging (DWI) shows some promise for nodal staging. Even more encouraging is the performance of contrast-enhanced MRI using blood-pool agents,[22] although both these and iron oxide MRI contrast agents have limited availability, reducing clinical uptake.

Tumour response evaluation after chemoradiotherapy is important; a proportion of patients have a complete response with no viable tumour at pathological examination after resection. MRI, in combination with clinical and endoscopic assessment, may be able to identify the patients who could forgo surgery and enter a 'wait-and-see' surveillance regime, particularly when DWI sequences are used.[23] This remains under investigation, and is not yet standard practice, but has a role in selected cases with particularly high operative risk.

MRI is also useful for imaging recurrent cancer, although FDG-PET/CT is probably superior. The key role for MR is to determine suitability for resection and guide the operative strategy (e.g. hemiclearance versus total pelvic exenteration) and the need for associated vascular reconstruction or sacral resection.

Anal Cancer

This rare tumour is increasing in prevalence, probably related to an increase in human papilloma virus (HPV), which is a leading aetiological factor. Squamous histology is typical. Tumours with an epicentre caudal to a point 2 cm above the dentate line should be staged as anal tumours. MRI is the test of choice for local staging, although endoanal US imaging may have a role. The T stage depends primarily on size and invasion of local organs (Fig. 5-20). Nodal drainage is usually to the inguinal region for tumours below the dentate line and the perirectal and internal iliac nodes for those above it. Metastases are best shown with FDG-PET/CT, although conventional CT is an alternative. MRI after standard chemoradiotherapy treatment can detect residual or recurrent tumour and facilitate selection for salvage surgery (abdominoperineal excision).

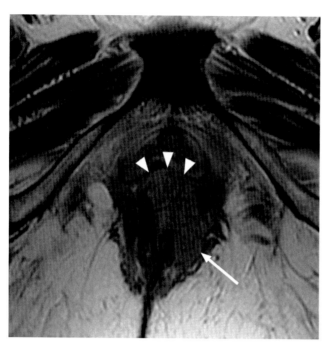

FIGURE 5-20 ■ Axial T2-weighted MRI showing an intermediate signal mass (arrow) in the mid-upper anal canal which abuts but does not invade the vagina (arrowheads).

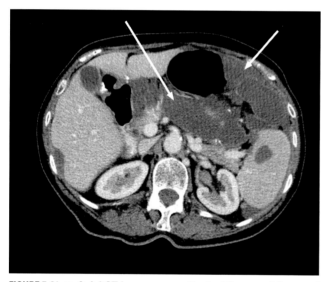

FIGURE 5-21 ■ Axial CT in a young patient with a past history of ruptured mucinous tumour of the appendix shows extensive low-density mucin deposition (arrows) around the liver, omentum and lesser sac.

Appendix Tumours

Around 1% of appendix specimens contain neoplasia, usually carcinoid or adenocarcinoma. Carcinoids are often small, incidentally detected, and adequately treated by the appendicectomy that led to their diagnosis. Conversely, mucinous adenocarcinomas may be problematic. Residual mucin can lead to pseudomyxoma peritoneii or retroperitoneii (Fig. 5-21).

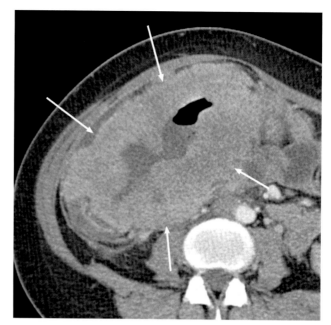

FIGURE 5-22 ■ Axial CT demonstrating marked symmetrical bowel wall thickening (arrows) secondary to a primary colonic lymphoma. Note the lumen remains patent.

Lymphoma

Large-bowel lymphoma is rare, accounting for less than 0.5% of colorectal malignancy. The classic radiological feature is aneurysmal dilatation of the affected segment (Fig. 5-22). There is often florid wall thickening without obstruction. Earlier manifestations are of a focal mass which may ulcerate. Perforation or intussusception may occur. Occasionally, there is diffuse large-bowel involvement, associated with peripheral T-cell lymphoma.

Secondary Cancers

The colon may be involved by direct invasion, along mesenteric planes, lymphatic permeation, intraperitoneal seeding or haematogenous spread. Serosal involvement causes mass effect and spiculated folds due to desmoplastic response to the tumour cells, causing wall contraction and tethering. Gastric cancer spreading via the gastrocolic ligament and pancreatic cancer via the transverse mesocolon are classical. Intraperitoneal seeding occurs in ovarian, gastric, pancreatic and colonic cancer, mainly affecting the surface of pelvic bowel loops, the right paracolic gutter and studding the colon. Omental caking is typical, predominantly involving the root of the omentum at its attachment to the transverse colon. During haematogenous dissemination tumour cells embolize in the capillaries of the vasa recta, growing into submucosal masses on the antimesenteric border. The metastases may be multiple, polypoid with a smooth surface due to their submucosal location, and are often umbilicated as a result of differential growth between the centre and the periphery. Carcinoma of the breast or lung, melanoma and lymphoma may all produce umbilicated metastases. Occasionally diffuse haematogenous submucosal deposition may produce a 'linitis plastica' appearance (Fig. 5-23).

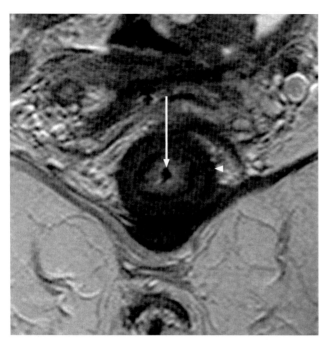

FIGURE 5-23 ■ **Coronal T2-weighted MRI shows florid wall thickening (from the lumen, arrow, to the muscularis propria, arrowhead) and a concentric ring pattern due to mural infiltration by metastatic gastric cancer.** (Image courtesy of Dr Velauthan Rudralingham, University Hospital of South Manchester.)

DIVERTICULITIS

Diverticular disease is a very common condition in older patients. The term describes a characteristic muscle abnormality most commonly in the sigmoid colon with typical 'out pouching' from the colonic wall – diverticula. Diverticulosis refers simply to the presence of diverticula, and diverticulitis to inflammatory changes within one or more diverticula. Deposition of elastin in the taeniae causes contraction and shortening of the bowel with corrugation of the mucosa and circular muscle layers, and is responsible for the thickened sigmoid with interdigitating folds. There are two rows of diverticula arising between the mesenteric and antimesenteric taeniae at points of weakness where the vasa recta penetrate the circular muscle layer. Each diverticulum consists of a pouch of mucous membrane with a very thin covering of longitudinal muscle. Diverticula are commonest in the sigmoid region, but may be scattered throughout the colon, or localised to the proximal colon in about 10% of cases. They have typical appearance on DCBE and CTC (Fig. 5-24). On CTC they often contain a high attenuation diverticulith which can mimic a polyp on 3D endoluminal view (Fig. 5-25). DCBE is able to provide a 'roadmap' of the disease distribution for surgical planning, although CTC is increasingly used for this purpose. Rectal diverticula are extremely rare. Diverticula in the right side of the colon tend to be larger and have wider mouths. Small intramural diverticula may be visible on the antimesenteric border.

Diverticulitis is the commonest complication of diverticular disease, occurring in about 10% of those affected. Its aetiology is thought to be due to faecal retention

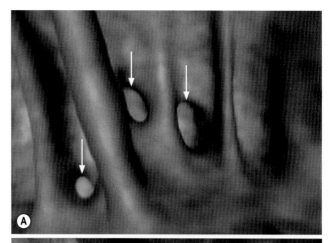

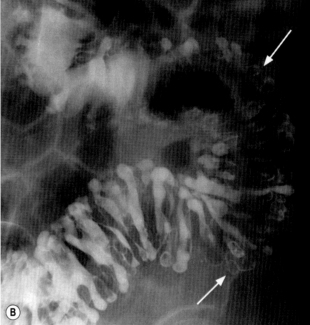

FIGURE 5-24 ■ (A) Endoluminal CTC shows the opening of three diverticula (arrows) between haustral folds in this segment of sigmoid. (B) Double-contrast barium enema in a different patient with florid diverticular change (arrows).

within the diverticulum, leading to ischaemic necrosis with microperforation, and so to the formation of a pericolic abscess, which is usually walled off within the pericolic fat. Adherence of such a chronic inflammatory mass may result in fistula formation (most commonly to the adjacent bladder). Rarely the abscess may perforate directly into the peritoneal cavity, causing faecal peritonitis. Bleeding from a diverticulum may be profuse and episodic, and is considered to be the result of intimal thickening of the vasa recta over the domes of the diverticula, with weakening of the wall leading to eccentric rupture and massive haemorrhage. The wider-mouthed diverticula in the proximal colon seem more predisposed to haemorrhage. CT is the most accurate radiological technique for determining the severity of diverticulitis. The hallmark of diverticulitis on CT is the combination of diverticular changes, colonic wall thickening and

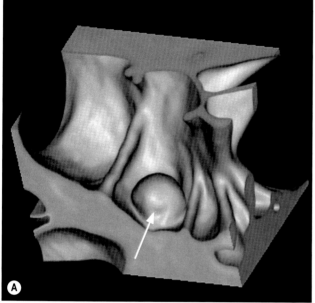

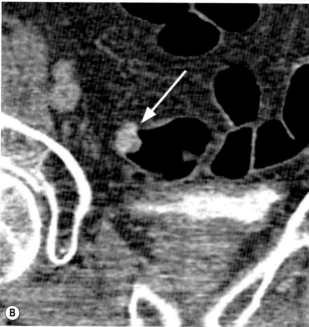

FIGURE 5-25 ▪ (A) CTC endoluminal view shows a large polypoid lesion (arrow) protruding between two haustral folds. (B) The corresponding 2D view shows this is a diverticulum filled by dense faeces (arrow).

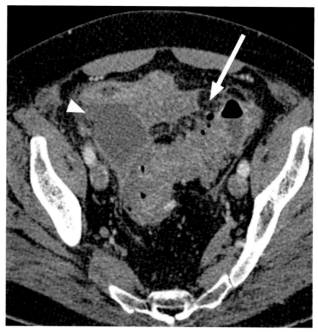

FIGURE 5-26 ▪ Axial CT shows acute diverticulitis manifest by a thickened sigmoid with diverticula and adjacent inflammatory fat stranding (arrow). A pelvic abscess (arrowhead) has formed next to the inflamed sigmoid.

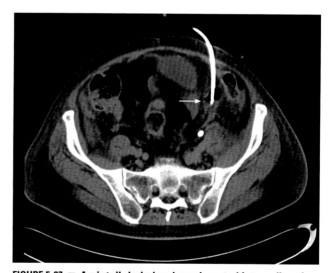

FIGURE 5-27 ▪ A pigtail drain has been inserted into a diverticular abscess (arrow) under CT control.

associated inflammatory reaction in the pericolic fat with 'fat stranding' and oedema producing a generalised increased attenuation. Fluid may track down the root of the sigmoid mesentery. An abscess (35%) is identified as a localised fluid collection (Fig. 5-26). Abscesses less than 3 cm are usually treated with antibiotics, although those larger than 4 cm often benefit from imaging-guided catheter drainage[24] (Fig. 5-27). Differentiation of acute diverticulitis from cancer can be problematic; cancer typically presents as a short segment of mass-like mural thickening, often with associated lymphadenopathy, and diverticulitis typically affects a longer colonic segment

(>10 cm) and is associated with vascular engorgement and mesenteric fluid. There is, however, clear overlap in imaging findings between the two. Perfusion CT parameters may have a role in distinguishing between cancer and diverticulitis.[25]

US is useful in episodes of mild diverticulitis with localised pain. Graded compression over the area of tenderness reveals the pericolic abscess as a low reflective collection related to the bowel wall and surrounded by reflective inflamed fat. MRI may also have a role.

Fistula formation most commonly involves the bladder. Conventionally a contrast enema is performed in cases

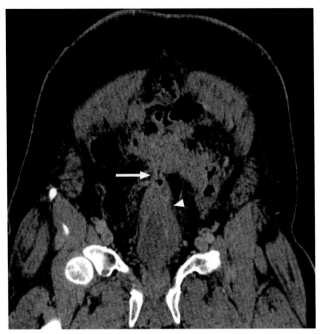

FIGURE 5-28 ■ Coronal oblique CT showing thickened sigmoid colon with a gas-filled track (arrow) extending towards the inflamed, thickened bladder dome (arrowhead). This was confirmed as a colovesical fistula at surgery.

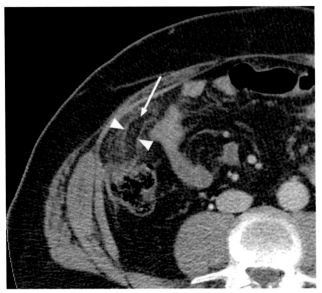

FIGURE 5-29 ■ Axial CT of epiploic appendagitis showing the typical, central ovoid fat-density mass (arrow) with peripheral enhancement (arrowheads).

of suspected colovesical fistula, although CT or MRI is increasingly the first-line investigation. The fistulous track may not always be seen, but the presence of gas in the bladder (in the absence of recent instrumentation), abscess related to the bladder wall, bladder wall thickening and/or adjacent adherent colon are highly suggestive (Fig. 5-28). Giant cyst formation is a rare complication, and represents a pseudocyst with no epithelial lining formed from expansion of a walled-off subserosal perforation. Its association with diverticular disease is apparent on CT or DCBE. The differential diagnosis includes a duplication cyst. Perforation or volvulus are rare complications.

EPIPLOIC APPENDAGITIS

Infarction of an epiploic appendage is most common either in the sigmoid or caecum where the appendages are most prominent, and causes acute pain and tenderness similar to diverticulitis or appendicitis. Most resolve spontaneously in about 2 weeks. The typical appearance on US is of a non-compressible pericolic hyperechoic ovoid mass immediately under the abdominal wall, and on CT focal hyperattenuation with a central area of fat density (Fig. 5-29).

COLITIS

Endoscopic techniques remain the primary diagnostic modality for colonic inflammation (colitis), facilitating direct mucosal inspection and histological sampling.

However, radiological imaging plays a large role, both in diagnosis and particularly in follow-up and detection of complications. Contrast enema (particularly using barium) can produce exquisite mucosal detail, but cross-sectional techniques are now widely used. There are numerous causes of colitis, and imaging features are often non-specific.

Imaging Features of Colitis

The hallmark of colitis on cross-sectional imaging is wall thickening (4 mm or more). Contrast enhancement is seen best in the enteric phase (typically 45–50 s post-IV contrast administration). The degree and pattern of contrast enhancement may give an indication of disease activity in inflammatory bowel disease (IBD),[26] although may not particularly reduce the differential diagnosis in unknown disease. For example a layered or striated pattern (central and peripheral enhancement with a central layer of relative reduced enhancement) may be seen in inflammatory bowel disease, infection and ischaemia, amongst others (Table 5-1). The ability to visualize extramural tissue is a significant advantage of cross-sectional techniques over luminal radiology; mesenteric oedema, abscesses, fistulation and lymphadenopathy are well seen. A phlegmon is an ill-defined inflammatory mass without overt abscess formation. These present as poorly defined focal masses of increased attenuation in adjacent omentum or mesentery. Abscesses are of low density (10–30 HU) and often contain gas bubbles either from gas-forming bacteria or a direct communication to bowel. On ultrasound the bowel wall is typically stratified in ulcerative colitis (UC) with differentiation between the submucosal and muscularis propria (Fig. 5-30), although in chronic Crohn's disease (CD) this may be lost. The surrounding fat is more reflective with acute inflammation.

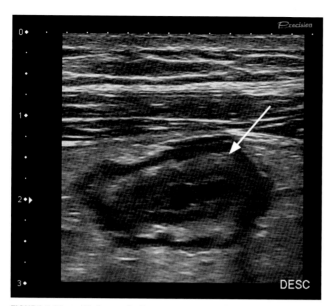

FIGURE 5-30 ■ **High-resolution transverse ultrasound image of the descending colon shows marked mural thickening and an exaggerated mural stratification pattern in keeping with colitis.** The arrow shows the echogenic submucosa.

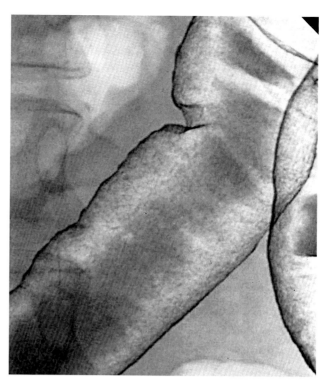

FIGURE 5-31 ■ **The granular mucosa typical of ulcerative colitis.** Note the intact mucosal line.

High-resolution isotropic cross-sectional images allow some appreciation of mucosal disease in well-distended bowel. High-definition thin-layer contrast studies, such as the DCBE, are, however, required to show superficial changes, although with the ubiquitous nature of endoscopy, the need for such detailed mucosal assessment is reducing in clinical practice. The rupture of crypt abscesses produces superficial erosions, which fill with barium to create the granular pattern typical of UC (Fig. 5-31). Crypt abscesses may erode through the muscularis mucosae to spread laterally in the loose submucosal tissue, creating undercut 'T'-shaped ulcers. Fissuring ulceration with thorn-like cuts into the bowel wall is a classic feature of CD. Aphthoid ulcers are very superficial so that there is no disruption of the mucosal line. Barium precipitates in the sloughed ulcer base, creating a dense amorphous pool *en face*. The edge of the ulcer is oedematous, slightly elevated and does not coat with barium, creating a surrounding black halo (Fig. 5-32). Aphthoid ulceration is typical of CD, does not occur in UC, but may be seen in amoebiasis, tuberculosis, Behçet's disease, and human immunodeficiency virus (HIV)-related infections. Reflux ileitis with a patulous ileocaecal valve and granular distal 10–15 cm of ileum is a typical feature of UC, and disappears rapidly following colectomy.

Extensive ulceration in acute colitis may virtually denude the mucosa, leaving oedematous remnants as pseudopolypoid elevations. With ulcer healing, mucosal tags may form sessile, filiform, adherent or bridging polyps, and are best called post-inflammatory polyps.

Inflammatory Bowel Disease

Inflammatory bowel disease usually refers to ulcerative colitis and Crohn's disease, although indeterminate colitis is also often included. Ulcerative colitis (UC) is a

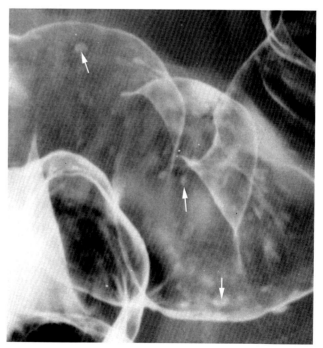

FIGURE 5-32 ■ **Aphthoid ulcers (arrows) in Crohn's disease.**

relapsing and remitting disease characterised by bloody diarrhoea. The rectum is always involved and the colitis is in continuity to its proximal extent.

The patient with CD presents with diarrhoea, abdominal pain and weight loss, with peak ages of onset at 20 and 50 years. Several classifications have been proposed: for example, the Montreal Classification, which takes into account age at diagnosis, disease location (ileal, colonic, ileocolonic or upper disease), stricturing, fistulation and anal involvement. Genetic status with NOD2 mutation may be relevant. Anal disease is associated with colonic involvement and affects 5% of individuals. The rectum is involved in only about half of cases and the disease is characteristically patchy and asymmetric.

Stool culture and laboratory tests are needed to exclude infective colitides and multiple biopsies are required to define the presence and nature of the colitis.

Differential Features

Ulcerative colitis and Crohn's colitis are different diseases, though they have some features in common. UC typically presents with a granular mucosa, rectal involvement and symmetrical disease that is in continuity to its proximal extent, with a shortened and narrowed bowel. Inflammatory changes are limited to the mucosa. In comparison, CD is asymmetrical with aphthoid ulceration. Inflammation is transmural, and deep fissuring ulceration may lead to fistula formation. The transmural nature of CD is reflected in the bowel wall thickness, which can be measured on CT, MRI, US or plain radiography where the properitoneal fat line demarcating the serosal edge is visible and the mucosa is outlined by barium/gas. The normal thickness is less than 3 mm; it may be 5–8 mm in UC, but can be grossly thickened in CD (on average 11 ± 5.1 mm). This tends to be greater in CD than UC (7.8 ± 1.9 mm).[27] Extraluminal manifestations of inflammatory bowel disease such as phlegmon, abscess and fistula formation suggest Crohn's disease. Small-bowel involvement in UC is limited to reflux ileitis.

Disease Activity in Inflammatory Bowel Disease

Disease activity assessment in inflammatory bowel disease is important with the widespread use of powerful anti-inflammatory medication such as anti TNF-α agents. Endoscopic scoring systems exist, mainly based on the presence and extent of ulceration, and the presence of stenosis. Histopathological features of inflammatory activity include ulcer formation, neutrophilic infiltration and crypt abscess formation. Cross-sectional imaging can help differentiate acute from chronic disease and assess treatment response. Increasing wall thickness and contrast enhancement, particularly in a layered pattern, are correlated with disease activity on CT, MRI and US,[28] as is mural T2 signal hyperintensity on MRI[29] (Fig. 5-33). Mesenteric vascular encouragement (comb sign), mesenteric oedema/fluid and lymphadenopathy are also associated with active disease. Fibrotic disease tends to exhibit moderate heterogeneous contrast enhancement, low signal on T2-weighted MRI and no adjacent mesenteric oedema or fluid. An increase in submucosal fat is characteristic of chronic UC and mesenteric fibrofatty proliferation accompanies chronic changes of CD. Fatty proliferation is responsible for widening the presacral space in rectal disease.

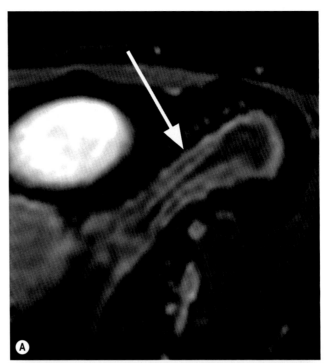

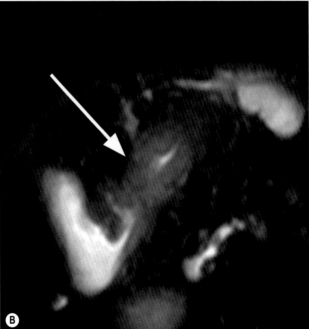

FIGURE 5-33 ■ (A) Post-gadolinum T1 high-resolution interpolated volumetric examination (THRIVE) fat-suppressed MRI at 3T shows a thickened sigmoid colon secondary to Crohn's colitis. The layered enhancement pattern suggests active disease. (B) T2-weighted MRI with fat suppression shows a thickened hepatic flexure in a different patient with Crohn's disease. The increased mural T2 signal (arrow) represents oedema and is also indicative of active inflammation.

Carcinoma in Colitis

There is an increased incidence of CRC in UC. Patients at risk are those with an extensive colitis of more than 10 years' duration. The carcinomas arise from dysplastic changes within the diseased epithelium and not from

TABLE 5-4   Common Location of Colitis According to Aetiology

Diffuse	Mainly Right-Sided	Mainly Left-Sided
Ulcerative colitis	Crohn's disease	Ulcerative colitis
CMV	*Salmonella*	Shigellosis
E. coli	TB	Lymphogranuloma venereum
Pseudomembranous colitis	*Yersinia*	Gonorrhoea
	Amoebiasis	Ischaemic colitis
	Neutropenic enterocolitis (typhlitis)	Radiation
	Immunosuppressive states (including AIDS)	Diverticulitis
	Ischaemic colitis	
	Hyopvolaemic states in young patients	
	Cocaine users	

adenomas as in the general population. The tumours are consequently frequently multiple and infiltrative. Colonoscopic surveillance with multiple biopsies is mandatory for patients with chronic UC, and imaging plays a limited role. Dysplasia is essentially a histological diagnosis, as it may be found in a flat mucosa and be unrecognisable radiologically. Dysplasia-associated lesions (DALMs), similar to villous adenomas, represent severe dysplasia and are occasionally visible radiologically.

OTHER COMMON CAUSES OF COLITIS

In general the imaging appearances of colitis are non-specific, but there are features which may narrow the differential diagnosis. Location is important (Table 5-4), but can only be used as a guide.

Ischaemic Colitis

Ischaemia is a common cause of colitis in the elderly (over 90% of those affected are over 60 years old), typically presenting with abdominal pain and rectal bleeding of sudden onset. There are a variety of causes: (A) mesenteric occlusion, arterial and venous; (B) mechanical, from strangulation or raised intracolonic pressure, such as proximal to an obstruction; or (C) low-flow states. In younger patients, hypercoaguable states, vasculitis, long distance running and use of cocaine are also causes. The region of the splenic flexure is most commonly affected (due to the watershed in vascular supply), but anywhere in the colon can be involved. Indeed, in low-flow states, the right colon is more commonly affected. The mucosa is most susceptible to vascular compromise but can repair, whereas necrosis of the submucosal and muscle layer creates more fibrosis, leading to stricture formation. Transmural necrosis or 'bowel infarction' is life threatening, requiring immediate surgical intervention. Plain radiographs may reveal narrowing and thumbprinting, and help exclude toxic megacolon, free perforation and intramural or portal venous gas. US may show a thickened wall (mean 7.6 mm) with stratification. On CT (Fig. 5-34) wall thickening is more marked with venous occlusion. A low-attenuation target sign is due to submucosal oedema. Wall thickness does not correspond to the extent of necrosis. The bowel may be relatively thin with transmural necrosis, or significantly thickened from

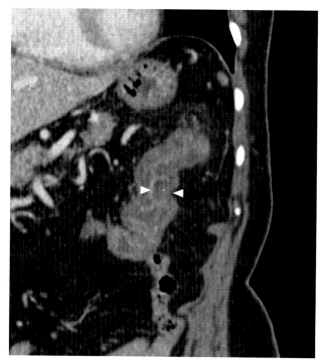

FIGURE 5-34 ■ Coronal CT shows mural thickening (arrowheads) due to acute ischaemic colitis extending from around the splenic flexure distally. The entire descending colon was affected (not shown). The mucosa retains brisk enhancement.

bacterial superinfection. Mesenteric fat stranding and free fluid may be seen with transmural necrosis, venous occlusion or superadded infection. Pneumatosis or portomesenteric gas indicates transmural necrosis.[30] Large vessel occlusion or aneurysm formation should also be looked for. Sacculation is common and is a feature of strictures due to either ischaemia or CD.

Radiation Colitis

Radiation-induced bowel damage is a late complication, often presenting years after otherwise successful therapy where the total dose has exceeded 45 Gy (4500 rad). The rectum is directly involved in treatment of rectal cancer, and may be indirectly affected following therapy for gynaecological or prostatic malignancy. The pathogenesis of radiation enteritis is occlusive endarteritis with thrombosis and fibrosis. In the early phase there is mucosal injury with an acute colitis, while the chronic changes involve a proctitis with possible ulceration, rectal stricturing, or fistula formation, usually to the vagina or bladder. Strictures may be smooth and symmetrical, but if there has been ulceration, these may be deformed with thick irregular folds. Perforation is rare. A barium enema will demonstrate the deformity or fistula. CT and MRI show generalised changes of rectal wall thickening, an increase in the mesorectal fat density, thickening of the mesorectal fascia and widening of the presacral space. Specific changes of complications such as fistula formation may also be seen.

Behçet's Syndrome

This is a chronic multisystem vasculitis that may affect the colon, usually the ileocaecal region in about 30% of cases. Deep discrete ulcers may lead to haemorrhage or perforation. CT shows a polypoid mucosa with wall thickening and marked enhancement. There is relatively little nodal enlargement or fibrofatty change, which helps distinguish the condition from CD. Also pericolonic inflammatory changes are minimal, unless there has been a perforation.

Infectious Colitis

Salmonella, *Shigella* and *Campylobacter* may all present as a localised or diffuse colitis, with a granular or ulcerated mucosa. There may be marked ileus in the acute stages of salmonellosis, and toxic megacolon has been reported.

Cytomegalovirus (CMV) causes a vasculitis with a thick wall, lymphadenopathy and large ulcers that may bleed, and is typically ileocolic in distribution. CT demonstrates wall thickening, serosal enhancement, mesenteric lymphadenopathy and often ascites. *Chlamydia trachomatis* causes lymphogranuloma venereum. A chronic proctitis is complicated by fistula formation, extensive fibrosis and eventual stricture formation.

Pseudomembranous Colitis

This colitis results from the effects of cytoplasmic endotoxins produced by overgrowth of *Clostridium difficile*, usually as a result of broad-spectrum antibiotic therapy. It is characterised endoscopically by yellowish plaques formed by sloughed mucosal cells that create the pseudomembrane. The presentation is with diarrhoea, pyrexia and leucocytosis, but may be fulminant with perforation from necrosis; hence, this is a potentially life-threatening condition. Plain radiographs may show a generalised ileus and nodular haustral thickening. CT, US and MRI may show gross wall thickening, with marked mucosal enhancement and extensive low attenuation from submucosal oedema.[31] This produces a very prominent target sign, often described as the 'accordion sign' (Fig. 5-35). This is typical of pseudomembranous colitis, but may be seen in acquired immunodeficiency syndrome (AIDS)-related or ischaemic colitis, and in severe oedema from cirrhosis. Pericolic stranding is minimal and ascites may be present.

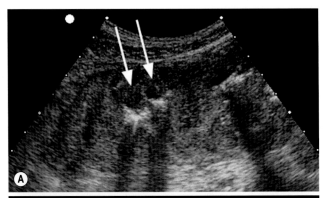
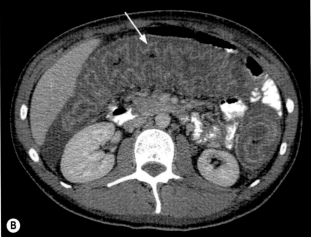

FIGURE 5-35 ■ (A) Ultrasound showing florid bowel wall and haustral fold thickening (arrows) secondary to pseudomembranous colitis. (B) The corresponding CT confirms marked colonic thickening and mucosal hyperenhancement (arrow).

Neutropenic Colitis

Neutropenia may be due to a number of causes, commonly chemotherapy with bone marrow transplantation. CT shows less bowel wall thickening than in pseudomembranous colitis, but pneumatosis is common (21%). Changes are typically right sided and may be limited to the caecum, which is why the term 'typhlitis' is often used.[32] Mesenteric stranding and small-bowel involvement are common.

Parasitic Colitis

In trichuriasis, the small, coiled worms may be seen on the mucosal surface on DCBE. *Strongyloides stercoralis* may simulate UC. In Chagas' disease, a megacolon results from the neurotoxic effect of the protozoon *Trypanosoma cruzi*. In schistosomiasis, ova are deposited in the submucosa of the large bowel. The inflammatory response results in the formation of numerous polyps. Fibrosis may later cause stricture formation and calcification may be visible in the bowel wall.

Tuberculosis

Most intestinal tuberculosis used to be secondary to pulmonary disease, but it is now more likely to be of primary

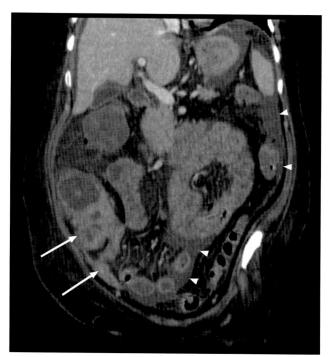

FIGURE 5-36 ■ Coronal CT of ileocaecal TB with caecal and terminal ileal thickening (arrows) and ascites (arrowheads).

bovine origin from drinking unpasteurised milk, with a normal chest radiograph. Ulcerative, hypertrophic or fibrotic forms are described. The ulcers tend to be large and circumferential with a shaggy edge, while the hypertrophic form presents with an inflammatory mass and stenosis of the bowel lumen.

Tuberculosis is commonest in the ileocaecal region, but may be seen in any part of the gastrointestinal tract, and may be indistinguishable from CD. It must always be considered in a patient from an endemic area, whatever the appearance of the colitis. Certain changes are suggestive of tuberculosis: a conical contracted caecum with a patulous ileocaecal valve and a dilated terminal ileum and transverse ulceration with a short hourglass stricture sharply demarcated from normal bowel. The hypertrophic form with a large exophytic mass may be difficult to distinguish from a lymphoma. Muscle involvement suggests TB, with actinomycosis as a differential. Wall stratification, increased vascularity and fibrofatty proliferation are not typical of TB and all favour CD, whereas ascites, peritoneal involvement, and lymphadenopathy favour TB (Fig. 5-36). Central caseous necrosis in lymph nodes creating a hypoechoic centre on US and peripheral enhancement on CT or MRI is highly suggestive of TB.

Amoebiasis

In endemic areas about 20% of the population harbour the cystic form of the protozoan *Entamoeba histolytica*. The radiological features of invasive amoebiasis include a segmental or diffuse colitis, with a granular or ulcerated mucosa. Aphthoid ulceration may be seen, and amoeboma formation occurs in about 10% of cases. These inflammatory masses comprising granulation cause an irregular stricture that may simulate a carcinoma; they are often multiple and are usually found at the flexures and the caecum. Embolic spread to the liver is seen in about 15% of cases. It is essential to examine fresh stools for trophozoites in all patients with colitis to exclude amoebiasis.

Acquired Immunodeficiency Syndrome

HIV infection and immunosuppression lead to a complex of intestinal infection and neoplasia, often superimposed on venereally acquired infections such as gonorrhoea, chlamydia and herpes simplex. CMV infection is common. *Cryptosporidium* and *Mycobacterium avium-intracellulare* cause nonspecific changes on barium enema. Kaposi's sarcoma most frequently involves the rectum with diffuse submucosal nodules that may coalesce into a mass. The lymph nodes are hyperaemic and show increased attenuation.

A specific diagnosis from imaging is difficult, even with typical changes, as multiple infections are common.

Defunctioned Colon

The defunctioned colon always has a low-grade bacterial colitis causing narrowing and loss of haustration. Barium may be retained for years and a water-soluble contrast agent is recommended for all examinations of defunctioned bowel.

Acute Fulminant Colitis

Any colitis including CD, ischaemic colitis, amoebiasis, antibiotic-associated colitis and salmonellosis can become fulminant where the inflammation becomes transmural and ulceration extends deeply into the muscle layer with neuromuscular degeneration, potentially leading to toxic dilatation and perforation. This complication is most commonly seen in UC, and accounts for most UC-related deaths.

The major signs of toxic megacolon are dilatation, loss of normal haustral contours and mucosal islands (Fig. 5-37). Plain radiography remains the mainstay in the diagnosis and monitoring of the condition, although cross-sectional techniques, particularly MRI, ultrasound and CT, have an increasing role. Dilatation of >5 cm is associated with ulceration deep into the muscle layer, and represents an initial stage of the process. In established cases the dilatation may be >8.5 cm. Haustration is always absent, and toxic megacolon should not be diagnosed if it is preserved. Changes are observed mostly in the transverse colon as in the supine position, this is the least dependent part of the colon where intraluminal gas will collect. Mucosal islands are oedematous remnants of mucosa and indicate the very extensive nature of the ulceration. The colon has the consistency of wet blotting paper and perforation is frequent.

The distinction between severe colitis and early toxic megacolon may be difficult and serial radiographs are helpful to monitor progress. MRI may have a role in staging and monitoring acute colitis—unprepared

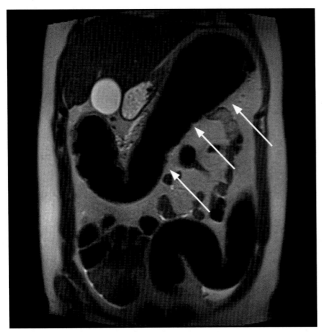

FIGURE 5-37 ■ **Coronal T2-weighted MRI showing gross dilatation of the transverse colon (arrows).** In the correct clinical setting, a haustral appearance and florid dilatation allows the diagnosis of toxic megacolon.

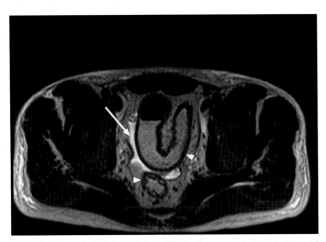

FIGURE 5-38 ■ **Axial T2-weighted MRI shows rectal and sigmoid mural thickening (arrowheads) and pelvic free fluid (arrow) in a patient with ulcerative colitis.**

T2-weighted axial and coronal images can efficiently image the colon and dilation, mural thickening, perimural mesenteric oedema and fluid are all easily appreciated as hallmarks of acute disease[33] (Fig. 5-38). Gaseous distension of the small bowel is a poor prognostic sign for successful medical treatment.

Perforation

Perforation is most likely to occur during an acute attack of UC, within the first year of onset of the disease. Perforation is the result of deep ulceration, which may be due to severe localised disease, or as part of toxic

TABLE 5-5   Causes of Large-Bowel Strictures

Physiological	Distended bladder, spasm
Surgical	Anastomosis, site of colostomy
Malignant	Annular, scirrhous, metastatic carcinoma, lymphoma
Diverticular disease	Pericolic abscess
Ischaemia	Sacculation common as with Crohn's strictures
Radiation colitis	In radiation field so usually rectosigmoid
Inflammatory bowel disease	Ulcerative colitis, Crohn's disease, tuberculosis, lymphogranuloma venereum, amoebiasis
Miscellaneous	Extrinsic mass, endometriosis, pelvic lipomatosis, trauma

megacolon. Free perforation is recognised by the presence of intraperitoneal gas, but sealed perforations cannot be reliably detected from plain radiographs. CT has high sensitivity for extraluminal gas in suspected perforation. Free perforation is rare in CD as, unlike in UC, the chronic transmural inflammatory nature of the disease causes adherence to adjacent structures. Cross-sectional imaging is required to demonstrate a localised pericolic abscess.

MISCELLANEOUS CONDITIONS

Large-Bowel Strictures

It is important to distinguish functional colonic narrowing from pathological causes (Table 5-5). The incidence of localised spasm is reduced by using a smooth-muscle relaxant, but it may still occur at one of the 'physiological sphincters' in the colon. There are seven such sites, of which Cannon's point in the mid-transverse colon is the best known. Spasm is easily abolished by further IV relaxants and gas insufflation.

The DCBE gives a purely luminal view with a positive predictive value of 96% for malignant and 86% for benign strictures.[34] Classically a fibrotic stricture has a smooth lumen with tapering ends, whereas a malignant one has an irregular lumen with shouldered ends. Scirrhous carcinoma is a rare exception, which may look more benign than malignant. Narrowing in diverticular disease is common. The retention of mucosal folds and the spiculated necks of compressed diverticula are important features in distinguishing a benign from a malignant stricture. In chronic UC there is considerable hypertrophy of the muscularis mucosae and submucosal thickening with fat. The smooth muscle changes are probably responsible for the generalised shortening of the colon, and may produce localised strictures in the left colon in 10–20% of patients with extensive long-standing UC strictures. Strictures in CD (Fig. 5-39) are usually asymmetrical with sacculation and secondary to ulceration on the antimesenteric border. As noted earlier, differentiation from malignancy can be problematic, particularly with cross-sectional techniques; any irregular raised area, shouldering or asymmetry suggests malignancy.

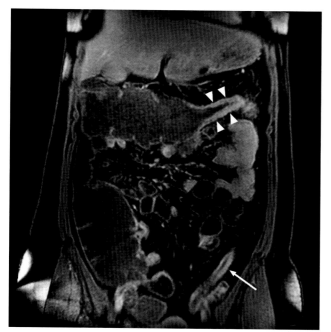

FIGURE 5-39 ■ **Post-gadolinum T1 high-resolution interpolated volumetric examination (THRIVE) fat-suppressed MRI shows dilated colon upstream of a distal transverse colonic stricture (arrowheads) in this patient with Crohn's disease.** There is also thickening of the descending colon (arrow).

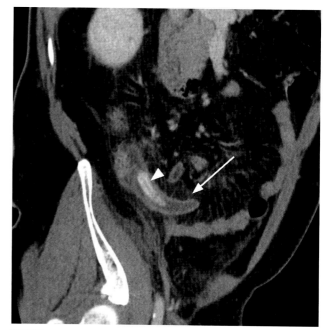

FIGURE 5-40 ■ **Coronal oblique CT showing a dilated, blind-ending appendix with surrounding inflammatory fat stranding (arrow) and an appendicolith (arrowhead) in the orifice.**

Cross-sectional imaging allows evaluation of the mural thickness, enhancement pattern and extracolonic findings which may help limit the differential diagnosis. The site of the stricture is also significant: radiation strictures are related to the field of therapy and so invariably affect the rectosigmoid colon; endometriosis usually involves the anterior wall of the rectosigmoid; ischaemic strictures are most common in the region of the splenic flexure.

Pseudodiverticula

Sacculation of the bowel wall is frequent in CD, secondary to fibrosis in healing eccentric ulceration. Pseudodiverticula may be seen in ischaemic strictures, but are rare in other forms of colitis and never occur in UC. Wide 'square'-shaped diverticula in focal areas of bowel wall weakness are seen in scleroderma.

Appendicitis

Appendicitis is the commonest abdominal emergency in the UK. Around 9% of men and 7% of women will have appendicitis at some point, typically adolescents or young adults. Imaging is only needed if the clinical diagnosis is uncertain. CT is probably the most sensitive and specific test, but a strategy based on initial ultrasound (with CT only if this is equivocal) has good positive and negative predictive value and reduces radiation exposure in this (often young) group (Fig. 5-40).[35] MRI (particularly with diffusion-weighted imaging) also shows substantial promise.

Lipomatous Disorders of the Large Bowel

Lipomatous disorders include lipomatous infiltration of the ileocaecal valve, solitary lipomas, or pelvic lipomatosis. Lipomatous infiltration of the ileocaecal valve causes diffuse enlargement of the valve, the surface of which may be smooth or lobulated. Two-thirds of all GI lipomas are in the colon, most being solitary lesions in the right colon. Those >4 cm may cause pain, bleeding, or intussusception. Lipomas are submucosal, so that the luminal surface is smooth, with no mucosal line at the edge of the lesion. The fat content, with a Hounsfield unit reading from −80 to −120 (around −100 HU), is apparent on CT, which is the optimum method for diagnosis.

Pelvic lipomatosis is a rare condition of unknown aetiology, in which there is proliferation of adipose tissue in the pelvis. The bladder and rectum are compressed. On plain radiographs, there is increased radiolucency of the pelvis and exceptionally good delineation of the sacrum. The presence on CT of a diffuse increase in pelvic fat is diagnostic.

Pneumatosis Coli

The origin of the gas cysts seen in this condition in the submucosal and subserosal layers of the bowel wall is uncertain. Small mucosal tears probably allow gas or gas-forming bacteria to enter the wall. Once a pocket is established in this way, diffusion into and out of the cyst may balance so that the lesion becomes self-perpetuating. Prolonged oxygen therapy alters these diffusion gradients, collapsing the cysts. Pneumatosis coli may be asymptomatic or present with diarrhoea or constipation, and rectal bleeding may result from superficial erosions.

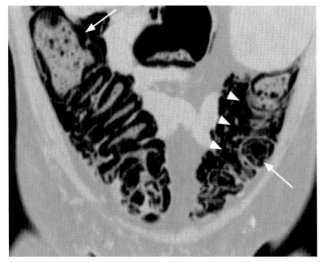

FIGURE 5-41 ■ Coronal CT demonstrates extensive bubbly mural (arrows) and mesenteric gas (arrowheads) in this asymptomatic patient (who was being imaged for an unrelated complaint).

Pneumoperitoneum from the rupture of a cyst is rare. The cysts are well-defined, closely packed, gas-filled lesions about 1–2 cm in diameter. A segment of the left colon is usually involved and the intramural location of the cysts is confirmed on imaging (Fig. 5-41). The plain radiographic changes are typical and should not be confused with those of other causes of gas in the bowel wall, such as necrotising enterocolitis, where there may be numerous minute foamy pockets of gas within a necrotic segment of bowel, or crescentic linear gas shadows running parallel to the bowel wall and portal venous gas in gross cases.

Volvulus

For volvulus to occur, the colon must be on a mesentery; thus the sigmoid is the commonest site. However, the caecum, transverse colon and splenic flexure are potential areas (Fig. 5-42), as is any part of the colon on a persistent dorsal suspending mesentery. Water-soluble contrast studies are useful for confirmation to show the 'bird's beak'-type twist. The 'whirl sign' on CT reflects the twisted bowel and mesentery and is proportional to the degree of rotation. Complicating features are bowel ischaemia and perforation. A formal DCBE or CTC is indicated with intermittent suspected volvulus when the patient is asymptomatic, to confirm abnormal redundancy of part of the colon and rule out any obstructing lesion.

Intussusception

Colonic intussusception in adults is almost always secondary to a tumour[36] and is perhaps more commonly seen on CT (Fig. 5-43) than barium enema, which may reduce the intussusception.

Endometriosis

Gastrointestinal involvement occurs in 12–37% of cases, mainly involving sigmoid and small-bowel loops in the

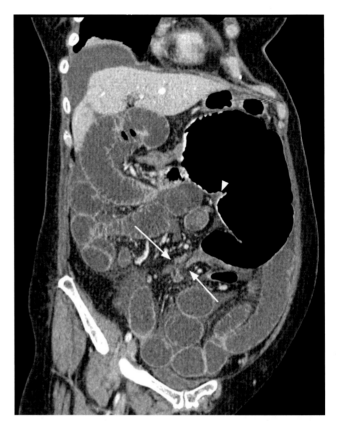

FIGURE 5-42 ■ Coronal oblique CT shows a dilated caecum in the left upper quadrant (arrowhead shows part of the ileocaecal valve). At the site of the twist there are two overlapping transition points (arrows), sometimes called the 'X-marks-the-spot' sign.

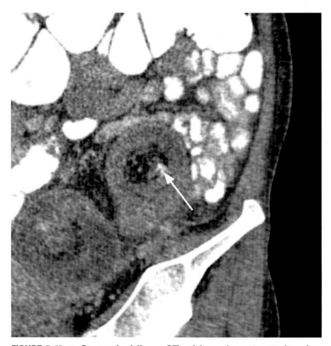

FIGURE 5-43 ■ Coronal oblique CT with oral contrast showing the typical 'target' appearance of intussusception. Dense oral contrast material (arrow) is present in the lumen of the intussusceptum which is surrounded by the indrawn mesenteric fat. This was colo-colic intussusception due to an adenocarcinoma serving as the lead-point.

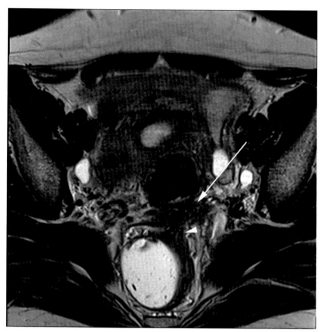

FIGURE 5-44 ■ Axial T2-weighted MR of the pelvis shows low signal obliteration of the pouch of Douglas (arrow) with tethering and angulation of the rectal wall (arrowhead) due to advanced endometriosis with deep colonic involvement.

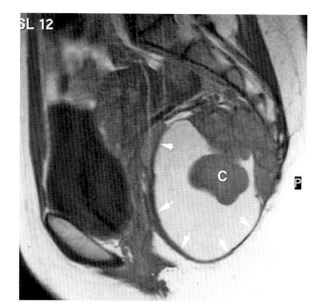

FIGURE 5-45 ■ Sagittal MRI of a large tailgut cyst (arrows) with cystic and solid (C) components, the latter due to the development of a carcinoid tumour within the cyst.

pelvis, though the caecum may also be affected. Serosal implants invade the muscularis propria, causing fibrosis with contraction of the wall and a mass effect. The mucosal surface remains intact, though rectal bleeding is a symptom. Contrast studies show a localised mass effect with characteristic contracted mucosal folds. MRI is increasingly used and can demonstrate the low signal fibrotic plaques which can obliterate the pouch of Douglas and involve the rectosigmoid (Fig. 5-44).[37]

Retrorectal Lesions

Tailgut cysts present as a mass that may be complicated by infection, bleeding, or malignant change. Most are developmental in origin[38] (Table 5-6). MRI provides the most complete examination to show the nature of the mass, signal characteristics of any cyst, any mural mass that might indicate malignancy, local infiltration and to exclude any meningocele or sacral lesion (Fig. 5-45).

FUNCTIONAL DISORDERS OF THE ANORECTUM

Hirschsprung's disease usually presents in infancy, and megarectum is mainly a childhood problem, but both may present in early adult life with a history of chronic intractable constipation. Plain radiographs demonstrate extensive faecal buildup, often outlining an enormously dilated rectosigmoid. A water-soluble contrast enema, without bowel preparation, will distinguish short-segment Hirschsprung's disease from megarectum. The lateral view of the pelvis in megarectum will show a dilated distal bowel (>6.5 cm in diameter) extending right down to the

TABLE 5-6   Retrorectal Mass

Developmental cysts	Epidermoid
	Dermoid
	Enteric (cystic hamartoma or rectal duplication)
Sacral lesions	Teratoma
	Anterior sacral meningocele
	Chordoma
	Lymphangioma
Anorectal lesions	Lipoma
	GIST
	Anal gland cyst

pelvic floor and often filling the entire pelvic cavity. There is a sudden transition proximally into colon of normal calibre. In Hirschsprung's disease there is a short abnormal segment, which is narrowed and may contract abnormally, leading into the funnel of the transition zone and dilated normal proximal bowel.

Constipation is a very common symptom and frequently due to slow colonic transit, which may be shown using radio-opaque markers with a plain film taken 6 days after the ingestion of 20 different geometric markers on days 1, 2 and 3. Retention of >4 of day 1, >5 of day 2 and >12 of day 3 markers is abnormal. Difficult defecation is also a component of constipation and may be due to anismus, which is the failure to relax the pelvic floor during attempted defecation. Evacuation proctography (using either barium or MRI) shows delayed and incomplete evacuation (<66% evacuated in >30 s).[39] An anterior bulge of the rectum is common during evacuation, particularly in women, but rectoceles are probably only functionally significant if there is retention within the rectocele at the end of evacuation (Fig. 5-46). Clinically, this is associated with perineal digitation to achieve complete emptying. Rectal prolapse starts with an infolding

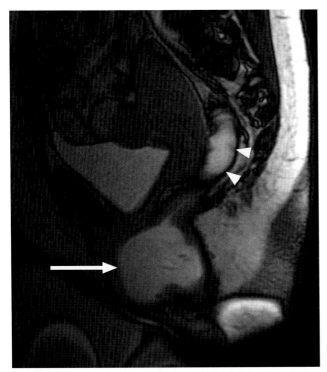

FIGURE 5-46 ■ Sagittal true fast imaging with steady-state precession (TrueFISP) MR defecography shows a large anterior rectocele (arrow) into which the rectally administered contrast material has entered and become 'trapped'. The rectum (arrowheads) itself is almost empty. This patient needed to digitate per vaginam to empty her rectum.

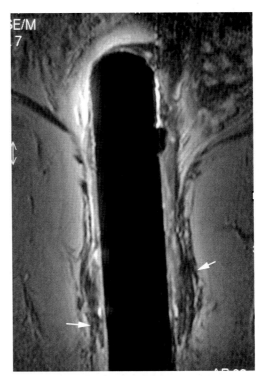

FIGURE 5-48 ■ Coronal sagittal MR image of diffuse atrophy with marked thinning of the external anal sphincter (arrows).

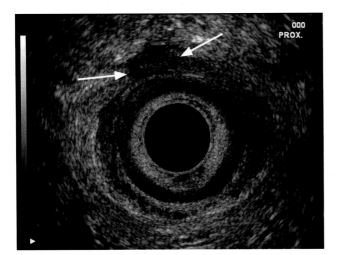

FIGURE 5-47 ■ Endoanal ultrasound shows an old scar (between arrows) at the site of an obstetric injury involving the external anal sphincter.

of the distal rectal wall entering the anal canal, an intra-anal intussusception. This is a typical finding in the solitary rectal ulcer syndrome. If the intussusception extends through the anal canal, it becomes an external prolapse.

Incontinence is a complex symptom, and, as with constipation, depends very much on the inter-relationship of the anorectum with the colon. Sphincter damage is best shown on endoanal US (Fig. 5-47) and striated muscle thinning or atrophy on endocoil MRI[40] (Fig. 5-48).

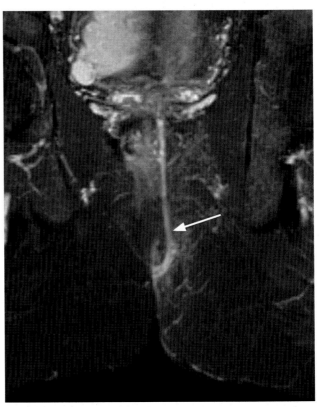

FIGURE 5-49 ■ Coronal STIR MRI shows an extrasphincteric fistula (arrow) running in the ischioanal fossa to the skin surface.

ANAL FISTULA

Anal fistulae are generally considered to be secondary to cryptogenic anal gland infection. Discharge of an abscess creates a track through part of the sphincter, usually the longitudinal layer, to the peri-anal skin. Discharge through the skin then completes the fistulous track from its internal opening in the anal canal out onto the skin. Fistulae are commonly classified according to the Parks classification based on their relationship to the muscles of the anal sphincter complex (trans-sphincteric, inter-sphincteric, suprasphincteric or extrasphincteric). MRI is the imaging modality of choice, although US has a role. On fat-suppressed T2-weighted sequences, fistulae appear as high signal against the lower signal sphincter complex and adjacent fat (Fig. 5-49).[41] Tracks may also link into abscesses, and into supralevator collections which are more difficult to detect clinically, but very well demonstrated on MRI. Preoperative MRI has been shown to reduce recurrence rates in complex fistula disease.[42]

Tracks within the sphincter and the internal opening are well shown on endosonography.

REFERENCES

1. Burton S, Brown G, Bees N, et al. Accuracy of CT prediction of poor prognostic features in colonic cancer. Br J Radiol 2008; 81(961):10–19.
2. Brown G, Kirkham A, Williams GT, et al. High-resolution MRI of the anatomy important in total mesorectal excision of the rectum. Am J Roentgenol 2004;182:431–9.
3. Burling D, Taylor SA, Halligan S, et al. Automated insufflation of carbon dioxide for MDCT colonography: distension and patient experience compared with manual insufflation. Am J Roentgenol 2006;186(1):96–103.
4. Taylor SA, Halligan S, Goh V, et al. Optimizing colonic distention for multi-detector row CT colonography: effect of hyoscine butylbromide and rectal balloon catheter. Radiology 2003;229: 99–108.
5. Thornton E, Morrin MM, Yee J. Current status of MR colonography. Radiographics 2010;30(1):201–18.
6. Mortele KJ, Fairhurst J. Dynamic MR defecography of the posterior compartment: Indications, techniques and MRI features. Eur J Radiol 2007;61(3):462–72.
7. Vogelstein B, Fearon ER, Hamilton SR, et al. Genetic alterations during colorectal-tumor development. N Engl J Med 1988;319(9): 525–32.
8. Yamaji Y, Mitsushima T, Ikuma H, et al. Right-side shift of colorectal adenomas with aging. Gastrointest Endoscopy 2006;63(3): 453–8.
9. Nusko G, Mansmann U, Partzsch U, et al. Invasive carcinoma in colorectal adenomas: multivariate analysis of patient and adenoma characteristics. Endoscopy 1997;29(7):626–31.
10. Zalis ME, Barish MA, Choi JR, et al. CT colonography reporting and data system: a consensus proposal. Radiology 2005;236(1): 3–9.
11. Snover DC. Update on the serrated pathway to colorectal carcinoma. Hum Pathol 2011;42(1):1–10.
12. Halligan S, Wooldrage K, Dadswell E, et al. Computed tomographic colonography versus barium enema for diagnosis of colorectal cancer or large polyps in symptomatic patients (SIGGAR): a multicentre randomised trial. Lancet 2013;381 (9873):1158–93.
13. de Haan MC, van Gelder RE, Graser A, et al. Diagnostic value of CT-colonography as compared to colonoscopy in an asymptomatic screening population: a meta-analysis. Eur Radiol 2011;21(8): 1747–63.
14. Hara AK, Blevins M, Chen M-H, et al. ACRIN CT colonography trial: does reader's preference for primary two-dimensional versus primary three-dimensional interpretation affect performance? Radiology 2011;259(2):435–41.
15. Halligan S, Mallett S, Altman DG, et al. Incremental benefit of computer-aided detection when used as a second and concurrent reader of CT colonographic data: multiobserver study. Radiology 2011;258(2):469–76.
16. Taylor SA, Iinuma G, Saito Y, et al. CT colonography: computer-aided detection of morphologically flat T1 colonic carcinoma. Eur Radiol 2008;18(8):1666–73.
17. Pickhardt PJ, Hassan C, Halligan S, Marmo R. Colorectal cancer: CT colonography and colonoscopy for detection–systematic review and meta-analysis. Radiology 2011;259(2):393–405.
18. Dighe S, Purkayastha S, Swift I, et al. Diagnostic precision of CT in local staging of colon cancers: a meta-analysis. Clin Radiol 2010;65(9):708–19.
19. Smith NJ, Bees N, Barbachano Y, et al. Preoperative computed tomography staging of nonmetastatic colon cancer predicts outcome: implications for clinical trials. Br J Cancer 2007;96(7): 1030–6.
20. Dighe S, Blake H, Koh M-D, et al. Accuracy of multidetector computed tomography in identifying poor prognostic factors in colonic cancer. Br J Surg 2010;97(9):1407–15.
21. Taylor FGM, Swift RI, Blomqvist L, Brown G. A systematic approach to the interpretation of preoperative staging MRI for rectal cancer. Am J Roentgenol 2008;191(6):1827.
22. Lambregts DMJ, Beets GL, Maas M, et al. Accuracy of gadofosveset-enhanced MRI for nodal staging and restaging in rectal cancer. Ann Surg 2011;253(3):539–45.
23. Lambregts DMJ, Vandecaveye V, Barbaro B, et al. Diffusion-weighted MRI for selection of complete responders after chemo-radiation for locally advanced rectal cancer: a multicenter study. Ann Surg Oncol 2011;18:2224–31.
24. Sarma D, Longo WE; NDSG. Diagnostic imaging for diverticulitis. J Clin Gastroenterol 2008;42(10):1139–41.
25. Goh V, Halligan S, Taylor SA, et al. Differentiation between diverticulitis and colorectal cancer: quantitative CT perfusion measurements versus morphologic criteria–initial experience. Radiology 2007;242(2):456–62.
26. Booya F, Fletcher JG, Huprich JE, et al. Active Crohn disease: CT findings and interobserver agreement for enteric phase CT enterography. Radiology 2006;241(3):787–95.
27. Gore RM, Balthazar EJ, Ghahremani GG, Miller FH. CT features of ulcerative colitis and Crohn's disease. Am J Roentgenol 1996;167:3–15.
28. Punwani S, Rodriguez-Justo M, Bainbridge A, et al. Mural inflammation in Crohn disease: location-matched histologic validation of MR imaging features. Radiology 2009;252(3):712–20.
29. Panés J, Bouzas R, Chaparro M, et al. Systematic review: the use of ultrasonography, computed tomography and magnetic resonance imaging for the diagnosis, assessment of activity and abdominal complications of Crohn's disease. Aliment Pharmacol Ther 2011;34(2):125–45.
30. Wiesner W, Mortele KJ, Glickman JN, et al. Pneumatosis intestinalis and portomesenteric venous gas in intestinal ischemia: correlation of CT findings with severity of ischemia and clinical outcome. Am J Roentgenol 2001;177:1319–23.
31. Thoeni RF, Cello JP. CT imaging of colitis. Radiology 2006; 240(3):623–38.
32. Kirkpatrick ID, Greenberg HM. Gastrointestinal complications in the neutropenic patient: characterization and differentiation with abdominal CT. Radiology 2003;226(3):668–74.
33. Hafeez R, Punwani S, Pendse D, et al. Derivation of a T2-weighted MRI total colonic inflammation score (TCIS) for assessment of patients with severe acute inflammatory colitis—a preliminary study. Eur Radiol 2011;21(2):366–77.
34. Blakeborough A, Chapman AH, Swift S, et al. Strictures of the sigmoid colon: barium enema evaluation. Radiology 2001;220: 343–8.
35. Toorenvliet BR, Wiersma F, Bakker RFR, et al. Routine ultrasound and limited computed tomography for the diagnosis of acute appendicitis. World J Surg 2010;34(10):2278–85.
36. Gollub MJ. Colonic intussusception: clinical and radiographic features. Am J Roentgenol 2011;196(5):W580–5.
37. Bazot M, Gasner A, Lafont C, et al. Deep pelvic endometriosis: limited additional diagnostic value of postcontrast in comparison with conventional MR images. Eur J Radiol 2011;80(3):e331–9.

38. Dahan H, Arrive L, Wendum D, et al. Retrorectal developmental cysts in adults: clinical and radiologic-histopathologic review, differential diagnosis, and treatment. Radiographics 2001;21: 575–84.

39. Halligan S, Bartram CI, Park HJ, Kamm MA. Proctographic features of anismus. Radiology 1995;197:679–82.

40. Stoker J. Magnetic resonance imaging in fecal incontinence. Semin Ultrasound CT MR 2008;29(6):409–13.

41. Halligan S, Stoker J. Imaging of fistula in ano. Radiology 2006;239(1):18–33.

42. Buchanan G, Halligan S, Williams A, et al. Effect of MRI on clinical outcome of recurrent fistula in-ano. Lancet 2002;360:1661–2.

CHAPTER 6

IMAGING OF THE PERITONEUM, MESENTERY AND OMENTUM

Nicholas Gourtsoyiannis • Panos Prassopoulos • Maria Daskalogiannaki

CHAPTER OUTLINE

ANATOMICAL CONSIDERATIONS

Introduction

The peritoneum is the largest serous membrane in the body. It consists of the parietal peritoneum, which lines the abdominal wall, and the visceral peritoneum, which envelops hollow and solid abdominal viscera. Between these two layers lies the peritoneal cavity. Peritoneal reflections interconnect the organs and viscera enclosed within the peritoneal cavity. The name of a particular ligament corresponds to the two major structures that it joins, e.g. hepatoduodenal, splenorenal ligament. Ligaments that attach the stomach to other structures are termed 'omenta'. The mesenteries connect a portion of bowel with the posterior abdominal wall. The fatty tissue enclosed by peritoneal folds is in anatomic continuity with the retroperitoneal and properitoneal tissues.[1] A potential space, termed the 'subperitoneal space' is enclosed within the peritoneal membrane of the mesenteries, bridges the peritoneal cavity with the retroperitoneum and represents a significant pathway for the spread of disease from the retroperitoneum to the peritoneal cavity and vice versa.[2]

The potential peritoneal spaces and the peritoneal reflections act as boundaries for pathological processes but may also become conduits for the spread of disease.[1] Typically, the peritoneal folds are not directly visible on cross-sectional imaging, but they can be identified by either their typical position or organ relationships or by the anatomical landmarks provided by their major constituent vessels. When they become thickened by oedema, inflammation or neoplastic infiltration, they can be directly recognised on computed tomography (CT) or magnetic resonance imaging (MRI).

Peritoneal Spaces

The peritoneal cavity is subdivided by peritoneal reflections into multiple compartments and recesses (Fig. 6-1). On cross-sectional imaging, the peritoneal spaces are not visualised unless they are distended by fluid (Fig. 6-2). The peritoneal cavity is divided into the supramesocolic and the inframesocolic compartments by the transverse colon and its mesentery.[3]

Supramesocolic Space

The supramesocolic space extends from the diaphragm to the transverse mesocolon. It is divided into right and left peritoneal compartments, which are arbitrarily subdivided into intercommunicating spaces.

The right supramesocolic space (Fig. 6-1A) includes the right perihepatic space and the lesser sac.[1] The right perihepatic space includes the subphrenic and subhepatic spaces. The subphrenic space extends over the diaphragmatic surface of the right lobe of the liver and it is limited on the left by the falciform ligament and posteromedially by the right coronary ligament, which forms the right lateral margin of the bare area of the liver. The subhepatic space, also called the hepatorenal fossa or Morison's pouch, consists of the posteromedial continuation of the subphrenic space, extending between the liver and the right kidney. Gallbladder infections or collections after gallbladder surgery tend to accumulate in this space.[2] The lesser sac is subdivided into a small superior recess and a larger inferior recess, by peritoneal reflection over the left gastric artery. The superior recess surrounds the caudate lobe of the liver and communicates with the right subhepatic space via the slit-like foramen of Winslow that is located between the inferior vena cava and portal vein. The larger inferior recess lies between the stomach, the visceral surface of the spleen and the pancreas. On the left it is bounded by the gastrosplenic ligament anteriorly and the splenorenal ligament posteriorly. Abnormalities of the transverse colon, pancreas, posterior wall of the stomach, duodenum and caudate lobe of the liver may extend into the lesser sac.

The left supramesocolic space is subdivided into four intercommunicating compartments.[1] The left anterior

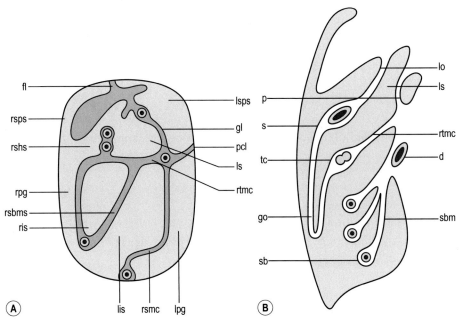

FIGURE 6-1 ■ (A) Coronal diagram showing division of the peritoneal cavity according to peritoneal attachments to the posterior abdominal wall. (B) Midsagittal diagram of the upper abdomen. Abbreviations: fl = falciform ligament; gl = gastrosplenic ligament; pcl = phrenicocolic ligament; ls = lesser sac; lsps = left subphrenic space; lpg = left paracolic gutter; lis = left infracolic space; rtmc = root of transverse mesocolon; rsbm = root of small-bowel mesentery; ris = right infracolic space; rpg = right paracolic gutter; rshs = right subhepatic space; rsps = right subdiaphragmatic space; smb = small-bowel mesentery; go = greater omentum; lo = lesser omentum; tc = transverse colon; sb = small bowel; s = stomach; p = pancreas; d = duodenum.

perihepatic space is bounded on the right by the falciform ligament, posteriorly by the liver surface and anteriorly by the diaphragm (Fig. 6-2A). It is mainly affected by lesions arising from the left lobe of the liver and the stomach.[2] The left posterior perihepatic space, also called the gastrohepatic recess, follows the posterior margin of the lateral segments of the left hepatic lobe. It is in close proximity to the lesser curve of the stomach, the anterior wall of the duodenal bulb and the anterior wall of the gallbladder. Abnormalities in any of these organs may extend into this space.[3] The left anterior subphrenic space lies between the anterior wall of the stomach and the left hemidiaphragm, communicating inferiorly with the left anterior perihepatic space. Fluid collections in this space may result from perforation of the stomach or the splenic flexure of the colon.[4] The left posterior subphrenic or perisplenic space is the posterior extension of the anterior subphrenic space (Fig. 6-2A).

Inframesocolic Space

The inframesocolic space is bordered superiorly by the transverse mesocolon and inferiorly by the pelvic rim. It contains the infracolic space and the paracolic gutters (Fig. 6-2B). The obliquely directed small-bowel mesentery, extending from the left upper midabdomen to the right iliac fossa, divides the infracolic space into a smaller right and a larger left space. The right infracolic space terminates at the ileocaecal junction. The left infracolic space is anatomically open to the pelvis except where it is restricted by the sigmoid mesocolon (Fig. 6-2C). The ascending and descending colon form the lateral

borders of the right and left inframesocolic space, respectively.

The paracolic gutters are located alongside the lateral borders of the ascending and descending colon. The right paracolic gutter is continuous with the right perihepatic space and with the intraperitoneal pelvic space. Cephalad continuation of the left paracolic gutter is partially restricted by the phrenicocolic ligament. The pelvic peritoneal cavity consists of the lateral paravesical spaces and the pouch of Douglas—the rectovesical space in men, the rectouterine space in women.

Peritoneal Reflections

The Mesenteries

The mesenteries are double-layered peritoneal folds enclosing either the small bowel or portions of the colon and connecting them to the posterior abdominal wall. They contain a variable amount of adipose tissue, the superior or inferior mesenteric arteries and their branches, the associated veins, lymphatic vessels and nerves.

The *small-bowel mesentery* is a broad fan-shaped fold that suspends the jejunum and ileum from the posterior abdominal wall and contains the intestinal branches of the superior mesenteric vessels, lymph nodes, nerves and abundant fat.[4] Its root originates at the duodeno-jejunal junction and extends downward in an oblique direction to the ileocaecal junction. The root is 15 cm long, while the intestinal border is 6–8 m in length. As a result, the mesentery has a pleated appearance along its intestinal border. The mesenteric folds are not

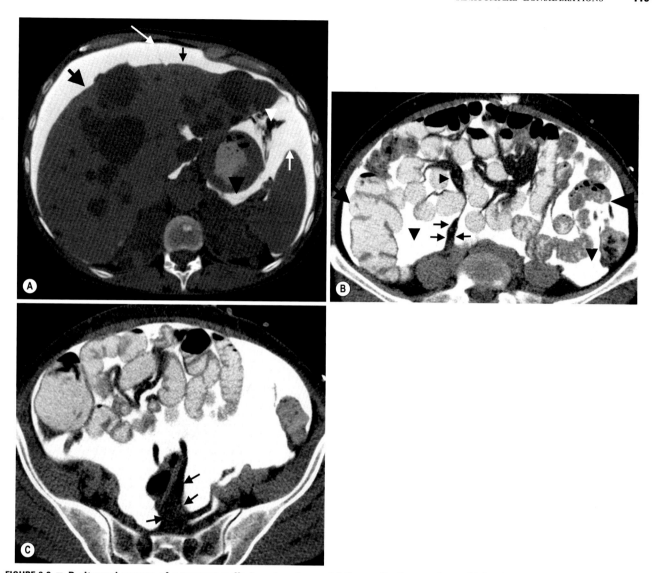

FIGURE 6-2 ■ **Peritoneal spaces of a woman suffering chronic renal failure, after intraperitoneal injection of water-soluble contrast material on CT.** (A) Contrast medium opacifies right subphrenic (large black arrow) and left posterior subphrenic (small white arrow) space. Left anterior perihepatic space (small black arrow) is bounded on the right by the falciform ligament (large white arrow). The lesser sac (black arrowhead) is delineated behind the stomach and its superior extension around caudate lobe of the liver is demonstrated. The gastrosplenic ligament (white arrowhead) is demonstrated as the fatty space between the lesser sac and the splachnic splenic surface. The bare area of the liver at reflection of the right coronary ligament is uncovered by contrast material. (B) Inframesocolic compartment. The opacified fluid delineates the right (large black arrow) and the left paracolic gutters. The right and the left inframesocolic spaces are also opacified (large arrowheads). A triangle-shaped opacified area (small arrowhead) intervenes between folds of small-bowel mesentery that are seen as lucent bands. The fat within the root of the small-bowel mesentery (small arrows) is outlined by fluid. (C) The opacified fluid in the left inframesocolic space is partly bounded by the sigmoid mesocolon seen as the fatty plane extending from the sigmoid colon to sacrum (arrows).

discernible, unless they are separated by intervening fluid (Fig. 6-2B) or peritoneal thickening. Vasa recta can be identified within the fatty mesenteric tissue radiating in relationship to the mesenteric borders of small-bowel loops.[3]

The *transverse mesocolon* suspends the transverse colon from the posterior abdominal wall and provides an important route for the spread of disease across the midabdomen. On cross-sectional imaging, the transverse mesocolon can be identified as the fat-containing area extending from the uncinate process, the inferior border of the body and tail of the pancreas to the ventrally positioned transverse colon, containing the middle colic vessels.

The *sigmoid mesocolon* attaches the sigmoid colon to the posterior pelvic wall (Fig. 6-2C) and contains sigmoid and haemorrhoidal vessels. It has an inverted V-shape configuration with its apex lying anterior to the bifurcation of the left common iliac artery.

The Omentum

The *greater omentum* is a four-layered fold that descends from the greater curvature of the stomach, before turning superiorly again to insert into the anterosuperior aspect of the transverse colon. It provides an important pathway of disease spread from the greater curvature of the stomach to the transverse colon and vice versa. It has also an important role in limiting the spread of infectious diseases and confining bowel injuries, whereas it is a common site of involvement in metastatic peritoneal disease. On cross-sectional imaging, the greater omentum is identified as a fatty area extending behind the anterior abdominal wall, sometimes descending deep into the pelvis. There are portions of the greater omentum that are referred to with special names. The gastrocolic ligament is the segment of the greater omentum that links the stomach with the transverse colon. The duodenocolic ligament connects the first portion of the duodenum and the transverse colon. The gastrosplenic ligament extends from the stomach to the splenic hilum (Fig. 6-2A).

The *lesser omentum* or gastrohepatic ligament extends from the lesser curvature of the stomach deep to the fissure for the ligamentum venosum, between the caudate and left hepatic lobes (Fig. 6-1B). It contains the left gastric artery, the coronary vein and the left gastric nodal chain. Disease processes from the stomach extending along the gastrohepatic ligament may invade the liver, as the areolar tissue within the ligament is continuous with the hepatic capsule.[1] The inferior edge of the gastrohepatic ligament, known as the hepatoduodenal ligament, bridges the upper duodenal flexure to the porta hepatis and contains the common hepatic duct, common bile duct, hepatic artery and portal vein.

PATHOLOGICAL CONSIDERATIONS

Ascites

The normal peritoneal cavity contains only a small amount of serous fluid—less than 100 mL. Free-fluid accumulation exceeding this amount is considered to be ascites. Accumulation of fluid in the peritoneal cavity is not a disease by itself, but it is the manifestation of a wide spectrum of processes that may involve intraperitoneal or extraperitoneal organs. Transudative collections may be associated with portal hypertension, cirrhosis, heart failure, nephrotic syndrome or obstruction of the inferior vena cava, hepatic vein or portal vein. Exudative fluid may be related to infection or peritoneal carcinomatosis. Blood collections may be the result of trauma, haemorrhagic diathesis or tumour rupture. Bile collections may follow rupture of the biliary tree; chylous collections may develop after lymphatic obstruction; pancreatic fluid collections may be the consequence of acute pancreatitis; urine collections may represent extension of a retroperitoneal urinoma; purulent collections may be the consequence of visceral inflammation, intestinal perforation or surgery. In general, haematoma, biliary, urinary or purulent collections may be limited by active peritoneal reaction; such reactions form adhesions which limit collections, isolate inflammatory processes and may plug perforations. Consequently, exudates may not move freely in the peritoneal cavity and are usually located or

isolated at the area where they develop compared with transudates, which diffuse throughout the peritoneal cavity with no significant peritoneal reaction.

Peritoneal fluid moves along predictable pathways that are influenced by body habitus, gravity, intra-abdominal pressure gradients, adhesions and mesenteric reflections and attachments.[3] At postmortem and at surgery ascites is mainly seen in the most dependent portion of the peritoneal cavity, namely the pouch of Douglas, which is the lowest and most posterior extension of the peritoneal reflections. In the intact abdomen, fluid migrates to the upper abdomen due to the lower hydrostatic pressure in the subdiaphragmatic related to respiratory movements. Fluid migration occurs along both the paracolic gutters and especially the right one, which is wider and deeper than the left, which in addition has an anatomical obstacle created by the phrenicocolic ligament at the level of the splenic flexure. Peritoneal fluid in the paracolic gutters is distinguished from retroperitoneal fluid by the preservation of the retroperitoneal fat posteriorly to the ascending or descending colon, provided there is not a complete ascending or descending mesocolon.

Ascites in the upper abdomen often accumulates in the pouch of Morison (or hepatorenal space, the most depended portion of the peritoneal cavity in the upper abdomen), the subdiaphragmatic spaces and the perihepatic and perisplenic spaces. Any amount of fluid that may be found in the inframesocolic compartment of the abdomen tends to move towards the lower pelvis; in the right inframesocolic compartment ascites flows along the surface of the small-bowel mesentery to a pouch at the ileocaecal conjunction and in continuation to the pelvis, while in the left inframesocolic compartment the fluid is directed to the surface of the sigmoid mesocolon and, thereafter, to the pelvis.

The CT attenuation values of ascites range from 0 to +30 HU. CT attenuation values are non-specific, although attenuation increases with increasing protein content as a general rule. Acute haemoperitoneum can be distinguished from other fluid collections by its high attenuation values (>30 HU), but lower values may be observed. In the presence of large ascites, the small-bowel loops are usually centrally positioned within the abdomen. However, in patients with very tense ascites, bowel loops can be displaced from the central position in the absence of intraperitoneal mass. Ascitic fluid under tension may result in extraperitoneal mass effect. Peritoneal fluid that becomes loculated due to benign or malignant adhesions may appear as a cystic lesion with mass effect.

Intraperitoneal Air

The most common location of free intraperitoneal air while the patient is in the supine position is anterior to the liver. CT is superior to plain radiographs in detecting minute quantities of pneumoperitoneum and negative window levels (lung settings) are very helpful in disclosing it. Free air demonstrated on CT can be distinguished from gas in the bowel because of its non-dependent location and lack of haustral or small-bowel folds. Perforation of the small bowel may be associated by inflammatory reaction in the mesentery in the form of streaky soft-tissue densities along with presence of extraluminal gas locally.

DEVELOPMENTAL/CONGENITAL ANOMALIES

Rotational Anomaly

Rotational anomalies of the small-bowel mesentery around the superior mesenteric artery occur when the normal process of fetal gut development is arrested. Intestinal malrotation in adults is generally asymptomatic. Reversal of the normal relationship between the superior mesenteric artery and vein, i.e. artery located to the right of vein, twisting of the mesentery around the artery and absence of the normal horizontal duodenum are characteristic findings.[5]

Developmental Defects

Internal hernias are formed by protrusion of a viscus through a peritoneal or mesenteric aperture. They include paraduodenal (53%), pericaecal (13%), foramen of Winslow (8%), transmesenteric and transmesocolic (8%), intersigmoid (6%) and retroanastomotic (5%) hernias. Internal hernias are often difficult to identify clinically. They are asymptomatic or cause symptoms ranging from intermittent and mild digestive complaints to acute intestinal obstruction. Imaging plays an important role in their diagnosis, with CT being the method of choice.

Paraduodenal, traditionally the most common type of internal hernias, result from congenital abnormalities in mesenteric peritoneal fixation. They are three times more frequent on the left side than on the right. Left paraduodenal hernias develop through the Landzert's fossa, which is present in approximately 2% of the population and is located at the duodenojejunal junction; the hernia sac lies posterior to the inferior mesenteric vessels. CT shows an abnormal cluster of dilated loops behind the stomach and pancreas, lateral to the duodenojejunal junction with anterior displacement of the stomach. Anterior displacement of the inferior mesenteric vein is a helpful sign.[5,6]

In right-sided paraduodenal hernias, bowel herniates through Waldeyer's fossa, behind the superior mesenteric artery and inferior to third portion of duodenum. It occurs most frequently in cases of a non-rotated small intestine. Imaging findings include encapsulated small-bowel loops in the right mid-abdomen with anterior displacement of the right colic vein, looping of the small intestine around the superior mesenteric vessels and abnormal position of the superior mesenteric vein relative to the artery.[5]

Transmesenteric hernias are increasing in incidence. They are more likely than other hernias to develop volvulus. In children, transmesenteric hernias are the most common type of internal hernia, related to congenital mesenteric defects. In adults, they are usually related to previous surgery, especially Roux-en-Y anastomoses. On CT, a cluster of dilated loops lying adjacent to the abdominal wall, without overlying omental fat lateral to the colon which is displaced centrally, provides an important clue (Fig. 6-3). The mesenteric vascular pedicle is characteristically engorged, stretched and crowded.[7]

Mesenteric Cysts

Lymphangioma is the most common mesenteric cystic lesion. Other mesenteric cysts like enteric duplication cyst, enteric cyst and mesothelial cyst are very uncommon.

Lymphangioma represents a congenital malformation of the lymphatic vessels arising from the bowel. The typical imaging appearance is that of a large, thin-walled,

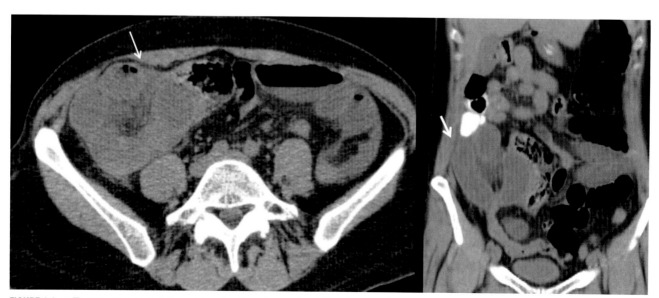

FIGURE 6-3 ■ **Transmesenteric internal hernia.** Unenhanced axial and coronal reformatted CT show a cluster of dilated, fluid-filled loops of small bowel lateral to ascending colon (arrows) beneath anterior abdominal wall, displacing omental fat. Engorged vessels and adjacent mesenteric haziness are also evident, reflecting strangulating obstruction.

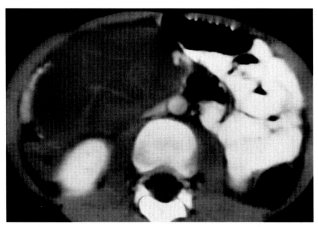

FIGURE 6-4 ■ **Cystic mesenteric lymphangioma.** Enhanced CT depicting a multilocular cystic mass with thin internal septa, occupying the small-bowel mesentery.

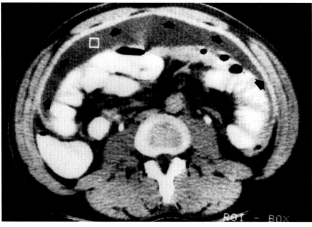

FIGURE 6-5 ■ **Peritoneal tuberculosis.** CT demonstrates marked thickening and enhancement of the parietal peritoneum (arrows). Note high-attenuation ascites (cursor).

single or multiloculated cystic mass, with contents of water-to-fat attenuation on CT (Fig. 6-4) and of high signal intensity on T2-weighted MR images. Enhancement of the cyst wall and septa is seen. It is frequently closely associated with the small bowel. US is helpful in demonstrating the internal septations of the cystic mass.[8]

Large mesenteric lymphangiomas can be differentiated from ascites by the presence of septa, compression on adjacent intestinal loops and lack of fluid in the dependent peritoneal recesses.

INFECTIONS–INFLAMMATIONS

Infective/inflammatory infection of the peritoneal cavity may be localised (abscess) or generalised (peritonitis).

The CT appearance of a peritoneal abscess is variable, depending primarily on its age. In the earliest stages it may appear as a mass displaying attenuation values approximating those of soft tissue. As the process advances, the abscess undergoes liquefactive necrosis. A definable wall that may exhibit contrast enhancement and a nearly water attenuation centre are features of a mature abscess on CT. Accompanying findings include thickening or obliteration of adjacent fat planes and displacement of adjacent structures. Gas within a loculated fluid collection is highly suggestive of abscess, but is not pathognomonic, because a necrotic non-infected tumour or a mass that communicates with the bowel may also contain air.

The CT features of abscesses may overlap with other pathological processes such as haematomas, bilomas, urinomas, necrotic tumours or pseudocysts. MRI is superior to CT in differentiating a haematoma from an abscess, but may miss a small amount of gas within an abscess. A percutaneous fine needle aspiration may reveal the nature of a fluid collection and is important for abscess diagnosis by aspirating pus.

Peritonitis is characterised by a generalised collection of intraperitoneal fluid occurring secondary to bacterial, granulomatous or chemical causes. Although bacterial peritonitis may be primary, it usually results from an intraperitoneal abscess or rupture of a hollow viscus. CT features include ascites in association with peritoneal and mesenteric thickening. Gadolinium-enhanced MR images may show smooth peritoneal enhancement.

Tuberculosis

Tuberculosis of the peritoneum is an uncommon manifestation of tuberculosis that can occur after rupture of a caseous lymph node, from direct GI tract involvement by the disease or by lymphatic or haematogenous spread.

Common findings include the combination of free or loculated ascites, thickened strands with crowded vascular bundles within mesentery, smooth uniform thickening of the peritoneum and a smudged pattern of omental involvement infiltrated by small ill-defined soft tissue (Fig. 6-5).[9] On CT, high-attenuation ascites (20–45 HU), reflecting its high protein content, may be seen. Lymphadenopathy is a common manifestation of abdominal tuberculosis and mesenteric nodes are frequently affected.

Peripheral enhancement with central low attenuation on CT may be seen and corresponds histologically to peripheral highly vascular inflammatory reaction around central liquefaction or caseous necrosis.[10] This appearance is suggestive but not pathognomonic of tuberculosis as low-attenuation mesenteric lymph nodes may also be seen with Whipple's disease, necrotic metastases, infection with *Mycobacterium avium-intracellulare*, the cavitating mesenteric lymph node syndrome of coeliac disease and occasionally lymphoma.[11]

Hydatid Disease

Hydatid disease is most commonly due to *Echinococcus granulosus*. Peritoneal hydatidosis is usually the result of traumatic or surgical rupture of hepatic hydatid disease and results in cystic, usually septated, thin-walled space-occupying lesions.[12] CT is the method of choice in peritoneal seeding (Fig. 6-6). A calcifying rim is a suggestive feature. Ultrasound is useful for the detection of membranes, septa and hydatid sand within the cyst.

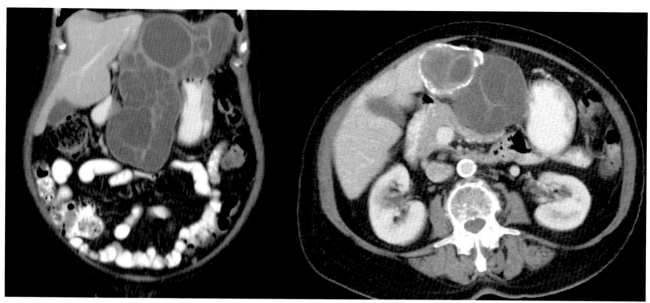

FIGURE 6-6 ■ **Peritoneal hydatidosis.** Enhanced CT shows a large multiseptated cystic peritoneal mass. Daughter cysts may be seen within the cyst, resulting in a septated, almost honeycomb, appearance. Rim calcification is characteristic.

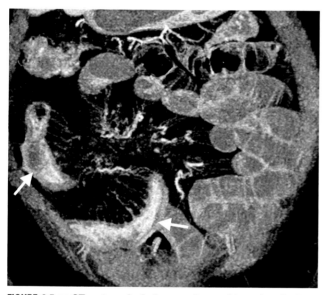

FIGURE 6-7 ■ **CT enteroclysis in a patient with active Crohn's disease.** Enhanced CT, MIP reconstruction, shows extensive ileal Crohn's disease (arrows) with fibrofatty proliferation of the mesentery and segmental hyperaemia.

Crohn's Disease

Mesenteric abnormalities are commonly seen in Crohn's disease. Hypertrophied mesenteric adipose tissue, known as fibrofatty mesenteric proliferation, constitutes a characteristic feature of Crohn's disease. On cross-sectional imaging it appears as an increased quantity of mesenteric fat, producing a mass effect on adjacent loops, predominantly along the mesenteric side of the bowel (Fig. 6-7). Fibrofatty proliferation remains present in clinically quiescent disease, while engorged vasa recta (the 'comb sign') indicate active inflammation. MDCT/MRI can provide excellent information concerning mesenteric involvement and complications of Crohn's disease.[13]

Mesenteric Lymphadenitis

This is an appendicitis-mimicking clinical diagnosis, with self-limited symptoms that relate to benign inflammation of lymph nodes within the ileal mesentery. US and CT may demonstrate clustered, moderately enlarged mesenteric lymph nodes in the right lower quadrant without any identifiable inflammatory process. The diameter usually does not exceed 10 mm in short axis. Occasionally, an underlying terminal ileitis may be the cause of mesenteric adenitis.[10]

Acute Pancreatitis

In acute pancreatitis, extravasated pancreatic enzymes may dissect along the mesenteric pathways.[1] An extrapancreatic acute fluid collection may spread along the root of transverse mesocolon and, at times, of small-bowel mesentery and extend along the vessels to the vasa recta of the transverse colon and small bowel (Fig. 6-8).[5]

Whipple's Disease

Whipple disease is a rare multisystemic infection caused by a Gram-positive bacillus. Low-attenuation mesenteric and retroperitoneal lymph nodes due to deposition of fat and fatty acids within the nodes are demonstrated on CT, in association with diffuse intestinal wall thickening (Fig. 6-9).[10,14]

Mesenteric Panniculitis–Sclerosing Mesenteritis

This complex disease entity is a rare, slowly progressive chronic inflammatory disorder of unknown origin

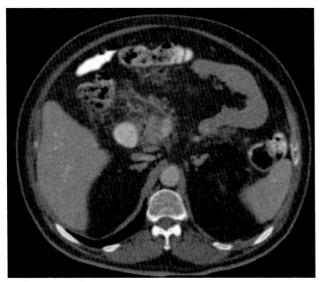

FIGURE 6-8 ■ **Spread of acute pancreatitis.** Enhanced CT shows the inflammatory changes spreading at the root of the transverse mesocolon toward the transverse colon.

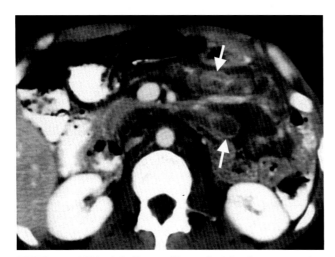

FIGURE 6-9 ■ **Whipple's disease.** Non-enhancing low-attenuation lymph nodes are seen within the small-bowel mesentery (arrows).

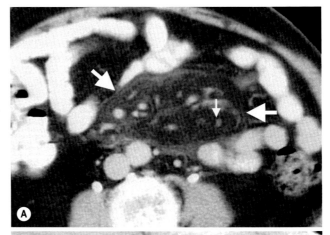

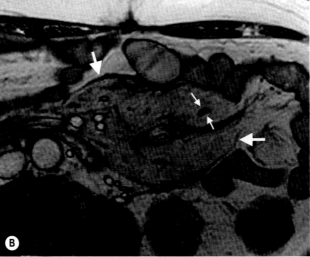

FIGURE 6-10 ■ **Mesenteric panniculitis.** Enhanced CT (A) and true-FISP MRI (B) in a patient who presented with abdominal pain show a well-delineated fatty mass (large arrows) extending from the root of the small-bowel mesentery towards the left abdomen, engulfing mesenteric vessels without distortion. Note the perivascular halo (small arrows).

involving the adipose tissue of the small-bowel mesentery and occasionally the mesocolon. It is now considered a single disease with two pathological subgroups. When inflammation and fatty necrosis are predominant components, it is known as mesenteric panniculitis. When fibrosis and retraction predominate, the disease is called sclerosing or retractile mesenteritis.

Various underlying causes, including prior abdominal surgery/trauma, autoimmune processes or malignancy, have been suggested. The disease is often asymptomatic. When present, symptoms are non-specific, including abdominal pain, diarrhoea, weight loss and fever of unknown origin.[15] While a definite diagnosis requires surgical excision biopsy, in the majority of cases the disease is suggested on the basis of imaging features.

A well-delineated, heterogeneous fatty mass at the mesenteric root, envelopment of mesenteric vessels, absence of adjacent bowel loops involvement, which may or may not be displaced, and low-attenuation halo surrounding vessels (Fig. 6-10) are the characteristic CT features of *mesenteric panniculitis*.[16] A hypointense capsule is demonstrated on T2-weighted MR images that shows contrast enhancement after intravenous gadolinium administration.

Retractile mesenteritis appears on CT as an infiltrative soft-tissue mass with associated radiating linear strands of soft-tissue attenuation (Fig. 6-11). These features may mimic those of fibromatosis or carcinoid tumours. MRI may help in the differentiation by showing low signal intensity on both T1- and T2-weighted images in sclerosing mesenteritis. Calcification may be present in the necrotic central portion of the mass (Fig. 6-12). The disease entity usually has a favourable prognosis and may be self-limiting.

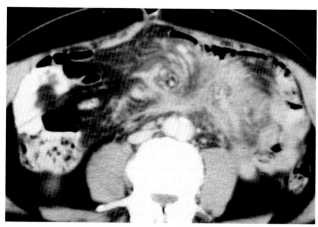

FIGURE 6-11 ■ **Fibrosing mesenteritis.** Enhanced CT in a patient who presented with fever of unknown origin demonstrates a fibrofatty mesenteric mass with irregular borders surrounding mesenteric vessels. Strands of soft-tissue density are seen radiating from the mass to the adjacent mesenteric fat.

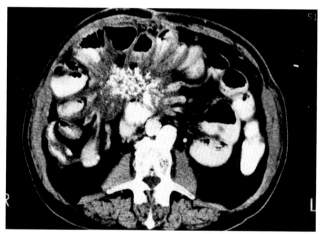

FIGURE 6-12 ■ **Fibrosing mesenteritis: CT appearances.** Enhanced abdominal CT demonstrating a large, ill-defined, soft-tissue mesenteric mass with extensive calcification. Note retraction and thickening of the adjacent bowel loops.

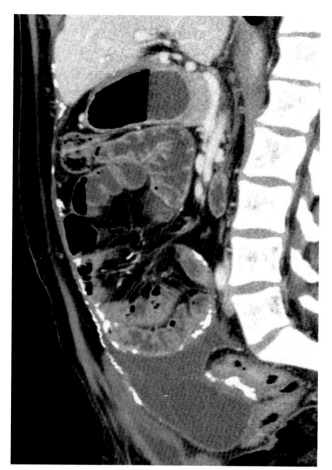

FIGURE 6-13 ■ **Sclerosing peritonitis.** Enhanced CT shows loculated fluid collection and extensive peritoneal calcification.

Sclerosing Peritonitis

Sclerosing peritonitis, also known as encapsulating peritoneal sclerosis, is a rare chronic inflammatory disorder of the peritoneum associated with significant morbidity and mortality that occurs most commonly in patients who undergo continuous ambulatory peritoneal dialysis. Other rare causes include abdominal tuberculosis, recurrent peritonitis, long-term β-blocker treatment (practolol), sarcoidosis, etc. Patients may be asymptomatic or have nausea, anorexia, malnutrition, weight loss and recurrent episodes of small-bowel obstruction. CT is the optimal investigation for disclosing sclerosing peritonitis. Smooth or irregular and nodular peritoneal thickening and calcification, marked enhancement of the peritoneum, loculated fluid collections and tethered, thick-walled small-bowel loops are considered characteristic CT features (Fig. 6-13).[17,18]

Non-inflammatory Oedema

Mesenteric oedema is defined as a diffuse increase in attenuation throughout the mesentery that obscures visualisation of the normally well-defined mesenteric vessels as they course to the bowel walls. It may be secondary to various causes, including hypoalbuminaemia, cirrhosis, nephrotic syndrome, right-sided congestive heart failure, mesenteric ischaemia, vasculitis or trauma. Increased attenuation of the mesenteric fat and abnormal signal is seen on CT and MRI, respectively. The extent and site of involvement may contribute to the differential diagnosis.

In systemic diseases, such as cirrhosis or heart failure, mesenteric oedema is manifested as a diffuse haziness extending from the root of the mesentery to the bowel surface, associated with congestion and blurring of the mesenteric vascular markings. It is usually accompanied by ascites and generalised subcutaneous and retroperitoneal fat haziness secondary to generalised oedema.

Hypoxia in acute mesenteric ischaemia causes a generalised increase in capillary permeability and consequently produces submucosal oedema. As ischaemia advances, venules in the mesentery become engorged with oedema and blood. If the ischaemic episode is not reversed, arterial flow to the involved segment becomes totally suspended. Mesenteric oedema secondary to

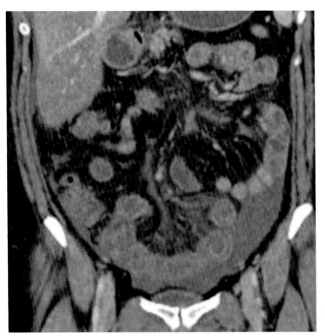

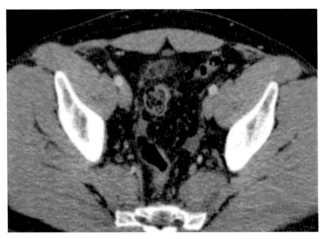

FIGURE 6-15 ■ **Epiploic appendagitis.** Enhanced CT shows the inflamed appendix epiploica as a fatty mass with hyperattenuating rim anterior to the sigmoid colon with some surrounding inflammation. The patient's symptoms subsided after anti-inflammatory therapy.

FIGURE 6-14 ■ **Thrombotic occlusion of superior mesenteric vein.** Enhanced CT shows localised haziness in the affected ileal mesentery with effacement of vascular markings as a result of occlusion of superior mesenteric vein and ileal branches. Mural thickening of the involved bowel loops is also seen.

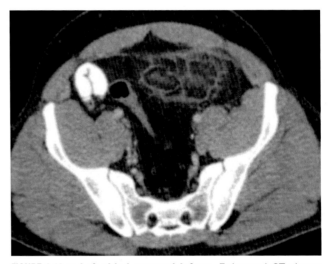

FIGURE 6-16 ■ **Left-sided omental infarct.** Enhanced CT shows an 8-cm-diameter heterogeneous fatty mass deep to the left rectus abdominal muscle and parietal peritoneum with surrounding inflammation.

mesenteric ischaemia may be focal or diffuse, depending on the site and extent of vascular compromise. As a result of oedema, increased attenuation of the mesenteric fat is seen on CT, together with poor definition of segmental mesenteric vessels (Fig. 6-14).

Epiploic Appendagitis

Epiploic appendagitis results from torsion or thrombosis of epiploic appendages. Clinical findings resemble acute diverticulitis or appendicitis. In the majority of cases, it is a self-limiting condition. CT findings of epiploic appendagitis are usually diagnostic, avoiding unnecessary surgery. The most common CT feature is an oval fatty lesion less than 5 cm in diameter surrounded by inflammatory changes and in contact with the serosal surface of the colon. A hyperattenuated rim that surrounds the mass and represents the inflamed visceral peritoneal lining may also be observed (Fig. 6-15). The lesion usually contains a central area of high attenuation corresponding to thrombosed vessels.[19,20] Mild reactive thickening of the adjacent colonic wall is often found.

Omental Infarction

Segmental omental infarction is an uncommon cause of acute abdominal pain resulting from vascular compromise of the greater omentum. Primary omental torsion, attributed to congenital or vascular variations that predispose to venous thrombosis, is right-sided. Obesity has especially been postulated as an important risk factor. Secondary omental infarction is related to pre-existing

abdominal pre-existing disease including surgery, abdominal inflammatory foci, tumours and hernial sacs and is located near the site of initial insult.

Typical CT findings include a large heterogeneous omental mass containing hyperattenuating streaks that is most often located in the right lower quadrant (Fig. 6-16). The mass is usually larger than 5 cm, differentiating it from epiploic appendagitis.[10,19,20] The appropriate treatment is conservative.

NEOPLASTIC DISEASES

Neoplastic Diseases of Peritoneum

Nearly all peritoneal masses neoplasms are malignant. Secondary neoplasms are the most common malignancies involving the peritoneum. They can disseminate through the peritoneum by four pathways: direct invasion, intraperitoneal seeding, lymphatic permeation and embolic haematogenous spread.[3] Although the imaging patterns of metastatic disease may coexist, many neoplasms metastasise predominantly by one particular route, indicating the primary site.

Direct Spread Along Mesenteric and Ligamentous Attachments

Malignant tumours of the stomach, colon, pancreas and ovary that have penetrated beyond the borders of these organs can spread directly along the adjacent visceral peritoneal surfaces to involve other structures. Early peritoneal invasion is manifested as linear strands in the fat adjacent to primary tumour. A mass contiguous with the primary neoplasm reflects more advanced dissemination. The mass may spread through the ligamentous attachments to involve other abdominal structures.[1] In this way, gastric malignancy may extend to the spleen via the gastrosplenic ligament or invade the superior margin of the transverse colon along the gastrocolic ligament and vice versa (Fig. 6-17). Biliary tumours spread along the gastrohepatic and hepatoduodenal ligaments. Retroperitoneal tumours, such as pancreatic carcinoma, may directly invade the liver via the hepatoduodenal ligament or spread along the transverse mesocolon to the inferior border of the transverse colon. Pancreatic carcinoma may also directly invade the splenic hilum through the

splenorenal ligament or the splenic flexure through the phrenicocolic ligament.[21] Ovarian carcinoma may spread diffusely through all adjacent peritoneal surfaces.

Intraperitoneal Seeding and Peritoneal Carcinomatosis

Peritoneal seeding is a common mechanism of metastatic dissemination in advanced gastrointestinal and gynaecological malignancies. *Peritoneal carcinomatosis* (PC) is the term given to malignant tumour seeding of the peritoneum with most common primaries being the ovarian (71%), gastric (17%) and colorectal (10%) cancers. When cancer cells from a growing primary neoplasm reach the peritoneal surface, they are carried out by the peritoneal fluid and disseminated throughout the peritoneal cavity. Distribution of disease in PC is related to peritoneal fluid circulation along predetermined anatomical routes as previously described in the section 'Ascites'. This peritoneal fluid circulation and the areas of temporal stasis of fluid explain the distribution of peritoneal seeding. Pooling of ascites favours the deposition and growth of seeded malignant cells. The most common seeding sites include the pouch of Douglas, the distal small-bowel mesentery near the ileocaecal junction, the sigmoid mesocolon, the right paracolic gutter, the pouch of Morison and the right subdiaphragmatic area.[3] In general, more aggressive neoplasms exhibit malignant peritoneal deposits closer to the primary tumour, as opposed to less aggressive neoplasms that tend to manifest deposits in remote areas in the abdominal cavity. Variable amounts of ascites may accompany peritoneal seeding but ascites is not always present. Ascitic fluid is sometimes locculated and/or septated, and therefore it may be absent in dependent areas such as the pelvis. Peritoneal deposits (Fig. 6-18) may appear as thickening or enhancement of the

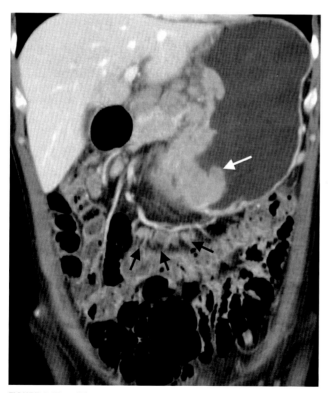

FIGURE 6-17 ■ **Direct extension of gastric carcinoma across the gastrocolic ligament.** Greater curvature carcinoma (white arrow) has spread inferiorly along the gastrocolic ligament to the anterior surface of the transverse colon (black arrows).

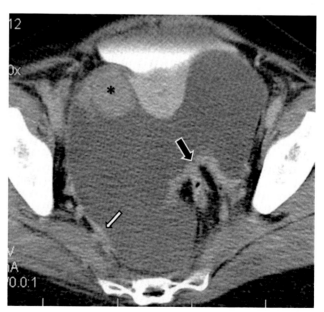

FIGURE 6-18 ■ **Malignant peritoneal implants in the form of (i) peritoneal thickening (white arrow), (ii) plaque (black arrow) and (iii) mass (asterisk).** The presence of ascites in the pelvis facilitates the demonstration of type (i) and (ii) lesions.

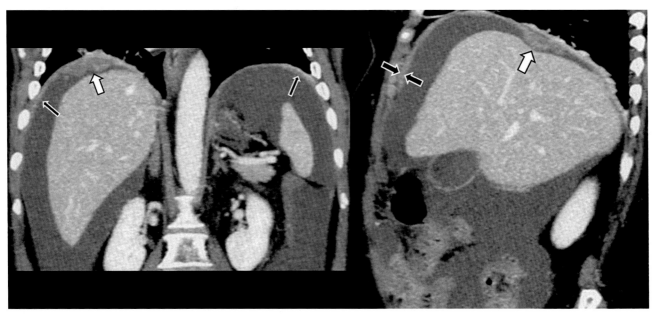

FIGURE 6-19 ■ **Coronal (left) and sagittal (right) reformations from axial MDCT images favour the visibility of peritoneal carcinomatosis.** Irregular thickening and mild enhancement of the parietal peritoneum underneath both hemidiaphragms (long black arrows) and presence of masses (white arrows) corresponding to extensive peritoneal carcinomatosis. A small nodular deposit is barely seen at the left paracolic gutter (small thick black arrows), close to the phrenicocolic ligament.

peritoneum, nodules or plaques on the peritoneal surfaces, masses or merely stranding of the mesenteric fat.

MDCT with coronal and sagittal reformations (Fig. 6-19) is considered the optimal technique for detecting the presence, location and extent of peritoneal carcinomatosis; overall diagnostic accuracy of 94%, specificity of 92% and sensitivities between 75 and 81% have been reported;[22] however, sensitivity for identifying small lesions by MDCT is significantly lower. Implantation of tumour deposits along the peritoneal surfaces of the diaphragm, liver and spleen results in smooth, nodular, or plaque-like thickening and contrast enhancement of the parietal peritoneal lining. However, these features are not specific for peritoneal carcinomatosis as they may be seen with other processes that seed the peritoneum, including tuberculosis, peritoneal mesothelioma and peritoneal lymphomatosis. Contrast-enhanced T1-weighted MR images with fat saturation can improve the detection of smaller or equivocal implants or of numerous very small implants that may be manifested as a contiguous 'line-type' enhancement along the peritoneal surfaces (Fig. 6-20). Peritoneal tumours often enhance slowly and are best seen on images obtained 5 min after injection of gadolinium. The combination of diffuse-weighted images (DWI) and conventional MRI improves the accuracy of MRI for depicting peritoneal implants;[23] therefore, DWI is suggested as an indispensable part of any MRI evaluation in patients suspected for PC.[23] DW-MRI and FDG-PET/CT are promising methods for the evaluation of peritoneal carcinomatosis,[23,24] but still have a limited role, especially for the identification of disease relapse after treatment. Calcification within peritoneal implants before chemotherapy suggests that the primary site is either serous papillary cystadenocarcinoma of the ovary, or, rarely, gastric carcinoma (Fig. 6-21).

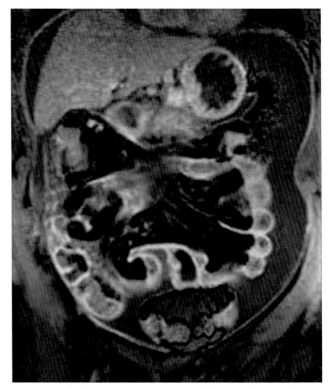

FIGURE 6-20 ■ Coronal T1-weighted MRI with fat saturation, after gadolinium administration demonstrating generalised thickening and enhancement of the parietal peritoneum and also of the peritoneal surface of the small-bowel mesentery, due to extensive peritoneal carcinomatosis. Ascites is also present.

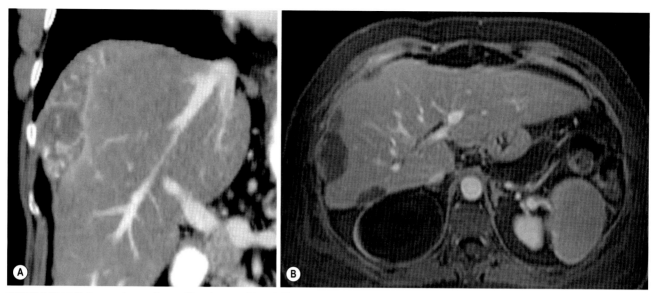

FIGURE 6-21 ■ **Subcapsular peritoneal implants with calcifications.** (A) Enhanced CT coronal reformatted image shows implants with calcifications that cause indentation on liver surface. (B) Corresponding axial T1-weighted post-gadolinium MRI exhibits implants of low signal intensity.

The evolution of *cytoreductive surgery* (CRS) has revolutionised the treatment of PC and is a challenge for imaging. Cytoreductive surgery aims at complete resection of tumour-bearing peritoneal surfaces and abdominal organs. Optimal CRS requires excision of any visible malignant peritoneal deposit. Complete CRS is often followed by *hyperthermic intraperitoneal chemotherapy* (HIPEC) to eliminate minimal residual PC. CRS with HIPEC is associated with significantly improved, progression-free and overall survival. Imaging techniques have an important role in the preoperative evaluation of PC and in the selection of candidates for CRS-HIPEC. Analysis of imaging findings should be performed on a site-by-site basis and the presence, type and size of peritoneal seeding should be reported in every region of the peritoneal cavity. Preoperative assessment of the overall disease burden and the extent of involvement in specific peritoneal areas are of decisive significance in the selection of patients that could benefit from CRS and in surgical planning.[25] For example, extensive involvement of the hepatoduodenal ligament or of the small-bowel mesentery may preclude a complete CRS, while infiltration of the ligaments suspending the stomach by PC may indicate the need for gastrectomy (Fig. 6-22).

Pseudomyxoma peritonei is a specific type of peritoneal neoplasia due to ruptured benign or malignant mucin-producing tumour of the appendix, ovary and, occasionally, pancreas, stomach, colorectal or urachus. Suggestive imaging findings include masses of low attenuation on CT and moderately high signal intensity on MRI, accompanied by ascites with septations representing the margins of mucinous nodules, scalloping of visceral surfaces especially the liver by adjacent mucinous peritoneal implants, and soft-tissue thickening of the peritoneal surfaces, reflecting the more solid components of the tumour.[26]

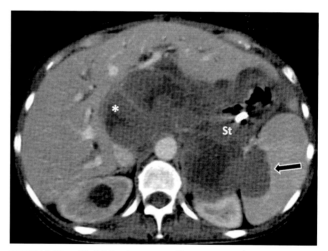

FIGURE 6-22 ■ **Multiple, large, confluent masses involving the region of the hepatoduodenal ligament (asterisk), infiltrating the spleen (arrow) and surrounding the stomach (St).**

Primary Neoplasms

Primary neoplasms of peritoneal origin are found less frequently than metastastic disease and include malignant mesothelioma, cystic mesothelioma, primary peritoneal serous carcinoma and desmoplastic small round cell tumour.

Malignant mesothelioma, most often seen in middle-aged men, is associated with asbestos exposure. Peritoneal involvement may occur, either alone or in association with pleural involvement. Imaging findings[27,28] include diffuse or nodular thickening of the peritoneum, omental thickening, a stellate mesenteric appearance or peritoneal and omental masses, with variable ascites, usually mild to moderate (Fig. 6-23). Local invasion of adjacent

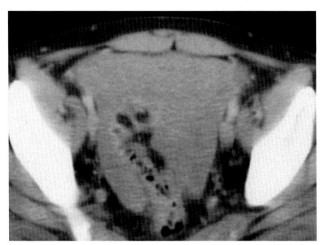

FIGURE 6-23 ■ **Peritoneal mesothelioma.** Enhanced CT shows a soft-tissue mass that obliterates pelvic peritoneal spaces and engulfs the sigmoid colon.

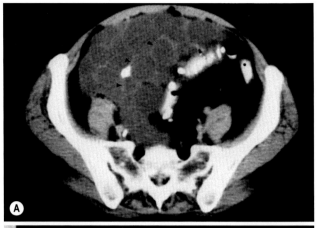

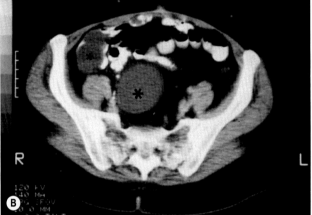

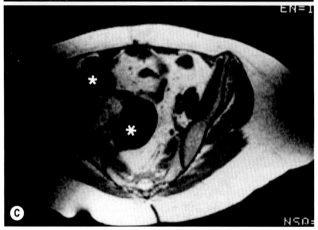

FIGURE 6-24 ■ **Cystic mesothelioma: CT and MRI findings.** (A) Enhanced CT demonstrates a well-defined, multilocular cystic mass with thin septations (arrowheads). (B) Sixteen months after resection, CT of the pelvis reveals two thin-walled cystic masses with serous contents (asterisks) representing local recurrence. (C) A corresponding T1-weighted MRI image reveals the watery nature of the fluid seen within the locules of the recurrent cystic mesothelioma (asterisks).

abdominal organs may be seen.[29] Enhancement of the peritoneal nodules or masses is typically seen on CT.[27] Diffuse malignant mesotheliomas are highly aggressive in contrast to localised mesotheliomas that usually have a good prognosis.[27] The differential diagnosis includes the more frequent peritoneal carcinomatosis and other abdominal processes such as tuberculous peritonitis, peritoneal lymphomatosis, peritoneal sarcomatosis, and pseudomyxoma peritonei. Malignant peritoneal mesothelioma appears similar to carcinomatosis but should be considered when sheet-like peritoneal thickening predominates. A smooth peritoneum with minimal thickening and marked enhancement suggests tuberculous peritonitis. Bulky mesenteric and retroperitoneal lymph node enlargement is the most prominent feature of lymphomatosis. Features suggesting sarcomatosis are heterogeneous bulky masses with hypervascularity, and variable ascites,[30] while liver scalloping and septate ascites should raise the possibility of pseudomyxoma peritonei; leiomyomatosis peritonealis disseminata should be considered if uterine leiomyomas are present.[27]

Cystic mesothelioma, also known as peritoneal inclusion cyst, is a rare non-malignant subtype of mesothelioma, most frequently found in the pelvis. It may be seen as a unilocular or complex cystic mass comprising cysts of 1 mm to 6 cm in size, simulating cystic lymphangioma or cystic epithelial neoplasms of the ovaries (Fig. 6-24).

Primary peritoneal serous carcinoma is derived from extraovarian mesothelium and occurs in postmenopausal women. It is histologically identical to serous ovary adenocarcinoma. Imaging findings include ascites, peritoneal and omental thickening and peritoneal and omental enhancing nodules; psammomatous calcification may be seen.[27]

Desmoplastic small round cell tumour is a rare aggressive malignancy occurring in adolescents and young adults. Bulky heterogeneous peritoneal masses usually originating in the omentum or paravesical region are characteristic.[31]

Neoplastic Diseases of Mesentery

Primary neoplasms arising in the mesentery are rare and usually of mesenchymal origin.[32] Benign primary mesenteric tumours such as desmoids, lipomas and neurofibromas are more common than malignant ones, such as fibrosarcoma (Fig. 6-25), liposarcoma or mesothelioma. Secondary neoplasms are more frequent than the primary malignancies and cystic tumours are more common than solid ones.

Primary Neoplasms

Primary neoplasms arising in the mesentery are rare and most are histologically benign, with fibromatosis being the commonest primary tumour.

Fibromatosis, or desmoid tumour, results from a benign proliferation of fibrous tissue. Although it can occur sporadically, desmoid tumours are especially common in patients with familial adenomatous polyposis (FAP), particularly those with Gardner's syndrome. They are often locally aggressive but do not metastasise. The imaging features reflect the relative abundance of collagen or myxoid stroma within the lesion.[33] On CT, lesions with highly collagenous stroma appear homogeneous, whereas those with myxoid stroma are hypoattenuated. A whorled appearance is described in lesions with both collagenous and myxoid areas. MRI shows low or intermediate signal intensity on T1-weighted images and variable signal intensity on T2 images (Fig. 6-26). The amount of hyperintensity on T2 images reflects the degree of cellularity and myxoid stroma.[34] Contrast material enhancement is variable on both CT and MRI.[33] It may be complicated by mesenteric ischaemia (Fig. 6-27) or intestinal obstruction. Fibromatosis accompanied by FAP (Fig. 6-28) is reported to be more invasive with higher local relapse rates.[33]

Lipomas are the second most common primary solid tumours of the mesentery, after fibromatosis. They appear as well-circumscribed homogeneous masses and are easy to diagnose on CT since they are composed entirely of low-attenuation fat. On MRI, they exhibit the characteristic high signal of fat on both T1- and T2-weighted images that turns to low signal when fat saturation techniques are applied. Internal septations are unusual.

Liposarcomas develop more frequently in the retroperitoneum than in the mesentery or peritoneum. Histologically, liposarcomas are classified, in increasing order of malignancy, as, myxoid, well-differentiated, pleomorphic, and round cell subtypes. They have variable CT and MR imaging appearances, reflecting their tissue composition, ranging from predominantly fat, fluid and soft-tissue elements to entirely soft-tissue density masses. Fat attenuation is less likely to be found in higher-grade liposarcomas such as the pleomorphic, and round cell subtypes (Fig. 6-29).[35]

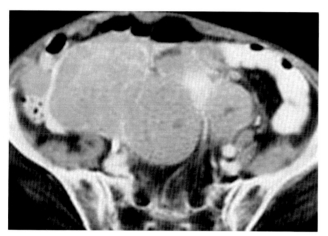

FIGURE 6-25 ■ **Mesenteric fibrosarcoma.** Enhanced CT shows an enhancing soft-tissue mass in the small-bowel mesentery compressing a neighbouring small intestinal loop.

Secondary Neoplasms

The most common malignancies spreading into the mesentery are secondary carcinoma, lymphoma and carcinoid tumour.

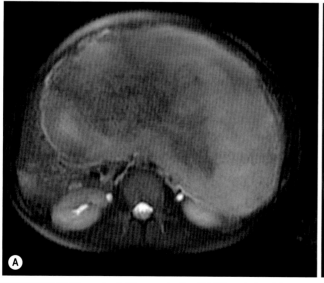
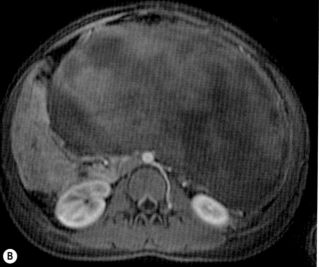

FIGURE 6-26 ■ **Mesenteric fibromatosis.** (A) T2-weighted fat-suppressed MR image shows a well-defined heterogeneous mass. The high signal intensity areas correspond to mucin within the mass. (B) Post-gadolinium T1-weighted fat-suppressed MR image demonstrates inhomogeneous enhancement of the mass.

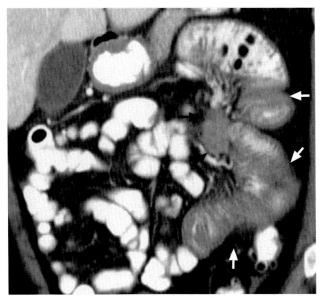

FIGURE 6-27 ■ **Mesenteric fibromatosis.** Enhanced CT shows a soft-tissue mass in the mesentery (black arrows), resulting in segmental jejunal ischaemia, manifested as symmetrical wall thickening (white arrows).

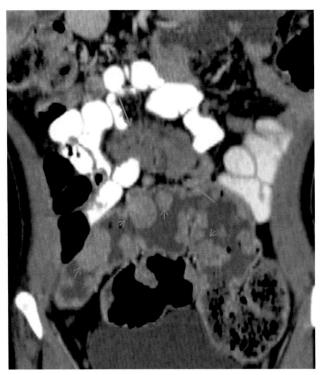

FIGURE 6-28 ■ **Mesenteric fibromatosis in familial adenomatous polyposis.** Enhanced CT shows homogeneous soft-tissue mass with ill-defined borders centred in the small-bowel mesentery (arrows) together with numerous polyps in sigmoid colon (small arrows).

Secondary Carcinoma. Primary neoplasms spread through mesentery by discrete pathways, producing characteristic imaging appearances.

Intraperitoneal Tumour Dissemination. The small-bowel mesentery is frequently involved by intra-peritoneally disseminated tumour. Common, although

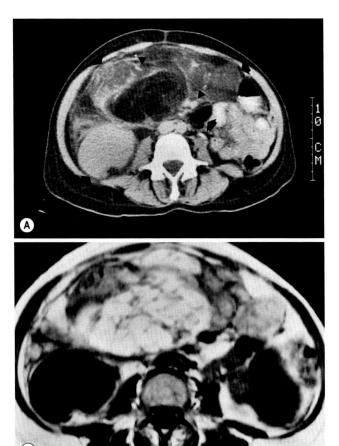

FIGURE 6-29 ■ **Liposarcoma: CT–MR pathological correlation.** (A) Enhanced CT of the abdomen demonstrates a large mesenteric mass (arrows) with both fat and soft-tissue densities, encasing large peripheral vessels (arrowheads). (B) T1-weighted spin-echo image demonstrating the multiple fibrous strands seen in this liposarcoma, as well as two components, one brighter centrally (corresponding to a fatty element) and a lower-intensity peripheral component (corresponding to an undifferentiated sarcomatous element).

non-specific, imaging findings include scattered nodules, rounded, ill-defined soft-tissue or cystic masses and mesenteric fixation and thickening of the mesentery. The latter may demonstrate either a stellate or a pleated form.[32] In the stellate appearance, a radiating configuration of the mesenteric folds with thickened rigid perivascular bundles and encased, straightened vascular structures is observed. A stellate pattern of infiltration has also been described in peritoneal lymphomatosis.[32] In the pleated appearance, sheets of soft tissue produce thickening of the mesenteric folds. As metastatic tumour deposits involve the surface of the mesentery, the mesenteric fat is compressed rather than invaded. There is usually associated fluid, at times loculated. When ascites is extensive, it tends to surround the bowel loops, which are tethered centrally by the rigid mesentery. Diffuse infiltration of the mesentery by metastatic tumour may result in appearances resembling mesenteric oedema in some cases. Fixation of mesenteric folds, more apparent on repeated CT in the lateral or prone position, may aid the differential diagnosis. Peritoneal seeding may result in metastatic

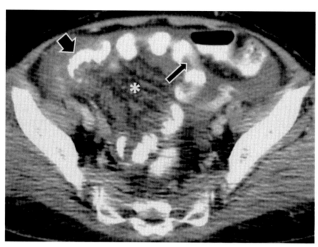

FIGURE 6-30 ■ **Extensive peritoneal seeding in the small bowel and its mesentery with a nodule (thin arrow), an irregular mural thickening with fixation (thick arrow) and mesenteric surface nodularity (asterisk).**

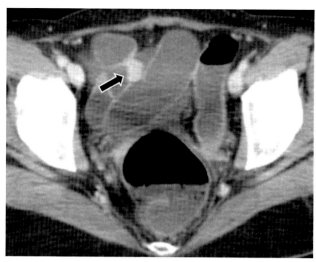

FIGURE 6-31 ■ **CT enteroclysis with distension of ileal loops.** A nodular peritoneal implant on the small-bowel surface is clearly visible (arrow).

tumour nodules in the visceral peritoneal surfaces adherent to the serosa of small-bowel loops (Fig. 6-30). Larger metastatic mesenteric lesions maintain their relationship with the distal small-bowel mesentery and they may cause inferior and medial displacement of ileal loops. In cases of severe desmoplastic response to the seeded metastases, the marked fixation and angulation of ileal loops may lead to obstruction.

Involvement of the small bowel (SB) and SB mesentery is considered an independent prognostic factor of survival in patients with peritoneal carcinomatosis. The extent of SB/SB mesentery involvement by peritoneal seeding is crucial in the selection process of candidates for CRS and it is also important for surgical planning. Furthermore, SB mesentery is a common location of suboptimally debulked disease after CRS. As opposed to the clinical significance of an accurate preoperative evaluation of peritoneal seeding affecting the SB/SB mesentery, cross-sectional imaging presents the lowest sensitivity and diagnostic accuracy in this specific area. CT enteroclysis with SB distension by negative contrast medium results in increased sensitivity and specificity in the diagnosis of the extent of SB/SB mesentery involvement by peritoneal carcinomatosis[36] and it has been proposed in the preoperative work-up in candidates for CRS (Fig. 6-31).

Embolic Metastases. Embolic metastases from melanoma and lung or breast carcinoma can spread via mesenteric arteries to locate along the anti-mesenteric border of the small bowel. CT manifestations include focal bowel wall thickening and thickening of the mesenteric folds.[29,32] Melanoma deposits may become large and ulcerated. Breast cancer deposits may cause multiple areas of small-bowel luminal narrowing with prestenotic dilatation.[37]

Lymphatic Dissemination. Lymphatic permeation plays a minor role in the spread of metastatic carcinoma but it is the main pathway of dissemination of lymphoma to mesenteric lymph nodes. Enlarged mesenteric lymph nodes occur at presentation in approximately 50% of patients with non-Hodgkin's lymphoma. Confluent lymphomatous nodes may surround the superior mesenteric vessels, producing a sandwich-like appearance. Coexistent lymphomatous mural involvement of the small-bowel loops affects their mesenteric border.[1]

Carcinoid. The small intestine is the commonest location for gastrointestinal carcinoid tumours. Approximately 40–80% of gastrointestinal carcinoids spread to the mesentery, either by direct extension or through the local lymphatics.[32] Since the primary tumour in the small bowel can be quite small, and occasionally occult, metastasis to the small-bowel mesentery is usually discovered first. Secondary involvement of the mesentery usually leads to a desmoplastic reaction incited by local release of serotonin and other vasoactive substances. On barium studies, desmoplastic reaction appears as angulation, tethering and fixation of the involved small-bowel loops. CT/MR enterography is a valuable tool for evaluating patients suspected of having carcinoid tumours, since it may depict not only characteristic appearance of infiltrated mesentery but also the primary mural nodule. Carcinoid metastatic in the small-bowel mesentery manifests as hypervascular enhancing soft-tissue masses with well-defined or spiculated borders (Fig. 6-32). Radiating linear bands in the mesenteric fat result from the intense fibrotic proliferation and desmoplastic reaction. The degree of radiating strands tends to increase with the degree of fibrosis seen histopathologically.[32,38] Segmental wall thickening of adjacent bowel loops resulting from chronic ischaemia or tumour infiltration as well as angulation can be seen. Dystrophic calcification is present in up to 40% of carcinoids on CT.[38]

On MRI the lesions exhibit low T1 signal intensity, high T2 signal intensity and moderately intense gadolinium enhancement.[39] Currently, somatostatin-receptor scintigraphy with ^{111}In-octreotide, ^{111}In-pentetreotide and ^{123}I-metaiodobenzylguanidine is the study of choice for imaging carcinoid and its metastatic spread.[40]

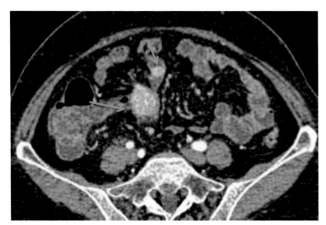

FIGURE 6-32 ■ **Carcinoid.** Enhanced CT shows a smoothly marginated enhancing mesenteric mass (large arrow) representing lymph node metastasis. An intensely enhanced mural nodule in ileum (small arrow) is seen corresponding to carcinoid tumour.

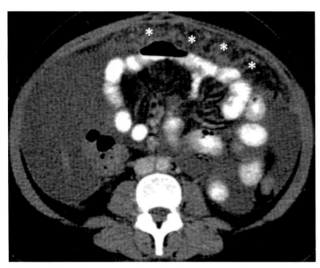

FIGURE 6-33 ■ **Omental infiltration by peritoneal carcinomatosis.** Thickening of the omentum and irregular soft-tissue permeation of the omental fat (asterisks).

Neoplastic Diseases of the Omentum

Primary neoplasms of the greater omentum, both benign and malignant, are similar to those that are also encountered in the mesentery. Benign neoplasms are usually well circumscribed and localised in the omentum. Malignant neoplasms frequently have indistinct margins and infiltrate surrounding structures.[21]

Secondary neoplasms of the omentum are more common than primary lesions. Secondary malignancies involving the omentum are similar to those responsible for peritoneal carcinomatosis, with the ovary being the most common source. The greater omentum is usually involved, since it is the site for re-absorption of the peritoneal fluid containing cancer cells. In addition, the greater omentum may be involved either by direct spread along the transverse mesocolon, the gastrosplenic, or gastrocolic ligaments or by peritoneal or haematogenous spread.

Early omental involvement is manifested on CT as omental thickening with increased attenuation values of the fat, fat stranding, nodules or irregular soft-tissue permeation of the omental fat (Fig. 6-33). In advanced seeding spread, the deposits range from discrete nodules to thick, confluent solid omental masses, the so-called omental 'cake'. At CT, metastatic implants may enhance and be more readily seen within the low attenuation omentum. However, inflammatory thickening of the omentum may be indistinguishable from neoplastic infiltration. On MRI, implants present with low signal intensity within the high signal omental fat on T1-weighted images and exhibit enhancement. Extensive involvement of the omentum is manifested by a crescent-shaped mass, intermediate in signal intensity, exhibiting diffuse enhancement after administration of gadolinium. Fat-suppression post-gadolinium T1-weighted MR images facilitate the depiction of omental involvement.

REFERENCES

1. Meyers MA, Oliphant M, Berne AS, Feldberg M. The peritoneal ligaments and mesenteries: Pathways of intraabdominal spread of disease. Radiology 1987;163:593–604.
2. Silverman PM. The subperitoneal space: Mechanisms of tumour spread in the peritoneal cavity, mesentery, and omentum. Cancer Imaging 2003;4:25–9.
3. Meyers MA. Intraperitoneal spread of malignancies. In: Meyers MA, editor. Dynamic Radiology of the Abdomen: Normal and Pathologic Anatomy. 5th ed. New York/London: Springer; 2000. pp. 131–263.
4. Pickhardt PJ. Peritoneum and retroperitoneum. In: Slone RM, editor. Body CT: A Practical Approach. New York: McGraw-Hill; 2000. pp. 159–77.
5. Okino Y, Kiyosue H, Mori H, et al. Root of the small-bowel mesentery: Correlative anatomy and CT features of pathologic conditions. Radiographics 2001;21:1475–90.
6. Martin LC, Merkle EM, Thompson WM. Review of internal hernias: Radiographic and clinical findings. Am J Roentgenol 2006;186:703–17.
7. Lassandro F, Iasiello F, Pizza NL, et al. Abdominal hernias: Radiological features. World J Gastrointest Endosc 2011;3:110–17.
8. Levy AD, Cantisani V, Miettinen M. Abdominal lymphangiomas: Imaging features with pathologic correlation. Am J Roentgenol 2004;182:1485–91.
9. Na-ChiangMai W, Pojchamarnwiputh S, Lertprasertsuke N, Chitapanarux T. CT findings of tuberculous peritonitis. Singapore Med J 2008;49:488–91.
10. Pickhardt PJ, Bhalla S. Unusual nonneoplastic peritoneal and subperitoneal conditions: CT findings. Radiographics 2005;25:719–30.
11. Lucey BC, Stuhlfaut JW, Soto JA. Mesenteric lymph nodes seen at imaging: Causes and significance. Radiographics 2005;25:351–65.
12. Gossios KJ, Kontoyiannis DS, Dascalogiannaki M, Gourtsoyiannis NC. Uncommon locations of hydatid disease: CT appearances. Eur Radiol 1997;7:1303–8.
13. Prassopoulos P, Papanikolaou N, Grammatikakis J, et al. MR enteroclysis imaging of Crohn disease. Radiographics 2001;21(Spec No):S161–72.
14. Balthazar EJ. Evaluation of the small intestine by computed tomography. In: Gourtsoyiannis NC, editor. Radiological Imaging of the Small Intestine Medical Radiology. Berlin/London: Springer; 2002. p. 87.
15. Papadaki HA, Kouroumalis EA, Stefanaki K, et al. Retractile mesenteritis presenting as fever of unknown origin and autoimmune haemolytic anaemia. Digestion 2000;61:145–8.
16. Daskalogiannaki M, Voloudaki A, Prassopoulos P, et al. CT evaluation of mesenteric panniculitis: Prevalence and associated diseases. Am J Roentgenol 2000;174:427–31.
17. Ti JP, Al-Aradi A, Conlon PJ, et al. Imaging features of encapsulating peritoneal sclerosis in continuous ambulatory peritoneal dialysis patients. Am J Roentgenol 2010;195:W50–4.

18. Courcoutsakis N, Souftas V, Thodis I, et al. Sclerosing peritonitis. Intern Med 2008;47:1441–2.
19. Singh AK, Gervais DA, Hahn PF, et al. Acute epiploic appendagitis and its mimics. Radiographics 2005;25:1521–34.
20. Pereira JM, Sirlin CB, Pinto PS, et al. Disproportionate fat stranding: A helpful CT sign in patients with acute abdominal pain. Radiographics 2004;24:703–15.
21. Raptopoulos V, Gourtsoyiannis N. Peritoneal carcinomatosis. Eur Radiol 2001;11:2195–206.
22. Marin D, Catalano C, Baski M, et al. 64-section multi-detector row CT in the preoperative diagnosis of peritoneal carcinomatosis: Correlation with histopathological findings. Abdom Imaging 2010;35:694–700.
23. Iafrate F, Ciolina M, Sammartino P, et al. Peritoneal carcinomatosis: Imaging with 64-MDCT and 3T MRI with diffusion-weighted imaging. Abdom Imaging 2012;37:616–27.
24. Soussan M, Des Guetz G, Barrau V, et al. Comparison of FDG-PET/CT and MR with diffusion-weighted imaging for assessing peritoneal carcinomatosis from gastrointestinal malignancy. Eur Radiol 2012;22:1479–87.
25. Tentes KA, Courcoutsakis N, Prasopoulos P. Combined cytoreductive surgery and perioperative intraperitoneal chemotherapy for the treatment of advanced ovarian cancer—clinical and therapeutic perspectives. In: Samir F, editor. Ovarian Cancer—Clinical and Therapeutic Perspectives. New York: InTech; 2012. pp. 143–67.
26. Sulkin TV, O'Neill H, Amin AI, Moran B. CT in pseudomyxoma peritonei: A review of 17 cases. Clin Radiol 2002;57:608–13.
27. Levy AD, Arnaiz J, Shaw JC, Sobin LH. From the archives of the AFIP: Primary peritoneal tumors: Imaging features with pathologic correlation. Radiographics 2008;28:583–607.
28. Park JY, Kim KW, Kwon HJ, et al. Peritoneal mesotheliomas: Clinicopathologic features, CT findings, and differential diagnosis. Am J Roentgenol 2008;191:814–25.
29. Gourtsoyiannis N, Bays D, Missas S, Gallis P. Solitary malignant mesothelioma of the small intestine: Radiological appearances. Abdom Imaging 1996;21:258–60.
30. Oei TN, Jagannathan JP, Ramaiya N, Ros PR. Peritoneal sarcomatosis versus peritoneal carcinomatosis: Imaging findings at MDCT. Am J Roentgenol 2010;195:W229–35.
31. Bellah R, Suzuki-Bordalo L, Brecher E, et al. Desmoplastic small round cell tumor in the abdomen and pelvis: Report of CT findings in 11 affected children and young adults. Am J Roentgenol 2005;184:1910–14.
32. Sheth S, Horton KM, Garland MR, Fishman EK. Mesenteric neoplasms: CT appearances of primary and secondary tumors and differential diagnosis. Radiographics 2003;23:457–73; quiz 535–6.
33. Levy AD, Rimola J, Mehrotra AK, Sobin LH. From the archives of the AFIP: Benign fibrous tumors and tumorlike lesions of the mesentery: Radiologic-pathologic correlation. Radiographics 2006; 26:245–64.
34. Azizi L, Balu M, Belkacem A, et al. MRI features of mesenteric desmoid tumors in familial adenomatous polyposis. Am J Roentgenol 2005;184:1128–35.
35. Pickhardt PJ, Bhalla S. Primary neoplasms of peritoneal and subperitoneal origin: CT findings. Radiographics 2005;25:983–95.
36. Courcoutsakis N, Tentes AA, Astrinakis E, et al. CT-enteroclysis in the preoperative assessment of the small-bowel involvement in patients with peritoneal carcinomatosis, candidates for cytoreductive surgery and hyperthermic intraperitoneal chemotherapy. Abdom Imaging 2013;38(1):56–63.
37. Gourtsoyiannis NC. Malignant small-intestinal neoplasms. In: Gourtsoyiannis NC, editor. Radiological Imaging of the Small Intestine. Berlin/London: Springer; 2002. pp. 399–425.
38. Levy AD, Sobin LH. From the archives of the AFIP: Gastrointestinal carcinoids: Imaging features with clinicopathologic comparison. Radiographics 2007;27:237–57.
39. Elsayes KM, Staveteig PT, Narra VR, et al. MRI of the peritoneum: spectrum of abnormalities. Am J Roentgenol 2006;186: 1368–79.
40. Modlin IM, Kidd M, Latich I, et al. Current status of gastrointestinal carcinoids. Gastroenterology 2005;128:1717–51.

CHAPTER 7

The Liver and Spleen

David J. Lomas • Lorenzo Mannelli

LIVER

ANATOMY[1-4]

The liver has a dome-shaped superior surface following the diaphragm contours extending anteriorly to the inferior edge of the liver. The major surface landmark is a sagittal groove containing the ligamentum teres (formerly umbilical vein), within the falciform ligament. The main feature of the inferior or visceral surface is the porta hepatis or hilum, a central depression conveying the portal vein, hepatic artery and common bile duct. The gallbladder fossa is positioned anterior to the hilum with the quadrate surface to the left. Posteriorly the caudate lobe separates the porta from the inferior vena cava (IVC). Several shallow surface impressions relate to adjacent organs, such as the right kidney. Normal liver volume, derived from postmortem studies of liver weight, ranges from 1 to 2.5 kg, and varies with gender, age and body mass. Liver weight is maximal in the fifth and sixth decades and subsequently declines rapidly. Riedel's lobe is an extension of the tip of the right lobe inferior to the costal margin based on clinical palpation; the term is misleading as it does not represent an anatomically discrete lobe or segment and is now considered part of the normal spectrum of liver shape and size (Fig. 7-1).

Subdivisions[1] (Fig. 7-2)

Studies of the vasculature demonstrate an internal craniocaudal principal plane (dividing the liver into left and right) not usually visualised on imaging techniques. The principal plane is defined by three key landmarks: the IVC groove, the middle hepatic vein and the gallbladder fossa. The liver is further subdivided into Couinaud segments based on the vascular supply. The caudate lobe or segment I has an autonomous blood supply from both left and right branches of the portal vein and hepatic artery along with independent venous drainage directly into the IVC.

Liver parenchyma has a lobular structure each comprising a central draining vein surrounded by sinusoids bounded peripherally by portal tracts, each a 'triad' of adjacent branches of the bile duct, portal vein and hepatic artery. At cellular level the liver is mainly composed of hepatocytes, stellate cells, and Kupffer cells, part of the reticulo-endothelial system. The liver receives approximately two-thirds of its blood supply from the portal vein and one-third from the hepatic artery. Blood drains via the hepatic veins to the IVC. During a meal, mesenteric blood flow volumes may double, increasing portal vein flow volumes correspondingly. The pressure difference between measurements in the wedged (occluded) hepatic vein and the IVC (the corrected sinusoidal pressure) is normally between 4 and 8 mmHg.

Lobar Agenesis/Atrophy[3]
(Figs. 7-3 and 7-4)

Right and left lobe agenesis has been reported but is controversial: the absence of supplying vasculature or dilated bile ducts is said to permit the diagnosis of true agenesis rather than early atrophy. Surgical hemihepatectomy or disease-related atrophy is more common. In normal livers compensatory hypertrophy of the remaining lobe often occurs with corresponding displacement of the gallbladder.

Vascular Anatomy Variation[5,6] (Fig. 7-5)

The common hepatic artery is one of the three major branches of the coeliac axis. After giving off the gastroduodenal artery, the main hepatic artery continues and

divides into the right and left hepatic arteries. Variations of the hepatic arterial supply are important for radiologists and hepatic surgeons. The portal vein divides into right and left branches and variations are infrequent, although early branches arising from the main trunk or close to the main division may create problems during liver resection. Three major hepatic veins drain into the

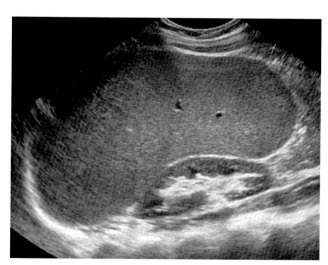

FIGURE 7-1 ■ **Riedel's lobe.** A normal variant where the right hepatic lobe extends anterior to the right kidney. On US the normal liver parenchyma is typically slightly more echo reflective than the renal cortex.

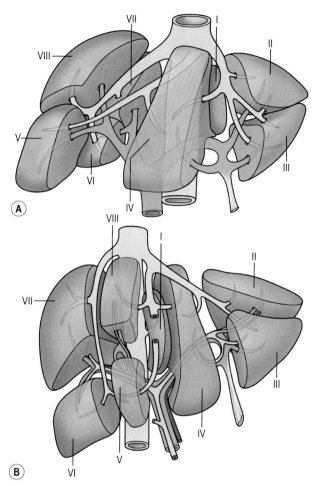

FIGURE 7-2 ■ **Segmental liver anatomy according to Couinaud's nomenclature.** Left and right anterior oblique views. (Reproduced with permission from Blumgart, in Surgery of the Liver and Biliary Tract, Churchill Livingstone, 1994.)

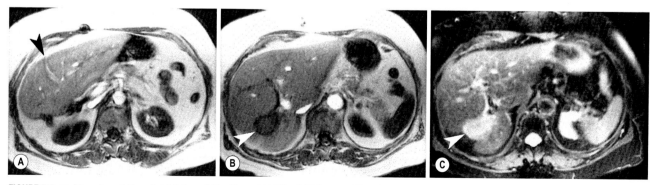

FIGURE 7-3 ■ **Atrophy of the right lobe of the liver.** (A) T1w MR image. The falciform ligament (black arrowhead) divides medial (IV) and lateral segments (II, II) of the left lobe; the right lobe is not present. (B) T1w and (C) T2w images immediately caudal to (A) demonstrate the atrophic right lobe (white arrowheads) with increased signal on T2w indicating confluent hepatic fibrosis.

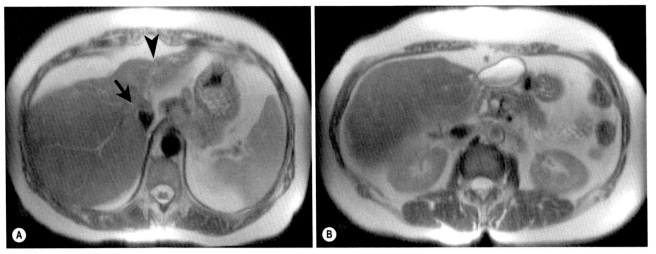

FIGURE 7-4 ■ **Atrophy of the left lobe.** (A) Cranial section on which the principal plane is marked by the arrow and the falciform liga-ment by an arrowhead. (B) Caudal section demonstrating the gallbladder displaced into the midline.

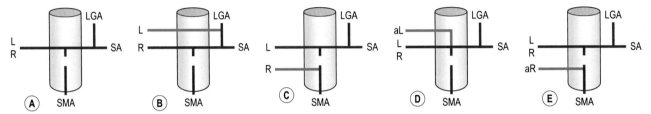

FIGURE 7-5 ■ **Normal variants of the hepatic artery.** The normal arrangement is shown in (A). The commonest four variations are replaced left hepatic artery (B), replaced right hepatic artery (C), accessory left hepatic artery (D) and accessory right hepatic artery (E). R = right hepatic artery, L = left hepatic artery, LGA = left gastric artery, SMA = superior mesenteric artery, SA = splenic artery, a = accessory.

IVC in 70% of cases, but in the remaining 30% accessory veins occur (19% having two left hepatic veins, 8% two right hepatic veins and 2% two middle hepatic veins). Absence of the IVC is rare and associated with complete situs inversus but may occur with partial situs and a right-sided liver. In this circumstance the hepatic veins drain direct to one of the cardiac atria with the azygos vein replacing the IVC, passing posterior to the diaphrag-matic crura into the chest. More commonly, aberrant gastric venous drainage of the posterior aspect of segment IV may occur and has been correlated with focal fat vari-ation. Accurate definition of the vascular and biliary anatomy is particularly important before live donor liver transplantation.

LIVER IMAGING TECHNIQUES

PLAIN RADIOGRAPHY

Plain radiographs are now rarely useful for liver evalua-tion, but may demonstrate gross hepatomegaly and hepatic calcification. The complex shape of the liver, limited soft-tissue contrast and projection acquisition of plain radiographs makes reliable identification of the liver boundaries difficult.

ULTRASOUND

Technique

Abdominal ultrasound (US) is routinely used with phased array transducers operating between 3 and 5 MHz, and Doppler capability, both spectral, colour and harmonic, is an integral part of the examination of the liver, allowing demonstration of hepatic blood flow and unequivocal bile duct identification. Contrast-enhanced US[9] is variably used to add an arterial and portal phase study comparable with CT and MRI.

Normal[7,8] (Fig. 7-6)

Normal liver parenchyma echo texture is homogeneous and slightly more reflective than adjacent renal cortex. Portal vein branches radiate from the hilum and have increased wall reflectivity. Hepatic veins converge on the IVC and right atrium and have walls indistinguisha-ble from the adjacent parenchyma. At Doppler examina-tion the normal hepatic vein waveform reflects the transmitted right heart pressure changes with transient flow reversal flow during the cardiac cycle (Fig. 7-7). The portal vein waveform is normally continuous antegrade (mean peak velocity approximately 15–25 cm/s) and may vary slightly with respiration and the cardiac cycle (Fig. 7-8).

COMPUTED TOMOGRAPHY

Technique[9–11] (Fig. 7-9)

Current volumetric CT systems allow complete isotropic data acquisition of the upper abdomen in a few seconds and choice of section thickness post acquisition. Unenhanced imaging remains valuable for assessing diffuse hepatic changes, such as fat infiltration and iron deposition, and for evaluating focal changes, in particular subtle calcification and haemorrhage. Dual energy systems may

in future remove the need for a separate unenhanced acquisition and provide new characterisation methods (Fig. 7-10). Multiphase contrast-enhanced imaging following IV administration of water-soluble iodinated contrast medium is routinely used for detection and characterisation of focal lesions. Many solid liver lesions have a predominantly arterial blood supply, whereas the liver parenchyma receives 75–80% of its blood supply via the portal vein. During contrast enhancement early and late arterial phase studies. Along with portal and delayed

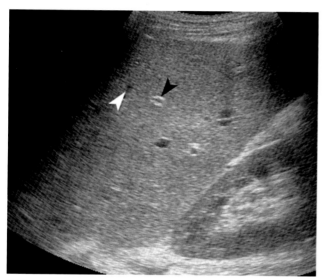

FIGURE 7-6 ■ **Normal liver US.** The hepatic parenchyma has an even texture with a reflectivity just above adjacent renal cortex. Portal vein branches have increased echo-reflectivity walls (black arrowhead) unlike hepatic vein branches (white arrowhead).

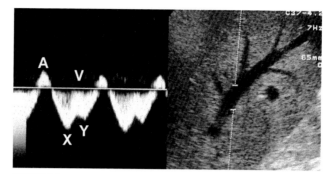

FIGURE 7-7 ■ **Normal hepatic vein on duplex Doppler US.** The spectral tracing reflects the normal right heart pressure changes leading to flow reversal occurring normally during the 'A' wave (right atrial contraction) and occasionally during the 'V' wave. The 'X' and 'Y' descents are also normally demonstrated.

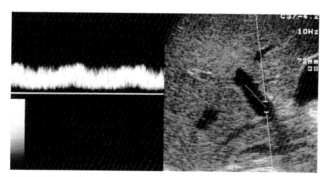

FIGURE 7-8 ■ **Normal portal vein on duplex Doppler US.** Flow is normally continuous towards the liver (hepatopetal) with slight undulation related to the cardiac cycle and respiration.

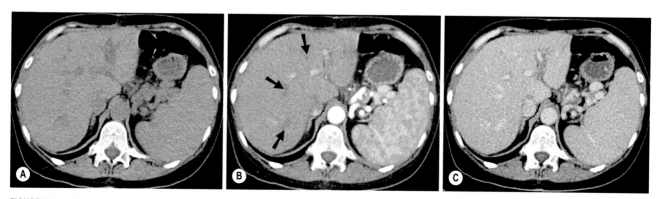

FIGURE 7-9 ■ **Normal liver multiphase CT examination.** Axial sections at the same location following a bolus of IV contrast medium demonstrating clearly the hepatic vessels and phases of enhancement: (A) unenhanced, (B) arterial phase and (C) portal phase. Note the hepatic veins are unenhanced (black arrows) on the arterial phase but opacify on the portal phase.

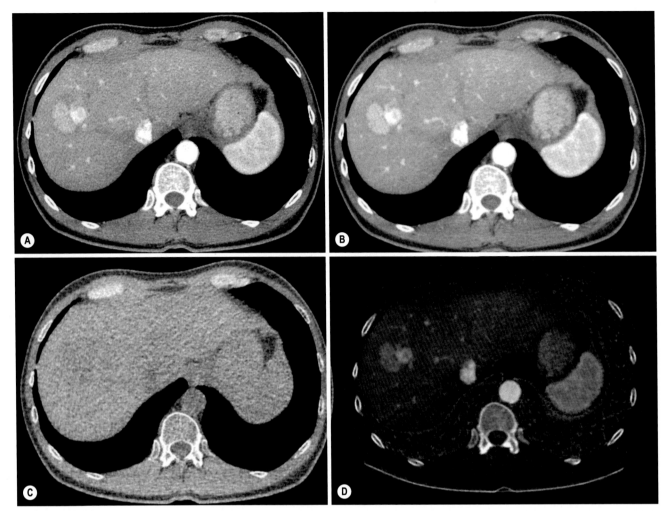

FIGURE 7-10 ■ **Dual energy CT images of a hepatocellular carcinoma.** (A) Arterial phase at 140 kV, (B) arterial phase at 70 kV, (C) reconstructed 'virtual' unenhanced image (comparable with an acquired unenhanced image) and (D) reconstructed 'iodine' image.

phase imaging, may be obtained. Optimising protocols and phase timing to maximise lesion-to-liver contrast varies with individual CT system but the minimum requirement for liver imaging is typically a relatively late arterial phase (e.g. centred 18 s post contrast medium arrival in the abdominal aorta) and a portal venous phase. Delayed CT imaging is used in selected cases, e.g. haemangiomas, and cholangiocarcinoma. CT arteriography (CTA) and CT arterioportography (CTAP) using direct hepatic artery injection during CT examination and Lipiodol CT are now rarely used.

Normal

Liver parenchyma is homogeneous with attenuation values of 54–60 Hounsfield units (HU), usually 8–10 HU greater than the spleen. Vascular structures can be identified by their location on the unenhanced images and confirmed by enhancement with IV contrast medium. The peripheral intrahepatic biliary tree is not normally visualised, although the main right and left hepatic ducts and the common hepatic and bile ducts are normally demonstrated.

MAGNETIC RESONANCE IMAGING

Techniques[12–14] (Fig. 7-11)

MRI has a wider range of contrast mechanisms than other imaging techniques and is increasingly used for lesion detection and characterisation. Biliary tract anatomy and hepatic vascular patency can be assessed during the same examination. A wide range of protocols is available because of the numerous combinations of field strength, pulse sequence implementation and interdependent sequence parameters, all of which can influence image quality. Multi-coil surface arrays are essential and most studies are mainly breath-hold examinations as rapid MRI sequences can rival CT, although they may have compromised contrast performance that may limit lesion detection sensitivity. This is traded off with improved anatomical definition of extrahepatic structures. A typical MRI protocol includes breath-hold T2- and T1-weighted (T2w and T1w) imaging, and chemical shift imaging for hepatic steatosis detection. High-quality T2w imaging can be obtained with respiratory-triggered multi-shot RARE sequences and pre- and

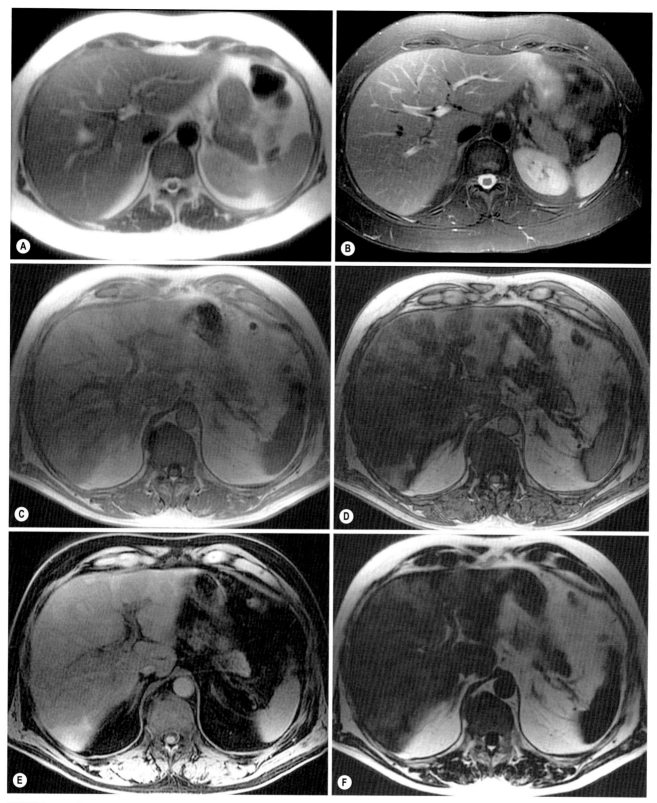

FIGURE 7-11 ■ **Normal liver on T2w MRI.** The spleen is normally higher signal than the liver. (A) Single-shot RARE (SSFSE/HASTE) TEeffective 60 ms, which is most useful for detecting long T2 value lesions (cysts/haemangiomas) and (B) fat-suppressed multi-shot RARE (FSE/TSE) TEeffective 60 ms, which is more sensitive to intermediate T2 value lesions such as metastases, benign tumours and HCC. T1w Dixon technique imaging is demonstrated in a different patient with multinodular hepatic fat deposition: (C) in-phase, (D) out of phase, (E) water only and (F) fat only. Modern techniques allow all four image sets to be generated from a single breath-hold 3D T1w acquisition. The signal reduction on the out-of-phase images indicates the presence of both water and fat in the same image voxels.

multiphase post-gadolinium imaging using rapid breath-hold 3D T1w volume imaging is now routine. Diffusion-weighted imaging (DWI) is increasingly used to improve liver lesion detection. MR-based quantification has been developed for the measurement of hepatic steatosis, iron and fibrosis using chemical shift imaging, T2 and T2* relaxometry and elastography. These techniques are undergoing standardisation and validation but are starting to enter routine clinical practice.

Intravenous Contrast Agents[12,15–17]
(Fig. 7-12)

Both non-specific intravenous gadolinium agents and liver-specific agents are in routine clinical use. Gadolinium-based agents that equilibrate rapidly with extracellular fluid include Gd-DTPA and GD-DOTA, as well as the more recent non-ionic agents gadodiamide, gadobutrol and gadoteridol. These agents provide enhancement on T1w images in a similar fashion to iodinated contrast media at CT examination. Breath-hold 3D T1w sequences allow the acquisition of multiphasic (arterial, portal, delayed) examinations as for CT. The enhancement characteristics for many focal lesions are, not surprisingly, similar to those for CT.

Hepatobiliary specific agents have been developed which target either the reticulo-endothelial system (RES) or hepatocytes. Iron oxide particles possess superpara-magnetic properties that create susceptibility-induced dephasing of protons, thereby shortening T2. A range of ultra-small paramagnetic iron oxide (USPIO) agents have been developed with varying sizes and properties targeting mainly the reticulo-endothelial cells but also capable of functioning as blood pool agents for vascular studies. The availability of the iron agents varies across the world and in some regions they have been withdrawn probably due to declining utilisation.

Mn-DPDP (mangafodipir trisodium), Gd-BOPTA (gadobenate dimeglumine) and most recently Gd-EOB-DTPA (gadoxetate) are all hepatocyte-specific paramagnetic agents which accumulate in hepatocytes followed by biliary excretion. They cause enhancement of the normal liver parenchyma and biliary tree on T1w imaging and indicate the presence of hepatocyte function. Mn-DPDP is no longer available but the other agents have been used for increasing the sensitivity of liver lesion detection, lesion characterisation and the study of the biliary tract.

Normal

The intensity of normal liver parenchyma is the same as, or slightly higher than, that of adjacent muscle. This holds for all sequence combinations except for inversion recovery techniques with inversion times that completely null liver signal. The appearance of vessels varies widely on MRI depending on pulse sequence, artefact suppression techniques and contrast media. In particular, intra-vascular signal on conventional spin-echo sequences may occur normally and should not be interpreted as throm-bus without confirmation using a reliable time-of-flight or contrast-enhanced technique. In routine practice liver–spleen differences are helpful as a simple guide to effective intrinsic T1 and T2 weighting. In general the spleen should be lower signal than the liver on effectively weighted T1w images and higher signal than the liver on T2w images.

SCINTIGRAPHY[18]

Radionuclide imaging of the liver for lesion characterisation has been largely superseded by the other techniques but is employed when they are unavailable or inappropriate. Studies typically use ^{99m}Tc-sulphur colloid or albumin colloid, which target the reticulo-endothelial system. Positron emission tomography (PET) combined with CT is increasingly used in oncology but, where FDG based, is rarely used for primary liver disease owing to the normal high liver uptake. This position may change as more selective radionuclides become available.

Technique

Liver/spleen imaging is usually performed following injection of a colloid agent such as ^{99m}Tc-sulphur colloid, injected intravenously. The majority of the colloid is taken up by the Kupffer cells in the liver and 5–10% is taken up by the spleen. A small portion is also absorbed by the bone marrow. Sulphur colloid is cleared rapidly from the bloodstream ($t_{1/2} = 2$ min) and in patients with normal liver function imaging may begin 5–10 min after injection but in those with compromised hepatic function and/or portal hypertension, optimal concentration of the sulphur colloid will take longer and imaging can be delayed to take account of this.

Gamma camera images are obtained in multiple projections and liver/spleen angiographic and blood flow phases can also be obtained at the start of a study by acquiring rapid sequential images during the first 30–60 seconds. Single-photon emission computed tomography (SPECT) imaging can be employed to evaluate suspicious areas for focal or diffuse space-occupying disease. PET and PET-CT imaging can provide both projection and tomographic images using a range of cyclotron-generated radionuclides with varying half-lives.

Normal

The evaluation of a sulphur colloid scintigram involves an assessment of liver size, shape, distribution of the radiopharmaceutical within the spleen, liver and bone marrow, and the homogeneity of uptake within the liver and spleen. Peripheral indentations on the liver are normally produced by the lateral rib margins, xiphoid process, gallbladder, right kidney and heart. The hepatic veins make a triangular impression on the superior, central margin of the liver, and the porta hepatis makes an impression on the inferomedial segment of the right lobe.

ANGIOGRAPHY[5,18,19]

Catheter-based intravascular angiography is dealt with in a separate chapter and its use in liver disease summarised

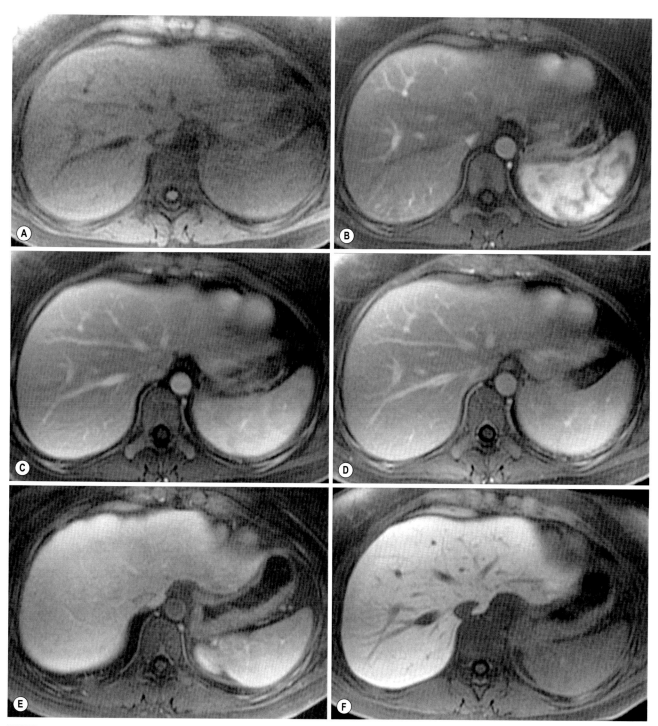

FIGURE 7-12 ■ **Normal liver with MRI contrast media.** (A) Pre, (B) arterial phase, (C) portal phase and (D) 5-min delayed phase post-intravenous gadolinium DTPA. The same patient had a follow-up examination with gadoxetic acid (a hepatocyte-specific agent) which has a similar appearance pre and in the arterial phase but the hepatocyte uptake changes the appearance in the portal phase (E) and 20-min delayed phase (F). Note the different appearance of the vessels in (E) and (F) compared with the conventional gadolinium chelate study.

here. Arteriography is best performed by selective catheterisation, and the arterial and parenchymal phases of the study are usually of most diagnostic value. The hepatic veins are seen routinely on digital subtraction angiography but the portal vein is not normally visualised on an arteriogram unless there has been flow reversal or an arterioportal shunt is present.

Portal venography is performed either directly or indirectly by portal vein or splenic pulp puncture. Indirect portography (arterioportography) is less hazardous than direct methods and combines an arterial study. Direct methods (including percutaneous splenic, transhepatic and transjugular approaches) are now used only when therapeutic procedures (e.g. transjugular intrahepatic portosystemic shunt (TIPSS)) or sampling techniques (e.g. direct portal venous pressure measurement) are being employed.

Hepatic venography is performed following retrograde catheterisation usually via the femoral or jugular veins. Filling of the small hepatic venous radicles is assisted if the patient performs a Valsalva manoeuvre. Hepatic venous wedge pressure measurement is performed by impacting an end-hole catheter in a small branch of an hepatic vein.

DIFFUSE DISEASE

Diffuse hepatic diseases are more difficult to detect than focal lesions as their effect on normal liver architecture may be minimal. Diagnoses are often made on the basis of clinical features with histological confirmation. Imaging can help assess extent and severity of diffuse disease by demonstrating liver abnormalities and sequelae such as portal hypertension changes. Recently MR techniques have been developed that provide quantification of hepatic steatosis, iron and fibrosis.

BENIGN DIFFUSE DISEASE

Hepatic Steatosis[20–22]

Diffuse steatosis is an increasingly common finding reflecting increased triglyceride loading of hepatocytes. It has a wide range of causes, including acute and chronic alcohol abuse, obesity, diabetes mellitus, insulin resistance, cystic fibrosis, malnourishment, total parenteral nutrition, tetracyclines, steroids and ileal bypass. Linkage to metabolic syndrome and cardiovascular disease make this formerly ignored condition the subject of much research interest. Focal fat variation is also common and discussed later.

US detects hepatic steatosis through increased parenchymal reflectivity, which obscures the portal vein margins (Fig. 7-13). Although this finding can be virtually diagnostic, further imaging may be required as fibrosis can also cause increased reflectivity. CT can demonstrate and quantify diffuse hepatic steatosis as the attenuation decreases by approximately 1.6 HU per mg of triglyceride increase per gram of liver substance. Confounding changes such as fibrosis, drug treatment and conditions such as haemochromatosis make this unreliable. The liver architecture is preserved, especially the vascular pattern and the liver enhances normally following IV contrast medium. With increasing fat infiltration the liver attenuation decreases, reversing, in turn, the normal liver–spleen difference and liver–blood difference (Fig. 7-14). MRI is the most sensitive and specific technique for demonstrating hepatic steatosis. Dixon-based (Fig. 7-11), 'chemical shift' or 'in- and out-of-phase' imaging (Fig. 7-15) allow both an accurate diagnosis and, with appropriate T2 and other corrections, accurate quantification. MRI is also the most accurate test for diagnosis of focal fat variation.

Cirrhosis[23–29]

Cirrhosis is the end stage of a wide variety of hepatic disease processes that cause hepatocellular inflammation and necrosis leading to hepatic fibrosis and nodular regeneration. Early changes may be detectable only on histological examination. As cirrhosis progresses, widespread fibrosis and nodular regeneration develop, along with macroscopic changes of liver morphology which can be detected on imaging. Liver stiffness also increases but the commonest anatomical finding in advanced cirrhosis is atrophy of the posterior segments (VI, VII) of the right

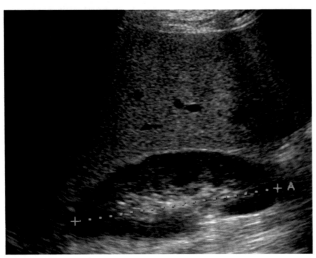

FIGURE 7-13 ■ **Diffuse hepatic steatosis US.** The liver is of abnormally increased echo-reflectivity when compared with the cortex of the adjacent right kidney.

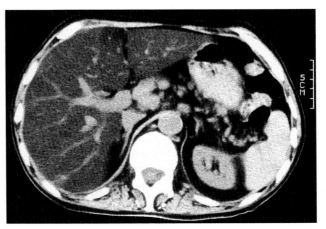

FIGURE 7-14 ■ **Diffuse hepatic steatosis CT.** Unenhanced CT in which the liver parenchyma is markedly reduced in attenuation, reversing the normal relationship with the spleen and blood vessels. The shape and vascular architecture of the liver are normal.

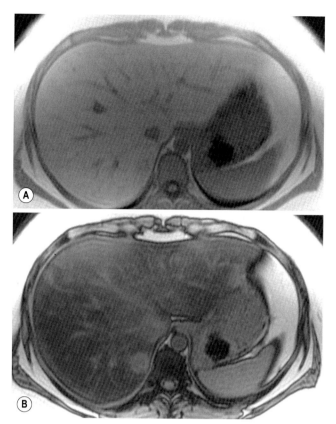

FIGURE 7-15 ▪ **Diffuse hepatic steatosis MRI.** Chemical shift or (A) in- and (B) out-of-phase gradient-echo imaging. The presence of steatosis leads to marked signal reduction on (B) owing to cancellation of the water and fat signal when present in the same voxel. There is moderate spatial variation in the degree of steatosis in the liver.

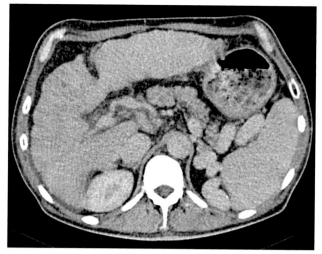

FIGURE 7-16 ▪ **Cirrhosis: portal phase CT study.** The nodular hepatic margin, atrophy of the right lobe and large splenorenal varices are all indicators of cirrhosis.

lobe. Hypertrophy of the caudate (I) lobe and of the lateral segments of the left lobe (II, III) is frequently seen. In primary sclerosing cholangitis caudate lobe hypertrophy is found in virtually all cases and the lateral segments of the left lobe (II, III) occasionally atrophy. The cause of these changes is uncertain but thought to be blood flow related. Hepatic and portal system dynamics may alter radically in cirrhosis, with both increased overall hepatic blood flow (through intrahepatic arteriovenous shunts) and decreased hepatic blood flow (resulting from increased intrahepatic vascular resistance) recognised in advanced disease.

US can demonstrate the nodularity of the liver margin in advanced cirrhosis, particularly when ascites is present and when using high-frequency transducers. Pure hepatic fibrosis increases reflectivity, resulting in loss of the margins of the portal vein branches, but is thought not to alter attenuation, a feature in the past used to discriminate steatosis from fibrosis but in practice the two often coexist making separation difficult. The liver texture becomes coarser or more heterogeneous as cirrhosis progresses, but this is difficult to quantify and subjective. As the liver atrophies in end-stage cirrhosis, the hepatic veins may become attenuated and difficult to visualise. Doppler US examination may reveal other non-specific features of cirrhosis: damping of the normal right heart

waveforms in the hepatic veins, reduced main portal vein blood flow (<10 cm/s mean peak) or hepatofugal flow. Occasionally increased flow in a large recanalised para-umbilical vein will 'steal' blood from the right portal vein branch, leading to reversed flow in the right portal vein but normal hepatopetal flow in the main and left portal veins. Hepatic arterial flow is usually increased in advanced cirrhosis as the portal contribution to hepatocyte perfusion decreases. This results in enlargement of the hepatic arterial system, which can be mistaken for enlarged bile ducts on US unless Doppler techniques are used to identify the vessels. Over the last decade several forms of ultrasound elastography have been developed that evaluate liver stiffness. These vary from a 1D non-imaging method 'transient' elastography to a pulsed shear wave method combined with 2D imaging 'acoustic radiation force imaging'. Several of these methods provide absolute quantification of liver stiffness and large trials suggest that these techniques may have a role in the detection and quantification of liver fibrosis although their exact role in patient management is not yet clear.

CT (Fig. 7-16) is insensitive to early fibrosis changes but demonstrates the nodular margin and lobar atrophy/hypertrophy changes of advanced disease. On unenhanced examinations regenerative areas have relatively normal attenuation but advanced fibrosis lowers attenuation, whereas the accumulation of iron in hepatocytes increases it. These features frequently coexist in many forms of cirrhosis, resulting in parenchymal heterogeneity both before and after enhancement with IV contrast medium. Portal phase imaging can be helpful in assessing portal vein patency, although flow volume and direction cannot be determined.

MRI is also insensitive to early fibrosis changes and there are no specific changes of parenchymal signal intensity on T1w or T2w imaging, although parenchymal heterogeneity (Fig. 7-17) may occur on T2w and delayed post-gadolinium T1w imaging, but is difficult to quantify. MRI delineates the morphological changes of advanced cirrhosis but can also provide non-invasive assessment of

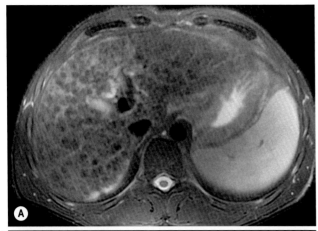

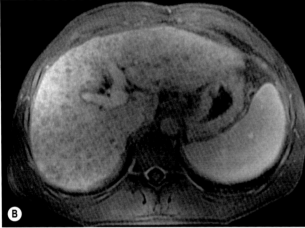

FIGURE 7-17 ■ **Cirrhosis.** On MRI marked heterogeneity may occur in cirrhotic livers on (A) multi-shot T2w FSE imaging due to the combination of increased signal from fibrosis and reduced signal from iron accumulation within nodules and for similar reasons on delayed post-gadolinium T1w imaging (B).

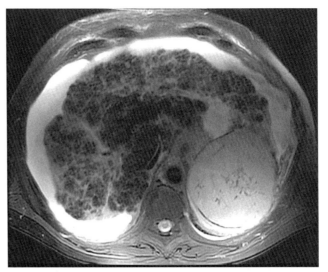

FIGURE 7-18 ■ **Haemochromatosis-related cirrhosis.** T2w MRI image demonstrating abnormally low liver signal parenchyma compared to adjacent muscle with linear fibrotic increased signal regions, nodular margins and moderate ascites.

portal vein patency along with flow direction and bulk flow volume estimation when other techniques have proved unhelpful. Studies using DWI and ^{31}P spectroscopy have given mixed results for trying to grade fibrosis. MR elastography is a relatively new technique quantifying liver stiffness in a similar fashion to US methods. This technique appears promising for detecting the relatively early stages of hepatic fibrosis and further research is ongoing.

Colloid scintigraphy is rarely used but in established cirrhosis demonstrates reduced, heterogeneous hepatic uptake and increased extrahepatic uptake. In advanced disease morphological changes may be detected. Angiography may be used to assess vascular complications such as variceal bleeding and portal hypertensive changes. Hepatic arteriography in cirrhotic liver demonstrates increased tortuosity of intrahepatic branches, so-called 'corkscrew vessels', which reflect lobar shrinkage.

Viral Hepatitis[30]

Viral hepatitis, including hepatitis B and hepatitis C, remains a major public health concern as it may lead to liver failure and primary liver cancer, often detected late. Diagnosis and monitoring based on serological tests and

imaging is relatively non-specific. In acute hepatitis, imaging excludes obstructive causes of jaundice. In chronic hepatitis with cirrhosis, imaging helps monitor disease progression, development of portal venous hypertension and complications such as hepatocellular carcinoma (HCC).

On US examination non-specific decreased reflectivity occurs in acute viral hepatitis, although the majority of cases have normal parenchyma. Gallbladder wall thickening is a common non-specific finding in acute hepatitis. On colloid scintigraphy the appearance of hepatitis is similar to the early stages of cirrhosis, with uneven and reduced uptake. In chronic hepatitis CT, MRI and angiography are of limited value until cirrhotic changes develop.

Haemochromatosis and Iron Overload[31,32]

Haemochromatosis and multiple transfusions may both result in iron deposition in the liver. Inherited genetic haemochromatosis causes hepatocyte iron accumulation (leading to subsequent cirrhosis) and iron accumulation in other organs, including myocardium, skin and endocrine glands. Affected individuals have an increased risk of developing malignancy in general and of hepatocellular carcinoma in particular. Initially the hepatic iron deposition is diffuse but the development of cirrhosis and regenerative changes often results in uneven distribution. By comparison hepatic iron overload from multiple transfusions (haemosiderosis) results in iron accumulation in the reticulo-endothelial system (Kupffer cells) in the liver, bone marrow and spleen. There is less risk of liver damage and the pattern of organ involvement can aid diagnosis.

MRI (Figs. 7-18 and 7-19) is the most specific imaging technique, as intracellular iron exerts a local susceptibility effect, reducing parenchymal T2 and T2*. This effect is

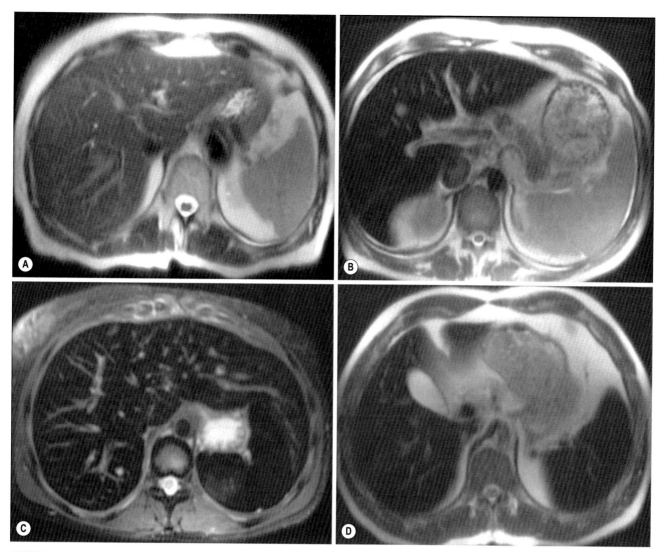

FIGURE 7-19 ■ **Patterns of hepatic iron accumulation on T2w MRI images.** (A) Normal liver, (B) haemochromatosis, (C) transfusion-related haemosiderosis and (D) variant haemochromatosis. Note the iron accumulation in the spleen in (C) and (D).

most sensitively detected by T2*w gradient-echo imaging although with significant accumulation the effect is easily seen on T2w spin-echo images, and when severe will affect T1w images. The liver signal is abnormally reduced (to less than that of adjacent muscle). Several studies have demonstrated that hepatic iron concentration correlates strongly with both T2* and T2 value, permitting accurate quantification. Abnormally reduced signal on T2w imaging is the main feature in other affected organs such as spleen and pancreas. Unenhanced CT demonstrates hepatic iron deposition through an increase in HU value (>75 HU) (Fig. 7-20) but this also occurs in amiodarone treatment and previous Thorotrast exposure. The changes are unreliable because of the confounding effect of steatosis. US may demonstrate increased parenchymal reflectivity but there are no specific features that characterise iron deposition.

Wilson's Disease

Wilson's disease is an autosomal recessive disorder in which copper is deposited in the liver, as cornea and lenticular nucleus of the brain. Copper is hepatotoxic and triggers inflammation that progresses to cirrhosis. Imaging demonstrates the generalised cirrhotic changes but the underlying cause is rarely evident. Copper accumulation rarely causes a detectable increase in hepatic attenuation on CT, and there is often coexistent steatosis counteracting the effect. On MRI there may be a subtle increased signal on T1w with a decrease on T2w images. There are no specific features on US studies.

MALIGNANT DIFFUSE DISEASE

Occasionally the liver is diffusely involved by malignancy, usually metastatic disease, e.g. breast carcinoma, which may give a diffusely increased echo-reflective and heterogeneous appearance on US. Some primary hepatic tumours, including hepatocellular carcinoma, may present with non-specific diffuse infiltrative changes. Lymphoma and leukaemia may also cause diffuse hepatic infiltration demonstrated by US as non-specific reduced echo reflectivity. In all these situations the diagnosis is

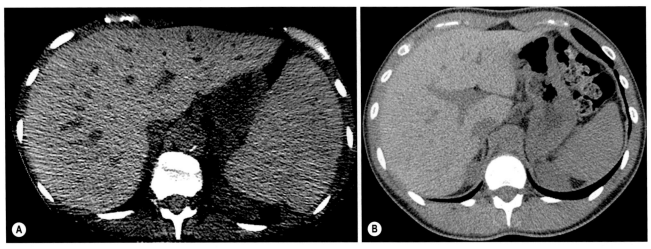

FIGURE 7-20 ■ **Haemochromatosis CT.** Unenhanced axial CT images. (A) Diffuse increased attenuation of the liver (91 HU) and spleen (81 HU) in a patient with haemosiderosis. (B) Increased liver attenuation following amiodarone therapy (B).

difficult to make although subtle heterogeneity that cannot be attributed to cirrhosis or fat infiltration is usually evident on most imaging techniques. The presence of other abnormalities (e.g. vascular thrombosis with HCC) may be helpful, but in the appropriate clinical context biopsy may be required to detect diffuse malignant involvement.

FOCAL DISEASE

Calcification[33]

Benign parenchymal calcification may occur following focal insults such as tuberculosis, *Pneumocystis* infection, sarcoidosis, pyogenic abscess and parenchymal haematoma. The calcification is well demarcated and surrounded by otherwise normal parenchyma. In *Pneumocystis carinii* infection widespread focal calcification may occur. Focal calcification also occurs within benign lesions (giant haemangioma) and malignant lesions, particularly mucin-secreting adenocarcinoma of the colon, where it is often relatively ill defined. Primary liver tumours such as hepatoblastoma and fibrolamellar hepatoma may also contain foci of calcification.

Plain radiographs demonstrate gross calcification, but unenhanced CT is more sensitive and detects subtle calcification, e.g. metastases (Fig. 7-21). US clearly demonstrates focal calcification, with increased reflectivity and a posterior acoustic corridor, but this feature alone does not always allow distinction from focal gas. Scintigraphy and MRI are insensitive to calcification.

Pneumobilia

Gas in the biliary tract may occur as a result of a sphincterotomy, or Roux loop procedure allowing reflux of intestinal gas into the biliary tree. It can be identified by the linear distribution radiating from the hilum and gravity dependence with air predominantly in the non-dependent parts of the biliary tree.

Both US and CT (Figs. 7-22 and 7-23) demonstrate clearly pneumobilia and its distribution. On US the ducts

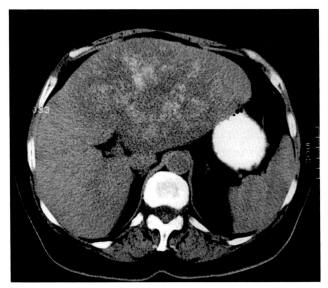

FIGURE 7-21 ■ **Liver calcification.** Unenhanced CT section, showing a large metastasis in the left lobe of the liver from a colonic adenocarcinoma. Faint calcification is visible in the metastasis. (Reproduced with permission from Blumgart, in Surgery of the Liver and Biliary Tract, Churchill Livingstone 1994.)

are increased echo-reflectivity linear structures that may be differentiated from calcification by the pattern and movement of the gas related to respiration, bowel peristalsis or patient position. CT is extremely sensitive to the presence of gas, which is easily demonstrated and localised.

Portal Vein Gas[34]

Portal vein gas is always abnormal and occurs when intestinal permeability increases and/or there is an increase in intestinal luminal pressure. These conditions are fulfilled in neonatal necrotising enterocolitis but also in adults with gastric emphysema, intestinal obstructions, infections and Crohn's disease. It has also been described in blunt abdominal trauma, invasive abdominal

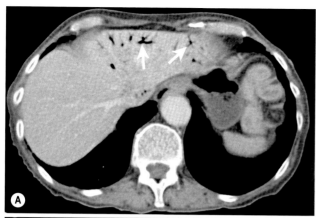

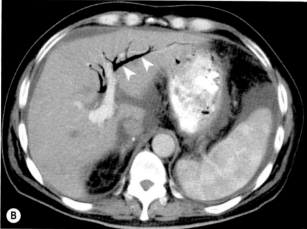

FIGURE 7-22 ▪ **Portal venous gas and pneumobilia.** Portal phase CT images (A) in a patient with portal vein gas (note the peripheral distribution (arrows)) and (B) in a patient with pneumobilia (arrowheads).

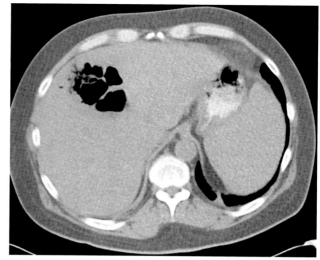

FIGURE 7-24 ▪ **Parenchymal gas.** Unenhanced CT demonstrates infarction and abscess formation, with intraparenchymal gas centrally in the liver following hepatic artery occlusion in a patient following liver transplantation.

malignancies (colon carcinoma, ovarian carcinoma), duodenal perforation at ERCP and in patients with colitis following a barium enema. The significance and outcome largely relates to the underlying aetiology. The gas typically radiates out from the hilum with less marked gravity dependence than pneumobilia and a more peripheral distribution (Fig. 7-22).

US sensitively detects moving gas bubbles in the main portal vein which can be visualised on B-mode images and detected by spectral Doppler as the gas bubbles reflect the sound beam overloading the system receivers giving rise to a characteristic high-pitched random bubbling sound with focal aliasing artefacts on the spectral display. The phenomenon occurs with both portal vein gas bubbles and microemboli. If sufficient gas accumulates it may become visible on CT peripherally in the portal vein branches and eventually becomes evident on plain radiographs.

Parenchymal Gas[35]

This is abnormal and results from a gas-forming organism in an abscess or infarct, or occasionally following trauma or hepatic arterial thrombosis following liver transplantation. It may be seen after embolisation or thermal ablation of liver tumours.

CT (Fig. 7-24) best delineates parenchymal gas collections and any related pathological changes. US will demonstrate gas collections but defining their extent may be difficult when they are large or peripheral and may be confused with adjacent bowel.

BENIGN CYSTIC LESIONS

Cysts[36]

True hepatic cysts arise from abnormal development of bile duct precursors (Meyenburg's complexes) and are

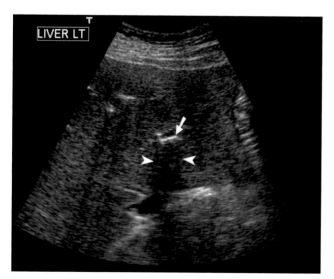

FIGURE 7-23 ▪ **Pneumobilia US.** Linear echo-reflective structures indicate gas in the bile ducts, radiating out from the hilum. Movement of the gas is often visible on real-time imaging and may help distinguish from calcification.

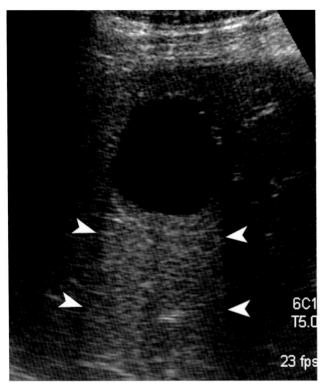

FIGURE 7-25 ■ **Simple liver cyst.** On US a simple cyst is well-defined with no internal echoes, no perceptible wall and posterior acoustic enhancement (arrowheads).

lined by cuboidal epithelium. The true incidence is unknown and they are indistinguishable from cysts that arise as the long-term sequelae of parenchymal haematomas or abscesses. Multiple cysts occur as part of adult polycystic disease. Hepatic cysts are rarely symptomatic, although large cysts may cause pain, become infected or suffer internal haemorrhage.

On US, hepatic cysts are spherical homogeneous structures with an imperceptible wall, posterior acoustic enhancement, lacking internal echoes and internal flow on Doppler (Fig. 7-25). A confident diagnosis may be made when these criteria are all met in a patient who does not have ovarian metastases or hydatid disease, as these conditions can mimic simple hepatic cysts. Internal echoes, thick septations, a perceptible wall or solid components should prompt further imaging (by CT or MRI) or aspiration as the differential diagnosis includes haemorrhage, abscess, cystic metastasis (e.g. ovarian), biliary cystadenoma or cystadenocarcinoma and hydatid disease. CT demonstrates cysts as homogeneous structures, with imperceptible walls, attenuation of 0–10 HU, and no enhancement following IV contrast medium. Difficulties arise with small lesions when partial volume effects may efface the characteristic features and US may be helpful to exclude a solid lesion. Occasionally cysts are of higher attenuation due to a high protein content in the fluid attributed to previous infection or haemorrhage. In these cases the lack of enhancement and features on other investigations help confirm the diagnosis. On MRI the fluid content of a cyst results in low signal on T1w imaging and very high signal on T2w imaging

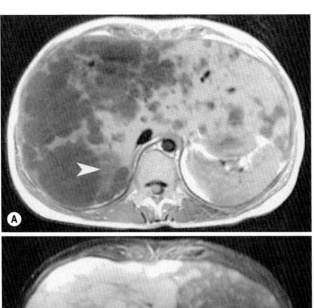

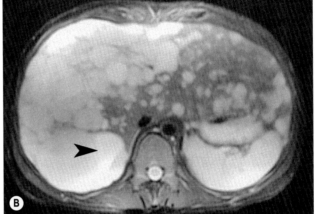

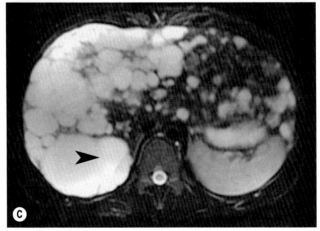

FIGURE 7-26 ■ **Polycystic liver disease MRI.** Multiple simple liver cysts are present and typically low signal on T1w (A), and increased signal (greater than that of the spleen) on T2w TE 60 ms (B) and T2w 120 ms (C). Confusion may occur in the presence of haemorrhage, as this may increase the signal on T1w (white arrowhead). In these circumstances the lack of enhancement following IV gadolinium DTPA may be diagnostic.

(particularly when using extended echo times or single shot echotrains), typically brighter than the spleen and comparable to the CSF or the gallbladder bile (Fig. 7-26). Cysts may be indistinguishable from haemangiomas on conventional T2w MRI but heavily T2w imaging (as used for MRCP) may help separate them. There is no enhancement with IV Gd-DTPA on T1w images. Scintigraphy will demonstrate large cysts as non-specific photopenic regions.

Hydatid Disease[37]

This is a hepatic infection with *Echinococcus granulosus*, a parasitic tapeworm present worldwide and transmitted from sheep, foxes and other wild animals to humans as part of its life cycle. Larvae migrate from the gut and embed in the liver, where they encyst and develop, slowly provoking a surrounding inflammatory reaction. The disease may remain occult for several years. On imaging there is a wide range of appearances, from a simple cyst indistinguishable from a true hepatic cyst to a complicated cyst with any or all of the following features: debris (hydatid 'sand' made up of dead scolices, which may calcify), daughter cysts, membrane separation, and wall calcification. The lesions may be multiple and vary widely in size. Serological testing confirms the presence of infection prior to any therapy or intervention. Although the risk of anaphylaxis following aspiration or surgery of these lesions is well recognised, it is less than previously thought, and uncomplicated aspiration following medical treatment has been described.

US demonstrates clearly not only the simple cyst form but also the more complex cyst features, such as the dependent debris, daughter cysts (cyst within a cyst appearance), membrane separation and wall calcification. CT defines all these features as well (Fig. 7-27) and is helpful where wall calcification obscures the view on US. MRI also defines the cystic structure and internal anatomy but is insensitive to the calcification.

Abscess[38]

Hepatic pyogenic abscesses usually arise from portal pyaemia. The increasing number of chronically and transiently immunocompromised patients has led to both fungal and mycobacterial abscesses becoming more common. An initial local inflammatory reaction is followed by progressive central liquefaction with a surrounding inflammatory margin or 'wall'. In the early stages abscesses may mimic solid tumours such as metastases on virtually all imaging techniques and aspiration or biopsy may be necessary for diagnosis. The mortality from hepatic abscess has decreased with more rapid diagnosis and prompt intervention. Modern management usually involves radiologically guided diagnostic aspiration and/or drainage combined with prolonged medical therapy; surgical intervention is now rarely required.

On US studies an early pyogenic abscess appears as a solid spherical lesion with an ill-defined margin and low reflectivity. As the abscess liquefies, a thickened and irregular wall appears and the necrotic centre contains sparse echoes from the debris (Fig. 7-28). On CT, abscesses are typically ill-defined, low attenuation and following IV contrast medium demonstrate rim enhancement (Fig. 7-29), although this may not occur if antibiotic treatment has started. These appearances are not specific and similar findings may be seen with metastatic deposits, particularly those with central necrosis or cystic

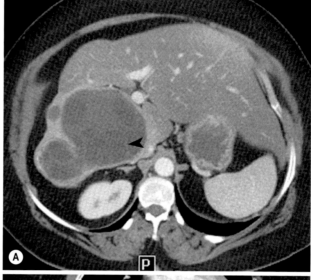

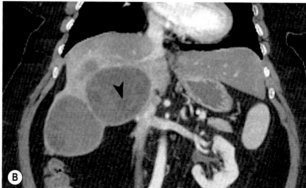

FIGURE 7-27 ■ **Hydatid disease.** Axial (A) and coronal (B) portal phase CT demonstrate a large cystic structure with a discrete wall, separate internal membranes and several 'daughter cysts' (arrowheads).

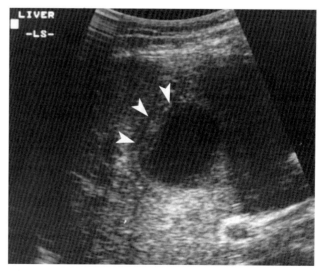

FIGURE 7-28 ■ **Liver abscess US.** A typical abscess, with reduced echo reflectivity and a thickened irregular wall (arrowheads).

components. The MRI findings also overlap with necrotic metastases with an ill-defined lesion on low signal on T1w and high signal on T2w, often with a higher signal outer margin. As the lesions liquefy, the central signal decreases on T1w and increases on T2w imaging.

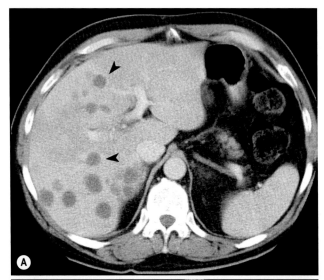

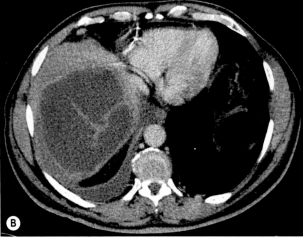

FIGURE 7-29 ■ **Liver abscess CT.** Portal phase examinations in two different cases. (A) Multiple low attenuation lesions with ring enhancement (arrowheads); these appearances are often non-specific on CT and often overlap with those of metastatic deposits. In (B) the presence of septae, central low attenuation along with a sympathetic pleural effusion aid the diagnosis.

MALIGNANT CYSTIC LESIONS

Metastases

Some metastatic lesions have a predominantly cystic appearance. This may occur with ovarian metastases, but has also been described with teratomas, colonic and metastatic squamous cell tumours.[29] Differentiation from an abscess may be impossible on imaging criteria alone and guided aspiration for cytology and microbiology examination may be required.

BENIGN SOLID LESIONS

Haemangioma[39–41]

Haemangiomas are the commonest benign hepatic tumours with a postmortem prevalence of 4–20% and may be multiple in 10% of these. They are composed of vascular channels of varying size (cavernous to capillary), lined with endothelium, often with intervening fibrous tissue. Most haemangiomas are asymptomatic incidental imaging findings. Haemangiomas between 2 and 4 cm in diameter are most likely to possess characteristic features that facilitate a confident imaging-based diagnosis.

MRI is the most sensitive and specific imaging examination for the diagnosis of haemangioma. Using extended echo time (e.g. TE of 120 to 160 ms) T2w spin-echo sequences at 1.5 T, haemangiomas appear as well-defined lesions with a lobular outline and homogeneously high signal on T2w, in excess of the spleen and approaching that of fluid (Fig. 7-30). Most malignant lesions, by comparison, have signal similar to that of the spleen and become less visible on longer echo time images, unlike haemangiomas. Single-shot RARE sequences with a T2 contrast response that emphasises long T2 values may prove even more accurate for evaluation. During the arterial phase following IV enhancement with Gd-DTPA haemangiomas have rapidly enhancing vessels at the periphery. Over a period of minutes the lesion will 'fill in' centripetally to become isointense or slightly hyperintense with the adjacent parenchyma (Fig. 7-31). CT examination demonstrates a well-defined, lobulated lesion with attenuation close to blood values before enhancement. The pattern of enhancement follows that for MRI, with centripetally infilling and eventually

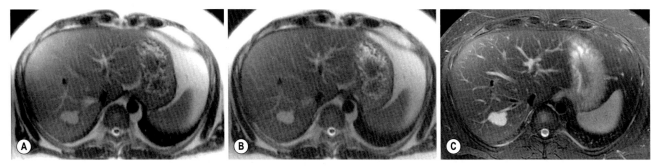

FIGURE 7-30 ■ **Haemangioma MRI.** Typical appearance on T2w sections: (A) TEeffective 60 ms single-shot RARE, (B) TEeffective 160 ms single-shot RARE and (C) TEeffective 60 ms multi-shot fat-suppressed RARE. On T2w imaging haemangiomas are well-defined homogeneous lesions of higher signal intensity than spleen and approaching that of fluid, particularly on the long echo time image (B).

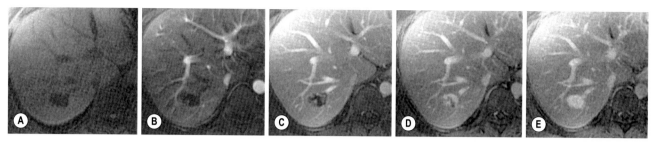

FIGURE 7-31 ■ **Haemangioma MRI.** The same case as 30 demonstrates the typical enhancement appearances following IV gadolinium-DTPA with initial peripheral nodular high signal followed by progressive infilling of the lesion. Images obtained pre (A) and at 40 s (B), 120 s (C), 5 min (D) and 15 min (E) following injection.

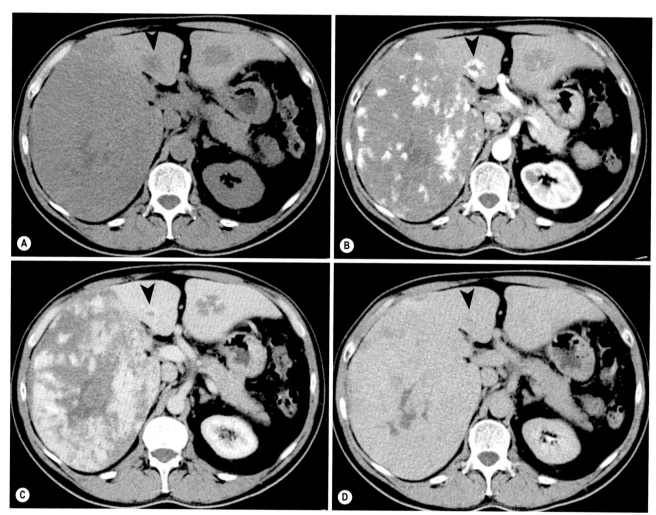

FIGURE 7-32 ■ **Haemangioma CT.** A patient with 3 haemangiomas. The smallest (arrowhead) demonstrates the typical features best: similar attenuation to blood before enhancement (A), peripheral nodular marked enhancement in the arterial phase (B), progressive infilling in the portal phase (C) and complete infilling and isoattenuation on the 10-min delayed phase (D).

merging with the background parenchyma (Fig. 7-32). Complete infilling has been applied as a diagnostic criterion, but is influenced by lesion size, with larger lesions taking 10 min or more to opacify. On US capillary haemangiomas are typically well-defined, lobular, homogeneous lesions with increased echo reflectivity (Fig. 7-33). There is usually no detectable Doppler signal within the lesion due to the slow flow, although signals may be detected in adjacent feeding vessels or within the lesion with more sensitive harmonic imaging techniques. Unfortunately some metastases, especially from neuroendocrine malignancies, may have a similar appearance. Some adult and most neonatal and infantile haemangiomas are of the cavernous type, with reduced echo reflectivity, probably due to the larger vascular channels found within them. In these lesions Doppler signals are usually

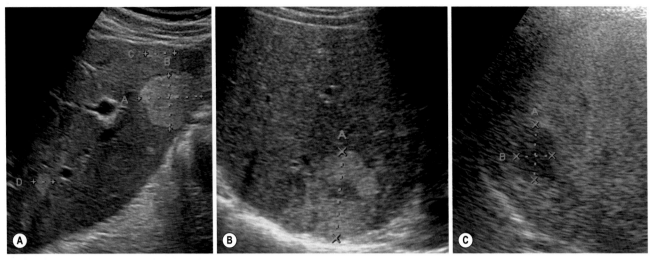

FIGURE 7-33 ■ **Haemangioma US.** Typical appearances of well-defined lobulated peripheral homogeneous increased echo-reflectivity lesions (A). Atypical haemangiomas with a fibrous central component (B) and a reduced echo-reflectivity lesion (C) resulting from a steatotic liver.

detectable due to more rapid flow rates. Haemangiomas appear as photopenic regions on liver sulphur colloid studies but show an increase in uptake on blood pool studies (e.g. [99mTc]-labelled red cells). This technique was widely used before the advent of MRI but is now only used where CT and MRI are unavailable.

Atypical Haemangiomas[39–41]

Small (<1.5 cm) lesions are frequently difficult to characterise and may fail to demonstrate either the characteristic signal changes on T2w MRI (partial volume effects) or the typical enhancement pattern on CT or MRI. Small lesions may fill in relatively rapidly and be confused with other arterial enhancing solid lesions. Larger lesions (>4 cm) often have atypical internal features such as an area of central fibrosis that does not enhance on MRI or CT and may cause discomfort, and rarely spontaneously rupture. On US atypical lesions may appear heterogeneous (Fig. 7-33). Neonatal or paediatric haemangiomas are more commonly of reduced echo reflectivity and diffuse hepatic steatosis in adults may also cause this appearance. Rarely, when the diagnosis is in doubt, core needle biopsy rather than aspiration should be considered. This is less likely to provoke serious haemorrhage than previously thought and can provide an unequivocal diagnosis.

Focal Nodular Hyperplasia[15,16,42–44]

This benign tumour occurs most commonly in women aged 20–50 years, but can occur in men and women at any age, with multiple lesions being found in 20% of cases. Focal nodular hyperplasia (FNH) is usually asymptomatic although rarely patients present with pain or hepatomegaly. It arises from an underlying congenital vascular malformation and enlarges in response to hormone stimulation, for example by oral contraceptives. Histologically, FNH is composed of normal liver elements including hepatocytes, bile ducts, Kupffer cells and

intervening fibrous septa. However, in FNH the biliary elements are not connected with the normal biliary tree; this characteristic aids discrimination from adenoma when using MRI with hepatocyte-specific contrast media. Up to 50% of FNH lesions have a typical central stellate fibrovascular scar, visible on at least one imaging technique. FNH lacks a true capsule and the presence of normal liver elements can make histological diagnosis difficult. Calcification, necrosis and haemorrhage are extremely rare, as even large FNH lesions do not usually outgrow their blood supply. Both the presence of Kupffer cell activity and the central scar have been used to characterise FNH, but even with these features present there is a small overlap with other lesions that may possess central scars (hepatocellular adenoma (HCA), hepatocellular carcinoma, haemangioma) and Kupffer cell activity (HCA, hepatocellular carcinoma). This may make histological confirmation crucial in young patients. Occasionally surgical excision is still required for symptomatic lesions or definitive diagnosis, especially when adenoma or well-differentiated hepatocellular carcinoma cannot be excluded on imaging and needle biopsy.

US findings are usually non-specific with subtle lesions of similar reflectivity to adjacent liver detectable mainly by their mass effect (Fig. 7-34). Central scars are rarely seen, although Doppler signals are often detected at the centre and edge of the lesion. Overall the features overlap substantially with those of other benign lesions such as adenoma and malignant vascular lesions such as hepatocellular carcinoma making further imaging studies necessary.

On unenhanced CT studies FNH are subtle and well defined and may exhibit mass effect, displacing adjacent vessels. Their attenuation is similar to surrounding liver parenchyma, and they may have a central focal low attenuation scar. They demonstrate marked homogeneous enhancement in the arterial phase of IV contrast enhancement, with the exception of the central scar, and large feeding vessels may be visible at the periphery. FNH often equilibrate and disappear in the portal and later phases although, if present, the scar may remain evident and may show enhancement on delayed phases. On MRI the lesions are also subtle, being either isointense or of minimally reduced signal on T1w and increased signal on T2w images (Fig. 7-35). The central scar is hypointense on T1w and hyperintense on T2w images, and may be visible on MRI when not visualised at CT and vice versa. Following IV gadolinium enhancement the features on T1w images are the same as described for CT (Fig. 7-36). Hepatocyte-specific contrast agents such as gadoxetic acid, taken up by hepatocytes and partially excreted into the biliary system, may differentiate FNH and adenoma (Fig. 7-36). On delayed phase T1w images using these agents, substantial hepatocellular enhancement occurs within the lesion, unlike most adenomas, and retention of the agent is related to the abnormal bile ducts.

Hepatic Adenoma[15,16,45–48]

Adenomas are rare benign tumours that may arise spontaneously or in association with anabolic steroid use, glycogen storage disease type 1, maturity-onset diabetes of the young and Klinefelter's syndrome when multiple lesions are commonly present. Oral contraceptives and androgenic/anabolic steroids are considered aetiological factors, but the overall increased risk (e.g. 4× risk from oral contraceptive use) remains extremely small. They are vascular lesions composed primarily of hepatocytes, with no portal tracts or bile ducts and no bilirubin excretion; this characteristic can be used to differentiate adenomas from FNHs by using hepatocyte-specific contrast agents. These hepatocytes also have a tendency to accumulate both fat and glycogen, which may influence their appearance on imaging. Kupffer cells are usually absent but some Kupffer cell activity has been observed in up to 20% of cases. Adenomas may have a fibrous pseudocapsule and a central scar, which can make differentiation from FNH difficult. They are frequently asymptomatic but as they enlarge have a tendency to outgrow their blood supply, resulting in haemorrhage, thrombosis and necrosis. Patients may present with pain or life-threatening haemorrhage. As there is a small (1–5%) but definite risk of malignant change, resection is usually preferred to conservative management. Studies of adenoma genetics are improving the understanding of the relationship between malignant transformation and other imaging features such as fat accumulation. The widely varying findings in large complex lesions can make it difficult to establish a definitive preoperative diagnosis.

On CT adenomas may be isointense with adjacent liver, or of slightly increased or decreased attenuation. This depends on both the amount of fat in the background liver (Fig. 7-37) and within the adenoma. Uncomplicated lesions are usually homogeneous with a well-defined margin and enhance markedly and uniformly during the arterial phase, then rapidly merge with surrounding liver during the portal phase. Necrosis following haemorrhage usually results in low attenuation

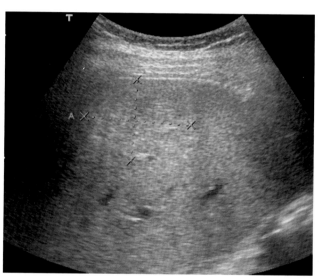

FIGURE 7-34 ■ **Focal nodular hyperplasia US.** A subtly increased echo-reflectivity lesion often difficult to define on real-time ultrasound.

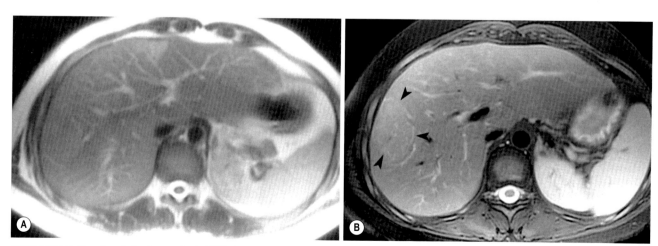

FIGURE 7-35 ■ **Focal nodular hyperplasia MRI.** On single-shot T2w FSE imaging the lesion is barely visible (A) but better demonstrated (arrowheads) on fat-suppressed multi-shot T2w FSE (B).

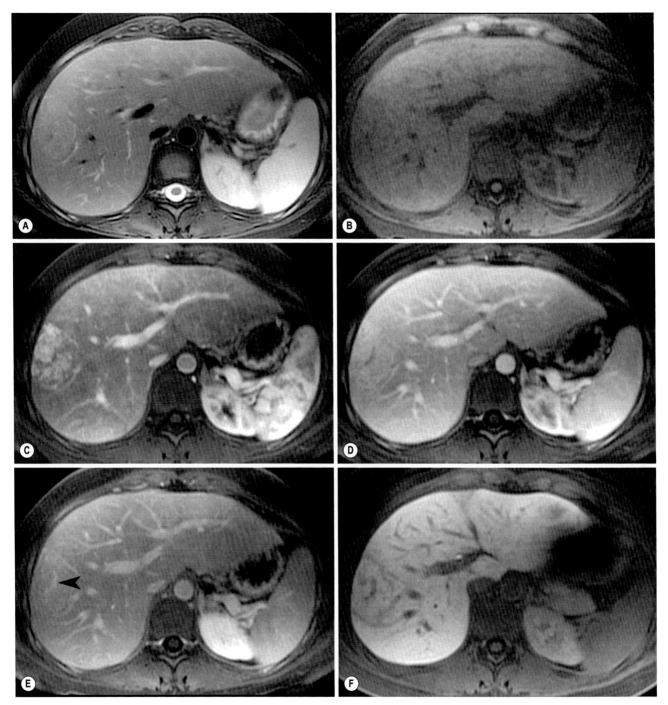

FIGURE 7-36 ■ **Focal nodular hyperplasia MRI.** A subtle lesion is demonstrated on fat-suppressed multi-shot T2w FSE (A) and unenhanced 3D T1w (B). There is avid arterial phase enhancement (C), becoming isointense in the portal (D) and delayed phases (E). A central scar is evident on some of the images (arrowhead), which enhances on the delayed image (E). On a separate occasion the lesion becomes isointense in the hepatobiliary phase following gadoxetic acid administration, typical of FNH (F).

regions within the lesion that enhance only slightly. On MRI examination, using conventional contrast agents, the appearances of uncomplicated lesions are similar to those of FNH (Fig. 7-38). The lesions are well-defined isointense or slightly hyperintense lesions on T2w and T1w images. They typically enhance markedly and uniformly during the arterial phase and disappear in the portal phase following gadolinium enhancement on T1w imaging. Adenomas that accumulate fat are well

demonstrated by MRI and may cause confusion with HCC (Fig. 7-39). Persisting delayed enhancement is described in the telangiectatic histological variant of adenoma (Fig. 7-40). In complex lesions with haemorrhage or necrosis the appearances are more heterogeneous. On delayed imaging following IV hepatocyte-specific contrast agents adenomas appear hypointense due to the absence of biliary ducts (Fig. 7-38H); this feature differentiates the majority of hepatic adenomas from FNH.

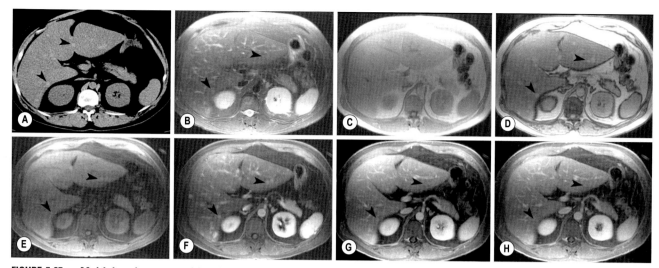

FIGURE 7-37 ▪ **Multiple adenomas with diffuse hepatic steatosis.** (A) Unenhanced CT reveals multiple foci of apparent focal fat sparing. (B) These appear as subtly increased lesions on fat-suppressed multi-shot T2w FSE. (C) They are not visible on in-phase gradient-echo imaging but become apparent on (D) the matching out-of-phase images. (E) They are subtly low signal lesions on the unenhanced T1w imaging which enhance avidly on the arterial phase (F), post gadolinium and persist subtly on the portal phase (G) and 5-min delayed phase (H). This patient was genetically XXY, a known association with multiple adenoma formation.

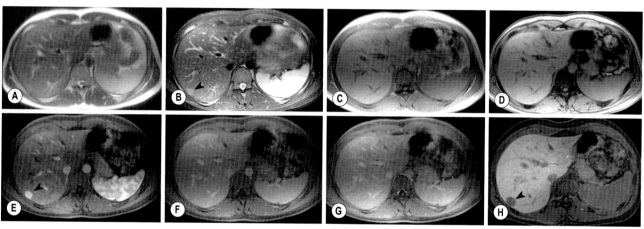

FIGURE 7-38 ▪ **Adenoma MRI.** A subtle posterior right lobe lesion is barely visible on single-shot T2w FSE (A) but more obvious (arrowhead) on the fat-suppressed multi-shot T2w FSE (B). (C) In- and (D) out-of-phase imaging demonstrate no fat accumulation. There is avid homogeneous enhancement in the arterial phase T1w imaging (E) and rapid equilibration in the portal (F) and delayed phase (G). On a separate occasion the lesion is low signal on the hepatobiliary phase following gadoxetic acid administration (H).

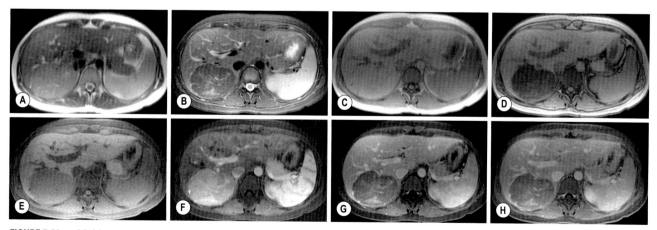

FIGURE 7-39 ▪ **Lipid-containing adenoma.** These lesions are associated with HNF1α and the fat results in increased signal on single-shot T2w FSE (A), decreased signal on fat-suppressed multi-shot T2w FSE (B) and marked signal reduction between (C) in- and (D) out-of-phase imaging. Following intravenous contrast enhancement the lesion appears to 'washout' in the later phases (E–H). This may lead to confusion with hepatocellular carcinoma. Because of the internal heterogeneity, this lesion was biopsied.

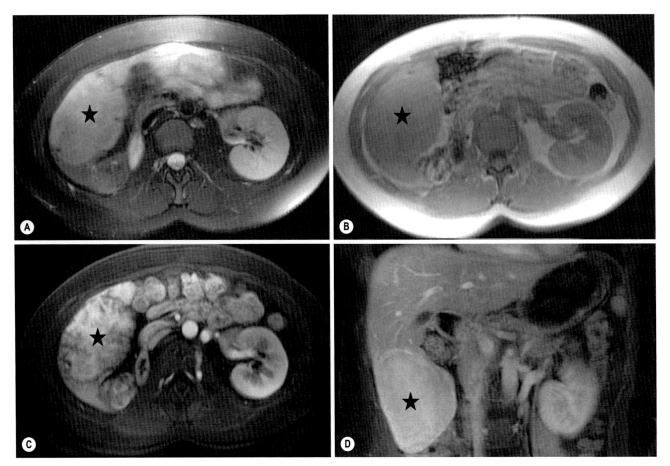

FIGURE 7-40 ■ **Telangiectatic adenoma.** These lesions (star) exhibit features similar to that of a typical adenoma on fat-suppressed (A) T2w and (B) T1w imaging, but demonstrate persistent enhancement in the delayed phase following contrast enhancement (C, D). Owing to the arterial heterogeneity and patient symptoms, the lesion was biopsied and then resected.

On US the lesions may be isoreflective with adjacent parenchyma or, if they accumulate fat, are well-defined increased echo-reflectivity lesions that mimic haemangiomas. Alternatively where there is hepatic steatosis and the adenoma does not accumulate fat they may be of reduced echo reflectivity and confused with metastases and other similar lesions.

Focal Fat[20–22]

Regional or focal variations (increase or decrease) of fat occur commonly and cause diagnostic confusion with tumours. The changes correlate with variations of local blood supply and venous drainage and commonly occur on either side of the falciform ligament, around the gallbladder fossa and in the posterior aspect of segment IV. Both focal fat accumulation (Fig. 7-41) and sparing (Fig. 7-42) are recognised in these locations. On both unenhanced CT and US, large regions of fat variation may have angular margins and a 'geographic' appearance that when combined with the lack of mass effect and preservation of the vascular architecture can be diagnostic. Focal lesions in unusual locations often preclude confident diagnosis with either CT or US, whereas MRI can be diagnostic and should be considered early in the imaging pathway when there is doubt at ultrasound. MRI using

Dixon methods (otherwise known as 'chemical shift' or 'in- and out-of-phase' imaging) is the most accurate non-invasive diagnostic test. This detects the presence of fat and water within the same image voxel as the water and fat signal combine on the in-phase image but cancel on the out-of-phase image, resulting in relative signal reduction. It should be noted that some subtle benign and malignant solid lesions such as adenomas, FNH and HCC may mimic focal fat sparing and a contrast-enhanced study may be required to exclude this possibility.

Focal Confluent Fibrosis[23,24]

This occurs in established cirrhosis, has a geographic shape and typically affects the anterior segments of the right lobe or the medial segments of the left lobe. Histologically there is massive confluent fibrosis and the affected region is atrophic.

On unenhanced CT the involved segment is low attenuation, with retraction of the overlying capsule. Following IV contrast (in the portal phase) the attenuation is the same or lower than that of adjacent liver. On MRI the same morphological features are evident and the lesions are typically of decreased signal on T1w images and increased signal on T2w images (Fig. 7-43). In the absence of any definite lobar or segmental atrophy these

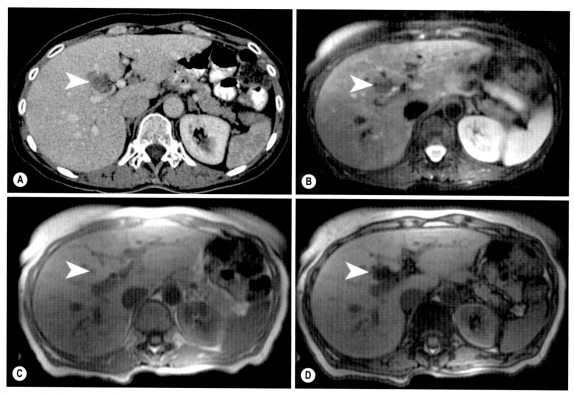

FIGURE 7-41 ■ **Focal fat deposition.** On portal phase CT (A) focal fat infiltration (arrowheads) in the posterior aspect of the left lobe medial segment (Couinaud IV) has a similar appearance to a metastasis. On fat-suppressed T2w imaging (B), the low signal makes metastasis unlikely but does not characterise the lesion. However, the demonstration of signal loss (relative to the spleen) on (C) in- and (D) out-of-phase gradient-echo imaging is diagnostic.

findings are relatively non-specific and overlap substantially with those of malignant lesions although they do not typically demonstrate arterial phase enhancement on either CT or MRI and this can be an important diagnostic feature.

Biliary Hamartomas[49] (Fig. 7-44)

Solitary and multiple biliary hamartomas occur and are typically small lesions of 3–5 mm with a combination of solid and cystic elements. They are increasingly of interest as they may be indistinguishable from small metastases on both US and CT and are probably the cause of some 'indeterminate' or 'too small to characterise' lesions. On US they are frequently overlooked unless large and predominantly cystic. When multiple they often range from 1–3 mm in size and hundreds of lesions may occur throughout the liver. In this form they are not clearly visualised as discrete lesions on US and often misinterpreted as diffuse malignant infiltration. CT often reveals their relatively cystic nature but as the lesions may have a solid component they can still masquerade as metastases and demonstrate nodular enhancement although they are usually low-attenuation lesions in the unenhanced and portal phases of a study. The MRI appearances of the multiple variant are often characteristic on heavily T2w imaging, which demonstrates more clearly the small irregular-shaped cystic components. Confident diagnosis may require biopsy and histological examination.

Atypical Regenerative Nodules

In chronic cirrhosis some regenerative nodules may become more prominent than others on imaging examinations, especially on US and MRI, causing diagnostic confusion, particularly with hepatocellular carcinoma (HCC). These atypical regenerative nodules are often not visualised on biphasic CT examination but may appear as well-defined, homogeneous lesions of reduced reflectivity on US. On MRI they are often of increased signal on T1w (owing to glycogen accumulation) and reduced signal on T2w resulting from focal iron accumulation (Fig. 7-45). The development of dysplastic and malignant foci within these nodules has been described; these may appear on T2w images as focal areas of high signal within the low signal of the nodule. Therefore, any heterogeneity within these lesions on T2w images should be viewed with suspicion.

MALIGNANT SOLID LESIONS

Hepatocellular Carcinoma[50–56]

HCC or hepatoma is the commonest primary malignant neoplasm of the liver. There are many predisposing factors, including direct carcinogens such as aflatoxin, chronic hepatitis and cirrhosis, particularly post-necrotic cirrhosis and haemochromatosis. There is wide geographical variation in incidence, which largely parallels

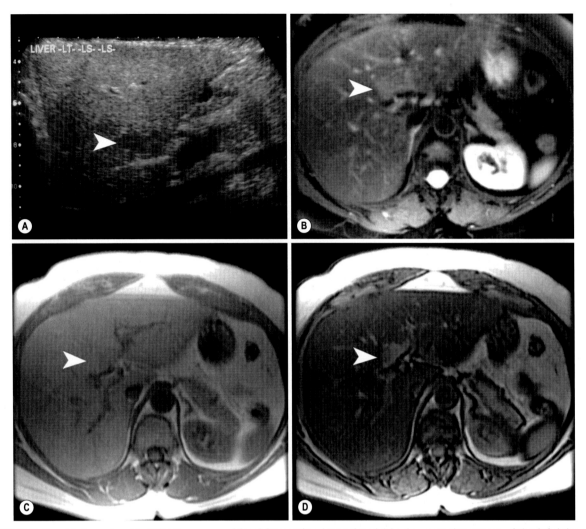

FIGURE 7-42 ■ **Focal fat sparing.** On US (A) an area of focal fat sparing (arrowheads) in the posterior aspect of the left lobe medial segment (Couinaud IV) in an otherwise fatty liver has an appearance similar to that of a metastasis. On fat-suppressed T2w imaging (B) this will appear of increased signal, suggesting a malignant lesion but the use of (C) in- and (D) out-of-phase gradient-echo imaging indicates that the 'lesion' is in fact normal liver surrounded by fatty liver that has reduced in signal on the out-of-phase image (D).

the prevalence of local predisposing conditions, in particular chronic hepatitis B and C. In Western countries incidence is increasing as a result of chronic hepatitis C infections, NASH and alcohol-related cirrhosis. Serum alpha-fetoprotein (AFP) can be helpful in diagnosis and when markedly elevated is diagnostic even in the absence of imaging confirmation. However, HCC may occur with a normal serum AFP value. HCC can be solitary, multifocal (in up to 40% of cases in the Far East) or, rarely, diffuse. Large lesions may demonstrate vascular invasive features, undergo haemorrhage (Fig. 7-46) and contain areas of fat, thrombosis and necrosis, complicating the imaging appearances. In cirrhotic livers all current imaging techniques have limited sensitivity (60–80%) for small hepatoma (≤1 cm) detection. As a result, combinations of imaging investigations are often employed to detect and diagnose small hepatomas: for example, before liver transplantation, as reflected in the AASLD criteria. Imaging techniques are more sensitive

at detecting HCC when the surrounding liver is normal. The overall 5-year survival of patients with HCC is low, at less than 30%.

US is widely used as a screening technique outside the USA and small hepatomas may be of increased or decreased reflectivity in relation to the adjacent parenchyma (Fig. 7-47). Any new solid lesion on US in a high-risk patient is considered a potential HCC. A reduced reflectivity outer margin is present in some cases and thought to represent the thin fibrous capsule. Large lesions may show internal heterogeneity, due to haemorrhage, necrosis, or fat and often cause portal vein thrombosis or tumour thrombus, which can expand the vein. High-velocity Doppler signals from within the lesion occur in the majority of cases as a result of arterioportal shunting.

Unenhanced CT may demonstrate focal or multifocal HCC as ill-defined low-attenuation lesions. Focal areas of internal calcification have been described in up to

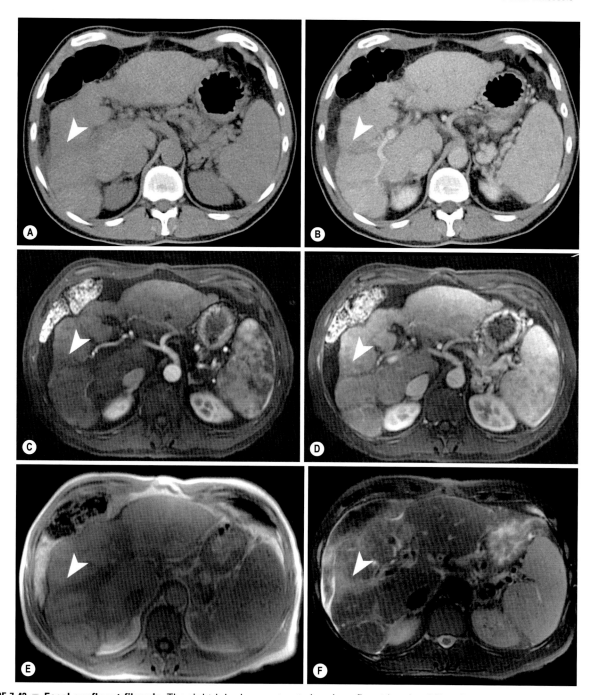

FIGURE 7-43 ■ **Focal confluent fibrosis.** The right lobe has contracted and confluent bands of fibrosis are present (arrowheads). On unenhanced (A) and portal phase CT (B), these appear of low attenuation and may mimic malignant lesions when focal. Unlike the majority of hepatocellular carcinomas on the arterial phase (C) and portal phase (D) T1w gadolinium-enhanced MRI and conventional T1w imaging (E), the fibrosis remains low signal but on T2w (F) the fibrosis is usually of increased signal and can mimic HCC.

7.5% of lesions but are rare in small lesions. Fat accumulation may also occur in HCC (Fig. 7-48). Most HCCs are hypervascular and enhance during the late arterial phase, with the majority demonstrating 'washout' in the portal phase and later phases. Some lesions may show a 'mosaic' pattern of enhancement on CT with an enhancing grid-like pattern as well as later rim enhancement. Multiphase CT with a late arterial phase is essential as many lesions are only visible during the arterial phase. Arterial infusion of Lipiodol followed 7–10 days later by

CT examination is widely used in Asia for the detection of HCC but not commonly used in other parts of the world, where arterial phase CT or MR predominates.

MRI is considered the most sensitive technique for HCC detection. Hepatoma is typically decreased signal on T1w and moderately increased signal on T2w with internal heterogeneity. However, 5–10% of HCC lesions have an atypical appearance, including being relatively avascular. Some HCC have increased T1w signal due to glycogen accumulation (Fig. 7-49) and a minority have

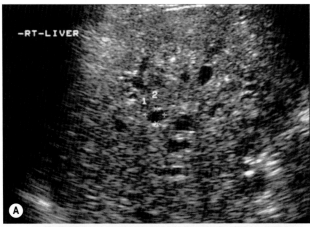

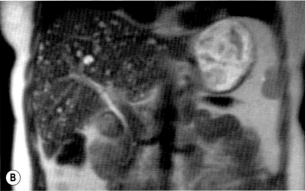

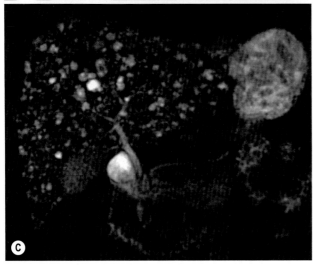

FIGURE 7-44 ■ **Multiple biliary hamartomas.** On US (A) only the larger cystic lesions are seen clearly and the background texture of the liver is heterogeneous and often misinterpreted as malignant infiltration. On conventional T2w (B) and MRCP-type T2w (C) imaging the extent and number of the multiple cystic lesions are more obvious. The solid components may be indistinguishable from métastases.

low signal on T2w. On contrast-enhanced T1w images the enhancement patterns with Gd-DTPA parallel those for enhanced CT examination, with typical lesions enhancing in the late arterial phase (Fig. 7-50) and demonstrating washout in the portal and/or delayed 5- to 10-min phases. Features of portal venous invasion include the development of thrombi and dilatation of the main

portal vein or its branches (Fig. 7-51). Atypical regenerative nodules or dysplastic nodules may cause confusion, as they may also enhance in the arterial phase but do not normally 'washout'. Often these are of increased signal on T1w and low signal on T2w, due to iron accumulation, but the presence of any heterogeneity should prompt further investigation and serial examinations may be necessary to monitor suspicious lesions. The presence of fat and iron either within HCC or background liver can substantially modify the typical arterial enhancement and subsequent washout pattern, causing false positives and negatives. The use of hepatocyte specific contrast agents (Fig. 7-52) and iron oxide agents may help improve sensitivity and specificity on MRI; however, well-differentiated HCC maintain some hepatocyte function and Kupffer cells may still be present, limiting the diagnostic utility of these contrast agents. DWI with restricted diffusion and low ADC values have been proposed as another method for improving the detection of small HCC on MRI (Fig. 7-52) but this is not yet universally accepted. Radionuclide imaging, including FDG-PET, is nonspecific for HCC and not widely used. The same applies to angiography, which may demonstrate dilated feeding arteries, abnormal tumour vessels and arteriovenous shunting.

Multiple locoregional therapies are now available for HCC and are discussed elsewhere. Contrast-enhanced US, CT and MRI have all been used to assess HCC treatment response based on residual enhancement. This is considered unreliable in the first 4–6 weeks post treatment but helpful on later follow-up studies where enhancing lesion components are considered viable. DWI and apparent diffusion coefficient (ADC) maps have also been successfully used in post-tumour treatment assessment. The ADC is increased in necrotic tissue, while it is restricted in viable tumour.

Fibrolamellar Carcinoma (FLC)[57]

(Fig. 7-53)

This lesion is now considered a separate entity to HCC that occurs in the 5–35 years' age group. It arises spontaneously with no known predisposing factors. FLC usually presents as a solitary, lobulated, well-defined large tumour containing a central fibrous scar. Punctate calcification is present in the scar in more than 50% of cases, which may aid diagnosis as calcification is relatively rare in HCC or FNH. Histologically FLC is composed of fibrotic lamellae and numerous eosinophilic hepatocytes. Treatment is resection where possible and 5-year survival is approximately 60%.

Unenhanced CT examination demonstrates a well-defined lobulated mass of low attenuation with an even lower attenuation central scar with radial linear components and, frequently, punctate calcification. The lesion demonstrates non-specific enhancement and delayed enhancement of the scar may occur, making differentiation from FNH difficult. MRI reveals a similar morphology with a low signal scar on T1w and T2w (in contrast to FNH, where the scar is typically high signal on T2w). The punctate calcification is rarely demonstrated. On US

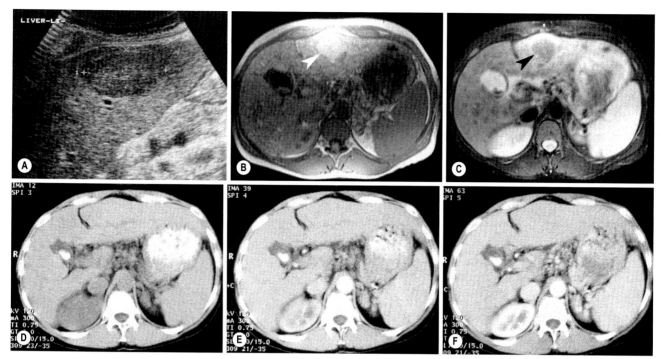

FIGURE 7-45 ■ **Atypical regenerative nodules.** Regeneration in cirrhosis often results in heterogeneity of the parenchyma. Occasionally nodules may become large, 'atypical' or 'dominant' as in this patient. US (A) demonstrates a reduced echo-reflectivity lesion in the left lobe, initially interpreted as probable tumour. However, on MRI the relatively homogeneous lesion (arrowheads) is of increased signal on T1w (B) and decreased signal on T2w (C). These appearances are not typical of malignancy and are recognised as a feature of regenerative nodules (in this case, confirmed on biopsy). Similar smaller nodules are widespread in the liver. Axial CT images (D) unenhanced, (E) arterial phase and (F) portal phase of the same patient demonstrating no differences in enhancement characteristics of the nodule when compared to the rest of the liver parenchyma.

the lesion is commonly increased reflectivity and the central scar and calcification may be evident.

Hepatoblastoma

This tumour occurs at any age but most commonly in children less than 3 years old. It is the third commonest abdominal childhood tumour, after neuroblastoma and Wilms' tumour, and is associated with markedly elevated serum AFP levels. Histologically it is composed of primitive hepatocytes, often with mesenchymal components.

On imaging the tumour presents as a large heterogeneous mass but may also appear composed of multiple confluent nodules. There may be central areas of necrosis, and enhancement may be seen in the arterial phase on CT. Punctate calcification is a common finding on US and CT.

Epithelioid Haemangioendothelioma[58]

This is a tumour of vascular origin occurring more commonly in adult women and is difficult to diagnose even with histology. Composed of 'epithelioid' endothelial cells, it occasionally contains areas of punctate calcification. On imaging, epithelioid haemangioendothelioma (EHE) presents as multiple peripheral nodules that often coalesce, causing capsular retraction, with compensatory hypertrophy of uninvolved liver segments. The lesions may cause and present with hepatic vein occlusion. On unenhanced CT, the lesions are visible as multiple peripheral heterogeneous areas of low attenuation (Fig. 7-54).

Enhancement of the rim of the nodules has been described, with a low-attenuation 'halo' outside the ring of enhancement. On US the tumours appear solid and of low reflectivity. On MRI the lesions are hypointense on T1w images, and moderately hyperintense on T2w images.

Hepatic Lymphoma[59]

Primary hepatic lymphoma is rare, although liver is a common site of secondary lymphomatous involvement. Primary lymphoma presents as a large, multilobulated mass on CT that enhances poorly following IV contrast medium, and central necrosis is common. Secondary lymphomatous involvement of the liver is commonly diffuse infiltration or micronodular, and imaging frequently demonstrates non-specific hepatomegaly with no focal lesions.

Angiosarcoma[60] (Fig. 7-55)

Angiosarcomas of the liver are rare tumours associated with polyvinyl chloride, arsenic or Thorotrast contrast medium exposure. These aggressive vascular hepatic neoplasms appear as infiltrating, contrast-enhanced masses on CT and occasionally present in a diffuse form not easily detected by imaging. Thorium, when present, is obvious on CT as it causes heterogeneously increased attenuation in the liver, perihepatic lymph nodes and spleen.

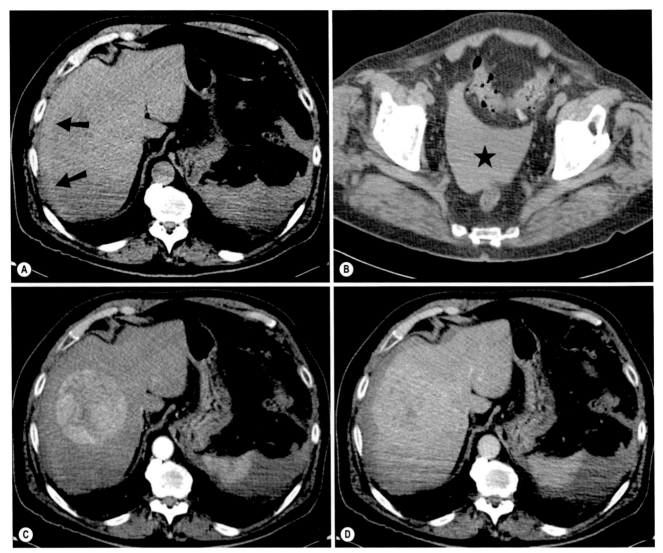

FIGURE 7-46 ■ **HCC presenting with spontaneous rupture.** A patient with acute abdominal pain. Unenhanced CT (A) demonstrates a rind of increased attenuation blood clot around the liver (arrows) and free blood in the pelvis (B). Arterial phase imaging (C) reveals a heterogeneous HCC which might have been overlooked on portal phase imaging alone (D).

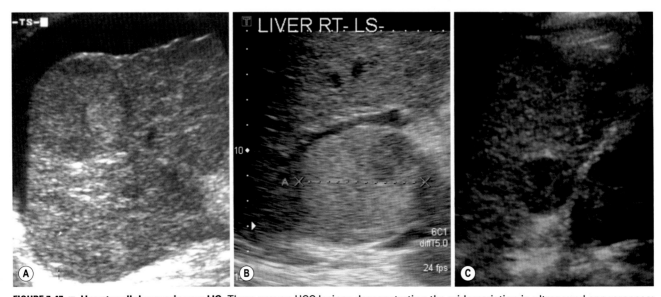

FIGURE 7-47 ■ **Hepatocellular carcinoma US.** Three proven HCC lesions demonstrating the wide variation in ultrasound appearances: (A) increased echo reflectivity; (B) a mixture with a 'nodule in a nodule' appearance; and (C) reduced echo reflectivity.

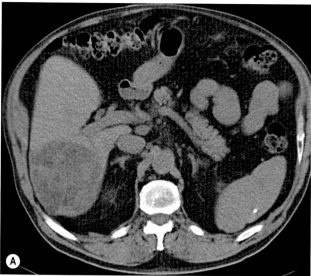

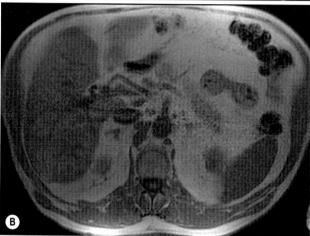

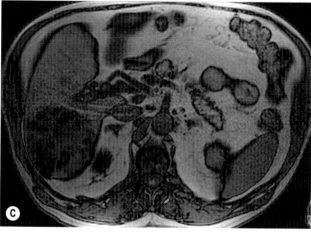

FIGURE 7-48 ■ **HCC containing fat.** In this patient a heterogeneous HCC is relatively well demonstrated on unenhanced CT (A) because of the presence of fat within the HCC, confirmed by (B) in- and (C) out-of-phase MRI.

Metastases[36,61–66]

Liver metastases are a common event in the natural history of many primary malignancies and most are haematogenous in origin. Gastrointestinal (GI) tract tumours metastasise to the liver via the portal vein, and tumours elsewhere via the hepatic artery.

Most imaging methods will not reliably detect and characterise hepatic lesions of less than 3–5 mm in diameter and cannot distinguish reliably between a small metastasis and a biliary hamartoma. Metastases have a wide range of appearances on imaging but usually share the features of growth on serial imaging, multiplicity and variation of size. They derive their blood supply from the hepatic artery but the majority are less vascular than adjacent liver parenchyma, a feature that influences their appearance with vascular enhancement techniques. Metastatic tumours that may have increased vascularity compared with normal liver parenchyma include breast, kidney, thyroid, neuroendocrine and melanoma. Increasingly, chemotherapeutic agents modify the imaging features of metastases, making post-treatment evaluation more complex.

Studies comparing the relative sensitivity and specificity of cross-sectional imaging techniques in the detection of hepatic metastases are difficult to evaluate because of variations in technique, validation and the rapid evolution of imaging technology. Overall, contrast-enhanced US, MR and CT are broadly similar in performance when performed with optimal techniques and equipment. Generally, specificity falls as sensitivity increases and the 'gains' in sensitivity with the newer MRI techniques such as DWI and hepatocyte-specific contrast media have been mainly in the detection of subcentimetre lesions. However, many subcentimetre lesions in patients with known malignancy are not in fact metastases, based on serial imaging and comparative histological studies. In clinical practice, the choice of imaging technique is influenced by the management implications, local availability and expertise.

On US metastases may be homogeneous and of increased or decreased reflectivity (Fig. 7-56). They may have a surrounding rim of reduced reflectivity, giving a target-type appearance. Central necrosis may result in a partly cystic appearance. Metastases of increased reflectivity can mimic haemangiomas and predominantly cystic metastases (e.g. ovary) can mimic simple cysts.

On CT most metastases are low attenuation on unenhanced images and portal phase images. Hypervascular tumours are often visible as low-attenuation lesions on unenhanced images and may enhance transiently in the arterial phase, some becoming invisible in the portal phase (Fig. 7-57). CT is the most sensitive method for detecting the subtle calcification that may occur within mucin-secreting metastases of GI tract origin. Central necrosis and rim enhancement can also be clearly demonstrated on CT examination.

On MRI most metastases are of low signal on T1w and high signal on T2w images, their signal approximately matching that of the spleen (Figs. 7-58 and 7-59). Contrast-enhanced MR studies give similar appearances to CT for the detection and demonstration of lesions in the unenhanced, arterial and portal phases although calcification is not usually visible. On T2w studies with paramagnetic iron oxide agents there is reduction of normal parenchymal signal due to Kupffer cell uptake, making the metastases (and any other lesions that do not take up the iron oxide) more obvious. Paramagnetic

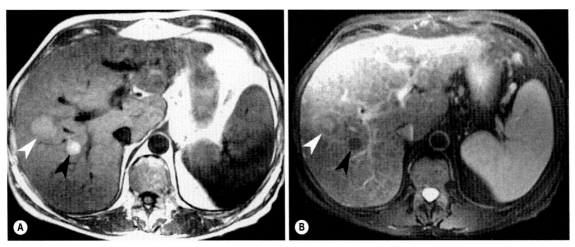

FIGURE 7-49 ■ **Hepatocellular carcinoma and regenerative nodule.** (A) T1w and (B) T2w MRI demonstrating a hepatocellular carcinoma (white arrowhead) and an adjacent atypical regenerative nodule (black arrowhead). Although the majority of hepatomas have decreased signal intensity on T1w, occasionally they have increased signal, thought to relate to fat or glycogen content. Note the heterogeneity in the hepatoma, particularly on T2w. The findings were confirmed at subsequent liver transplantation.

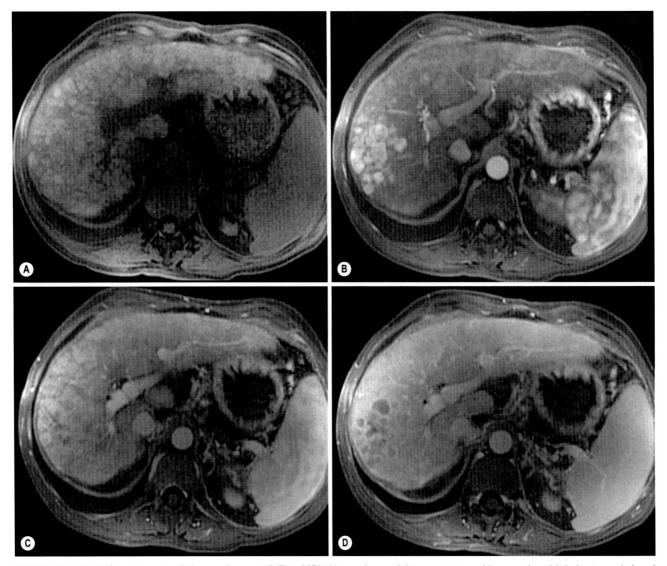

FIGURE 7-50 ■ **Multifocal hepatocellular carcinoma.** 3D T1w MRI (A) unenhanced demonstrates widespread multiple increased signal nodules, (B) arterial enhancing multifocal HCC is clearly visible in the right lobe, (C) the HCC lesions become isointense in the portal phase and (D) the HCC demonstrates washout on the 5-min delayed image. Note that a protocol providing only (A) and (C) would likely result in the diagnosis being missed.

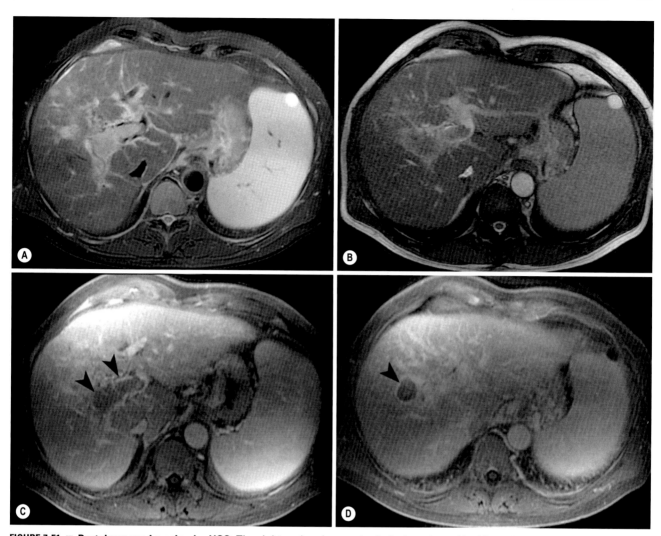

FIGURE 7-51 ■ **Portal venous invasion by HCC.** The right and main portal vein is thrombosed in this patient with HCC. (A) Multi-shot T2w FSE is not reliable as intravascular signal may be due to slow flowing blood. The thrombus is more clearly visualised on the balanced gradient-echo imaging (B) and most reliably in the portal phase following intravenous contrast medium (C, D). Note how the thrombus expands the portal vein (arrowheads) and extends cranially towards the underlying tumour (not shown).

hepatocyte-specific contrast media increase the normal liver signal on T1w imaging, whereas metastases (and other lesions) are unable to metabolise hepatocyte specific contrast agents and appear hypointense on delayed phases (Fig. 7-60). Recently the use of DWI with intermediate b-values has demonstrated high sensitivity for small metastases. This technique is relatively fast, avoids contrast administration and relies on increased cellular density in metastases (compared to normal liver parenchyma) restricting water molecule diffusion, resulting in high signal intensity on intermediate b-values and reduced ADC values (Fig. 7-60). On colloid radionuclide imaging, the majority of metastases appear as areas of reduced activity due to a lack of Kupffer cells.

VASCULAR LESIONS

Budd–Chiari Syndrome[67,68]

Obstruction of the hepatic veins secondary to obstruction of the IVC by a membrane or thrombus, or occlusion of

the major hepatic vein branches (usually by thrombus) is termed Budd–Chiari syndrome (BCS). In most cases there is preservation (and early hypertrophy) of the caudate lobe, which drains via separate veins directly into the IVC. BCS is frequently idiopathic but also associated with oral contraceptive use, coagulopathies (polycythaemia, thrombotic thrombocytopenic purpura) and congenital membranes or webs in the IVC (rare in Western practice). BCS may also occur secondary to compression of the hepatic veins by tumours, or following hepatic vein trauma or surgery. BCS may present acutely with hepatomegaly, abdominal pain and ascites, as the liver becomes congested and swells, or more insidiously with features of secondary portal hypertension. Over time the periphery of the affected segments atrophy and the preserved caudate lobe and unaffected segments demonstrate compensatory hypertrophy. Findings are often variable, as only one or two major veins may be affected and collateral venous channels permit regeneration to occur in the peripheral liver as well as the caudate lobe. Although all imaging techniques may demonstrate some features of BCS, core needle biopsy is frequently required

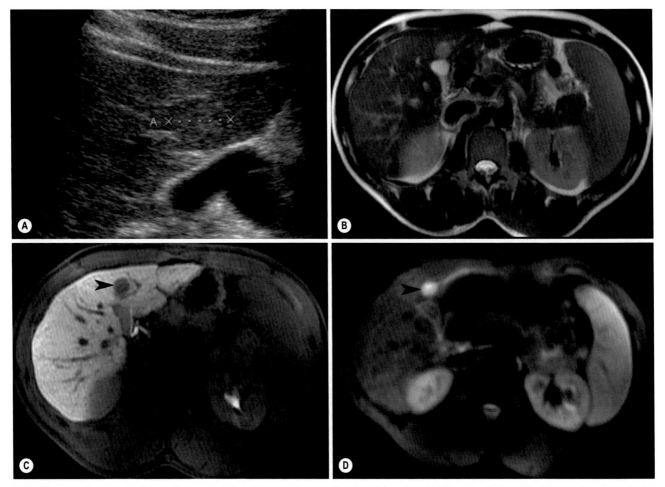

FIGURE 7-52 ■ **Hepatocellular carcinoma.** In this patient with a small well-differentiated HCC, detected on US (A), an adequate arterial phase at MRI was not possible but the lesion was just visible on single-shot FSE (B) and has the low signal features of HCC in the hepatocyte phase post gadoxetic acid (C) and restricted diffusion on DWI (D), b500 image.

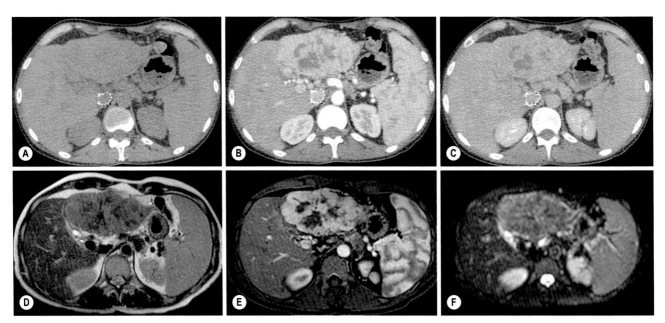

FIGURE 7-53 ■ **Fibrolamellar carcinoma.** The large heterogeneous lesion with a fibrous central region with limited enhancement post contrast medium is demonstrated on CT pre (A), arterial (B) and delayed phase (C), as well as on MR single-shot T2w FSE (D), arterial phase T1w (E) and on DWI b500 imaging (F).

to exclude the presence of tumour and confirm central venous congestion or venous thrombi.

US by an experienced operator can lead to unequivocal diagnosis in acute BCS by identifying acute thrombus in the major veins. More commonly US will demonstrate abnormally curved collateral veins passing between the major hepatic veins, or continuous reversal of flow in a main hepatic vein. The inability to demonstrate the

hepatic veins or related flow is highly suspicious but this should be interpreted with caution in the presence of cirrhosis. Damping of the normally pulsatile hepatic vein waveform may occur but is non-specific. On unenhanced CT the enlarged, congested peripheral liver is lower attenuation than normal, with reduced and heterogeneous uptake following enhancement which may outline a hepatic vein branching pattern, whereas the caudate is often preserved with a normal attenuation and enhancement pattern (Fig. 7-61). In chronic cases peripheral liver atrophy, with compensatory hypertrophy of the caudate is common along with collateral venous channel formation (Fig. 7-62). However, as the appearance of the peripheral liver is variable and heterogeneous following contrast enhancement, BCS is not infrequently mistaken for extensive tumour involvement. This situation is complicated as BCS can occur secondary to malignancy and be the presenting feature. Rarely CT may directly demonstrate hepatic vein thrombus in acute cases.

MRI demonstrates similar morphological features to CT, and in the acute stages hepatic vein thrombus may be identified, along with collaterals (Fig. 7-61). MR angiography techniques are helpful in assessing vascular patency and may be used to identify the direction of flow. The congested peripheral liver is often heterogeneous on both T1w and T2w images in contrast to the relatively normal or hypertrophied caudate lobe. Radionuclide imaging with sulphur colloid will demonstrate normal or increased caudate lobe activity and reduced activity in the remainder of the liver. On angiography the venographic appearances are characteristic and said to resemble a spider's web as a result of numerous small interconnecting collateral vessels.

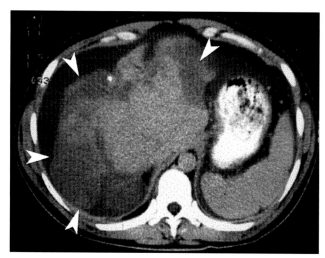

FIGURE 7-54 ■ **Epithelioid haemangioendothelioma.** CT demonstrates peripheral low-attenuation lesions (arrowheads) that have coalesced to form a rind of tumour enclosing the central normal liver parenchyma. The patient presented with Budd–Chiari syndrome secondary to the tumour, diagnosed on needle biopsy and confirmed at subsequent liver transplantation.

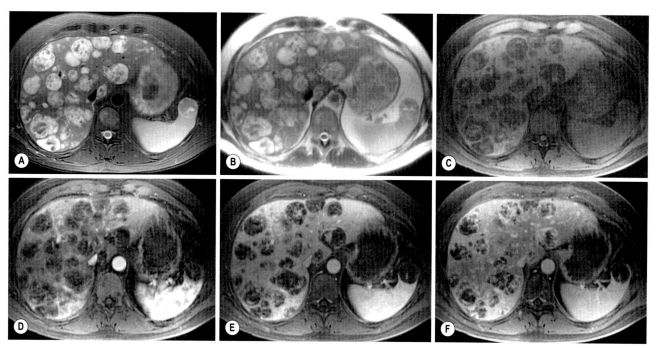

FIGURE 7-55 ■ **Hepatic angiosarcoma.** Multifocal well-defined heterogeneous lesions are clearly demonstrated on (A) fat-suppressed multi-shot T2w FSE, (B) single-shot T2w FSE and (C) unenhanced 3D T1w. They demonstrate progressive heterogeneous enhancement following gadolinium (D–F). The lesions had trebled in diameter over an 8-week period.

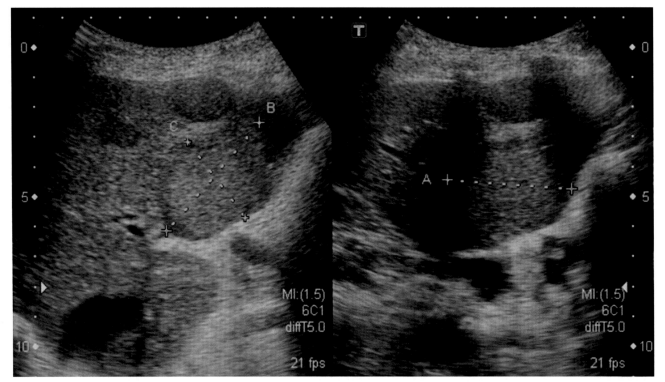

FIGURE 7-56 ■ **Hepatic metastases US.** Metastases may have widely varying appearances on US. Here there are both increased and decreased echo-reflectivity lesions present.

Veno-Occlusive Disease

Veno-occlusive disease (VOD) results from obliteration of the central draining veins of the hepatic lobules by an inflammatory fibrotic process that often leads to secondary portal hypertension. Causes include Jamaican bush-tea drinking, but more commonly VOD follows chemotherapy in bone marrow transplantation. The diagnosis is made by biopsy, although coagulation markers may prove to be an effective alternative.

The main role of imaging is to exclude other causes of abnormal liver function and frequently demonstrates non-specific hepatomegaly but the major hepatic veins usually remain patent.

Portal Venous Hypertension

The pressure difference between the wedged hepatic vein and the IVC is normally 4–8 mmHg; higher pressures indicate portal hypertension (PH). This results from many different disease processes that increase resistance to portal venous flow. Ascites is a common general finding in PVH. Typically the mesenteric veins are distended and the walls of the gallbladder, stomach and small bowel are oedematous. Splenomegaly is not always present and dependent on the degree and distribution of portosystemic shunting elsewhere in the portal venous system. A portal vein diameter in excess of 15 mm is suggestive of PVH, but a normal portal vein diameter does not exclude the diagnosis and there is little agreement on a repeatable site for measurement. Portosystemic venous collaterals support a diagnosis of PVH and may occur at many sites, including splenogastric,

gastro-oesophageal, splenorenal and recanalised paraumbilical veins. Treatment may involve shunt creation and typical surgical locations are splenorenal and portocaval. Radiologically placed transjugular portosystemic stent shunts (TIPSSs) are widely used for palliating portal venous hypertension.

US provides reliable assessment of the major hepatic vasculature, confirming size, patency and flow direction in the main portal vein. Main portal vein mean peak velocity values of less than 10 cm/s are considered abnormal and another indicator of portal venous hypertension. In severe cases portal vein flow may become stationary or oscillating with a pattern related to respiration and/or arterial pulsation before leading to flow reversal and continuous hepatofugal flow (Fig. 7-63). In the presence of a recanalised paraumbilical vein unusual flow patterns may emerge such as 'stealing' from the right portal vein having reversed flow with normal hepatofugal flow in the left portal vein. CT provides a rapid abdomino-pelvic overview and accurately detects portosystemic shunts, and oedema of the small bowel and gastric wall. On MRI balanced gradient-echo breath-hold techniques can demonstrate gastrointestinal tract changes, assess the portal vein and detect shunt vessels. These may be confirmed on multiphase gadolinium-enhanced T1w volumetric studies. Both CTA and MRA are routinely used when US proves technically inadequate.

Portal Vein Thrombosis[69]

This may be idiopathic but usually has an underlying aetiology such as hepatic cirrhosis, infection (portal pyaemia, acute cholecystitis), inflammation (pancreatitis,

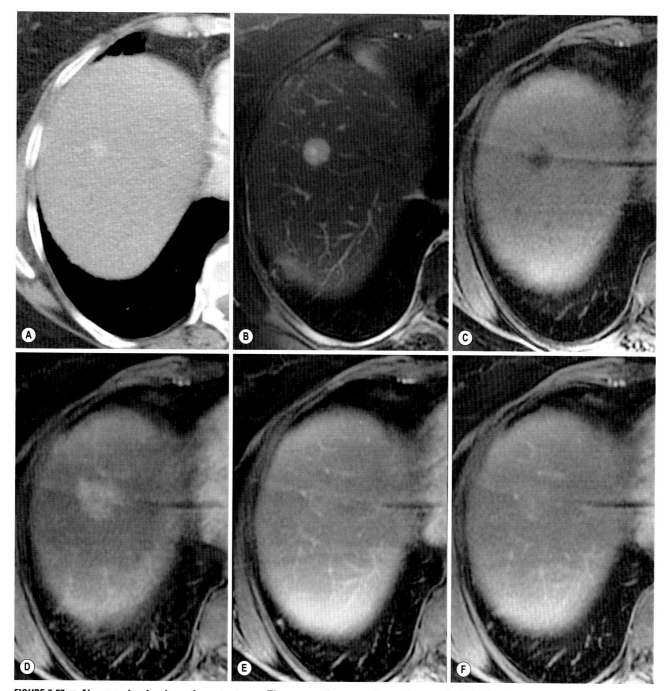

FIGURE 7-57 ■ **Neuroendocrine hepatic metastases.** These are often vascular and may mimic both HCC and haemangiomas. In this patient a subtle lesion only visible in the arterial phase was detected at CT (A) and subsequent MRI demonstrated a well-defined lesion on multi-shot T2w FSE (B) which was hypointense to the liver parenchyma on pre-contrast T1w image (C) and enhanced in the arterial phase (D) and persisted in the later phases (E-F).

necrotising colitis), tumour (HCC, pancreatic carcinoma, gastric carcinoma), trauma, coagulopathy, or surgery (liver transplantation). Acute thrombosis presents with abdominal pain or secondary complications of acute portal venous hypertension, such as bowel infarction and ascites. In patients with established cirrhosis, portal hypertension and portosystemic shunt vessels, PVT may be occult. Imaging in the early stages of an acute thrombosis demonstrates an avascular solid thrombus occluding and often expanding the portal vein. In more

established thrombosis the portal vein is small, and frequently becomes fibrotic or calcified with multiple surrounding collateral vessels (cavernous transformation). A thrombosed portal vein or branch vein that remains enlarged or increases in size is suspicious for underlying tumour.

US is the most useful technique for assessing thrombosis of the main portal vein branches (Fig. 7-64). Acute thrombus may be of low reflectivity, making it difficult to detect on B-mode imaging and Doppler studies are

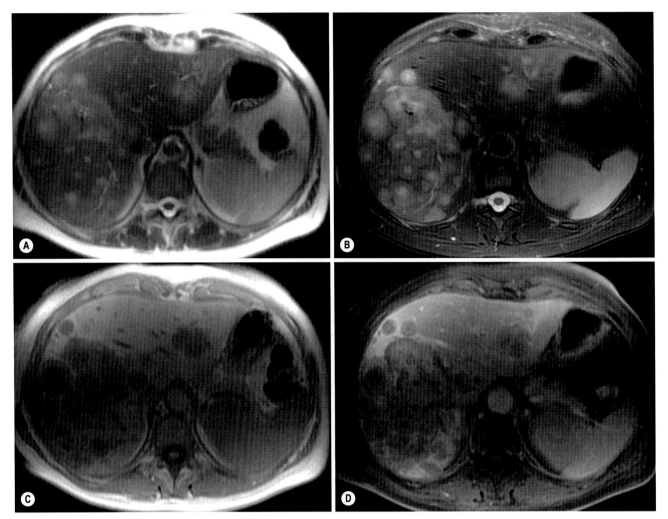

FIGURE 7-58 ■ **Hepatic metastases MRI.** Multiple 'target'-type metastases from breast cancer on single-shot T2w FSE (A), multi-shot T2w FSE (B), T1w (C) and portal phase post-gadolinium enhancement (D). Note the improved lesion contrast on the multi-shot FSE and the similar signal intensity to the spleen.

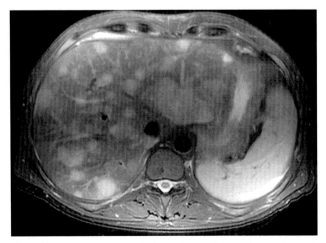

FIGURE 7-59 ■ **Hepatic metastases MRI.** Fat-suppressed multi-shot T2w FSE, adenocarcinoma metastases from a bowel tumour of similar intensity to the spleen.

essential for confident diagnosis. Arterial signals within an apparent thrombus suggest the presence of tumour but may reflect recanalisation as a thrombus evolves. In the presence of severe cirrhosis or hepatic steatosis the acoustic beam can become too attenuated to allow reliable Doppler imaging and other techniques should be used.

Contrast-enhanced MRI and CT techniques can provide accurate demonstration of portal vein thrombosis (Fig. 7-65) which on CT may be hyperdense in the acute stage, and they are particularly useful for demonstrating aetiologies such as tumour or pancreatitis.

Arterioportal Shunts

These are often caused by a penetrating injury of the liver, including percutaneous diagnostic and interventional procedures, and may be misinterpreted as malignant lesions. In addition, shunts occur in cirrhosis, portal hypertension and tumours, particularly large hepatocellular carcinomas.

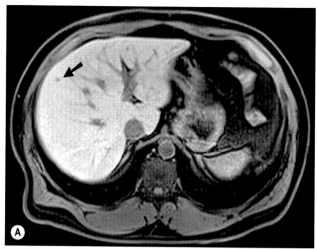

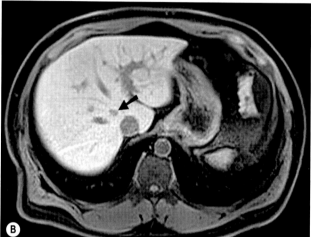

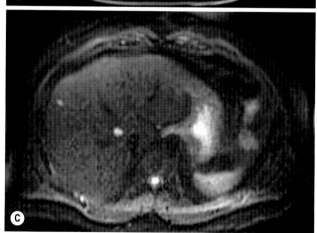

FIGURE 7-60 ■ **Hepatic colorectal cancer metastases MRI.** (A, B) Two small (arrows) low signal metastases on adjacent thin sections of 3D T1w imaging in the hepatobiliary phase following gadoxetic acid. (C) Both lesions are clearly shown on DWI imaging (b = 500).

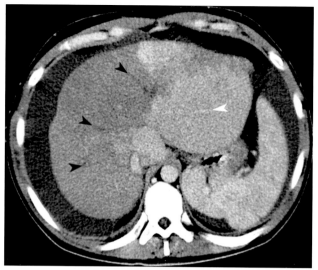

FIGURE 7-61 ■ **Acute Budd–Chiari syndrome.** On portal phase CT most of the caudate and left lobe of the liver has enhanced normally and the left hepatic vein can just be seen (white arrowhead) but the right lobe is abnormally low attenuation and the middle and right hepatic vein branches are attenuated and have failed to opacify (black arrowheads). Ascites is present.

Intrahepatic Portosystemic Shunts[70]

Intrahepatic portosystemic shunts occur in association with cirrhosis and portal hypertension but also arise congenitally. Most congenital cases have multiple small portovenous shunts (1–2 mm diameter) in the periphery of an otherwise normal liver and may present with unexplained hepatic encephalopathy. In patients with portal hypertension and cirrhosis the shunts are often larger. Small shunts may only be detectable on angiography, whereas larger shunts are demonstrated on US, CT and MR.

Arteriovenous Shunts

These also occur as a result of trauma and tumours but also as part of hereditary haemorrhagic telangiectasia (Osler–Weber–Rendu disease) where multiple small intrahepatic arteriovenous shunts occur. These are often asymptomatic but large shunts lead to heart failure, and through vascular dilatation (Fig. 7-67) cause biliary obstruction and recurrent cholangitis. Ultimately hepatic necrosis and liver failure may occur. This process is usually exacerbated by any attempt at arterial embolisation. Larger lesions and enlargement of the supplying arteries can be demonstrated using Doppler US and demonstrated with arterial phase contrast-enhanced CT and MRI.

HEPATIC TRAUMA[71,72]

Blunt or penetrating trauma may cause intraparenchymal laceration and haematoma (Fig. 7-68), subcapsular haematoma or capsular rupture with intraperitoneal haemorrhage. Intraparenchymal lacerations and haematomas are

These lesions appear as areas of increased flow on colour Doppler and arterialisation of portal venous flow occurs with large shunts (Fig. 7-66) which may cause regional hepatic atrophy. During arterial phase CT examination, an early enhancing focal lesion may be demonstrated along with early filling of the portal vein.

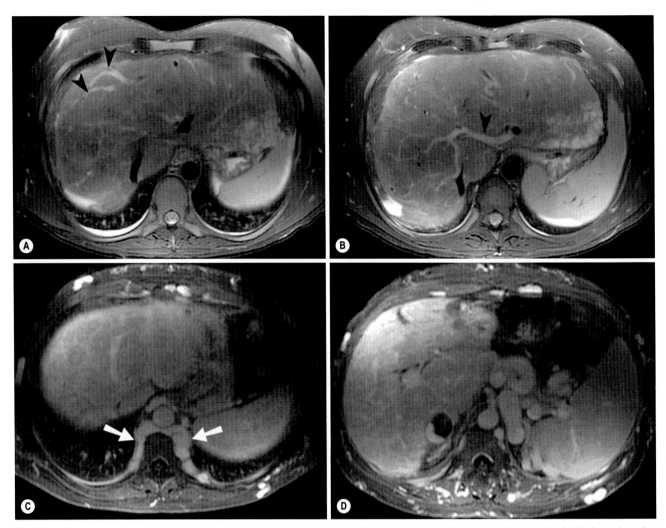

FIGURE 7-62 ■ **Chronic Budd–Chiari syndrome.** Changes in a patient with previous occlusion of the right and middle hepatic veins include hypertrophy of the left lobe and numerous abnormal curved venous channels (arrowheads) shown on multi-shot T2w FSE imaging at two different levels (A, B). In a separate patient following occlusion of the IVC by thrombus (C, D) there are enlarged retroperitoneal and azygos system veins (arrows) as well as numerous superficial collateral veins shown on post-gadolinium T1w MRI.

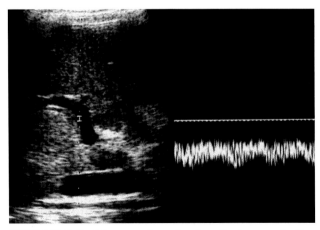

FIGURE 7-63 ■ **Portal venous hypertension.** Duplex examination demonstrates continuous reversed (hepatofugal) flow in the portal vein, usually reflecting underlying severe cirrhosis and portal venous hypertension with varices.

usually elliptical or linear in shape. Lacerations directly involving the major branches of the major vessels are relatively rare (Fig. 7-69) but may lead to life-threatening haemorrhage. Secondary problems may develop, including ischaemia, necrosis of part of the liver, abscess formation, haemobilia, focal fibrosis, calcification and lobar or segmental atrophy. In recent years liver trauma has been conservatively managed with less surgical resection. Imaging plays an important role in the assessment of the nature and extent of hepatic trauma except where injuries are immediately life threatening and require emergency surgery. Information regarding the type of lesion and its anatomical location in relation to the major hilar structures and the confluence of the hepatic veins and IVC can be rapidly obtained and used to guide subsequent management.

Prompt multiphase CT is the diagnostic technique of choice for evaluating upper abdominal trauma. Unenhanced images may reveal large lacerations as low-attenuation regions, and both subcapsular and free

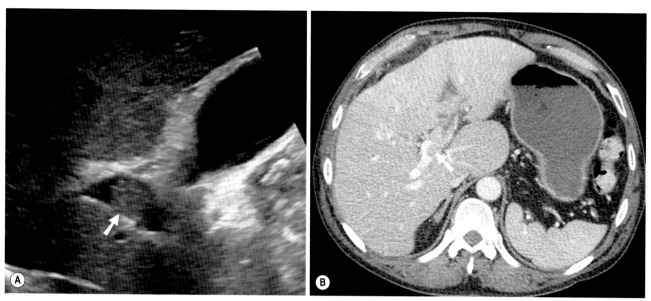

FIGURE 7-64 ■ **Portal vein thrombosis.** A partial thrombosis is visible on ultrasound (A) as echo-reflective material within the portal vein (arrow). (B) This is shown as a filling defect on the matching portal phase CT.

intraperitoneal blood. The location of fresh thrombus (typically higher attenuation than normal blood) may indicate the source of haemorrhage is nearby. Arterial and portal phase imaging with IV contrast medium are mandatory for the detection of arterial injuries, subtle lacerations and evaluation of hila involvement (Fig. 7-70). Angiography is usually reserved for therapeutic embolisation. US may demonstrate free intraperitoneal fluid or thrombus but does not reliably identify all liver lacerations. Parenchymal lacerations with related haematoma may be seen as elliptical or irregularly shaped areas of mixed low and high reflectivity. Subcapsular haematomas are well demonstrated and US is useful mainly for the follow-up of known lesions and detecting later complications such as abscess formation. MRI is not normally employed for acute hepatic trauma but may be used to monitor established parenchymal or subcapsular haematomas in which methaemoglobin increases the signal intensity on T1w images (Fig. 7-71).

LIVER TRANSPLANTATION

Background and Indications[73–75]

Orthotopic liver transplantation is an established treatment for end-stage liver disease from a wide range of causes, most commonly cirrhosis secondary to infective hepatitis, autoimmune disease or alcohol but also rare inherited conditions such as Alagille's syndrome. The procedure has a survival rate of 90% at 1 year and 80% at 5 years. Improvements in outcome have resulted from selection of patients most likely to benefit, optimisation of surgical techniques and new therapies for controlling immune system rejection. Most procedures use cadaveric organs but demand exceeds supply; this led to the development of split-graft procedures, where a single donor organ benefits two or more patients and living donors.

Imaging plays an important role in the assessment of patients and living donors prior to transplantation as well as during the immediate perioperative period and subsequent follow-up of the graft for the diagnosis and treatment of complications.

Recipient Assessment[76,77]

Imaging is employed to detect and characterise focal liver lesions, demonstrate patency of the portal vein and IVC, and delineate relevant anatomical variants including varices that may cause problems at surgery. Hepatomas are a common problem and, when present, the Milan criteria are currently used to restrict transplantation to cases with a single lesion measuring 5 cm or less or three lesions measuring 3 cm or less. These criteria, based on an outcome analysis during the 1990s, are being reviewed and extended to take into account the 'aggressiveness' of a lesion through growth rate and the impact of locoregional therapies. Most centres avoid biopsy of likely hepatomas prior to transplantation to avoid the risk of 'seeding' the tumour outside the liver, so the detection and characterisation of focal liver lesions relies primarily on imaging.

CTA and MRA are used to detect any variant hepatic artery supply (Fig. 7-5) and evaluate the hepatic veins and IVC. Portal vein patency is assessed primarily with Doppler US and, where needed, CTA or MRA. If the portal vein is occluded, evaluation includes the extent of thrombus and whether the confluence of the superior mesenteric vein and the splenic vein is involved. Vascular reconstructions can be used to 'jump' an occluded main portal vein and connect to this confluence if patent.

Living Donor Assessment[78–81]

Most liver transplant living donors undergo left lobe resection, although increasingly right lobe segments are

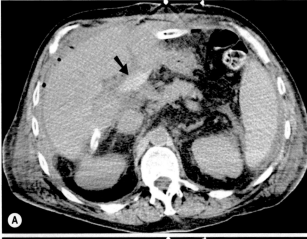

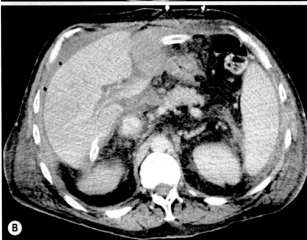

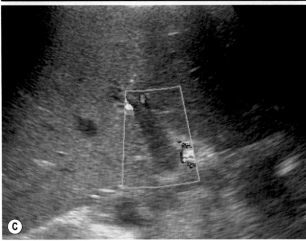

FIGURE 7-65 ■ Acute portal vein thrombosis. This patient deteriorated 48 h after liver transplantation. Unenhanced CT (A) demonstrates a hyperdense thrombus filling the main portal vein (arrow). This became isointense (and undetectable) with the remainder of the portal vein in the portal phase (B) following intravenous contrast enhancement and was confirmed on Doppler ultrasound (C).

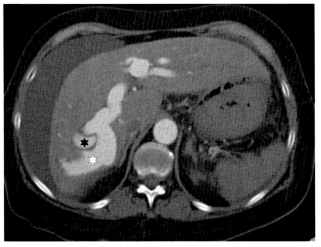

FIGURE 7-66 ■ Arterioportal shunt. Portal phase CT demonstrates ascites and an atrophic right liver lobe. The enlarged artery is visible (black *) which connected almost directly into the portal vein (white *), creating a large volume shunt. The portal venous system has enlarged as a result and the shunting led to the right lobe atrophy and liver failure.

hepatic venous and biliary systems that might complicate the procedure or make it impractical. Anomalies that cross the planned surgical division plane are the most important and may lead to complications for both the donor and the recipient. US can demonstrate clearly the portal and hepatic venous anatomy, but both contrast-enhanced CT and MR provide more information regarding the artery and can be combined with biliary studies.

Perioperative Imaging

The detection of early complications such as haemorrhage, haematoma, abscess formation and anastomotic breakdown is usually performed with imaging and guided interventional drainage or aspiration performed, if appropriate. In high-risk groups such as paediatric transplants, or those with more complex vascular reconstructions, surveillance US is often performed regularly during the early postoperative period to detect complications such as hepatic artery occlusion that might respond to immediate intervention.

Graft Failure[82,83]

Early graft failure may be due to primary non-function where hepatocyte function fails to recover in the newly perfused graft, despite vascular patency and apparently good perfusion at implantation. Other causes of early graft loss are major vessel occlusion and overwhelming sepsis. Portal vein thrombosis and IVC occlusions are relatively rare but hepatic artery thrombosis (HAT) occurs in 3–5% of adults and 5–15% of children. HAT may present in three main ways: (A) catastrophic liver failure with infarction and abscess formation (Fig. 7-24); (B) biliary complications such as leak or stricture formation; and (C) silently with no obvious sequelae. Doppler US has been the mainstay of diagnosis, although CTA and MRA are often used for confirmation. Acute rejection is

being donated, despite several related donor deaths occurring. Before donation, cross-sectional and three-dimensional (3D) imaging techniques are essential for evaluating residual liver and donated lobar volumes, and for detecting variants of the arterial, portal venous,

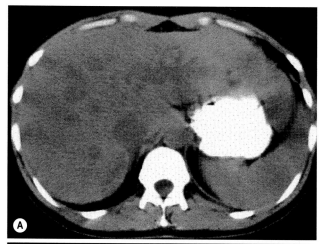

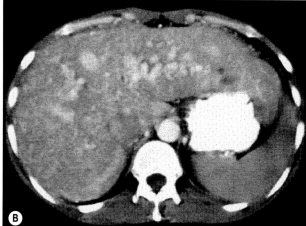

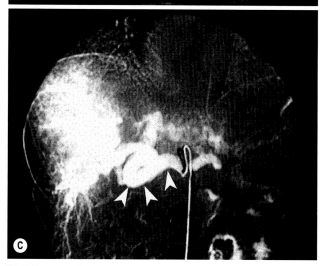

FIGURE 7-67 ■ **Hereditary haemorrhagic telangiectasia.** Arteriovenous shunts result in enlarged vascular channels throughout the liver at CT (A), which enhance rapidly (B). The increased volume of shunted blood results in further enlargement of the vessels (C), including the supplying hepatic artery (arrowheads).

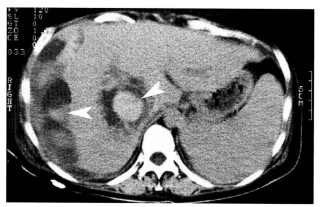

FIGURE 7-68 ■ **Intrahepatic haematoma CT.** Recent intraparenchymal haemorrhage following a liver biopsy is evident on unenhanced CT where sequestered blood has formed thrombi that undergo contraction increasing globin density. This results in areas of subtly increased attenuation (arrowheads).

now a relatively infrequent complication of early transplantation due to improved immunosuppression.

Late graft failure may be the result of chronic rejection, chronic ischaemia, biliary anastomotic failure or diffuse biliary disease due to sepsis, or increasingly recurrence of the underlying disease such as primary sclerosing cholangitis or hepatitis C infection. In many cases the diagnosis of late failure is made on biopsy, but imaging is used to assess the biliary tree for anastomotic strictures or diffuse cholangiopathy changes.

LIVER BIOPSY

Liver Biopsy, Aspiration and Drainage

Liver biopsy is widely used for diagnosis of focal and diffuse liver disease, and monitoring chronic liver disease progression. Imaging guidance is particularly appropriate in the presence of coagulopathy, ascites, obesity, colonic interposition, segmental (rather than whole) liver transplantation, chronic liver disease with severe right lobe atrophy (typically placing the gallbladder superficially in the mid-axillary line) and failed previous traditional 'blind' liver biopsy. Aspiration and drainage procedures require imaging guidance and are widely used in the management of liver abscess and perihepatic collections.

Devices

A wide range of core needle biopsy devices are available, categorised by method of operation as well as needle diameter. Most use either suction (Menghini), or cutting sheath action, and may be spring-powered or manually operated. Disposable spring-powered cutting sheath biopsy devices are widely used and collect more consistent core biopsies with less crush artefact than older manually operated systems. There is wide variation across the world in the relative utilisation and accuracy of cytological and histological examination for the diagnosis of liver disease, which directly influences the choice of biopsy device. Aspiration is performed using a wide range of hollow needles and cannulas. Drainage procedures where a catheter is left in place typically utilise pigtail drainage catheters with multiple side holes and may include locking devices to prevent displacement.

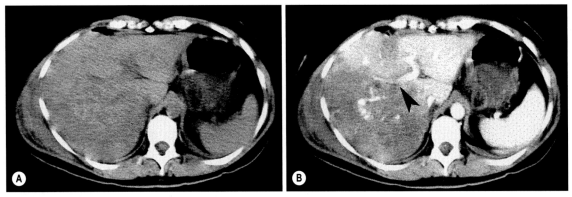

FIGURE 7-69 ■ **Portal vein trauma.** This patient sustained liver trauma during a road traffic accident. (A) Unenhanced and (B) portal phase CT sections demonstrate probable disruption of the right main portal vein (arrowhead) and failure of enhancement in the right lobe of the liver.

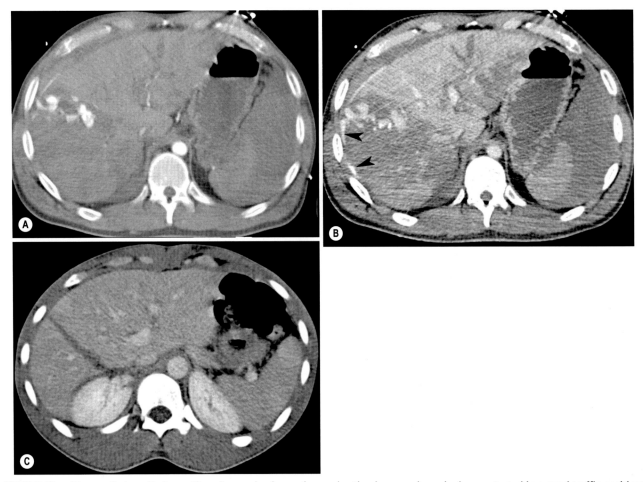

FIGURE 7-70 ■ **Traumatic hepatic laceration.** A complex laceration and active haemorrhage is demonstrated in a road traffic accident patient on (A) arterial phase and (B) portal phase. Note the ongoing accumulation of contrast medium in the laceration and around the liver capsule (arrowheads). The patient went to immediate laparotomy. In a separate patient stabbed with a 15-cm knife a deep laceration is clearly demonstrated on portal phase imaging (C). Remarkably no major vessel was damaged and there was minimal haemorrhage.

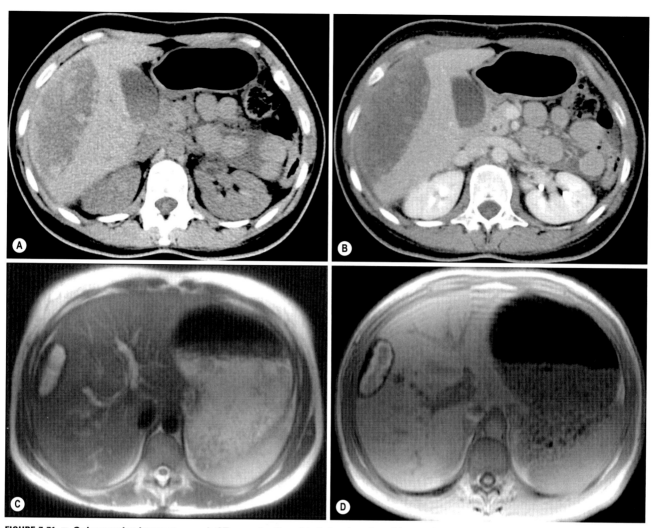

FIGURE 7-71 ■ **Subcapsular haematoma.** A CT examination 4 h following liver biopsy demonstrating a heterogeneous appearance with mixed solid and fluid components that fail to enhance pre (A) and portal phase (B) post contrast medium. Six months later the haematoma has largely organised and reduced in size with fluid signal on single-shot T2w FSE (C) and a low signal rim (haemosiderin) and increased signal inner margin (residual methaemoglobin) on T1w gradient-echo imaging (D).

Approach Routes

The traditional route for liver intervention uses a horizontal right lateral intercostal approach but imaging guidance allows the use of other approaches. An anterior subcostal approach that does not traverse the pleura is less likely to cause pulmonary complications and, where practical, may be preferred in patients with respiratory compromise. Liver lesion biopsy using a route through intervening normal liver probably reduces the risk of haemorrhage, although there is no scientific evidence to support this. The planned approach to the lesion should take into account adjacent vulnerable structures, including the hilum, gallbladder, hepatic flexure, stomach, duodenum, mesenteric vessels, pericardium, pleura, lung and diaphragm.

In the authors' practice, US guidance is primarily used as the real-time capability allows faster positioning of the needle or catheter. US also allows selection of an oblique approach, which can be particularly useful for targeting lesions near the diaphragm or heart.

CT is limited to axial imaging and is therefore suited to orthogonal biopsy approaches in the plane of the image. Angulated approaches are possible but require careful planning to obtain the desired results. In the authors' practice CT is employed mainly for lesions inaccessible to US biopsy. The intermittent nature of the imaging makes CT more dependent on repeatable breath-holding by patients. CT fluoroscopy can overcome this problem at the expense of a larger dose of radiation.

Practical Procedural Issues

In obese patients it is important to identify the rib space clearly during needle insertion and to achieve adequate anaesthesia of the parietal peritoneum and liver capsule. In patients with chronic cirrhosis the liver parenchyma may be quite stiff, making instrument manipulation difficult. Choice of imaging technique is occasionally dictated by whether the lesion is visible using that technique. Problems arise with subtle hepatomas, and benign lesions

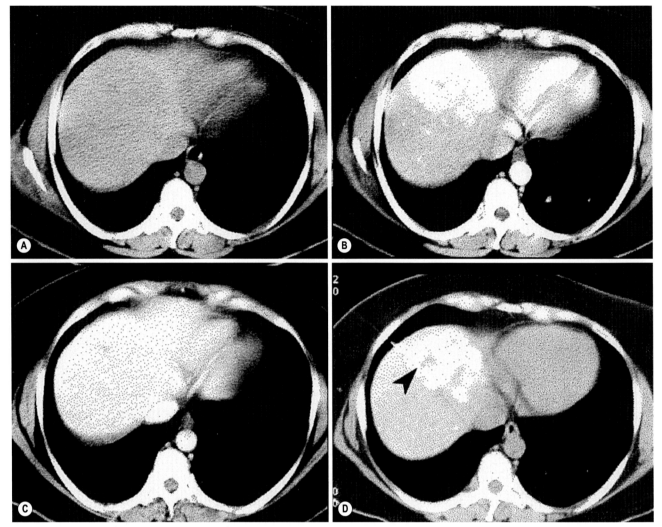

FIGURE 7-72 ■ **Lipiodol marking of a focal nodular hyperplasia lesion with CT for biopsy.** (A) Unenhanced. (B) Arterial phase. (C) Portal phase. Transient enhancement is seen during the arterial phase, and a possible central scar. Intra-arterial Lipiodol was injected to 'mark' the lesion for subsequent CT-guided biopsy (D), performed 6 h after arterial injection.

such as FNH and adenoma, which may not be visible on US and may be only transiently visualised on CT (during the arterial phase). Delayed phase CT may be helpful; alternatively, intra-arterial Lipiodol may be useful to mark vascular lesions prior to biopsy (Fig. 7-72).

Complications and Safety[84–88]

A wide range of complications have been reported, including haemorrhage (Fig. 7-71), pneumothorax, biliary peritonitis, perforation of bowel and gallbladder, haemobilia and arterioportal shunt formation. In a review of more than 68,000 biopsies the mortality rate was estimated at approximately 1 : 10,000, with all the deaths in patients being either cirrhosis or malignant disease. Serious complications requiring treatment (haemorrhage, pneumothorax, biliary peritonitis) were three times more common with cutting sheath (3/1000) when compared with suction systems (1/1000). Of these complications, 61% occurred within the first 2 h and 96% within 24 h of biopsy. There is no correlation between the number of passes made with the biopsy needle and mortality and the presence of ascites is not a contraindication to biopsy. There is good evidence from animal studies that increasing needle calibre correlates positively with increased risk of haemorrhage.

SPLEEN

ANATOMY[89–91]

The spleen has a smooth lateral convex surface conforming to the adjacent abdominal wall and left hemidiaphragm, whereas the medial surface is concave. Prominent lateral and inferior clefts are often present and may simulate splenic lacerations. There are wide variations in normal spleen size, but a 12-cm maximal

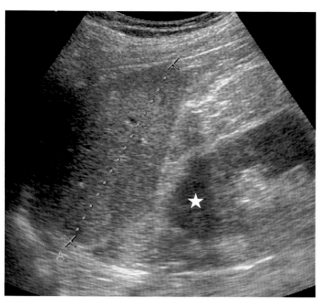

FIGURE 7-73 ■ **On ultrasound the normal spleen is positioned immediately superior to the left kidney (star).** The parenchyma is homogeneous and measures less than 12 cm in oblique craniocaudal length.

craniocaudal length is commonly used as a threshold for splenomegaly. The splenic artery is a branch of the coeliac artery and the splenic vein drains into the portal vein.

On US, the spleen is homogeneous with intermediate to low echo reflectivity (Fig. 7-73). On unenhanced CT the spleen is homogeneous with density values 5–10 HU lower than normal liver. Following IV contrast medium administration (on both CT and MRI) the spleen has a characteristic striped pattern of enhancement during the early parenchymal phase. This results from fast and slow vascular channels in the cords of red pulp in the spleen. During the venous and later phases the spleen has a uniform, homogeneous appearance (Fig. 7-9). At MR the normal signal intensity of the spleen is less than that of hepatic parenchyma on T1w images, and slightly greater than that of muscle, whereas on T2w images the spleen demonstrates higher signal intensity than liver (Fig. 7-12).

CONGENITAL VARIATIONS

Accessory Spleen or Splenunculus[90]
(Fig. 7-74)

An accessory spleen is normal splenic tissue discrete from the main splenic body. Splenunculi are common and vary in size from a few millimetres to several centimetres and occur most frequently at the splenic hilum. In atypical locations, accessory spleens may be mistaken for tumours but may be detected by the similar (to the normal spleen) tissue contrast and enhancement pattern, although usually lacking the arterial phase heterogeneous appearance. Splenunculi also occur post-splenectomy, and may enlarge, although they usually retain a spherical shape.

Polysplenia and Asplenia[89,91] (Fig. 7-75)

Polysplenia (the presence of multiple small spleens instead of a single large spleen) is more common in women and associated with situs ambiguous. The absence of a spleen is associated with situs inversus and occurs more commonly in male patients. Both polysplenia and asplenia are rare and often associated with other congenital rotational and symmetry abnormalities involving the mesentery, heart, liver and the IVC.

ACQUIRED DISEASES

Trauma[71,72] (Fig. 7-76)

The spleen is frequently injured in abdominal trauma. Both acute and delayed splenic rupture may cause life-threatening haemorrhage making detection, staging and follow-up of splenic trauma essential. In recent years management has become more conservative, preserving splenic tissue where possible to avoid the increased severity of pneumococcal infection following splenectomy. Multiphase contrast-enhanced CT has a sensitivity and specificity above 95%, and is the established imaging technique for splenic injury diagnosis and grading. Splenic trauma may manifest as parenchymal laceration or haematoma. On unenhanced CT acute haematomas may be hyperdense or isodense to normal parenchyma but fail to enhance post intravenous contrast administration. Focal areas of enhancement within a haematoma may indicate active bleeding. Splenic lacerations are linear low-attenuation parenchymal defects, and almost always associated with a haemoperitoneum. Where a laceration traverses two splenic capsular surfaces, it is termed a fracture. Even in the absence of a parenchymal defect a significant splenic injury is indicated by a perisplenic or subcapsular haematoma, which are crescentic well-defined lesions along the splenic margin. On US, haematoma has a similar appearance to that described in relation to the liver and when organised appears as well-defined, hypoechoic areas, but US is not considered sensitive enough to reliably exclude significant splenic injury following trauma although haematoma resolution may be followed by US or CT. MRI is rarely used in acute trauma but will demonstrate haematomas and the imaging characteristics depend on the phase of blood product degradation.

Infections[89,91,92] (Fig. 7-77)

Solitary or multiple abscesses occur in the spleen and occur more frequently in immunocompromised patients. Trauma (15%) and splenic infarction (10%) may also predispose to splenic abscesses. On unenhanced CT images, splenic abscesses are spherical or lobulated hypodense lesions, which rarely contain gas. Post IV contrast administration no capsular rim of enhancement is visualised unlike liver abscesses. Fungal infections are also more common in the immunocompromised population and large fungal abscesses may have a target appearance which relates to their structure: (1) a central nidus of necrotic hyphae, hypoechoic at US and hypodense at

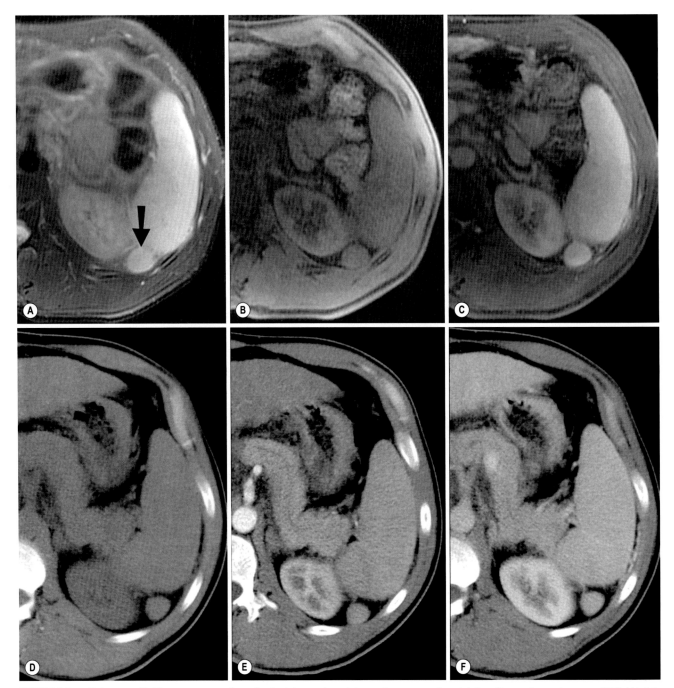

FIGURE 7-74 ■ **Splenunculi.** These are usually spherical (arrow) and have the same signal intensity as the spleen on MRI (A) fat-suppressed T2w multi-shot FSE, (B) unenhanced 3D T1w, (C) portal phase 3D T1w and the same attenuation on CT (D) unenhanced, (E) late arterial and (F) portal phase.

CT; (2) a concentric band of viable fungal elements, hyperechoic at US and hyperdense at CT; and (3) a surrounding circular area of inflammation, hypoechoic at US and hypodense at CT. At MR, fungal deposits are round-shaped T1-hypointense and T2-hyperintense masses. The peripheral area of inflammation may demonstrate enhancement on CT or MR after contrast administration.

Splenic involvement is common in patients with disseminated tuberculosis (TB) and other granulomatous infections. It is usually widely distributed in a fine miliary pattern and TB lesions may appear on CT as tiny low-density foci scattered throughout the whole spleen. On ultrasound they may present with numerous increased echo-reflectivity foci creating a 'bright spleen' or 'pepper pot' pattern which may persist after treatment. Splenic TB may also present with larger focal lesions as pseudo-tumours or tuberculomas and this may occur without overt pulmonary or gastrointestinal tract involvement. There is splenomegaly with multiple small masses

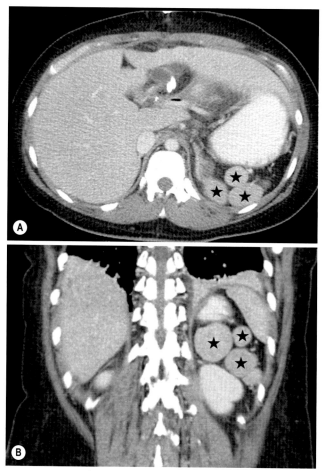

FIGURE 7-75 ■ **Polysplenia.** (A) Axial and (B) coronal portal phase CT demonstrates multiple spleens in the left upper quadrant (black stars). This may be associated with situs inversus.

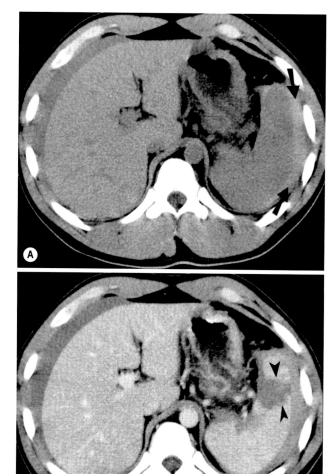

FIGURE 7-76 ■ **Splenic trauma.** On the unenhanced CT (A) a rind of high-attenuation material (blood clot) is visible adjacent to the spleen (arrows), indicating the likely source of haemorrhage in this trauma patient. Only on the portal phase (B) is the splenic 'fracture' clearly visible (arrowheads).

(1–3 cm in size), hypoechoic at US and hypodense at CT, scattered throughout the spleen. Large chronic tuberculoma lesions often calcify.

Infarction[89,91] (Figs. 7-78 and 7-79)

The splenic artery is an end artery, so branch occlusions commonly cause splenic infarction. This may result from emboli related to vascular atheroma, acute pancreatitis, coagulopathies, and following hepatic arterial embolisation. Venous infarction also occurs in portal venous hypertension or splenic vein occlusion. Splenic infarcts may become infected or rupture and the imaging appearance depends on the time after onset. Hyperacute (day 1) infarcts appear on US as decreased echo-reflectivity areas with ill-defined margins and on unenhanced CT ill-defined areas of decreased attenuation, although a heterogeneous pattern of increased attenuation foci occurs in the case of haemorrhagic infarcts. Acute (days 2–4) and subacute (days 4–8) infarcts appear as wedge shaped well-demarcated areas which are hypoechoic but not cystic at US and which are low attenuation with no enhancement at CT. After 2–4 weeks, infarcts may decrease in size, and their attenuation may return to

normal on CT images obtained both before and after IV contrast medium. In the long term, infarcts may completely disappear, result in a residual contour deformity or calcify. MR characteristics depend on the stage of infarction but also any haemorrhagic component: subacute or chronic arterial infarcts intensity on T1w images and high signal intensity on T2w images. In cases of venous infarction there is often eventual haemosiderin deposition visible as foci of low signal on T1w and T2w imaging which demonstrate 'blooming' effects (enlargement) on gradient-echo imaging owing to susceptibility effects.

BENIGN LESIONS

Benign lesions demonstrate signal characteristics similar to cysts, with low signal.

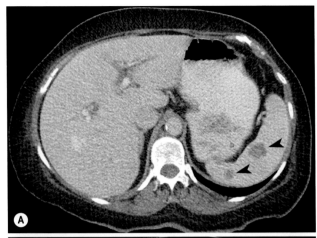

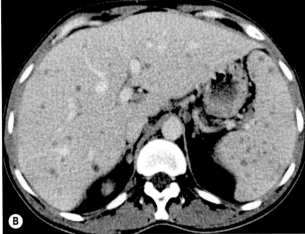

FIGURE 7-77 ■ **Splenic abscess.** (A) An immunocompromised patient with 'target'-type fungal abscesses (arrowheads). In (B) a patient with disseminated TB there are multiple small, low-attenuation abscesses in both the liver and spleen.

Cysts[89,91] (Fig. 7-80)

Splenic cysts may be congenital true cysts with an epithelial lining or acquired pseudocysts. True cysts are developmental in origin, probably due to infolding of peritoneal mesothelium in splenic sulci. Pseudocysts account for 80% of splenic cysts; they lack an epithelial lining and their aetiology is most likely post-traumatic, post infarction, or post infective. True cysts and pseudocysts appear identical at imaging, being characteristically unilocular well-defined anechoic masses at ultrasound, and homogeneous water density lesions with no discernible wall, and no enhancement following IV contrast administration at CT. MR images demonstrate a well-defined round hyperintense lesion on T2w and a low-signal lesion in T1w which does not enhance following IV contrast administration.

Parasitic splenic cysts are typically caused by *Echinococcus*. These cysts appear at CT and US as sharply marginated, round/ovoid water density masses and may have ring-like calcification and small daughter cysts may be present at the periphery of the main cyst. *Echinococcus*

cysts may be heterogeneous secondary to internal debris and hydatid sand.

Haemangioma[93] (Fig. 7-81)

Splenic haemangiomas consist of vascular channels of varying size lined by a single layer of endothelium; they are commonly single asymptomatic lesions, unless part of a generalised angiomatosis, such as Klippel–Trénaunay–Weber syndrome. Imaging characteristics vary depending on the gross morphology and range from solid to mixed (with cystic and solid components) to cystic. At US, small cystic areas are often seen within an increased echo-reflectivity mass and calcification may occur with echo-reflective foci with acoustic shadowing. Colour Doppler flow US may demonstrate blood flow within the solid portions. On CT images, splenic haemangiomas are solid, homogeneous, hypoattenuating or multicystic masses often containing foci of calcification. After administration of intravenous contrast medium these lesions demonstrate enhancement and appear similar to the normal splenic tissue. At MR, splenic haemangiomas are hypointense on T1w images and markedly hyperintense on T2w images; however, haemangiomas may be heterogeneous on T2w images when there are mixed cystic and solid components. Areas of haemorrhage or proteinaceous fluid within haemangiomas may appear hyperintense on T1w images.

Hamartomas and Lymphangiomas[89,91]
(Fig. 7-82)

Splenic hamartomas are solitary low-attenuation splenic masses which may be solid or cystic and, when solid, have imaging characteristics similar to splenic parenchyma. Splenic lymphangiomas are composed of a single cyst or multiple cysts of varying size lined by endothelium and filled with proteinaceous fluid. Lymphangiomas have US and CT imaging characteristics similar to simple cysts; they are single or multiple homogeneous lesions with a sharply marginated thin wall and do not enhance. Small marginal linear calcifications may be present. At MR these lesions are also very similar to simple cysts: homogeneously hypointense on T1w and hyperintense on T2w images, although areas of high signal intensity on T1w images may be present related to proteinaceous fluid.

MALIGNANT LESIONS

Angiosarcoma[93–95] (Fig. 7-83)

Primary angiosarcomas of the spleen are rare and have a poor prognosis. They may present as multiple nodules of varying size, solitary complex masses of cystic and solid components with a variable degree of contrast enhancement, well-defined haemorrhagic nodules or as diffuse splenic involvement. CT may demonstrate hypodense lesions on unenhanced images associated with focal areas of high density representing acute haemorrhage or haemosiderin. The enhancement pattern can be similar

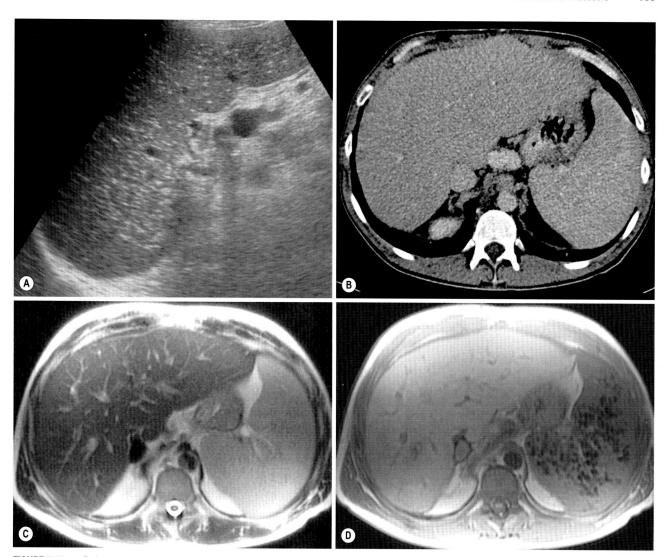

FIGURE 7-78 ■ **Splenic venous infarcts.** On ultrasound (A) multiple increased echo-reflectivity lesions may occur following granulomatous infections such as TB and histoplasmosis but may also be caused by small focal haemorrhages arising in portal venous hypertensions (Gandy-Gamna bodies). They are often not well visualised on CT (B) unless they calcify and are also overlooked on spin-echo-based T2w imaging (C) but 'bloom' owing to their susceptibility effect on gradient-echo imaging (D).

to hepatic haemangioma and evidence of distant metastases may be the only indication of malignancy. On MR they are nodular masses with hypointense margins on T1w and T2w images, representing haemorrhagic nodules. The signal intensity on T1w of the central portion varies, depending on the age of haemorrhage and the presence of necrosis.

Lymphoma[89,91] (Fig. 7-84)

Secondary splenic involvement is common in many lymphomas, whereas primary splenic lymphoma is relatively uncommon. Spleen size alone is not a reliable sign of lymphomatous involvement although splenomegaly is present in most patients with non-Hodgkin's lymphoma. Up to a third of patients with splenomegaly have no evidence of splenic lymphoma at histological examination. In addition, up to a third of patients with lymphoma of any kind have histological involvement of the spleen without splenomegaly. Splenic lymphomas may present at US with three different patterns: (1) diffusely heterogeneous with disruption of the normal splenic ultrasound appearance; (2) small, nodular, hypoechoic lesions; and (3) large, focal, hypoechoic lesions that may be cyst like. Cyst-like lesions may be markedly hypoechoic and resemble simple cysts; however, they lack posterior acoustic enhancement. A cystic appearance may also be due to necrosis. CT is unreliable in the diagnosis of splenic lymphoma because a normal-appearing spleen may still contain tumour cells. Demonstration of splenic hilum adenopathy and focal splenic enhancing defects, in addition to splenomegaly, are more reliable CT indicators of lymphomatous involvement. At MR, areas of lymphoma involvement appear as slightly hypointense foci on T1w and hyperintense foci on T2w images. In similar fashion to CT, MR imaging cannot reliably depict

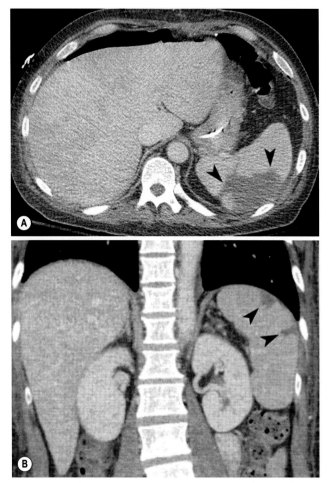

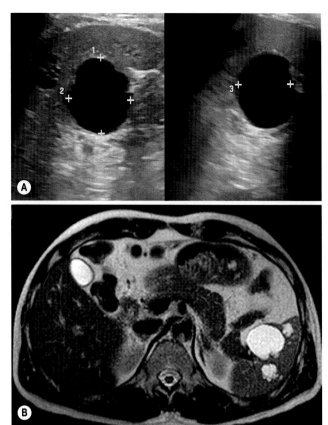

FIGURE 7-80 ■ **Splenic cysts.** These are well-defined lesions with no perceptible walls and no internal echoes on (A) US and well-defined homogeneous high signal lesions on (B) T2w imaging.

FIGURE 7-79 ■ **Splenic arterial infarcts.** Arterial emboli commonly result in peripheral well-defined wedge-shaped lesions, as shown here on an axial (A) and coronal (B) portal phase CT study (arrowheads).

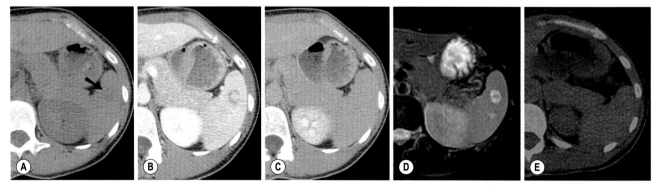

FIGURE 7-81 ■ **Splenic haemangioma.** Unenhanced CT (A) demonstrates a subtle low-attenuation lesion (arrow) that partially enhances on the arterial phase (B) and equilibrates in the portal phase (C). It is high signal on fat-suppressed T2w FSE imaging but heterogeneous (D). A PET-CT confirms the lack of metabolic activity and excludes a malignant lesion (E).

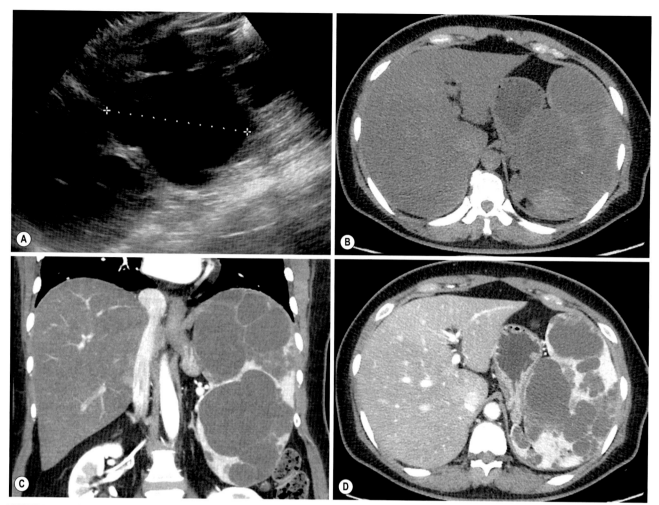

FIGURE 7-82 ■ **Splenic lymphangioma.** A complex predominantly cystic lesion with multiple subdivisions and septations expanding the spleen is demonstrated at US (A) and CT unenhanced (B) and portal phase coronal (C) and axial (D) imaging.

infiltrative lymphoma, because both normal spleen and lymphomatous infiltrated spleen may have similar T1w and T2w signal intensity. When necrosis is present, imaging differentiation from other cystic entities is difficult.

Metastases[89,91] (Fig. 7-85)

Splenic metastases are relatively uncommon, but melanoma metastases account for 50% of all cases; the remaining 50% are mainly due to adenocarcinoma of breast, lung, colon, ovary, endometrium, and prostate. At US, metastatic lesions are mainly reduced echo reflectivity, although increased echo-reflectivity lesions can occur. In cystic metastases low-level echoes may be present, secondary to the presence of internal debris. At CT, metastases are demonstrated as ill-defined, low-density foci or as well-delineated, unilocular or septate lesions with attenuation similar to water. The CT features of a cystic splenic metastasis can be identical to those of a benign cyst. MR images demonstrate hypointense on T1w and hyperintense T2w lesions. The presence of blood

products from haemorrhage or of other paramagnetic substances, such as melanin within melanomas, may result in high signal intensity on T1w images. On CT and MR enhancement may be present in the periphery and within viable internal septa. Aspiration or biopsy may be required to confirm the diagnosis.

Leukaemia

Patients with leukaemia may present with a homogeneous markedly enlarged spleen which otherwise has a normal imaging appearance on US, CT and MRI.

OTHER PROBLEMS

Portal Hypertension/Splenic Vein Thrombosis[91,96]

Portal hypertension is a frequent cause of splenomegaly. At CT and MR the presence of gastro-oesophageal varices

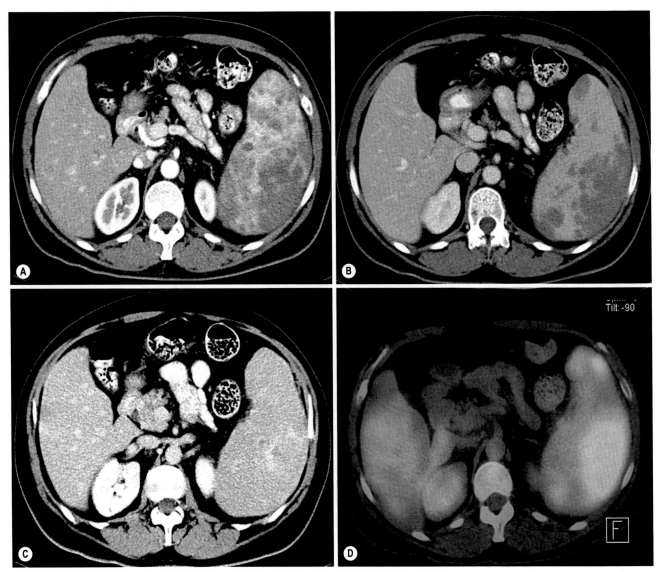

FIGURE 7-83 ■ **Splenic angiosarcoma.** A heterogeneously enhancing mass expands the spleen on CT (A) arterial phase, (B) portal phase and equilibrates on the delayed phase (C). FDG PET-CT demonstrates the associated increased metabolic activity (D).

and perisplenic collateral vessels are better demonstrated after contrast administration. Gandy–Gamna bodies are present in about 10% of patients with portal hypertension. These are deposits of hemosiderin related to small intraparynchymal haemorrhages and are seen at MR as tiny foci of low signal intensity on both T1w and T2w images, which 'bloom' on gradient-echo imaging (Fig. 7-78).

Sarcoidosis

Sarcoidosis may cause splenomegaly and, on CT, a pattern of homogeneous splenomegaly on unenhanced images associated with heterogeneous enhancement in the later phases. This pattern is due to poorly enhancing multiple 2- to 3-cm nodular lesions. Splenic sarcoidosis may also present as a necrotic mass with focal calcification. On

MR, sarcoidosis may be low signal intensity on both T1w and T2w images. The lesions are most conspicuous on T2w or early-phase images following IV contrast enhancement where they are low signal.

Amyloidosis

Two main patterns of splenic involvement occur in amyloidosis: a nodular form involving the lymphoid follicles and a diffuse form infiltrating the red pulp. CT patterns of splenic amyloidosis include discrete low-attenuation masses within an enlarged spleen and a diffuse low-attenuation spleen with poor IV contrast enhancement. Splenomegaly correlates poorly with the degree of involvement. The vascular fragility and acquired coagulopathy associated with amyloidosis are thought to explain the associated high incidence of splenic rupture.

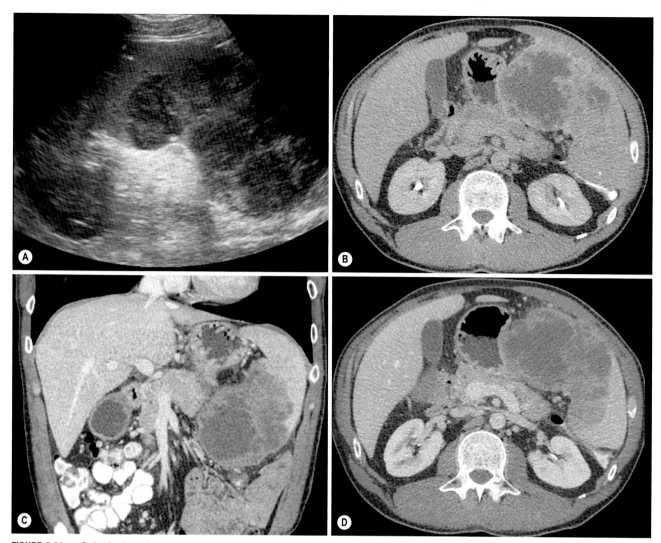

FIGURE 7-84 ■ **Splenic lymphoma.** A heterogeneous expanding irregular lesion with regions of reduced echo reflectivity on US (A) and corresponding heterogeneity and low attenuation on post contrast CT (B). Partial enhancement of the lesion is evident on the delayed coronal (C) and axial images (D).

Haemosiderosis

In haemosiderosis CT demonstrates increased splenic attenuation due to accumulation of iron in the reticulo-endothelial cells. Haemosiderin decreases signal intensity on T2w and T1w MR images.

Extramedullary Haematopoiesis

Extramedullary haematopoiesis of the spleen is mainly associated with myeloproliferative disorders, such as myelofibrosis and chronic haemolytic anemias. Other associations with splenic haematopoiesis include disseminated carcinomatosis, multiple myeloma and Albers–Schönberg disease. Splenic haematopoiesis has also been demonstrated in patients with cirrhosis and in healthy individuals. Splenic extramedullary haematopoiesis is usually diffuse, resulting in splenomegaly; however, focal masses of haematopoietic tissue may occur and mimic the

appearance of tumours at CT and MR. The signal intensity of the mass depends on the evolution of the haematopoiesis. Active lesions demonstrate intermediate signal intensity on T1w images, high signal intensity on T2w images, and contrast enhancement. Older lesions may be hypointense on T1w and T2w images and may not show any contrast enhancement.

Gaucher's Disease[97]

Gaucher's disease is a lysosomal disorder leading to accumulation of glucocerebroside in the reticuloendothelial cells and causes marked hepatosplenomegaly. Splenic infarcts and fibrosis commonly occur. On MR the spleen demonstrates low signal intensity on T1w images, secondary to glucocerebrosides; on T2w images, the splenic signal intensity is intermediate except for hypointense foci representing clusters of Gaucher's cells.

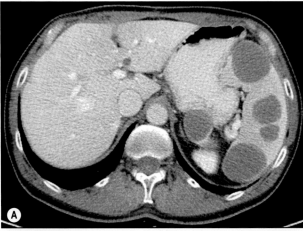

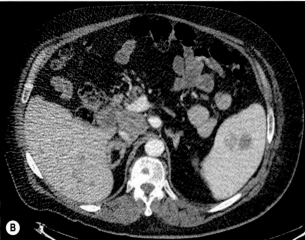

FIGURE 7-85 ■ Portal phase CT in two different patients (A, B) with splenic melanoma metastases demonstrates relatively non-specific multiple low attenuation lesions within the spleen.

REFERENCES

1. Lafortune M, Madore F, Patriquin H, et al. Segmental anatomy of the liver: a sonographic approach to the Couinaud nomenclature. Radiology 1991;181:443–8.
2. Gillard JH, Patel MC, Abrahams PH, et al. Riedel's lobe of the liver: fact or fiction? Clin Anat 1998;11:47–9.
3. Makanjuola D, al Smayer S, al Orainy I, et al. Radiographic features of lobar agenesis of the liver. Acta Radiol 1996;37:255–8.
4. Ludwig J. Normal weights and measurements. Current Methods of Autopsy Practice. Philadelphia: WB Saunders; 1979. pp. 343–7.
5. Matsui O, Takahashi S, Kadoya M, et al. Pseudolesion in segment IV of the liver at CT during arterial portography: correlation with aberrant gastric venous drainage. Radiology 1994;193:31–5.
6. Coulden RA, Lomas DJ, Farman P, et al. Doppler ultrasound of the hepatic veins: normal appearances. Clin Radiol 1992;45:223–7.
7. Martínez SM, Crespo G, Navasa M, et al. Noninvasive assessment of liver fibrosis. Hepatology 2011;53:325–35.
8. Simonovsky V. The diagnosis of cirrhosis by high resolution ultrasound of the liver surface. Br J Radiol 1999;72:29–34.
9. Kopp AF, Heuschmid M, Claussen CD. Multidetector helical CT of the liver for tumor detection and characterization. Eur Radiol 2002;12:745–52.
10. Ma X, Samir AE, Holalkere NS, et al. Optimal arterial phase imaging for detection of hypervascular hepatocellular carcinoma determined by continuous image capture on 16-MDCT. AJR Am J Roentgenol 2008;191:772–7.
11. Miller FH, Butler RS, Hoff FL, et al. Using triphasic helical CT to detect focal hepatic lesions in patients with neoplasms. AJR Am J Roentgenol 1998;171:643–9.
12. Goodwin MD, Dobson JE, Sirlin CB, et al. Diagnostic challenges and pitfalls in MR imaging with hepatocyte-specific contrast agents. Radiographics 2011;31:1547–68.
13. Lomas DJ. Optimization of sequences for MRI of the abdomen and pelvis. Clin Radiol 1997;52:412–28.
14. Rosenkrantz AB, Mannelli L, Mossa D, et al. Breath-hold T2-weighted MRI of the liver at 3.0T using the BLADE technique: impact upon image quality and lesion detection. Clin Radiol 2011;66:426–33.
15. Ringe KI, Husarik DB, Sirlin CB, et al. Gadoxetate disodium-enhanced MRI of the liver: part 1, protocol optimization and lesion appearance in the noncirrhotic liver. AJR Am J Roentgenol 2010;195:13–28.
16. Cruite I, Schroeder M, Merkle EM, et al. Gadoxetate disodium-enhanced MRI of the liver: part 2, protocol optimization and lesion appearance in the cirrhotic liver. AJR Am J Roentgenol 2010;195:29–41.
17. Seneterre E, Taourel P, Bouvier Y, et al. Detection of hepatic metastases: ferumoxides-enhanced MR imaging versus unenhanced MR imaging and CT during arterial portography. Radiology 1996;200:785–92.
18. Welch TJ, Sheedy PFD, Johnson CM, et al. Focal nodular hyperplasia and hepatic adenoma: comparison of angiography, CT, US, and scintigraphy. Radiology 1985;156:593–5.
19. Kim BM, Cho JH, Won JH, et al. Altered findings of hepatic arteriography after radiofrequency ablation of hepatocellular carcinoma: comparison of pre-ablation and post-ablation angiograms. Abdom Imaging 2007;32:332–8.
20. Mitchell DG. Focal manifestations of diffuse liver disease at MR imaging [see comments]. Radiology 1992;185:1–11.
21. Ducommun JC, Goldberg HI, Korobkin M. The relation of liver fat to computed tomography numbers: a preliminary experimental study in rabbits. Radiology 1979;180:311.
22. Reeder SB, Cruite I, Hamilton G, et al. Quantitative assessment of liver fat with magnetic resonance imaging and spectroscopy. J Magn Reson Imaging 2011;34:729–49.
23. Ohtomo K, Baron RL, Dodd GDD, et al. Confluent hepatic fibrosis in advanced cirrhosis: appearance at CT. Radiology 1993;188:31–5.
24. Ohtomo K, Baron RL, Dodd GD, et al. Confluent hepatic fibrosis in advanced cirrhosis: evaluation with MR imaging. Radiology 1993;189:871–4.
25. Muthupillai R, Lomas DJ, Rossman PJ, et al. Magnetic resonance elastography by direct visualization of propagating acoustic strain waves. Science 1995;269:1854–7.
26. Castéra L, Vergniol J, Foucher J, et al. Prospective comparison of transient elastography, Fibrotest, APRI, and liver biopsy for the assessment of fibrosis in chronic hepatitis C. Gastroenterology 2005;128:343–50.
27. Rouvière O, Yin M, Dresner MA, et al. MR elastography of the liver: preliminary results. Radiology 2006;240:440–8.
28. Mannelli L, Godfrey E, Graves MJ, et al. Magnetic resonance elastography: feasibility of liver stiffness measurements in healthy volunteers at 3T. Clin Radiol 2012;67:258–62.
29. Bolondi L, Li Bassi S, Gaiani S, et al. Liver cirrhosis: changes of Doppler waveform of hepatic veins. Radiology 1991;178:513–16.
30. Giorgio A, Amoroso P, Fico P, et al. Ultrasound evaluation of uncomplicated and complicated acute viral hepatitis. JCU J Clin Ultrasound 1986;14:675–9.
31. Chandarana H, Lim RP, Jensen JH, et al. Hepatic iron deposition in patients with liver disease: preliminary experience with breath-hold multiecho T2*-weighted sequence. AJR Am J Roentgenol 2009;193:1261–7.
32. Wood JC, Enriquez C, Ghugre N, et al. MRI R2 and R2* mapping accurately estimates hepatic iron concentration in transfusion-dependent thalassemia and sickle cell disease patients. Blood 2005;106:1460–5.
33. Hale HL, Husband JE, Gossios K, et al. CT of calcified liver metastases in colorectal carcinoma. Clin Radiol 1998;53:735–41.

34. Hong JJ, Gadaleta D, Rossi P, et al. Portal vein gas, a changing clinical entity. Report of 7 patients and review of the literature. Arch Surg 1997;132:1071–5.

35. Shapiro RS, Gendler R, Garten AJ. Intrahepatic gas formation without abscess after hepatic artery thrombosis in the setting of liver transplantation. Clin Imaging 1994;18:12–15.

36. Federle MP, Filly RA, Moss AA. Cystic hepatic neoplasms: complimentary roles of CT and sonography. AJR Am J Roentgenol 1981;136:345.

37. Ustunsoz B, Akhan O, Kamiloglu MA, et al. Percutaneous treatment of hydatid cysts of the liver: long-term results. AJR Am J Roentgenol 1999;172:91–6.

38. Barakate MS, Stephen MS, Waugh RC, et al. Pyogenic liver abscess: a review of 10 years' experience in management. Aust N Z J Surg 1999;69:205–9.

39. Karhunen PJ. Benign hepatic tumors and tumor-like conditions in men. J Clin Pathol 1986;39:183–8.

40. Stark DD, Felder RC, Wittenberg J, et al. Magnetic resonance imaging of cavernous hemangioma of the liver: tissue-specific characterization. AJR Am J Roentgenol 1985;145:213–22.

41. Ashida C, Fishman EK, Zerhouni EA, et al. Computed tomography of hepatic cavernous hemangioma. J Comput Assist Tomogr 1987;11:455–60.

42. Rummeny E, Weissleder R, Sironi S, et al. Central scars in primary liver tumors: MR features, specificity, and pathologic correlation. Radiology 1989;171:323–6.

43. Mahfouz AE, Hamm B, Taupitz M, et al. Hypervascular liver lesions: differentiation of focal nodular hyperplasia from malignant tumors with dynamic gadolinium-enhanced MR imaging. Radiology 1993;186:133–8.

44. Vilgrain V, Flejou JF, Arrive L, et al. Focal nodular hyperplasia of the liver: MR imaging and pathologic correlation in 37 patients. Radiology 1992;184(3):699–703.

45. Paradis V, Champault A, Ronot M, et al. Telangiectatic adenoma: an entity associated with increased body mass index and inflammation. Hepatology 2007;46:140–6.

46. Casarella WJ, Knowles DM, Wolff M, et al. Focal nodular hyperplasia and liver cell adenoma: radiologic and pathologic differentiation. AJR Am J Roentgenol 1978;131:393–402.

47. Ronot M, Bahrami S, Calderaro J, et al. Hepatocellular adenomas: accuracy of magnetic resonance imaging and liver biopsy in subtype classification. Hepatology 2011;53:1182–91.

48. Dokmak S, Paradis V, Vilgrain V, et al. A single-center surgical experience of 122 patients with single and multiple hepatocellular adenomas. Gastroenterology 2009;137:1698–705.

49. Lev-Toaff AS, Bach AM, Wechsler RJ, et al. The radiologic and pathologic spectrum of biliary hamartomas. AJR Am J Roentgenol 1993;165:309–13.

50. Miller WJ, Baron RL, Dodd GD 3rd, et al. Malignancies in patients with cirrhosis: CT sensitivity and specificity in 200 consecutive transplant patients. Radiology 1994;193:645–50.

51. Addley HC, Griffin N, Shaw AS, et al. Accuracy of hepatocellular carcinoma detection on multidetector CT in a transplant liver population with explant liver correlation. Clin Radiol 2011;66:349–56.

52. Matsuzaki K, Sano N, Hashiguchi N, et al. Influence of copper on MRI of hepatocellular carcinoma. J Magn Reson Imaging 1997;7:478–81.

53. Rosenkrantz AB, Mannelli L, Kim S, et al. Gadolinium-enhanced liver magnetic resonance imaging using a 2-point Dixon fat-water separation technique: impact upon image quality and lesion technique. J Comput Assist Tomogr 2011;35:96–101.

54. Mannelli L, Kim S, Hajdu CH, et al. Assessment of tumor necrosis of hepatocellular carcinoma after chemoembolization: diffusion-weighted and contrast-enhanced MRI with histopathologic correlation of the explanted liver. AJR Am J Roentgenol 2009;193:1044–52.

55. Peterson MS, Baron RL, Murakami T. Hepatic malignancies: usefulness of acquisition of multiple arterial and portal venous phase images at dynamic gadolinium-enhanced MR imaging. Radiology 1996;201(2):337–45.

56. Park MS, Kim S, Patel J, et al.. Hepatocellular carcinoma: Detection with diffusion-weighted vs. contrast-enhanced MRI in pre-transplant patients. Hepatology 2012;56:140–8.

57. Wong LK, Link DP, Frey CF, et al. Fibrolamellar hepatocarcinoma: radiology, management, and pathology. AJR Am J Roentgenol 1982;139:1172–5.

58. Miller WJ, Dodd GDD, Federle MP, et al. Epithelioid hemangioendothelioma of the liver: imaging findings with pathologic correlation. AJR Am J Roentgenol 1992;159:53–7.

59. Sanders LM, Botet JF, Straus DJ, et al. CT of primary lymphoma of the liver. AJR Am J Roentgenol 1989;152:973–6.

60. Silverman PM, Ram PC, Korobin M. CT appearance of abdominal Thorotrast deposition and Thorotrast-induced angiosarcoma of the liver. J Comput Assist Tomogr 1983;7:655–8.

61. Hardie AD, Naik M, Chandarana H, et al. Diagnosis of liver metastases: value of diffusion-weighted MRI compared with gadolinium-enhanced MRI. Eur Radiol 2010;20:1431–41.

62. Desai AG, Park CH, Schilling JF. 'Streaming' in portal vein. Its effect on the spread of metastases to the liver. Clin Nucl Med 1985;10:556–9.

63. Delbeke D, Martin WH, Sandler MP, et al. Evaluation of benign vs malignant hepatic lesions with positron emission tomography. Arch Surg 1998;133:510–15.

64. Albrecht T, Holmann J, Oldenburg A, et al. Detection and characterisation of liver metastases. Eur Radiol 2004;14(Suppl. 8):25–33.

65. Schwartz LH, Gandras EJ, Colangelo SM, et al. Prevalence and importance of small hepatic lesions found at CT in patients with cancer. Radiology 1999;210:71–4.

66. Oliver JH 3rd, Baron RL, Federle MP, et al. Hypervascular liver metastases: do unenhanced and hepatic arterial phase CT images affect tumor detection? Radiology 1997;205(3):709–15.

67. Valla DC. The diagnosis and management of the Budd-Chiari syndrome: consensus and controversies. Hepatology 2003;38:793–803.

68. Iwai M, Kitagawa Y, Nakajima T, et al. Clinical features, image analysis, and laparoscopic and histological liver findings in Budd-Chiari syndrome. Hepatogastroenterology 1998;45(24):2359–68.

69. Imaeda T, Yamakawi Y, Hirota K, et al. Tumor thrombus in the branches of the distal portal vein: CT demonstration. J Comput Assist Tomogr 1989;13:262–8.

70. Mori H, Hayashi K, Fukuda T, et al. Intrahepatic portosystemic venous shunt: occurrence in patients with and without liver cirrhosis. AJR Am J Roentgenol 1987;149:711–14.

71. Weishaupt D, Grozaj AM, Willmann JK, et al. Traumatic injuries: imaging of abdominal and pelvic injuries. Eur Radiol 2002;12:1295–311.

72. Orwig D, Federle MP. Localized clotted blood as evidence of visceral trauma on CT: the sentinel clot sign. AJR Am J Roentgenol 1989;153:747–9.

73. European Liver Transplant Registry Website: http://www.eltr.org.

74. Dodd GD 3rd, Baron RL, Oliver JH 3rd, et al. End-stage primary sclerosing cholangitis: CT findings of hepatic morphology in 36 patients. Radiology 1999;211:357–62.

75. Odorico JS, Hakim MN, Becker YT, et al. Liver transplantation as definitive therapy for complications after arterial embolization for hepatic manifestations of hereditary hemorrhagic telangiectasia. Liver Transpl Surg 1998;4:483–90.

76. Cucchetti A, Cescon M, Bigonzi E, et al. Priority of candidates with hepatocellular carcinoma awaiting liver transplantation can be reduced after successful bridge therapy. Liver Transpl 2011;17:1344–54.

77. Mazzaferro V, Regalia E, Doci R, et al. Liver transplantation for the treatment of small hepatocellular carcinomas in patients with cirrhosis. N Engl J Med 1996;334:693–9.

78. Sahani D, D'souza R, Kadavigere R, et al. Evaluation of living liver transplant donors: method for precise anatomic definition by using a dedicated contrast-enhanced MR imaging protocol. Radiographics 2004;24:957–67.

79. Schroeder T, Malago M, Debatin JF, et al. 'All-in-one' imaging protocols for the evaluation of potential living liver donors: Comparison of magnetic resonance imaging and multidetector computed tomography. Liver Transpl 2005;11:776–87.

80. Sahani D, Mehta A, Blake M, et al. Preoperative hepatic vascular evaluation with CT and MR angiography: implications for surgery. Radiographics 2004;24:1367–80.

81. Catalano OA, Singh AH, Uppot RN, et al. Vascular and biliary variants in the liver: implications for liver surgery. Radiographics 2008;28:359–78.

82. Yerdel MA, Gunson B, Mirza D, et al. Portal vein thrombosis in adults undergoing liver transplantation: risk factors, screening, management and outcome. Transplantation 2000;69:1873–81.

83. Glockner JF, Forauer AR. Vascular or ischaemic complications after liver transplantation. AJR Am J Roentgenol 1999;173:1055–9.

84. Cacho G, Abreu L, Calleja JL, et al. Arterioportal fistula and hemobilia with associated acute cholecystitis: a complication of percutaneous liver biopsy. Hepatogastroenterology 1996;43:1020–3.

85. Piccinino F, Sagnelli E, Pasquale G, et al. Complications following percutaneous liver biopsy. A multicentre retrospective study on 68,276 biopsies. J Hepatol 1986;2:165–73.

86. Maharaj B, Bhoora IG. Complications associated with percutaneous needle biopsy of the liver when one, two or three specimens are taken. Postgrad Med J 1992;68:964–7.

87. Little AF, Ferris JV, Dodd GD 3rd, et al. Image-guided percutaneous hepatic biopsy: effect of ascites on the complication rate. Radiology 1996;199:79–83.

88. Lundstedt C, Stridbeck H, Andersson R, et al. Tumor seeding occurring after fine-needle biopsy of abdominal malignancies. Acta Radiol 1991;32:518–20.

89. Elsayes KM, Narra VR, Mukundan G, et al. MR imaging of the spleen: spectrum of abnormalities. Radiographics 2005;25:967–82.

90. Unver Dogan N, Uysal II, Demirci S, et al. Accessory spleens at autopsy. Clin Anat 2011;24:757–62.

91. Freeman JL, Jafri SZ, Roberts JL, et al. CT of congenital and acquired abnormalities of the spleen. Radiographics 1993;13:597–610.

92. Semelka RC, Kelekis NL, Sallah S, et al. Hepatosplenic fungal disease: diagnostic accuracy and spectrum of appearances on MR imaging. AJR Am J Roentgenol 1997;169:1311–16.

93. Abbott RM, Levy AD, Aguilera NS, et al. From the archives of the AFIP: primary vascular neoplasms of the spleen: radiologic-pathologic correlation. Radiographics 2004;24:1137–63.

94. Oztürk E, Mutlu H, Sönmez G, Sildiroğlu HO. Primary angiosarcoma of the spleen. Turk J Gastroenterol 2007;18:272–5.

95. Vrachliotis TG, Bennett WF, Vaswani KK, et al. Primary angiosarcoma of the spleen: CT, MR, and sonographic characteristics—report of two cases. Abdom Imaging 2000;25:283–5.

96. Mannelli L, Godfrey E, Joubert J, et al. Magnetic Resonance Elastography (MRE): spleen stiffness measurements in healthy volunteers. Preliminary experience. AJR Am J Roentgenol 2010;195:387–92.

97. Poll LW, Koch JA, vom Dahl S, et al. Gaucher disease of the spleen: CT and MR findings. Abdom Imaging 2000;25:286–9.

CHAPTER 8

THE BILIARY SYSTEM

Robert N. Gibson • Thomas Sutherland

BILIARY ANATOMY

The intrahepatic pattern of bile duct branching is best described according to the system of Healey and Schroy, to which can be applied the Couinaud system for numbering segments. The typical pattern and its variations are shown in Figs. 8-1 and 8-2. The confluence of the bile ducts is a bifurcation in about 60% of individuals and a trifurcation in about 12% (Fig. 8-3).[1,2] A right sectoral duct crosses to the left to join the left hepatic duct in 28% of cases (22% right posterior sectoral, 6% right anterior sectoral) (Fig. 8-4).[1] Occasionally a right posterior sectoral or segmental duct (more often posterior than anterior) courses inferiorly and either enters the common hepatic duct directly or cystic duct (Fig. 8-5).

Other uncommon left branching variations are shown in Figs. 8-2 (E and F).

The cystic duct typically joins the common hepatic duct in the middle third of the extrahepatic bile duct—often referred to as the 'common duct' on ultrasound (US) for convenience—which then continues as the common bile duct (CBD). The cystic duct usually joins the right side of the common duct but can pass behind or in front of the common duct to join it from the left. The cystic duct can join the common duct at a very low level, in which case it may be mistaken for the common duct on imaging. Uncommonly it may join a right-sided duct, which is usually a low, aberrant right sectoral or

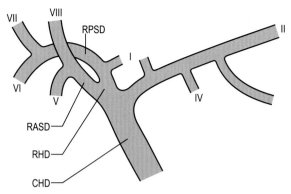

FIGURE 8-1 ■ **Typical pattern of intrahepatic biliary branching.** Segments are numbered according to the system of Couinaud. CHD = common hepatic duct, RHD = right hepatic duct, LHD = left hepatic duct, RPSD = right posterior sectoral duct, RASD = right anterior sectoral duct. (From Blumgart L H, Fong Y (eds) 2000 Surgery of the Liver and Biliary Tract, 3rd edn. WB Saunders, London, p 365, with permission.)

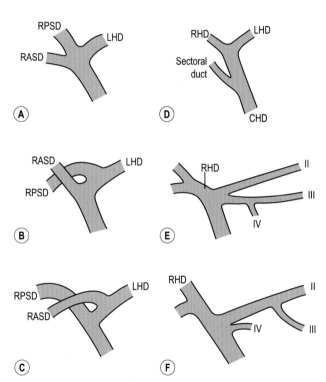

FIGURE 8-2 ■ **Variations of biliary branching patterns.** The more common are A, B and C. Segments are numbered according to the system of Couinaud. CHD = common hepatic duct, RHD = right hepatic duct, LHD = left hepatic duct, RPSD = right posterior sectoral duct, RASD = right anterior sectoral duct. (From Blumgart L H, Fong Y (eds) 2000 Surgery of the Liver and Biliary Tract, 3rd edn. WB Saunders, London, p 365, with permission.)

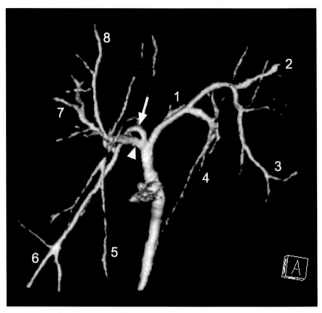

FIGURE 8-3 ■ **Biliary duct anatomy.** CT-IVC (surface-rendered maximum intensity reformat) shows trifurcation at the biliary confluence and segments numbered according to Couinaud. Arrowhead shows right anterior sectoral duct; arrow shows right posterior sectoral duct.

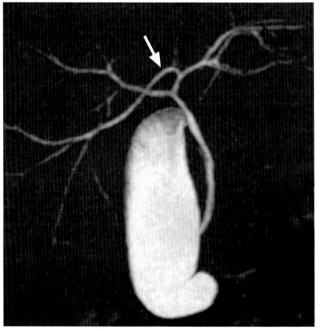

FIGURE 8-4 ■ **Biliary duct anatomy.** CT intravenous cholangiography (CT-IVC) (maximum intensity reformat). Right posterior sectoral duct (arrow) passes to the left to drain into left hepatic duct.

segmental duct (Fig. 8-5). Some of these variations predispose patients to duct injury at cholecystectomy.

Other variations include ducts of Luschka or subvesical ducts, and cystohepatic ducts. There is some confusion over nomenclature but it seems that the terms subvesical duct and duct of Luschka both describe an intrahepatic duct running adjacent to the gallbladder fossa, unaccompanied by a portal vein branch, and emptying into either the right hepatic or common hepatic

duct. The term 'cystohepatic duct' is probably best reserved for small ducts that drain directly into the gallbladder or cystic duct. The significance of these variants is their proximity to the gallbladder and the potential for injury at cholecystectomy resulting in a bile leak.[3]

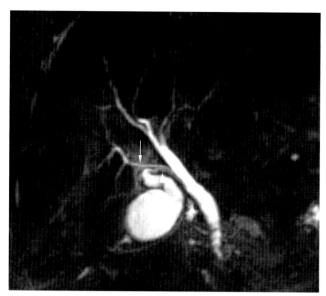

FIGURE 8-5 ■ **Biliary duct anatomy.** Coronal oblique MRCP showing the cystic duct (arrowhead) running with a low right posterior sectoral duct (arrow) and the two joining prior to the common duct. This ductal configuration can predispose to inadvertent duct injury.

It is important to remember that the anterior position of the left intrahepatic ducts affects the pattern of filling at direct cholangiography. During percutaneous transhepatic cholangiography (PTC) or T-tube cholangiography it may be necessary to roll the patient to the left to ensure good left-duct filling. Conversely the left ducts fill first

at endoscopic retrograde cholangiopancreatography (ERCP) with the patient in the prone position. Furthermore, as the patient is usually oblique during ERCP, the left-sided ducts are often projected to the right and may be misinterpreted as being right-sided ducts if there is incomplete filling of intrahepatic ducts.

GALLBLADDER ANATOMICAL VARIANTS

Agenesis of the gallbladder is extremely rare, with a prevalence of 0.03–0.07%. A double gallbladder occurs in about 0.03%, usually with a shared cystic duct, and the accessory gallbladder is often diseased.

True gallbladder septa are uncommon and when occurring at the fundus form a Phrygian cap. Frequently, an apparent septum is merely gallbladder wall folding, which can vary with patient position.

The gallbladder can be abnormal in position, being retrohepatic, suprahepatic, left-sided or intrahepatic, the latter potentially presenting as a liver abscess if complicated by acute cholecystitis. A number of forms of left-sided gallbladder exist:

1. The gallbladder lies under the left hepatic lobe to the left of the falciform ligament
2. Independent development of a second gallbladder from the left hepatic duct with regression or failure of development of a right gallbladder
3. Herniation of the gallbladder through the foramen of Winslow
4. Transposition of the viscera.

METHODS OF INVESTIGATION

ULTRASOUND

Transabdominal ultrasound is frequently the first imaging technique employed for patients presenting with hepatobiliary-type symptoms as it is more accurate than CT for diagnosing acute biliary disease.[4] Imaging is usually performed following a 4-hour fast, allowing the gallbladder to fill and reducing obscuring upper abdominal gas. The wall of a normal non-contracted gallbladder is <3 mm thick and is smooth. Ultrasound allows a dynamic assessment and by moving the patient helps differentiate stones, sludge and polyps. Doppler ultrasound allows assessment of vascularity, while focal gallbladder tenderness can be determined using probe pressure. The normal cystic duct may not be visible; however, the extrahepatic bile duct can be seen as a tubular structure anterior to the portal vein and lacking blood flow on Doppler.

Contrast-enhanced ultrasound (CEUS) using second-generation microbubble agents can be performed at transabdominal, endoscopic and intraoperative ultrasound. CEUS is useful in selected patients: for example, in differentiating sludge from tumour, identifying

perforation in cholecystitis and better demonstrating hilar cholangiocarcinoma.

COMPUTED TOMOGRAPHIC CHOLANGIOGRAPHY

Computed tomographic (CT) cholangiography relies on either oral or intravenous (IV) contrast agents that are excreted preferentially by the liver, to opacify the bile ducts. Most centres now use IV contrast agents for CT cholangiography, so-called CT-intravenous cholangiography (CT-IVC). This technique involves the IV infusion of an agent such as sodium ipodate with helical CT performed about 30 minutes later. Multislice helical CT allows high-resolution imaging and multiplanar reformatting. Prone imaging can be performed after supine imaging if there is substantial intraductal gas or contrast layering.

Sodium iotroxate is safer than older IV biliary agents, with reported complications in 3.5% of patients (3.0% minor, 0.3% moderate and 0.2% severe)[5] and an estimated mortality rate of 0.005%.[6]

Adequate contrast excretion relies on near-normal hepatocyte function, so the technique is of no value in the investigation of jaundice, and usually fails if bilirubin levels are more than about two times normal.

Since CT-IVC relies on the excretion and subsequent passage of a contrast agent, it provides a functional dimension not obtained with conventional magnetic resonance cholangiography (MRC), allowing the direct demonstration of bile leaks, biliary communication with cysts and segmental obstruction.

MAGNETIC RESONANCE CHOLANGIOPANCREATOGRAPHY

Magnetic resonance cholangiopancreatography (MRCP) has substantially replaced diagnostic PTC and ERCP. It relies on heavily T2-weighted sequences that display stationary water as high signal. Multiplanar thin and thick section acquisitions are obtained using fast spin-echo techniques. Since conventional MRCP is not reliant on contrast excretion it is suitable for jaundiced patients, a clear advantage compared with CT-IVC.

More recently MR has been combined with hepatobiliary contrast agents. These agents, which include mangafodipir trisodium, gadobenate dimeglumine and gadoxetic acid disodium, shorten T1 relaxation, providing positive contrast images on T1-weighted sequences. Imaging is performed at least 30 minutes after IV infusion to allow hepatocyte uptake and biliary excretion. It therefore provides functional as well as anatomical information but, as with CT-IVC, depends on near-normal excretory hepatocyte function.[7] Since T1-weighted MR sequences are used it is possible to use near-isotropic three-dimensional gradient echo acquisitions. Contrast-enhanced MR cholangiography using hepatobiliary contrast agents has similar applications to CT-IVC, except that it is not as sensitive as conventional MRCP for the detection of choledocholithiasis.

Diagnostic pitfalls with MRCP include localised signal voids caused by surgical clips, and intraductal gas or blood. Bile flow voids may mimic small stones but the former are centrally placed and have less well-defined margins than stones. Acquisition times are longer for MRCP than CT-IVC and therefore more prone to motion artefacts.

ENDOSCOPIC RETROGRADE CHOLANGIOPANCREATOGRAPHY

ERCP provides direct opacification of bile ducts and pancreatic ducts, with success rates of 92–97%, and provides dynamic information during contrast medium introduction and drainage. It allows visual assessment of the duodenum and ampulla of Vater and enables biopsy and brushings, as well as interventional procedures such as sphincterotomy and stone extraction, biliary stenting and biliary stricture dilatation. Complication rates vary depending on the indication for the procedure, the presence of coexisting disease and the experience of the endoscopist, with severe complication rates of 0.9 to 2.3%, and total complication rates of 8.4–11.1%, the most common significant complication being acute pancreatitis.[8] The main diagnostic pitfall with ERCP is the underfilling of ducts above a stricture.

PERCUTANEOUS TRANSHEPATIC CHOLANGIOGRAPHY

PTC has been substantially replaced by ERCP and MRCP. Its role now is mostly as part of transhepatic biliary intervention. A 22G Chiba needle is used to puncture the right or left intrahepatic ducts from the right flank or, for left ducts, from an epigastric approach. The epigastric approach is used if the left ducts cannot be opacified from the right or as part of a left-lobe approach to biliary drainage. Any coagulation disorder should be reversed prior to the procedure, which is performed with broad-spectrum IV antibiotic cover and conscious sedation or occasionally general anaesthesia.

If the ducts are dilated, the needle is withdrawn gradually with suction applied and when bile is aspirated contrast medium is injected to opacify the biliary tree. If the ducts are not dilated, or if initial passes fail to opacify them, small injections of contrast medium are made as the needle is gradually withdrawn until bile ducts are opacified. Samples should be taken for microbiology and, if malignant obstruction is suspected, cytological examination. Care should be taken to opacify the entire biliary tree, especially in cases of lobar or segmental biliary obstruction. A common pitfall is the failure to fill the left hepatic ducts from a right-sided approach and this should be suspected if no ducts are opacified in the midline. The aspiration of some bile during the procedure reduces the risk of bile leak and endotoxaemia by reducing intraductal pressure.

Success rates are close to 100% if the ducts are substantially dilated and about 75% if they are non-dilated or only slightly dilated, the latter group usually requiring multiple needle passes. US guidance may be used if a particular segment is to be opacified and some operators use it routinely for PTC or percutaneous transhepatic biliary catheterisation. The major complication rate is about 4% and includes haemobilia, bacteraemia and bile leak.[9]

INTRAOPERATIVE CHOLANGIOGRAPHY

Intraoperative cholangiography (IOC) is performed routinely or selectively during cholecystectomy to detect choledocholithiasis, confirm duct stone clearance and delineate anatomy to minimise risk of bile duct injury.

T-TUBE CHOLANGIOGRAPHY

If the CBD has been explored at cholecystectomy a T-tube is usually left in place and cholangiography performed via this tube after about 7 days, prior to its removal. Cholangiography should confirm stone clearance and the free passage of contrast medium into the duodenum. Care must be taken to avoid the injection of air bubbles.

HEPATOBILIARY SCINTIGRAPHY

Hepatobiliary iminodiacetic acid (HIDA) scintigraphy uses a derivative of iminodiacetic acid, a bilirubin analogue, labelled with ^{99m}Tc. It is injected intravenously and serial gamma camera images are obtained over 2–4 hours. It relies on near-normal bilirubin levels, although some agents can be excreted with moderate elevations of bilirubin. Serial image acquisitions show accumulation of the isotope in the liver, bile ducts, duodenum, small bowel and gallbladder (providing it is present and the cystic duct is patent).

ENDOSCOPIC ULTRASOUND

Biliary endoscopic ultrasound (EUS) provides high-frequency grey-scale imaging, colour Doppler and contrast-enhanced ultrasound for evaluation of the extrahepatic biliary tree and pancreas. EUS has similar sensitivity and specificity to MRCP in diagnosing causes of biliary obstruction.[10] Though relatively invasive, advantages are that it allows direct visualisation of the duodenum, fine-needle aspiration cytology and potentially biliary drainage. More sophisticated and expensive systems of 'mother-daughter' probes allow intraductal examination of the CBD, but are not routinely available.

DISORDERS OF THE GALLBLADDER

GALLBLADDER STONES

The prevalence of gallbladder stones in adults in Western communities is approximately 15%. They are asymptomatic in about 80% but in this group about 15% will develop symptoms over 15 years and they confer a small lifetime risk of gallbladder carcinoma. About 70% of gallbladder stones are solely or predominantly cholesterol in type, with up to 30% being black pigment stones composed mainly of calcium bilirubinate.[11]

Less than 10% of stones are opaque on plain radiographs, the larger stones showing laminated or peripheral calcification. On CT a minority of gallbladder stones are visible, being hyperdense, hypodense, or of mixed density.

US is the most accurate investigation for the diagnosis of gallbladder stones, which appear as echogenic foci producing acoustic shadows (Fig. 8-6). Stone mobility is frequently identifiable (Fig. 8-7), though is not essential for diagnosis. The sensitivity of US is > 95%.[12] False-negative diagnoses are commoner than false-positive ones, and are usually due to small stones in patients in whom there is poor acoustic access to the gallbladder because of obesity or other unfavourable anatomy. False-negative diagnoses are reduced by careful US technique. Small stones are differentiated from small polyps by the demonstration of mobility or the presence of an acoustic shadow.

Non-visualisation of the gallbladder on US can be due to a previous cholecystectomy, non-fasting state, an abnormal gallbladder position, emphysematous cholecystitis, or because the gallbladder is filled with stones. The latter can be recognised by identifying the so-called 'double-arc shadow' sign in the gallbladder fossa, consisting of two parallel curved echogenic lines separated by a thin anechoic space with dense acoustic shadowing distal to the deeper echogenic line (Fig. 8-8).

SLUDGE

Sludge is commonly seen on US and appears as fine, non-shadowing dependent echoes. It is composed of calcium bilirubinate granules, cholesterol crystals and glycoproteins.[13] It is more commonly seen in chronic fasting states, critically ill patients, those receiving total parenteral nutrition and in pregnancy. Sludge resolves spontaneously in 50% of patients and gallstones will develop in 5–15%.[14]

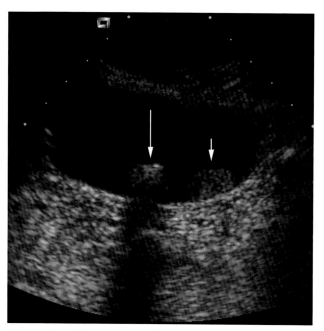

FIGURE 8-6 ■ Gallstone and polyp. Ultrasound showing a non-shadowing polyp (short arrow) just to the right of a shadowing calculus (long arrow).

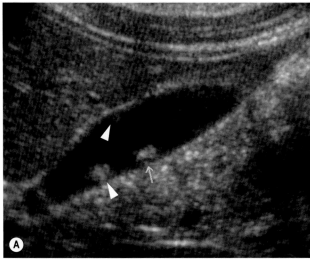

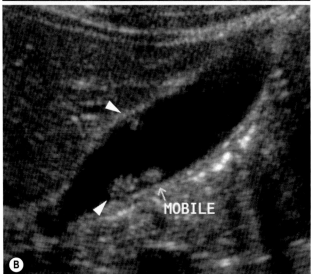

FIGURE 8-7 ■ **Mobility of gallstones.** Ultrasound demonstrates two dependent intraluminal non-shadowing structures (A). The patient was rolled and reimaged (B) and the lesion marked with an arrow proved to be mobile in keeping with a stone while the fixed dependent and antidependent lesions are polyps (arrowheads).

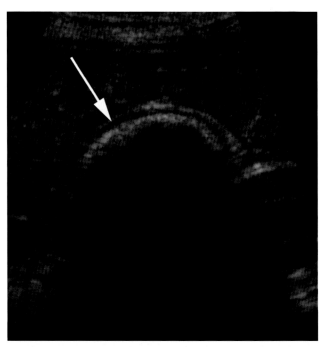

FIGURE 8-8 ■ **Gallbladder filled with stones producing the 'double-arc' sign; hypoechoic line between two echogenic lines (arrow) and a distal acoustic shadow.**

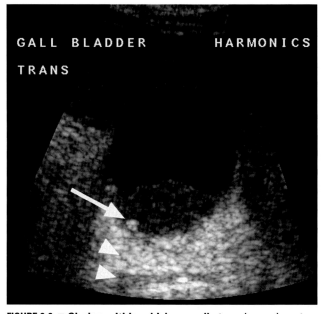

FIGURE 8-9 ■ **Sludge within which a small stone (arrow) casts a subtle acoustic shadow (arrowheads).**

Small stones are difficult to locate within sludge, so careful imaging through sludge is important (Fig. 8-9). Usually sludge layers in a dependent fashion but occasionally it mimics a tumour mass, i.e. 'tumefactive sludge'. Sludge can usually be differentiated from tumour by its mobility, lack of internal blood flow on Doppler examination, lack of focal gallbladder wall abnormality, or lack of enhancement on CEUS.

Blood (haemobilia) and pus (empyema) may have a similar appearance to sludge and the clinical setting aids in their differentiation. Sludge, blood and pus can also occur in the bile ducts.

MILK OF CALCIUM BILE

Milk of calcium bile, or limy bile, is an uncommon condition in which the gallbladder bile becomes viscous, probably as a result of stasis, and contains a high concentration of calcium bilirubinate. On US it causes diffuse echoes, similar to sludge, but is more echogenic (Fig. 8-10A) with a tendency to layer out and produce an acoustic shadow. On CT (Fig. 8-10B) and, occasionally, on plain radiographs it is visible as layering high-density material.

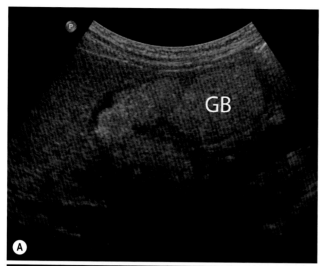

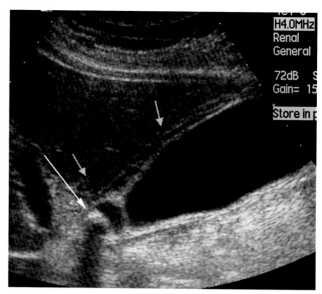

FIGURE 8-11 ■ **Acute cholecystitis.** The gallbladder has an oedematous wall (short arrows) with an impacted shadowing stone in the neck (long arrow).

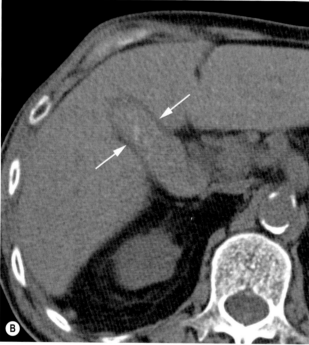

FIGURE 8-10 ■ Milk of calcium bile producing fine echoes within the gallbladder lumen (GB) on ultrasound (A) and being hyperdense on non-contrast CT (arrows) (B).

CHOLECYSTITIS

Acute Calculous Cholecystitis

US is the best initial imaging investigation in patients with suspected acute cholecystitis, which, in 90–95% of cases, is due to gallstones (acute calculous cholecystitis). The positive predictive values of stones combined with either tenderness localised to the gallbladder (positive sonographic Murphy's sign), or the presence of a gallbladder wall thickness of >3 mm, are 92 and 95%, respectively (Fig. 8-11). The negative predictive value of the absence of gallbladder stones and a negative sonographic Murphy's sign is 95%. US can be definitive in about 80% of cases.[15] Gallstone(s) may be impacted in the gallbladder neck and this region must be carefully

examined. Other US signs are gallbladder distension (diameter >5 cm), pericholecystic fluid, gallbladder wall striations and, occasionally, wall hyperaemia on Doppler examination. Fine echoes within the gallbladder may be due to sludge or pus (gallbladder empyema). If liver function tests suggest duct obstruction, a careful evaluation of the CBD should be made for choledocholithiasis.

CT is less accurate than US for acute cholecystitis, but is widely used to evaluate patients with acute abdominal pain. The CT findings in acute cholecystitis include gallbladder wall thickening, subserosal oedema, gallbladder distension, high-density bile, pericholecystic fluid and inflammatory stranding in pericholecystic fat (Fig. 8-12). Gallstones are identifiable in the minority. Gallbladder wall enhancement is variable and not a reliable predictor of cholecystitis since normal gallbladders can show wall enhancement. Transient pericholecystic liver rim enhancement may be seen.[16]

Hepatobiliary scintigraphy has a high diagnostic accuracy for acute cholecystitis. A positive result is non-visualisation of the gallbladder, which results from cystic duct obstruction. Although its accuracy is similar to US, it is more time consuming and does not allow assessment of related organs. It can be helpful, however, when diagnostic uncertainty remains after US.

Gallbladder wall thickening may result from many causes other than cholecystitis. These include non-fasting state, generalised oedematous states, hepatitis, pancreatitis, gallbladder wall varices, adenomyomatosis and carcinoma, though the latter two usually cause focal rather than diffuse thickening.

Gangrenous Cholecystitis

This condition is suggested on US by pronounced irregularity or asymmetrical thickening of the gallbladder wall, internal membranous echoes resulting from

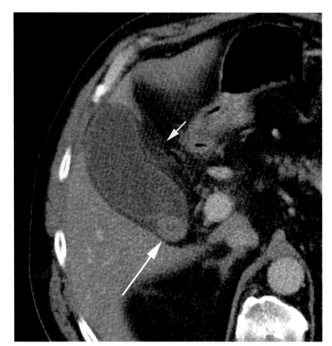

FIGURE 8-12 ■ Acute cholecystitis on CT. The gallbladder wall is thickened with oedema in the adjacent fat (short arrow) and a stone located in the neck (long arrow). There is no abnormal contrast enhancement in this case.

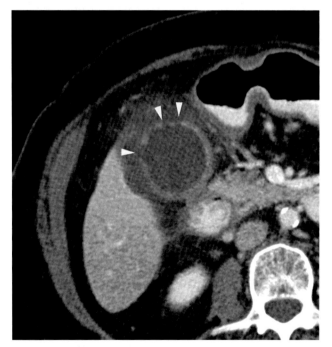

FIGURE 8-13 ■ Gangrenous cholecystitis. Portal venous CT with incomplete mucosal enhancement (arrowheads) in a distended gangrenous gallbladder with pronounced pericholecystic fatty inflammation.

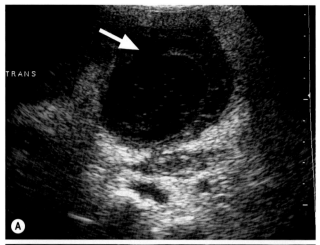

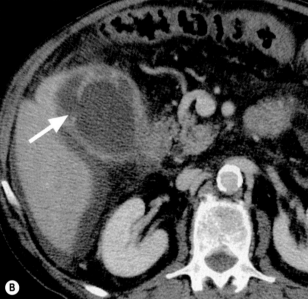

FIGURE 8-14 ■ Acute cholecystitis with localised perforation on (A) US and (B) CT. The thickened gallbladder wall shows a local defect (arrow) and on CT there is small amount of intraperitoneal fluid and oedema of adjacent fat.

internal membranes and pericholecystic abscess. Of these, interrupted wall enhancement is the most sensitive sign (70.6%) and is highly specific (100%).[17]

Gallbladder perforation, occurs in 5–10% of patients with acute cholecystitis.[16] It is suggested by pericholecystic fluid and the features of gangrenous cholecystitis. Localised disruption of the gallbladder wall is seen on US in 40% and on CT in 80% (Fig. 8-14). Less often, generalised peritoneal fluid may be present.[18] CEUS can help identify perforation by showing local absence of gallbladder wall enhancement.

Emphysematous Cholecystitis

This condition accounts for only 1% of acute cholecystitis but has a relatively high mortality rate. It is more common in men (the reverse of the usual female predominance in cholecystitis), about 50% are diabetics, and stones are present in <50%.[16] The diagnosis may be evident on plain

sloughed mucosa and pericholecystic fluid. The clinical findings, paradoxically, may diminish with progression to gangrenous change. CT signs suggesting gangrenous cholecystitis are gas in the wall or lumen, discontinuous and/or irregular mucosal enhancement (Fig. 8-13),

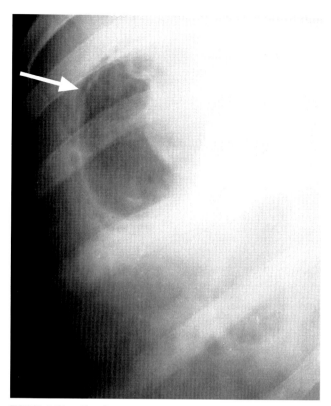

FIGURE 8-15 ■ **Emphysematous cholecystitis.** Image showing intramural (arrow) as well as intraluminal gallbladder gas.

radiographs (Fig. 8-15) and is readily made on CT (Fig. 8-16A), which shows intramural and/or intraluminal gas caused by gas-forming organisms. On US intramural gas appears as focal or diffuse bright echogenic lines. Intra-luminal gas, in the non-dependent portion of the gallbladder, causes a curvilinear, brightly echogenic band with shadowing (Fig. 8-16B), which can make recognition of the gallbladder difficult and lead to a false-negative US result. Small foci of intramural gas may cause ring-down artefact and mimic adenomyomatosis.

Acalculous Cholecystitis

Acute acalculous cholecystitis is most often seen in critically ill patients, and the clinical presentation is usually one of sepsis. The US signs are gallbladder distension, gallbladder wall thickening, echogenic contents and, occasionally, sloughed membranes/mucosa and peri-cholecystic fluid. Positive diagnosis is often difficult as sludge and gallbladder distension may occur without cholecystitis in this group. All investigations—US, CT and biliary scintigraphy—are less accurate than in acute *calculous* cholecystitis. Biliary scintigraphy is possibly the most accurate technique. Gallbladder aspiration has been used to aid diagnosis but is often unhelpful.[19] Localised gallbladder tenderness is a good predictive sign when present but is frequently difficult to assess in this cohort.

Chronic acalculous cholecystitis is a controversial entity as there are no clear clinical, pathological or imaging criteria for its diagnosis. The clinical setting is usually unexplained biliary-type pain, and patients have

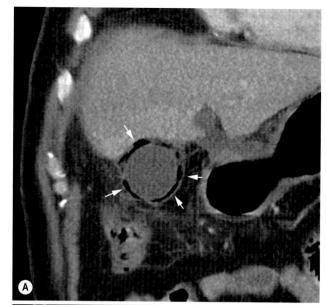

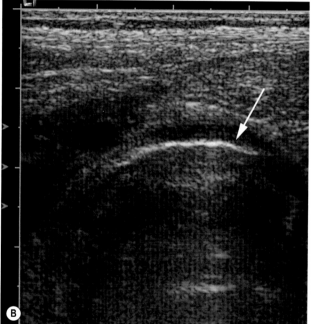

FIGURE 8-16 ■ **Emphysematous cholecystitis.** (A) Coronal CT—intramural gas (arrows); (B) US—intraluminal gas appears as a bright curvilinear echogenic band (arrow) with 'dirty' shadowing.

often previously undergone numerous other negative investigations. US may show gallbladder wall thickening and, by definition, no stones. Cholescintigraphy followed by the IV infusion of cholecystokinin (CCK), or one of its analogues, can be used to assess gallbladder contractibility. An ejection fraction <35% on CCK-cholescintigraphy is generally taken to be an indicator of gallbladder dysfunction and helps select patients who may benefit from cholecystectomy.

Xanthogranulomatous cholecystitis is an unusual form of chronic cholecystitis that may mimic malignancy. It usually presents with the clinical features of cholecystitis or biliary obstruction (a variant of Mirizzi's syndrome). It is characterised by focal or diffuse gallbladder wall thickening, which can be marked. Stones are present in the majority, and in a small percentage there is associated gallbladder carcinoma.[20]

GALLBLADDER MUCOCELE

Gallbladder mucocele, also known as gallbladder hydrops, is the result of chronic gallbladder obstruction, without superimposed infection, allowing accumulation of large volumes of sterile mucinous fluid. It is usually caused by impacted stones and less often by polyps, tumours or adjacent adenopathy. The gallbladder is markedly distended, fluid filled and may present as a mass.

GALLBLADDER FISTULAE

Gallbladder fistulae are rare. The great majority are due to chronic stone disease rather than neoplasm. Most communicate with the duodenum and most of the remainder to the colon. Cholecystoduodenal fistulae may result in bowel obstruction due to the impaction of larger stones in the distal small bowel, so-called gallstone ileus, a condition associated in a minority of patients with a visible gallstone on plain radiographs or CT, and gas in the biliary tract.

PORCELAIN GALLBLADDER

Porcelain gallbladder is an uncommon condition occurring in 0.2% of cholecystectomy specimens[21] and consisting of complete or scattered mural calcification. There is an association with gallbladder carcinoma, although the incidence of coexisting carcinoma is less than previously thought at <5%.[21] However, prophylactic cholecystectomy is often advocated, due to the high morbidity and mortality of gallbladder carcinoma. The calcification follows the contour of the gallbladder wall, may be focal or diffuse, and may be visible on CT (Fig. 8-17B) or plain radiography. On US (Fig. 8-17A) it can mimic emphysematous cholecystitis or gallstones but the 'double-arc shadow' sign of stones is absent.

ADENOMYOMATOUS HYPERPLASIA

This condition is known by several names, including adenomyomatosis and cholecystitis glandularis proliferans. It occurs in up to 9% of cholecystectomy specimens and in 90% of cases there are associated gallstones. It is characterised by thickening of the gallbladder wall due to epithelial and smooth muscle hyperplasia, with cystic epithelial invaginations into the wall (Rokitansky–Aschoff sinuses) and these spaces may contain small stones. Its distribution is fundal (most common), segmental (usually in mid-body) or diffuse. On US it appears as gallbladder wall thickening with secondary luminal narrowing (Fig. 8-18). The affected segment often contains bright echoes arising from the cystic spaces, often associated with 'comet-tail'

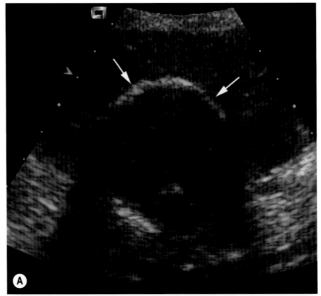

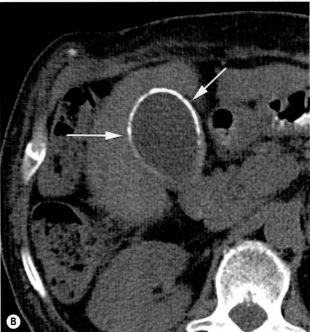

FIGURE 8-17 ■ **Porcelain gallbladder.** (A) US—echogenic wall with marked shadowing (arrows); (B) non-contrast CT with continuous mural calcification (arrows).

ring-down artefacts. CT shows wall thickening. Contrast gallbladder studies and T2-weighted MR may show the intramural cystic spaces (Fig. 8-19).[20] Adenomyomatous hyperplasia is usually asymptomatic, yet it is important to recognise, to avoid misdiagnosis as gallbladder carcinoma. Differentiation of focal forms of adenomyomatosis from small gallbladder carcinomas can be difficult with CT, and ultrasound is usually more reliable.

GALLBLADDER POLYPS

The great majority of polyps are composed of cholesterol and less often are adenomatous. Cholesterol polyps are

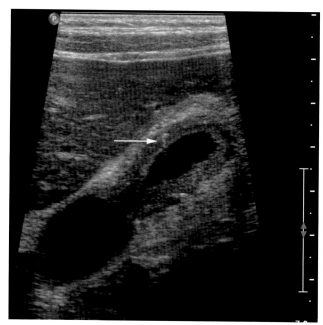

FIGURE 8-18 ■ **Adenomatous hyperplasia.** Ultrasound showing mural thickening of the fundus producing an hourglass configuration of the gallbladder with comet-tail artefact (arrow).

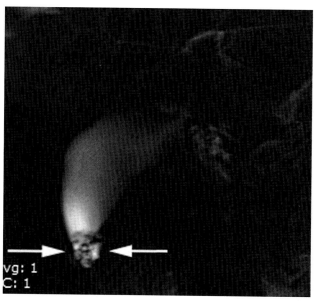

FIGURE 8-19 ■ **Adenomyomatous hyperplasia.** Coronal MRCP of multiple T2 hyperintense cyst-like structures in the deformed gallbladder fundus (arrows).

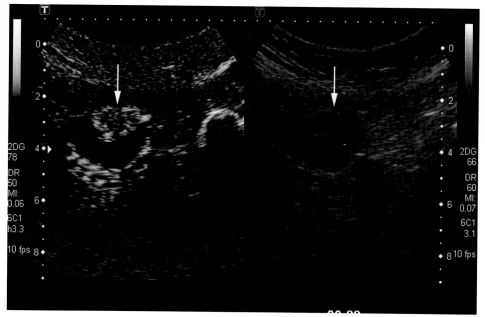

FIGURE 8-20 ■ **Gallbladder polyp.** B mode image (right image) showing a polypoid lesion (arrow) that contains vascularity with ultrasound contrast (left image).

usually 2–10 mm in size, whereas adenomas can be up to 2 cm. They both appear as small echogenic non-shadowing foci (Fig. 8-6) adherent to the gallbladder wall, often in a non-dependent portion. The main differential diagnosis is small stones and careful US technique can show the subtle, thin, acoustic shadowing diagnostic of a stone. Lack of mobility favours a polyp rather than a stone (Fig. 8-7). True malignant polyps are rare,[22] and predictors for neoplastic polyps include age over 60 years, a diameter of >10 mm, or local disruption of the adjacent gallbladder wall.[20,23,24] Single polyps are

no more likely to be neoplastic than multiple polyps.[24] Polyp growth rate of <0.6 mm per month has a negative predictive value of 90% for neoplastic polyps.[24] Doppler flow within an echogenic lesion differentiates it from sludge but does not distinguish reliably between benign and malignant polyps. CEUS (Fig. 8-20) shows promise at differentiating malignant gallbladder lesions from benign polyps by demonstrating wall destruction and rapid washout;[25] however, more studies are required to determine if it can accurately differentiate neoplastic from non-neoplastic polyps.

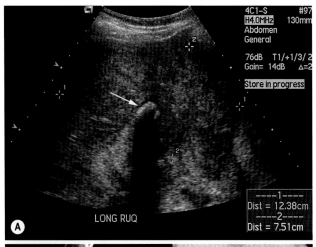

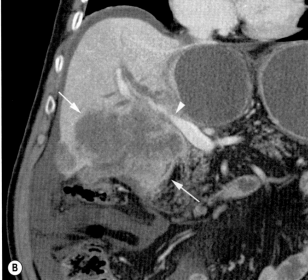

FIGURE 8-21 ■ **Gallbladder carcinoma.** US (A) shows a mass filling the gallbladder bed with a shadowing stone buried within the mass (arrow). Coronal CT (B) in the same patient shows hepatic invasion (arrows) and attenuation of the portal vein (arrowhead).

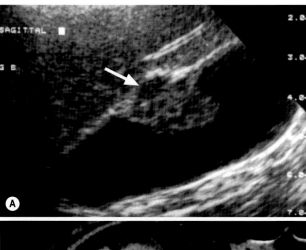

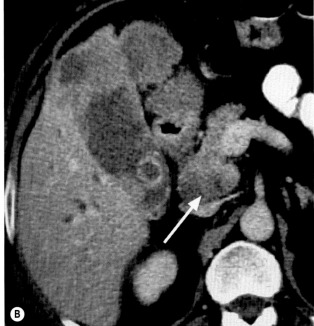

FIGURE 8-22 ■ **Gallbladder carcinoma.** (A) Ultrasound shows a polypoid lesion in the wall of the gallbladder with breach of continuity of the underlying wall (arrow). (B) Advanced carcinoma extending outside the fundus, with a nodal metastasis posterior to the pancreatic head (arrow). An associated stone can be seen in the gallbladder neck.

GALLBLADDER CARCINOMA

Gallbladder carcinoma is an uncommon malignancy, often with a poor prognosis. A minority will be detected early as a polypoid intraluminal mass or incidentally at cholecystectomy. Usually, however, presentation is late stage with right upper-quadrant pain, often presenting as hilar biliary obstruction. In addition to findings of biliary obstruction, carcinoma may be seen as focal or diffuse irregular gallbladder wall thickening or as a large gallbladder fossa mass with little or no gallbladder lumen identifiable. Gallbladder stones are present in the majority and may appear 'buried' in the mass (Fig. 8-21).

The disease tends to spread to lymph nodes around the portal vein relatively early and at presentation there may be nodal masses extending down to the head of pancreas. It also spreads to the adjacent liver (segments 4 and 5). Doppler blood flow can frequently be shown within the mass, and contrast enhancement may occur on CT and MR which, in the larger masses, is in the periphery around areas of central necrosis.[16] Malignant polypoid lesions show destruction of the gallbladder wall (Fig. 8-22), allowing differentiation from benign pathologies, while MRI with diffusion-weighted imaging also shows promise in differentiating polypoid gallbladder carcinomas from non-malignant asymmetric wall thickenings.[26]

GALLBLADDER METASTASES AND LYMPHOMA

Gallbladder metastases are rare, with most due to melanoma, although renal cell carcinoma, gastrointestinal malignancy and hepatocellular carcinoma metastases have also been described.[27] They may be single or multiple broad-based protrusions into the lumen. Most patients have widely disseminated disease at the time of diagnosis and although the gallbladder lesion is frequently asymptomatic, they may cause acute cholecystitis or extrahepatic biliary obstruction.

ROLE OF RADIOLOGY IN INVESTIGATION OF JAUNDICE

The principal role of imaging in the jaundiced patient is the identification and detailed assessment of major bile duct obstruction. Of patients with obstructive jaundice, 64% are due to malignancy, the bulk of which are pancreatic carcinomas, followed by cholangiocarcinoma and metastases, and then gallbladder carcinoma. Sixty-five per cent of benign causes are due to choledocholithiasis.[28] US is the preferred initial imaging investigation, but will usually be supplemented with a combination of CT, MRCP, direct cholangiography and, in some centres, endoscopic and/or intraoperative US.

The questions that need to be addressed are:
1. Is bile duct obstruction present?
2. What is the anatomical level of obstruction?
3. What is the cause of the obstruction?
4. If the obstruction appears to be malignant:
   a. Is there evidence of non-resectability?
   b. In those patients with malignant hilar obstruction who are unsuitable for surgical resection, what approach should be taken to palliative stenting?

Attention to these questions at the initial US allows targeted use of the supplementary investigations.[29]

First, determine whether there is intrahepatic and/or extrahepatic duct dilatation as a marker of duct obstruction. The intrahepatic ducts should measure no more than 2–3 mm centrally; more peripherally they are usually only just visible on US and should be smaller than the adjacent portal vein branches. Mild dilatation of the intrahepatic ducts may occur without duct obstruction in the elderly.

Selection of a single common duct diameter to predict distal bile duct obstruction is problematic. The maximum diameter of the normal common duct (includes the common hepatic and CBD) is influenced by age and where the duct is measured. A diameter of >7 mm is commonly used as a predictor of bile duct obstruction in jaundiced patients but is only a guide.[30] Lower values should be used in younger adults and, in the elderly, values of 8 mm or more are not unusual. The upper limit of 'normal' is also less well-defined post-cholecystectomy, when the duct is commonly up to 10 mm. Further investigation in these instances is guided by the pretest probability of obstruction.

The authors' practice is to attempt to visualise the entire duct and measure the largest internal diameter, which tends to be in the suprapancreatic portion. If only the very upper end of the common duct is seen and is not dilated, this does not totally exclude pathological dilatation of the distal portion. Conversely, if there is mild dilatation of the suprapancreatic portion but the duct tapers to a normal size in its pancreatic portion, further imaging is not mandatory and should be guided by the clinical picture.[30] Hilar biliary obstruction will produce only intrahepatic duct dilatation, whereas more distal obstruction will result in extrahepatic dilatation followed by intrahepatic dilatation.

Approximately 95% of patients with bile duct obstruction have biliary dilatation. In the remaining 5% there are usually sufficient clinical/biochemical indicators of duct obstruction to suggest that cholangiography is warranted. Most cases of biliary obstruction without duct dilatation are due to choledocholithiasis, primary sclerosing cholangitis or postoperative stricturing.

If duct obstruction (i.e. duct dilatation) is present, the anatomical level should be determined: namely, whether it is hilar/perihilar or low/mid common duct (Fig. 8-23). This aids the differential diagnosis (see Table 8-1) and selection of further imaging tests.

At ultrasound, if choledocholithiasis is demonstrated, patients can proceed to endoscopic sphincterotomy or cholecystectomy. If choledocholithiasis is not demonstrated but stones are highly likely on clinical grounds (e.g. pain and fever associated with jaundice), most patients should proceed to ERCP, particularly in the presence of sepsis. In patients with comorbidities that contraindicate ERCP or surgery, MRCP is helpful in providing confirmatory evidence of stones or suggesting another cause of obstruction.

US detects the level of obstruction in up to 95% and cause in up to 88%.[29] If the cause is not evident, and stones are not considered the most likely diagnosis, CT is usually the next most useful test, although MRCP and MRI may be substituted depending on local access and expertise.

MRCP identifies the presence of obstruction in up to 99%, the level of obstruction in 96% and detects tumour in 88% of patients with a malignant cause.[31] CT is highly

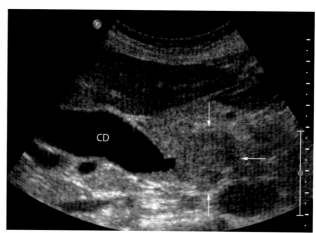

FIGURE 8-23 ■ Low biliary obstruction. Longitudinal US shows a very dilated bile duct and a large pancreatic head carcinoma (arrows).

TABLE 8-1   **Causes of Major Bile Duct Obstruction**

Anatomical Location	Malignant	Benign
Hilar	Gallbladder carcinoma*** Hepatocellular carcinoma**	
Low/mid duct	Pancreatic carcinoma**** Ampullary carcinoma**	Pancreatitis (acute or chronic)**
Either	Cholangiocarcinoma*** Metastases*** Lymphoma* Benign biliary tumors*	Stones**** Mirizzi's syndrome** Postoperative strictures*** Primary sclerosing cholangitis*** Other cholangiopathy* Haemobilia* Parasites*

Asterisks indicate approximate relative incidence (**** = most common). Low/mid-duct obstruction is more common than hilar obstruction.

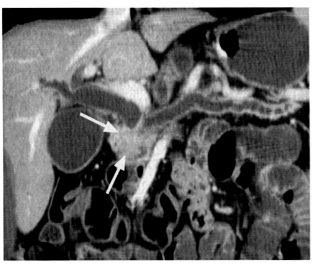

FIGURE 8-24 ■ **Low biliary obstruction.** Multislice CT with curved coronal reformat displaying a pancreatic head tumour (arrows) obstructing the common bile duct and pancreatic duct.

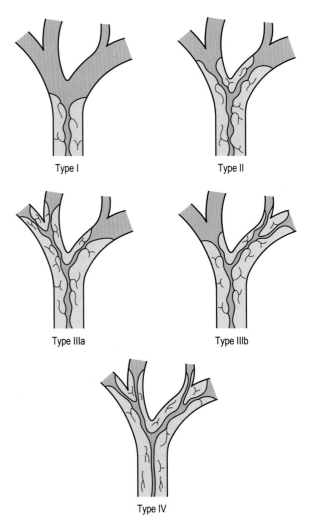

FIGURE 8-25 ■ **Modified Bismuth classification of malignant hilar biliary obstruction based on proximal extent of tumour.**

accurate for identifying the level and cause of obstruction, having similar accuracy to MRI and MRCP, especially with use of multiplanar and cholangiography-type CT reformats (Fig. 8-24),[32,33] the exception being that MRCP has a higher accuracy for detection of choledocholithiasis.

The next questions with presumed malignant obstruction relate to tumour resectability and biliary decompression options. In malignant hilar obstruction, evaluation should assess the proximal extent of stricturing into the right and left hepatic ducts, the presence of lobar atrophy, the patency of the portal veins (main, right and left branches) and the presence of any intrahepatic or local extrahepatic metastases. The proximal extent of stricturing is classified according to the modified Bismuth classification (Fig. 8-25).[34] In malignant low obstruction, usually due to pancreatic carcinoma, the main factors to assess are tumour size, vascular involvement (portal vein, superior mesenteric vein and superior mesenteric artery, coeliac trunk, common hepatic artery), lymph node metastases and hepatic metastases.

Even with modern imaging techniques it can be difficult to accurately differentiate benign from malignant strictures. Serum bilirubin levels have an association with malignancy, with levels over 100 μmol/L being 71.9% sensitive and 86.9% specific, while levels over 250 μmol/L are 97.1% specific for malignancy.[35]

Further information concerning pancreatic lesions giving rise to biliary obstruction may be found in Chapter 33, The Pancreas.

US (including Doppler), CT, MRI (including MRCP and MRA) and EUS can all provide information about tumour resectability, replacing angiography and direct cholangiography (PTC and ERCP) in most centres for this purpose. Positron emission tomography (PET) imaging is more helpful in identifying metastases than in identifying primary biliary tumours.[36]

Resectability assessment should, ideally, identify signs of non-resectability without excluding appropriate patients from potentially curative surgery. CT has a good overall accuracy for assessment of resectability. For hilar tumours MRCP allows assessment of the proximal extent of the lesion and determination of its Bismuth classification. EUS allows the assessment of the portal veins, superior mesenteric vessels and coeliac trunk for involvement by pancreatic head or periampullary tumours.

Core biopsy or fine-needle aspiration of suspected malignant obstructing lesions can be guided by US (transabdominal or endoscopic) or CT. If surgical resection is considered, a preoperative biopsy is not usually appropriate. If palliative stenting is being performed, biopsy is preferable *after* decompression to reduce the risk of a bile leak.

BENIGN BILE DUCT PATHOLOGY

CHOLEDOCHOLITHIASIS

At least 90% of bile duct stones originate in the gallbladder, so-called secondary stones. Primary stones are those that arise in the bile duct and these are pigment stones. For patients younger than 60 years undergoing cholecystectomy, 8–15% have duct stones, the figure increasing substantially in older patients.[37]

Ultrasound

Ultrasound sensitivity varies greatly, with the upper range being 50–80% and is better in jaundiced patients. The specificity is, however, about 95%. Duct dilatation and acoustic shadowing are each absent in about 30% of cases.[38] Positive stone diagnosis depends on the demonstration of an intraductal echogenic focus in both the longitudinal and transverse planes (Fig. 8-26A). Conditions that may mimic stones on US are:
1. *Intraductal gas*—usually recognisable by its linear nature and movement.
2. *Haemobilia and sludge*—they produce more diffuse echoes than stones.
3. *Surgical clips, hepatic artery calcification and duodenal diverticula*—these do not lie within the duct lumen.
4. Parasites.

As bile duct diameter increases, the likelihood of duct stones also increases.[39] In patients with previous cholecystectomy the correlation is less well established but a duct diameter of <4 mm carries a high negative predictive value for choledocholithiasis.

Endoscopic US (Fig. 8-26B) is more accurate than transcutaneous US, with a sensitivity of >90% and an even higher specificity.[40,41]

Unenhanced CT

The reported sensitivity of unenhanced helical CT in detection of choledocholithiasis varies. Two studies report sensitivities of 88 and 80%, and specificities of 97 and 100%, respectively.[42,43] Another study, however, reported a sensitivity of only 60%,[44] which is probably closer to what is achieved in routine practice. Stones usually appear as a ring density or soft-tissue density surrounded by lower-density bile, or sometimes as uniformly high density (Fig. 8-27).

Cholangiography

ERCP has a high accuracy for the diagnosis of choledocholithiasis but it does not detect all stones and in one study its sensitivity was 89% in comparison with EUS.[41]

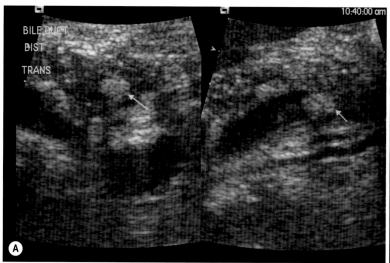
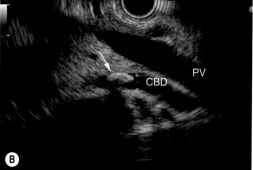

FIGURE 8-26 ■ **Choledocholithiasis.** (A) Two orthogonal transabdominal US images of a stone in the common duct (arrows). (B) Endoscopic ultrasound of a stone (arrow) in the CBD (common bile duct). PV = portal vein.

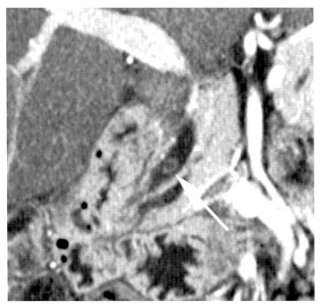

FIGURE 8-27 ■ **Choledocholithiasis.** Coronal portal venous CT. A distal common bile duct stone (arrow) is slightly dense compared with the surrounding low-density bile.

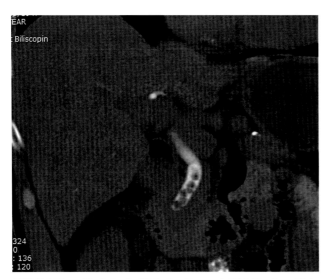

FIGURE 8-28 ■ **Choledocholithiasis.** Coronal CT-IVC of multiple small stones in the distal common duct.

The sensitivity and specificity of CT-IVC for detection of CBD stones is 85–96% and 88–98%, respectively.[44–47] A strength of this technique is the diagnosis of stones <5 mm in diameter with high accuracy (Fig. 8-28)[46] and a weakness is the low diagnostic yield if bilirubin is more than twice normal.

MRCP (Fig. 8-29) is highly accurate in the diagnosis of choledocholithiasis with meta-analyses reporting pooled sensitivities of 92[31] and 94%,[48] and specificity of 99%.[48] However, for stones under 3 mm the sensitivity is less than 50%,[49] with small stones accounting for most false-negative results. MRCP quality, however, is independent of bilirubin level. Potential causes of false-positive diagnoses for MRCP are gas, haemobilia and

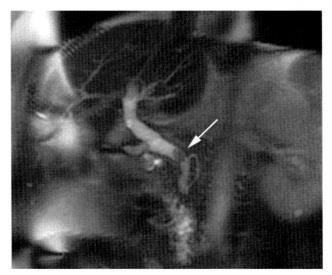

FIGURE 8-29 ■ **Choledocholithiasis.** Single common duct stone (arrow) on thick-section, oblique, coronal MRCP.

flow voids. Well-defined intraluminal signal voids should be visible in two thin-section orthogonal planes to reduce false-positive diagnoses for small stones.

The investigation of choice for suspected choledocholithiasis depends on the clinical likelihood of stones. Ultrasound should be performed first, as it has a high positive predictive value. High pretest probability patients should proceed to endoscopic US or ERCP, especially if they have cholangitis, as that will allow prompt intervention and stone extraction. Intermediate-to-low probability patients can proceed to either MRCP or CT-IVC.

The differential diagnosis of stones on cholangiography is similar to that on ultrasound.

HEPATOLITHIASIS

In Western populations the majority of duct stones are extrahepatic. Intrahepatic stone formation, or hepatolithiasis, may occur in association with common duct stones but is often associated with other pathology including benign strictures; primary sclerosing cholangitis (PSC); postoperative strictures; recurrent pyogenic cholangitis and Caroli's disease. The imaging features are similar to extrahepatic stones.

BENIGN BILIARY STRICTURES

Postoperative Strictures

Postoperative strictures most often result from cholecystectomy. They are usually <10 mm in length and are commonly only 1–2 mm (Fig. 8-30) and involve the common duct, but can involve the right and left hepatic ducts, or aberrant ducts, especially low right sectoral or segmental ducts. Biliary strictures following liver transplantation are common and are divided into anastomotic strictures (8.9% of transplants)[50] and non-anastomotic strictures (16% of transplants).[51] Duct stones may develop

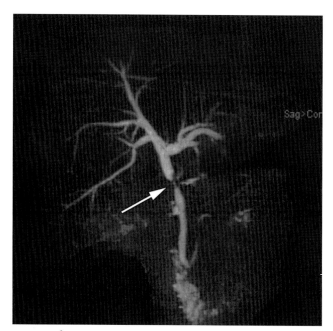

FIGURE 8-30 ■ **MRCP shows a post-cholecystectomy stricture (arrow) that characteristically, is short.**

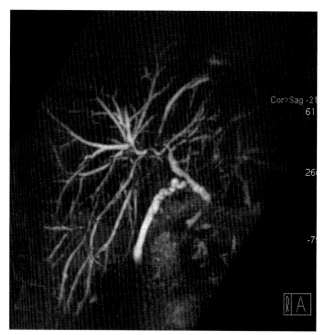

FIGURE 8-32 ■ **Primary sclerosing cholangitis.** Thick-slab oblique coronal MRCP shows multiple intrahepatic and extrahepatic segments of stricturing.

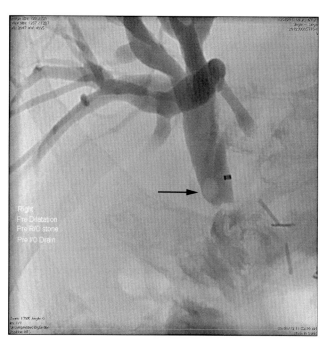

FIGURE 8-31 ■ **Postoperative stricture.** PTC following hepaticoje-junostomy showing a stone (arrow) immediately above a tight anastomotic stricture.

proximal to any stricture (Fig. 8-31). Good-quality cholangiography is required for assessment, particularly of hilar strictures, to define their anatomy. MRCP has the advantage over ERCP of demonstrating ducts above a complete stricture while CT-IVC can show bile leaks. A common artefact on MRCP is pseudostricture of the common hepatic duct caused by the hepatic artery or its right branch as it crosses the duct.

Primary Sclerosing Cholangitis

The most common form of cholangitis causing stricturing is PSC, 70% of patients having a background of chronic inflammatory bowel disease, usually ulcerative colitis. PSC is characterised on cholangiography by multiple segments of stricturing involving intrahepatic and/or extrahepatic ducts (Fig. 8-32). A characteristic feature in the common duct is diverticula-like outpoachings (Fig. 8-33). On ultrasound, PSC is characterised by bile duct wall thickening, particularly at sites of stricturing (Fig. 8-34), and the diverticula-like outpoachings may be seen as local echogenic foci in the duct wall. Well-established PSC is associated with areas of atrophy and hypertrophy within the liver, best seen with CT or MRI. Bile duct stones occur in about 10% of patients with PSC and tend to be high density on CT and cast-like on US.[52]

Cholangiocarcinoma complicates about 10% of PSC and is a notoriously difficult and late diagnosis (Fig. 8-35). It should be suspected if there is progressive duct dilatation proximal to a stricture, or if a nodule >1 cm in diameter is identified. Dual-phase, contrast-enhanced CT, especially when correlated with cholangiography, can improve cholangiocarcinoma detection.[53] PET may prove helpful, though results at present are mixed.[54,55] A current screening recommendation[56] is for annual hepatic MRI and MRCP, recognising the greater sensitivity than ultrasound without the radiation burden of CT.

Mirizzi's Syndrome

Mirizzi's syndrome is characterised by common duct narrowing by inflammation and fibrosis related to chronic gallstone disease. Typically a stone is impacted in the neck of the gallbladder, the cystic duct, or cystic duct

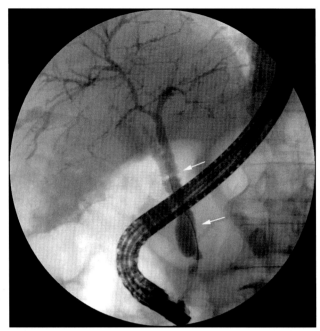

FIGURE 8-33 ■ **Primary sclerosing cholangitis.** ERCP shows strictures and characteristic diverticula-like outpouchings affecting the common duct.

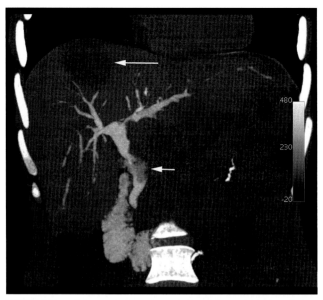

FIGURE 8-35 ■ **Primary sclerosing cholangitis and cholangiocarcinoma.** CT-IVC MIP showing multiple intrahepatic strictures in a patient with PSC. A polypoid cholangiocarcinoma (short arrow) is present as an irregular filling defect in the common hepatic duct extending into the proximal CBD. A hepatic metastasis is present (long arrow).

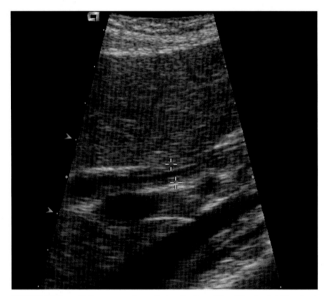

FIGURE 8-34 ■ **Primary sclerosing cholangitis.** Typical bile duct wall thickening on US (calipers).

remnant (Fig. 8-36). A fistula may develop between the gallbladder or cystic duct and the common duct and the stone may partially or totally pass into the common duct. The level of stricturing varies, being most common in the upper and middle common duct, but it can be lower if the cystic duct has a low entry. On cholangiography the stricture is usually smooth, 2–3 cm in length, and often with a rightward concavity. Fistula formation is most readily appreciated at ERCP. The diagnosis should be suspected on US when there is ductal dilatation down to the level of a stone that is not clearly within the common

duct. The diagnosis can be challenging preoperatively but is important as it can mimic malignant stricturing, especially that due to gallbladder carcinoma, and surgery can be difficult with a high rate of bile duct injury.

Pancreatitis

Pancreatitis, both acute and chronic, can produce biliary stricturing caused by fibrosis and/or an inflammatory mass. Cholangiographically the strictures are typically smooth and tapered, and tend to extend over a few centimeters (Fig. 8-37).

IgG4-related Sclerosing Disease

IgG4-related sclerosing disease is an immune-mediated multisystem disease most frequently presenting as autoimmune pancreatitis. Extrapancreatic disease is common with hilar adenopathy in 80% and bile duct lesions in 74% of patients.[57] This may mimic pancreatic carcinoma, cholangiocarcinoma or PSC;[58] IgG4 serum levels are typically elevated.

HIV Cholangiopathy

Human immunodeficiency virus (HIV) cholangiopathy (or acquired immune deficiency syndrome [AIDS] cholangiopathy) typically occurs in patients with a CD4 T-lymphocyte count below 100/mm³, and is usually caused by opportunistic infection, most commonly *Cryptosporidium* and cytomegalovirus. US can exclude other causes of pain and cholestasis with a high sensitivity for identifying cholangiopathy. The findings include bile duct wall thickening and enhancement, focal strictures

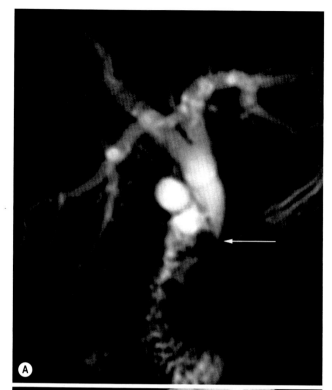

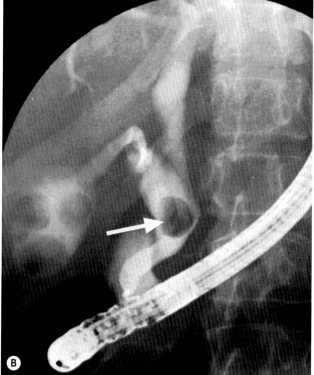

FIGURE 8-36 ■ **Mirizzi's syndrome.** MRCP (A) shows a stricture of the lower common duct caused by a stone (arrow) lying in an expanded cystic duct on ERCP (B). Multiple gallbladder stones are also seen.

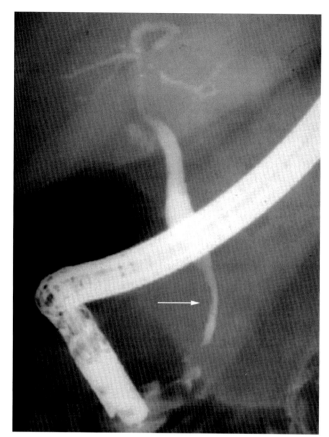

FIGURE 8-37 ■ **Chronic pancreatitis.** Typical smooth, elongated, incomplete stricture of the lower common bile duct.

(intrahepatic and/or extrahepatic) resembling PSC, and duct dilatation, the latter sometimes due to papillary stenosis.[59] Gallbladder wall thickening is common. Cholangiography shows corresponding changes and endoscopic drainage may be required.

Acute Bacterial Cholangitis

Acute bacterial cholangitis is almost always associated with at least partial bile duct obstruction, most often secondary to choledocholithiasis. Patients present with some or all features of Charcot's triad: fever, right upper quadrant pain and jaundice. Typically it is polymicrobial and caused by Gram-negative enteric organisms, and requires IV broad-spectrum antibiotics, urgent imaging to identify the underlying pathology and appropriate biliary tract drainage, either endoscopic or transhepatic. Imaging should include US and sometimes CT, especially if hepatic abscesses are suspected, and these may require transhepatic drainage. MRCP may identify obstructing pathology but if the clinical likelihood is choledocholithiasis then patients require urgent ERCP and sphincterotomy.

Recurrent Pyogenic Cholangitis

Recurrent pyogenic cholangitis (RPC) occurs mainly in South-East Asia or its emigrants and is characterised by recurrent episodes of cholangitis, bile duct stones, biliary dilatation and strictures. Infection is due to enteric bacteria that are thought to be responsible for stone formation, although parasites, in particular *Clonorchis sinensis*, may play a role. The parasite is rarely identified at imaging.[60] The stones are mostly intrahepatic, often very

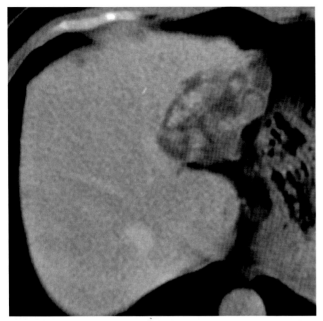

FIGURE 8-38 ■ **Recurrent pyogenic cholangitis.** Multiple high-density stones lie in dilated ducts within an atrophic left lobe.

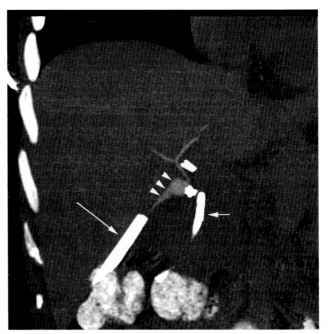

FIGURE 8-39 ■ **Postoperative bile leak.** Coronal CT-IVC post-cholecystectomy showing contrast agent external to the biliary tree (arrowheads) at the cystic duct stump passing towards a drain tube (long arrow). Note plastic stent (short arrow) in the distal common duct.

extensive, and composed of calcium bilirubinate, and therefore frequently visible on CT as high densities within dilated intrahepatic ducts (Fig. 8-38). US shows duct dilatation and stones that may not shadow. Cross-sectional imaging identifies segmental distribution, complicating abscesses and atrophy. Cholangiography shows duct dilatation and multiple stones, which may be widespread or segmental, and duct strictures are common. Ductal dilatation may be disproportionately prominent in the extrahepatic ducts and central intrahepatic ducts, sparing the smaller peripheral ducts.[61] Management usually involves a combination of surgery, endoscopic and percutaneous techniques. Long-term complications include liver fibrosis, portal hypertension and cholangiocarcinoma.

PARASITIC INFECTIONS

Ascaris lumbricoides

Ascaris lumbricoides is a parasitic roundworm 20–30 cm in length and about 5 mm in diameter, which may enter the bile duct through the duodenal ampulla. This can be asymptomatic or result in cholangitis, cholecystitis or pancreatitis. The worm may be visible on US or cholangiography as a tube-like structure.

Hydatid

A small proportion of hepatic hydatid cysts will rupture into the biliary tree and potentially obstruct it. The ruptured membranes may be seen as curvilinear structures on US or cholangiography. Communication between the ruptured cyst and the bile ducts may be shown on ERCP or CT-IVC.

Fascioliasis

Fascioliasis is caused by the liver fluke *Fasciola hepatica*, which is leaf-shaped and measures 1–2 mm. The infestation comprises two stages: hepatic and biliary. The hepatic stage results in multiple small abscesses and, sometimes, subcapsular haemorrhage. The biliary stage results in bile duct wall thickening and sometimes the flukes are visible within the bile ducts or gallbladder.[62]

BILIARY LEAKS AND BILE DUCT INJURIES

Bile leaks usually occur following cholecystectomy, or trauma. US or CT may detect collections, though CT provides a more reliable examination of all subphrenic spaces. ERCP is useful post-cholecystectomy as there is a high likelihood of a retained stone and stone extraction and/or temporary stenting may be required. Both HIDA scintigraphy and CT-IVC can demonstrate biliary leaks (Fig. 8-39), the former being more sensitive whereas the latter provides more anatomical information. MRCP shows fluid collections arising from bile leaks, but cannot differentiate these from other causes of fluid collections and cannot usually identify the source unless hepatocyte-specific contrast agents and T1-weighted MRCP are employed.

If a major bile duct injury is suspected in the early postoperative period, the most important imaging investigation is high-quality cholangiography to demonstrate the duct anatomy above the injury. For this reason ERCP may not be sufficient if there is complete transection or

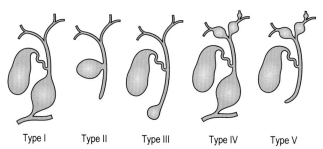

FIGURE 8-40 ■ **Biliary cystic disease classification (after Todani).**

ligation of a duct. MRCP or CT-IVC may provide sufficient information but sometimes PTC is necessary before surgical repair.

BILIARY CYSTIC DISEASE

Biliary cystic disease, which is quite rare, is described by the Todani classification (Fig. 8-40).[63] The approximate relative incidences of cysts are: Type I choledochal cyst 79%, Type IV 13%, Type III (choledochocoele) 4%, Type II 3% and Type V (Caroli's disease) 1%. Types I and IV are characterised by a long common channel shared with the pancreatic duct. There is a high incidence of stone development in the affected ducts and an association with various biliary tumours, most commonly cholangiocarcinoma, with a 20-fold increased incidence. Type I cysts commonly present in childhood with jaundice and a right upper-quadrant mass. Otherwise, the presentation is similar to gallstone disease, including pain, cholangitis, jaundice and pancreatitis.

The diagnosis may be suspected on cross-sectional imaging but the cysts are best evaluated with cholangiography (Fig. 8-41). Their cholangiographic appearance is similar regardless of the technique used, though ERCP, CT-IVC, PTC and contrast-enhanced MRCP are able to demonstrate directly the communication between the bile ducts and the cysts (Fig. 8-41), whereas conventional MRCP cannot. MRCP and ERCP are best able to demonstrate the long common channel seen with Types I and IV. Other less common cysts such as duodenal duplication cysts may communicate with the distal bile duct and this feature is well demonstrated by CT-IVC.

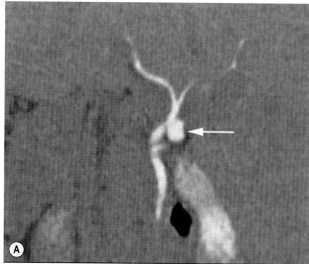

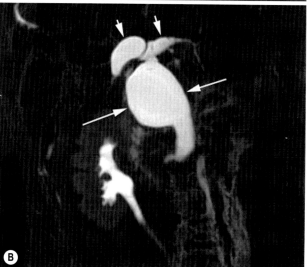

FIGURE 8-41 ■ **Choledochal cyst.** (A) Curved CT-IVC reformat of a Type II choledochal cyst (arrow). (B) Oblique coronal thick-slab MRCP of a Type IV choledochal cyst demonstrating marked dilatation of the common hepatic duct (long arrows) and central intrahepatic ducts (short arrows) with no stricture or peripheral dilatation.

NEOPLASTIC BILE DUCT PATHOLOGY

CHOLANGIOCARCINOMA

Cholangiocarcinoma is an uncommon tumour arising from the bile duct epithelium, which tends to spread by local infiltration. Approximately 60% arise in the perihilar region (Klatskin tumours), <30% arise in the distal common duct and <10% are diffuse or multifocal.[64] Approximately 10% are classified as peripheral, arising within the liver and presenting as an hepatic mass; these are discussed in Chapter 31, The Liver and Spleen.

Pathologically, cholangiocarcinomas are usually 'infiltrating stenotic' or 'exophytic masses',[65] with 'intraluminal polypoid' and 'mucin-secreting' types being uncommon. Their appearance on imaging varies with size and pathological type. Most of the exophytic tumours are <5 cm and the infiltrating stenotic tumors are usually <1–2 cm in diameter.

On US the tumours appear as nodules or focal bile duct wall thickening, which are usually slightly hyperechoic. On CT the nodules are usually isodense or slightly hypodense compared with liver and are more easily seen on dual-phase contrast-enhanced imaging; the infiltrating stenotic type tends to enhance in the arterial phase and the exophytic are more conspicuous on portal-phase imaging, being hypodense to liver.[65] On MRI the tumours are hypointense on T1 and hyperintense on T2 and show some progressive enhancement on dynamic imaging greater than normal liver, indistinct margins, luminal irregularity and asymmetry.[66] The proximal extent of the stricturing, which critically affects treatment options, is well shown with MRCP, which performs better than US and CT and is comparable to direct cholangiography (Fig. 8-42).[67] The majority of hilar

cholangiocarcinomas are hyper- to isoenhancing at ultra-sound contrast studies, and demonstrate rapid washout to be hypoenhancing by the portal venous phase.[68] PET/CT is relatively insensitive for the detection of cholangi-ocarcinoma, with its role largely confined to preoperative detection of nodal and distant metastases.[69] The uncom-mon mucin-secreting type of tumour tends to produce duct expansion, which can be pronounced and is caused by the volume of mucin secreted rather than by tumour obstruction alone.

The criteria for resectability depend on individual surgical approaches but imaging should assess the proxi-mal extent of stricturing, any tumour involvement of

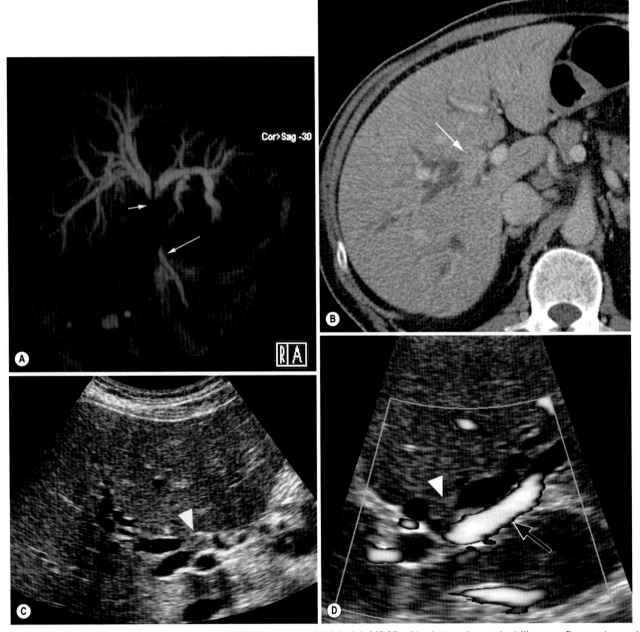

FIGURE 8-42 ■ **Small hilar cholangiocarcinoma.** (A) Oblique coronal thick-slab MRCP with obstruction at the biliary confluence (arrow). Note non-distended distal CBD (long arrow) in a Bismuth Type II cholangiocarcinoma. (B) Portal venous axial CT in a different patient, showing distended ducts passing to a small hilar mass (arrow) that is isodense to liver. A different patient with (C) longitudinal US and (D) transverse colour Doppler US showing a small hilar carcinoma (arrowheads) (open arrow: normal left portal vein).

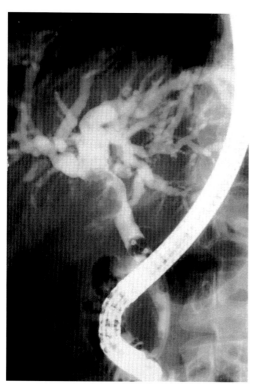

FIGURE 8-43 ■ **Gallbladder carcinoma producing a tight hilar stricture on balloon occlusion ERCP.** The impression from the right side suggests either gallbladder carcinoma or Mirizzi's syndrome.

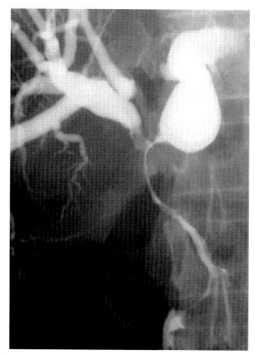

FIGURE 8-44 ■ **Metastatic adenocarcinoma.** PTC shows a long stricture of the common duct involving the hilar confluence. The stricture has a characteristic scalloped appearance.

the portal vein (main and right and left branches), the presence of lobar liver atrophy and intrahepatic and extrahepatic tumour spread. Some surgeons also require information about any tumour involvement of the hepatic artery and caudate ducts. MRI with MRCP has a similar accuracy to MDCT combined with direct cholangiography for determination of resectability, with an accuracy of between 74 and 77.8%,[70] while other studies show that high-resolution dual-phase CT has a negative and positive predictive value of 92 and 85%, respectively, for resectability.[71]

Gallbladder carcinoma can present with bile duct obstruction that tends to be hilar, and may mimic cholangiocarcinoma or Mirizzi's syndrome (Fig. 8-43).

METASTASES AND LYMPHOMA

Metastases and lymphoma may result in hilar or mid/low biliary obstruction. Cholangiographically they mimic other malignant causes of obstruction. The strictures may be long and have a characteristic scalloped appearance on cholangiography (Fig. 8-44), and on cross-sectional imaging abnormal soft tissue is usually evident. Intraductal metastases are rare.

PANCREATIC AND AMPULLARY TUMOURS

Pancreatic and ampullary tumours are discussed further in Chapter 33, The Pancreas.

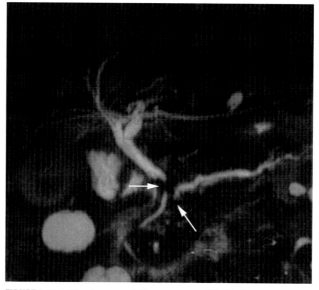

FIGURE 8-45 ■ **Carcinoma of the pancreas.** MRCP shows adjacent strictures (arrows) of the common bile duct and pancreatic duct ('double-duct sign').

On cholangiography, pancreatic carcinoma produces a tight stricture that is often shouldered, but may have a blunt cut-off that is straight or convex upward or downward. The differential diagnosis for malignant low/mid duct obstruction includes cholangiocarcinoma, metastases and ampullary and periampullary carcinomas. Adjacent strictures of both bile duct and pancreatic duct ('double-duct sign') are highly suggestive of pancreatic carcinoma (Fig. 8-45) or, less often, periampullary

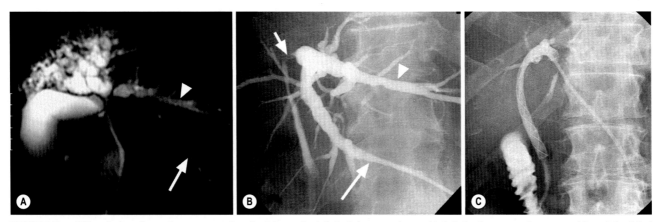

FIGURE 8-46 ■ **Hilar cholangiocarcinoma associated with marked right-lobe atrophy and left-lobe hypertrophy, treated by a left-sided transhepatic metal stent.** (A) MRCP shows a Bismuth Type II stricture with very dilated and crowded ducts in a small atrophic right lobe. Arrowhead = segment II; long arrow = segment III (partially out of section). (B) Left-sided PTC and catheterisation of segment III (long arrow), with short stricture of first-order left hepatic duct (short arrow). (C) A metal biliary stent has been placed across the hilar stricture.

carcinoma. Groove pancreatitis, a variant of chronic pancreatitis, can sometimes produce a double-duct sign but there are usually other imaging signs to suggest the diagnosis.

MISCELLANEOUS BILIARY TUMOURS

Various uncommon tumours are recognised, most of them described as polyps, papillomas, adenomas and cystadenomas.

These are benign, occur most often in the CBD, typically in the ampullary region, and present with jaundice. The rarer entity of multiple biliary papillomatosis has malignant potential, usually presents with jaundice and may cause the secretion of large volumes of mucin.

LIVER ATROPHY

Lobar and segmental liver atrophy may be associated with lobar or segmental bile duct obstruction due to malignant or benign causes. Cholangiocarcinoma is the commonest malignant cause, while the main benign causes are postoperative strictures and PSC. Malignant obstruction is frequently associated with ipsilateral portal vein branch occlusion or narrowing.[72] Lobar atrophy is frequently associated with contralateral lobar hypertrophy (Fig. 8-46). The pattern of lobar and segmental liver

atrophy is influenced by hilar biliary anatomical variants.[73]

LOBAR OR SEGMENTAL DUCT OBSTRUCTION

Lobar or segmental duct obstruction may present with cholangitis but can be relatively asymptomatic. Serum bilirubin is usually normal, but usually gammaglutamyl transferase and alkaline phosphatase are elevated. Causes include stones, postoperative strictures, PSC and lobar or segmental cholangiocarcinoma. The condition is usually more easily recognised on cross-sectional imaging or MRCP than on direct cholangiography.

HAEMOBILIA

Most bleeding into the biliary tree results from trauma, including iatrogenic injury from liver biopsy, percutaneous biliary procedures, or surgery. Other causes include hepatic artery aneurysms, tumours and cholecystitis. On US haemobilia appears similar to sludge in either the gallbladder or bile ducts, and on CT it may appear as slightly high-density material. An underlying aneurysm may be visible on Doppler US or contrast-enhanced CT, though angiography more reliably identifies underlying vascular lesions and allows selective arterial embolisation. On cholangiography haemobilia appears as a cast-like filling defect in the bile ducts.

INTERVENTIONAL TECHNIQUES

PERCUTANEOUS CHOLECYSTOSTOMY

This procedure is performed in two main groups: those with acute calculous cholecystitis and comorbidities presenting unacceptable surgical risk, and the critically ill

with presumed acalculous cholecystitis. Patients may recover to a stage of being suitable for cholecystectomy. Others may require the percutaneous extraction of gallbladder stones using a variety of techniques including irrigation, forceps removal, basketing, or lithotripsy.

A catheter such as a 6 or 8Fr pigtail is inserted under US guidance using either a coaxial or trocar technique and, if stone removal is required, the track is subsequently dilated to the required size. The gallbladder may be punctured via the fundus in a transperitoneal approach or via a transhepatic approach into the gallbladder body in an attempt to avoid transgressing the peritoneum. The authors' preference is a transperitoneal approach as there is no evidence of higher complication rates and it provides a more favourable approach for any subsequent stone removal.

If stones cannot be cleared, and cholecystectomy is not possible, the catheter can be removed after 2–3 weeks' drainage. Before removal, contrast studies should demonstrate cystic duct patency and determine whether there are any bile duct stones requiring treatment by endoscopic sphincterotomy. In patients with acalculous cholecystitis, catheters should not be removed earlier than 3 weeks.[74]

PERCUTANEOUS TRANSHEPATIC BILIARY CATHETERISATION

Percutaneous transhepatic biliary catheterisation is performed as part of a range of interventional procedures. Common applications are the relief of malignant obstruction (usually followed by stent insertion), the dilatation of benign strictures, transhepatic duct stone treatment, drainage of infected bile ducts and, occasionally, as part of a combined procedure for endoscopic intervention ('rendezvous procedure'), though this is now used infrequently. The complications of the method are similar to those for PTC, but up to twice as common.

MALIGNANT DISEASE

The major role of percutaneous transhepatic biliary drainage and stent insertion is the palliation of malignant biliary obstruction in patients with non-resectable tumour or who are medically unfit for surgery, which constitutes the majority of patients. Preoperative biliary drainage is not routinely of benefit, though it is still used by some surgeons and is valuable if there is life-threatening biliary sepsis.

The non-surgical palliation of malignant biliary obstruction can be transhepatic or endoscopic. Endoscopic stenting, with either plastic or metal stents, is preferred for low biliary obstruction. For hilar obstruction the advantage of avoiding a transhepatic track can be offset by inappropriate stent positioning. Careful positioning of stents is especially important for Bismuth Types II–IV strictures.

Transhepatic drainage can be achieved by permanent catheters or indwelling stents. Catheters can be inserted across malignant strictures in 80–90% of cases, establishing internal as well as external drainage, although 20% remain jaundiced.[9] Generally, internal stents are preferable to percutaneous catheters as they avoid the ongoing discomfort and inconvenience associated with catheters. Percutaneous catheters can be used as access

for brachytherapy using ^{192}Ir in combination with metal stent insertion; there is some evidence that this improves stent patency and, possibly, survival.[75]

Expanding metal stents are preferable to plastic stents as they have larger lumens, longer patency rates, lower early complication rates and require fewer reinterventions, which make them cost-effective at least in those patients expected to live for a number of months. One prospective study reported that for metal and plastic stents 30-day mortality rates were 10 and 24%, obstruction rates 19 and 27%, median patency 272 and 96 days and median time to death or obstruction 122 and 81 days, respectively. Hospital stay was shorter with the metal stents (10 days compared with 21 days) and their placement cost was lower.[76]

For strictures below the biliary confluence, the approach can be via either the right or left lobe. The authors' preference is to use the right flank approach as the anatomy provides a less-angled pathway at the biliary confluence, and may result in less haemobilia.[77]

Hilar Strictures—Special Considerations

With hilar strictures that separate the right and left hepatic ducts (Bismuth Types II–IV) accurate stent placement is critically important. Many believe that careful placement of a unilateral stent provides results at least as good as routine bilateral stents. Given that endoscopic bilateral stent placement is achievable in only about 30% of the cases in which it is attempted,[78] and that percutaneous bilateral stents require bilateral transhepatic tracks, the authors' preference is for a carefully placed single stent (either endoscopic or percutaneous). The stent must be placed so that it drains the largest possible volume of non-atrophic and tumour-free liver.[79–81] This assessment is best made with CT and MRCP before intervention to assess the proximal extent of the stricturing and the presence of atrophy (Fig. 8-46). Contralateral stenting is required if the opposite lobe contains infected bile as revealed by contralateral fine-needle bile aspiration in patients with suspected cholangitis.

BENIGN DISEASE

Transhepatic procedures may be performed for benign strictures or stones to:
1. *Drain an obstructed infected system* (including lobar or segmental obstruction), which is not amenable to endoscopic drainage.
2. *Dilate benign strictures* when surgery or endoscopic treatment is not possible. Such strictures are usually due to cholecystectomy injury, biliary-enteric anastomotic strictures, or sclerosing cholangitis. Balloon dilatation should be followed by 2 weeks (and sometimes much longer) of biliary drainage catheter placed across the stricture.
3. *Treat intrahepatic or extrahepatic ductal stones* that are not amenable to endoscopic or surgical management. Stones may be removed by basketing, or

lithotripsy. Creation of a large-calibre, mature transhepatic track is usually necessary.

Transhepatic techniques may be combined with operative approaches in complex benign biliary problems, with transhepatic access created by the placement of a transhepatic tube at operation.[82]

Percutaneous Transjejunal Biliary Intervention

This technique was developed to provide endoscopic stone clearance via a stoma in recurrent pyogenic cholangitis and was subsequently modified to allow percutaneous radiological access without a stoma to treat benign strictures and stones.[83,84] The afferent or efferent limb of the Roux-en-Y loop is fixed to the anterior parietal peritoneum at the time of creation of a biliary-enteric anastomosis. The fixation site is marked with surgical clips to allow subsequent percutaneous puncture under fluoroscopy. Percutaneous transjejunal cholangiography (PTJC) can be performed via the loop with stricture dilatation and stone extraction performed as needed. The procedure is safe, well-tolerated, requires minimal hospitalisation and can be repeated without the need for long-term indwelling catheters or transhepatic catheterisation. The approach has been extended to treat malignant strictures following attempted resection, allowing transjejunal brachytherapy and/or stent insertion.[84]

Gallstone Extraction Via T-Tube Track

Percutaneous extraction of post-cholecystectomy retained bile duct stones can be performed via a T-tube track that has matured for 5–6 weeks and has a high success rate but has been largely replaced by endoscopic sphincterotomy and stone extraction as this avoids the inconvenience of a longer period with a T-tube.

BIOPSY TECHNIQUES

Cytological or histological diagnosis of suspected malignant disease involving the bile ducts can be attempted by percutaneous needling using a fine needle (e.g. 22G) for cytology or a slightly larger needle for histology (e.g. 18G). In one review the sensitivity of fine-needle aspiration cytology (FNAC) for extrahepatic bile duct tumours was 62%, and for pancreatic cancer 76%. For the latter group a higher sensitivity appears possible with histological samples. The total complication rate for FNAC of liver, biliary tract and pancreas was less than 0.2% and included bleeding, bile leak, pancreatitis and infection (each reported as being less than 0.08%). Needle track seeding was reported in up to 0.05% of cases and deaths in 0.006–0.03%.[85] Gallbladder masses can be biopsied if they are large, but the biopsy of polypoid masses is not reliable and carries a substantial risk of biliary leakage. The cytological examination of bile or of biliary brushings yields a sensitivity of about 55%, but a positive result is helpful.[86,87] In the setting of biliary obstruction, biopsy should be delayed until after biliary

decompression, and is not generally recommended if resection will be attempted.

Guidance for biopsy is usually by US, CT, EUS or fluoroscopy with cholangiography; the choice is determined by which best shows the target, and operator preference.

ERCP provides a direct means of undertaking a biopsy of tumours involving the ampulla or duodenum. Extrahepatic biliary masses can be biopsied at EUS with relatively high success rates, and less concern of tumour seeding in potential resection candidates.

REFERENCES

1. Healey JE Jr, Schroy PC. Anatomy of the biliary ducts within the human liver; analysis of the prevailing pattern of branchings and the major variations of the biliary ducts. AMA Arch Surg 1953;66(5):599–616.
2. Couinaud C. Le foie. Paris: Masson; 1957.
3. Albishri SH, Issa S, Kneteman NM, et al. Bile leak from duct of Luschka after liver transplantation. Transplantation 2001;72(2):338–40.
4. Harvey R, Miller W. Acute biliary disease: initial CT and follow-up US versus initial US and follow-up CT. Radiology 1999;213(3):831–6.
5. Nilsson U. Adverse reactions to iotroxate at intravenous cholangiography. A prospective clinical investigation and review of the literature. Acta Radiol 1987;28(5):571–5.
6. Biliscopin—Meglumine iotroxate, Schering. Berlin: SBU Diagnostics; 1997. pp. 9–10.
7. Goodwin MD, Dobson JE, Sirlin CB, et al. Diagnostic challenges and pitfalls in MR imaging with hepatocyte-specific contrast agents. Radiographics 2011;31(6):1547–68.
8. Freeman ML, DiSario JA, Nelson DB, et al. Risk factors for post-ERCP pancreatitis: a prospective, multicenter study. Gastrointest Endosc 2001;54(4):425–34.
9. Gibson R. Percutaneous transhepatic cholangiography and biliary drainage. In: Adam A, Gibson R, editors. Practical Interventional Radiology of the Hepatobiliary System and Gastrointestinal Tract. London: Edward Arnold; 1994.
10. Fernández-Esparrach G, Ginès A, Sánchez M, et al. Comparison of endoscopic ultrasonography and magnetic resonance cholangiopancreatography in the diagnosis of pancreatobiliary diseases: a prospective study. Am J Gastroenterol 2007;102(8):1632–9.
11. Bouchier IAD. Gallstones: formation and epidemiology. In: Surgery of the Liver and Biliary Track. 2nd ed. London: Churchill Livingstone; 1994.
12. Hessler PC, Hill DS, Deforie FM, et al. High accuracy sonographic recognition of gallstones. Am J Roentgenol 1981;136(3):517–20.
13. Allen B, Bernhoft R, Blanckaert N, et al. Sludge is calcium bilirubinate associated with bile stasis. Am J Surg 1981;141(1):51–6.
14. Ko CW, Sekijima JH, Lee SP. Biliary sludge. Ann Intern Med 1999;130(4 Pt 1):301–11.
15. Ralls PW, Colletti PM, Lapin SA, et al. Real-time sonography in suspected acute cholecystitis. Prospective evaluation of primary and secondary signs. Radiology 1985;155(3):767–71.
16. Gore RM, Yaghmai V, Newmark GM, et al. Imaging benign and malignant disease of the gallbladder. Radiol Clin North Am 2002;40(6):1307–23, vi.
17. Wu C, Chen CC, Wang CJ, et al. Discrimination of gangrenous from uncomplicated acute cholecystitis: accuracy of CT findings. Abdom Imaging 2011;36(2):174–8.
18. Kim PN, Lee KS, Kim IY, et al. Gallbladder perforation: comparison of US findings with CT. Abdom Imaging 1994;19(3):239–42.
19. Mirvis SE, Cornwell EE 3rd, Rodriguez A, et al. The diagnosis of acute acalculous cholecystitis: a comparison of sonography, scintigraphy, and CT. Am J Roentgenol 1986;147(6):1171–5.
20. Levy AD, Murakata LA, Abbott RM, et al. From the archives of the AFIP. Benign tumors and tumorlike lesions of the gallbladder and extrahepatic bile ducts: radiologic-pathologic correlation. Armed Forces Institute of Pathology. Radiographics 2002;22(2):387–413.

21. Khan ZS, Livingston EH, Huerta S. Reassessing the need for prophylactic surgery in patients with porcelain gallbladder: case series and systematic review of the literat ure. Arch Surg 2011; 146(10):1143–7.
22. Ito H, Hann LE, D'Angelica M, et al. Polypoid lesions of the gallbladder: diagnosis and followup. J Am Coll Surg 2009;208(4): 570–5.
23. Cha BH, Hwang JH, Lee SH, et al. Pre-operative factors that can predict neoplastic polypoid lesions of the gallbladder. World J Gastroenterol 2011;17(17):2216–22.
24. Shin S, Lee JK, Lee KH, et al. Can the growth rate of a gallbladder polyp predict a neoplastic polyp? J Clin Gastroenterol 2009;43(9): 865–8.
25. Xie XH, Xu HX, Xie XY, et al. Differential diagnosis between benign and malignant gallbladder diseases with real-time contrast-enhanced ultrasound. Eur Radiol 2010;20(1):239–48.
26. Sugita R, Yamazaki T, Furuta A, et al. High b-value diffusion-weighted MRI for detecting gallbladder carcinoma: preliminary study and results. Eur Radiol 2009;19(7):1794–8.
27. Barretta ML, Catalano O, Setola SV, et al. Gallbladder metastasis: spectrum of imaging findings. Abdom Imaging 2011;36(6): 729–34.
28. Björnsson E, Gustafsson J, Borkman J, et al. Fate of patients with obstructive jaundice. J Hosp Med 2008;3(2):117–23.
29. Gibson RN, Yeung E, Thompson JN, et al. Bile duct obstruction: radiologic evaluation of level, cause, and tumor resectability. Radiology 1986;160(1):43–7.
30. Bowie JD. What is the upper limit of normal for the common bile duct on ultrasound: how much do you want it to be? Am J Gastroenterol 2000;95(4):897–900.
31. Romagnuolo J, Bardou M, Rahme E, et al. Magnetic resonance cholangiopancreatography: a meta-analysis of test performance in suspected biliary disease. Ann Intern Med 2003;139(7): 547–57.
32. Zandrino F, Benzi L, Ferretti ML, et al. Multislice CT cholangiography without biliary contrast agent: technique and initial clinical results in the assessment of patients with biliary obstruction. Eur Radiol 2002;12(5):1155–61.
33. Ahmetoglu A, Koşucu P, Kul S, et al. MDCT cholangiography with volume rendering for the assessment of patients with biliary obstruction. Am J Roentgenol 2004;183(5):1327–32.
34. Bismuth H, Nakache R, Diamond T. Management strategies in resection for hilar cholangiocarcinoma. Ann Surg 1992;215(1): 31–8.
35. Garcea G, Ngu W, Neal CP, et al. Bilirubin levels predict malignancy in patients with obstructive jaundice. HPB (Oxford) 2011; 13(6):426–30.
36. Khan SA, Thomas HC, Davidson BR, et al. Cholangiocarcinoma. Lancet 2005;366(9493):1303–14.
37. National Institutes of Health Consensus Development Conference Statement on Gallstones and Laparoscopic Cholecystectomy. Am J Surg 1993;165(4):390–8.
38. Vilgrain V, Palazzo L. Choledocholithiasis: role of US and endoscopic ultrasound. Abdom Imaging 2001;26(1):7–14.
39. Hunt DR, Reiter L, Scott AJ. Pre-operative ultrasound measurement of bile duct diameter: basis for selective cholangiography. Aust N Z J Surg 1990;60(3):189–92.
40. de Ledinghen V, Lecesne R, Raymond JM, et al. Diagnosis of choledocholithiasis: EUS or magnetic resonance cholangiography? A prospective controlled study. Gastrointest Endosc 1999;49(1): 26–31.
41. Prat F, Amouyal G, Amouyal P, et al. Prospective controlled study of endoscopic ultrasonography and endoscopic retrograde cholangiography in patients with suspected common-bileduct lithiasis. Lancet 1996;347(8994):75–9.
42. Neitlich JD, Topazian M, Smith RC, et al. Detection of choledocholithiasis: comparison of unenhanced helical CT and endoscopic retrograde cholangiopancreatography. Radiology 1997;203(3): 753–7.
43. Jimenez Cuenca I, del Olmo Martinez L, Perez Homs M. Helical CT without contrast in choledocholithiasis diagnosis. Eur Radiol 2001;11(2):197–201.
44. Cabada Giadas T, Sarría Octavio de Toledo L, Martínez-Berganza Asensio MT, et al. Helical CT cholangiography in the evaluation of the biliary tract: application to the diagnosis of choledocholithiasis. Abdom Imaging 2002;27(1):61–70.
45. Polkowski M, Palucki J, Regula J, et al. Helical computed tomographic cholangiography versus endosonography for suspected bile duct stones: a prospective blinded study in non-jaundiced patients. Gut 1999;45(5):744–9.
46. Gibson RN, Vincent JM, Speer T, et al. Accuracy of computed tomographic intravenous cholangiography (CT-IVC) with iotroxate in the detection of choledocholithiasis. Eur Radiol 2005;15(8): 1634–42.
47. Takahashi M, Saida Y, Itai Y, et al. Reevaluation of spiral CT cholangiography: basic considerations and reliability for detecting choledocholithiasis in 80 patients. J Comput Assist Tomogr 2000; 24(6):859–65.
48. Medical Services Advisory Committee (MSAC). Magnetic Resonance Cholangiopancreatography, Department of Health and Aging. Canberra, ACT: Commonwealth of Australia; 2005.
49. Nandalur KR, Hussain HK, Weadock WJ, et al. Possible biliary disease: diagnostic performance of high-spatial-resolution isotropic 3D T2-weighted MRCP. Radiology 2008;249(3):883–90.
50. Verdonk R, Buis CI, Porte RJ, et al. Anastomotic biliary strictures after liver transplantation: causes and consequences. Liver Transpl 2006;12(5):726–35.
51. Buis CI, Verdonk RC, Van der Jagt EJ, et al. Nonanastomotic biliary strictures after liver transplantation, part 1: Radiological features and risk factors for early vs. late presentation. Liver Transpl 2007;13(5):708–18.
52. Dodd GD 3rd, Niedzwiecki GA, Campbell WL, et al. Bile duct calculi in patients with primary sclerosing cholangitis. Radiology 1997;203(2):443–7.
53. Campbell WL, Peterson MS, Federle MP, et al. Using CT and cholangiography to diagnose biliary tract carcinoma complicating primary sclerosing cholangitis. Am J Roentgenol 2001;177(5): 1095–100.
54. Rajaram R, Ponsioen CY, Majoie CB, et al. Evaluation of a modified cholangiographic classification system for primary sclerosing cholangitis. Abdom Imaging 2001;26(1):43–7.
55. Prall RT, Wiesner RH, La Russo NF. Primary sclerosing cholangitis. In: Blumgart LH, Fong Y, editors. Surgery of the Liver and Biliary Tract. 3rd ed. London: WB Saunders; 2000.
56. Razumilava N, Gores GJ, Lindor KD. Cancer surveillance in patients with primary sclerosing cholangitis. Hepatology 2011; 54(5):1842–52.
57. Hamano H, Arakura N, Muraki T, et al. Prevalence and distribution of extrapancreatic lesions complicating autoimmune pancreatitis. J Gastroenterol 2006;41(12):1197–205.
58. Nakazawa T, Ohara H, Sano H, et al. Schematic classification of sclerosing cholangitis with autoimmune pancreatitis by cholangiography. Pancreas 2006;32(2):229.
59. Bilgin M, Balci NC, Erdogan A, et al. Hepatobiliary and pancreatic MRI and MRCP findings in patients with HIV infection. Am J Roentgenol 2008;191(1):228–32.
60. Leung JW, Sung JY, Chung SC, et al. Hepatic clonorchiasis—a study by endoscopic retrograde cholangiopancreatography. Gastrointest Endosc 1989;35(3):226–31.
61. Heffernan EJ, Geoghegan T, Munk PL, et al. Recurrent pyogenic cholangitis: from imaging to intervention. Am J Roentgenol 2009;192(1):W28–35.
62. Aksoy DY, Kerimoglu U, Oto A, et al. Infection with *Fasciola hepatica*. Clin Microbiol Infect 2005;11(11):859–61.
63. Todani T, Watanabe Y, Narusue M, et al. Congenital bile duct cysts: Classification, operative procedures, and review of thirty-seven cases including cancer arising from choledochal cyst. Am J Surg 1977;134(2):263–9.
64. Nakeeb A, Pitt HA, Sohn TA, et al. Cholangiocarcinoma. A spectrum of intrahepatic, perihilar, and distal tumors. Ann Surg 1996;224(4):463–73.
65. Tillich M, Mischinger HJ, Preisegger KH, et al. Multiphasic helical CT in diagnosis and staging of hilar cholangiocarcinoma. Am J Roentgenol 1998;171(3):651–8.
66. Kim J, Lee JM, Han JK, et al. Contrast-enhanced MRI combined with MR cholangiopancreatography for the evaluation of patients with biliary strictures: differentiation of malignant from benign bile duct strictures. J Magn Reson Imaging 2007;26(2):304–12.
67. Manfredi R, Masselli G, Maresca G, et al. MR imaging and MRCP of hilar cholangiocarcinoma. Abdom Imaging 2003;28(3):319–25.
68. Xu HX, Chen LD, Xie XY, et al. Enhancement pattern of hilar cholangiocarcinoma: contrast-enhanced ultrasound versus

contrast-enhanced computed tomography. Eur J Radiol 2010;75(2): 197–202.

69. Li J, Kuehl H, Grabellus F, et al. Preoperative assessment of hilar cholangiocarcinoma by dual-modality PET/CT. J Surg Oncol 2008;98(6):438–43.

70. Park HS, Lee JM, Choi JY, et al. Preoperative evaluation of bile duct cancer: MRI combined with MR cholangiopancreatography versus MDCT with direct cholangiography. Am J Roentgenol 2008;190(2):396–405.

71. Aloia TA, Charnsangavej C, Faria S, et al. High-resolution computed tomography accurately predicts resectability in hilar cholangiocarcinoma. Am J Surg 2007;193(6):702–6.

72. Ham JM. Lobar and segmental atrophy of the liver. World J Surg 1990;14(4):457–62.

73. Friesen B, Gibson RN, Speer T, et al. Lobar and segmental liver atrophy associated with hilar cholangiocarcinoma and the impact of hilar biliary anatomical variants: a pictorial essay. Insights Imaging 2011;2:525–31.

74. Boland GW, Lee MJ, Leung J, et al. Percutaneous cholecystostomy in critically ill patients: early response and final outcome in 82 patients. Am J Roentgenol 1994;163(2):339–42.

75. Bruha R, Petrtyl J, Kubecova M, et al. Intraluminal brachytherapy and selfexpandable stents in nonresectable biliary malignancies—the question of long-term palliation. Hepatogastroenterology 2001;48(39):631–7.

76. Lammer J, Hausegger KA, Flückiger F, et al. Common bile duct obstruction due to malignancy: treatment with plastic versus metal stents. Radiology 1996;201(1):167–72.

77. Rivera-Sanfeliz GM, Assar OS, LaBerge JM, et al. Incidence of important hemobilia following transhepatic biliary drainage: left-sided versus right-sided approaches. Cardiovasc Intervent Radiol 2004;27(2):137–9.

78. Tytgat GN, Bartelsman JF, Den Hartog Jager FC, et al. Upper intestinal and biliary tract endoprosthesis. Dig Dis Sci 1986;31(9 Suppl):57S–76S.

79. Cowling MG, Adam AN. Internal stenting in malignant biliary obstruction. World J Surg 2001;25(3):355–9; discussion 359–61.

80. Hii MW, Gibson RN, Speer AG, et al. Role of radiology in the treatment of malignant hilar biliary strictures 2: 10 years of single-institution experience with percutaneous treatment. Australas Radiol 2003;47(4):393–403.

81. Inal M, Akgül E, Aksungur E, et al. Percutaneous placement of biliary metallic stents in patients with malignant hilar obstruction: unilobar versus bilobar drainage. J Vasc Interv Radiol 2003;14(11): 1409–16.

82. Gibson RN, Adam A, Czerniak A, et al. Benign biliary strictures: a proposed combined surgical and radiological management. Aust N Z J Surg 1987;57(6):361–8.

83. Hutson DG, Russell E, Yrizarry J, et al. Percutaneous dilatation of biliary strictures through the afferent limb of a modified Roux-en-Y choledochojejunostomy or hepaticojejunostomy. Am J Surg 1998; 175(2):108–13.

84. McPherson SJ, Gibson RN, Collier NA, et al. Percutaneous transjejunal biliary intervention: 10-year experience with access via Roux-en-Y loops. Radiology 1998;206(3):665–72.

85. Soreide O. Fine needle biopsy and aspiration cytology. In: Blumgart LH, Fong Y, editors. Surgery of the Liver and Biliary Tract. 3rd ed. London: WB Saunders. 2000.

86. Ferrari Junior AP, Lichtenstein DR, Slivka A, et al. Brush cytology during ERCP for the diagnosis of biliary and pancreatic malignancies. Gastrointest Endosc 1994;40(2 Pt 1):140–5.

87. Jin YH, Kim SH, Park CK. Diagnostic criteria for malignancy in bile cytology and its usefulness. J Korean Med Sci 1999;14(6): 643–7.

CHAPTER 9

THE PANCREAS

Wolfgang Schima • E. Jane Adam • Robert A. Morgan

EMBRYOLOGY

The pancreas develops in two parts, both of which arise from the endoderm of the primitive duodenum. The dorsal part or anlage is the first to appear, as a diverticulum from the dorsal wall of the duodenum. This eventually forms the whole of the neck, body and tail of the gland, together with part of the head. The ventral anlage develops more caudally as a diverticulum from the developing bile duct at the point where the latter opens into the duodenum. Soon after the appearance of the two parts, the duodenum undergoes partial rotation and they approximate each other and fuse. Until this stage the dorsal duct, the duct of Santorini, opens into the duodenum proximal to the major papilla (ampulla of Vater) at the minor papilla, whereas the ventral duct, the duct of Wirsung, which is joined with the lower common bile duct, opens into the major papilla. In the majority of cases, fusion of the two ducts occurs at the junction of the head and body of the gland (Fig. 9-1). Thus the main pancreatic duct opens into the major papilla.

THE NORMAL PANCREAS

The pancreas lies in the most anterior of the three retroperitoneal compartments, the anterior pararenal space. Ventrally, this is bounded by the posterior parietal peritoneum. Dorsally, the space is bounded by the anterior renal or Gerota's fascia and more laterally by the lateroconal fascia (Fig. 9-2). Other structures occupying the anterior pararenal space include the duodenal loop and ascending and descending colon. The pancreas is surrounded by retroperitoneal fat (Fig. 9-3). The position, size and configuration of the pancreas are very variable, depending on body habitus and the size and shape of adjacent organs and this inherent variation makes it

difficult to define the normal size of the pancreas. The gland is relatively larger in adolescents than adults and becomes smaller with increasing age.

CONGENITAL ANOMALIES

Several congenital anomalies of the pancreas may occur secondary to failure of normal embryological development.

Pancreas Divisum

Pancreas divisum is the commonest congenital pancreatic anomaly, characterised by the failure of normal fusion of the dorsal and ventral anlagen in the fetal period in approximately 5% of the population. The dorsal and ventral ducts fail to fuse (Fig. 9-4), with the duct of Wirsung (duct of the ventral anlage) draining only the head of the pancreas via the major papilla and the duct of Santorini (dorsal anlage) draining the body and tail via the more cranially and anteriorly positioned minor papilla. This anomaly may result in functional stenosis and pancreatitis (Fig. 9-5). In an ERCP-based study, of the 94 patients identified to have pancreas divisum, 57% had evidence of chronic pancreatitis.[1] The prevalence of pancreas divisum was much higher in patients with chronic/recurrent 'idiopathic' pancreatitis (43%/33%) than in the general population (2.6%).[2] An increased incidence of pancreatic malignancy has been described,[3] possibly based on the increased prevalence of chronic pancreatitis in this group. Magnetic resonance cholangiopancreatography (MRCP) reliably enables visualisation of panceas divisum. Stimulation of pancreatic secretions with secretin-enhanced MRCP allows visualisation of functional stenoses at the minor papilla.

Annular Pancreas

Annular pancreas is the second most common congenital anomaly and is the result of failure of normal rotation during development. This results in pancreatic tissue partially or completely encircling the duodenum. The anomaly may cause proximal duodenal dilatation and symptomatic duodenal narrowing. The diagnosis may be suspected if barium studies show narrowing of the duodenum at the level of the major papilla or pancreatic tissue is seen surrounding the second part of the duodenum on CT. ERCP or MRCP can confirm the diagnosis by demonstrating a segment of pancreatic duct encircling the duodenum (Fig. 9-6A). With contrast-enhanced CT a circumferential rim of pancreatic tissue is demonstrated (Fig. 9-6B).

Pancreatic Agenesis, Hypoplasia and Ectopic Pancreas

Agenesis of the whole pancreas is exceptionally rare, but agenesis or hypoplasia of the dorsal anlage may occur.[4]

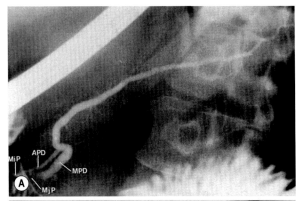

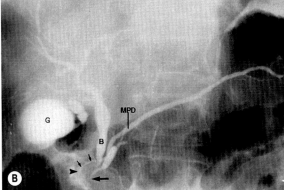

FIGURE 9-1 ■ **Normal pancreatic duct.** (A) Normal ERCP shows the accessory pancreatic duct (APD) draining separately into the minor papillary (MiP) and the major pancreatic duct (MPD) draining into the major papilla (MjP). (B) ERCP shows filling of the main pancreatic duct (MPD), common bile duct (B) and gall bladder (G). The MPD and CBD drain into the major papillary (large arrow). The small accessory pancreatic duct (small arrows) drains separately into the minor papilla (arrowhead).

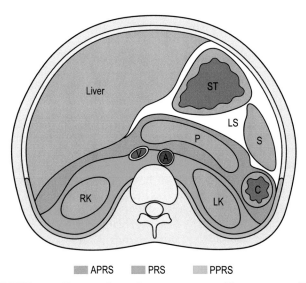

FIGURE 9-2 ■ **Retroperitoneal compartments.** The pancreas (P) lies in the anterior PRS perirenal space (APRS), together with the ascending and descending colon (C) and duodenum. ST = stomach, S = spleen, RK = right kidney, LK = left kidney, A = aorta, V = inferior vena cava, LS = lesser sac, PRS = pararenal space, PPRS = posterior pararenal space.

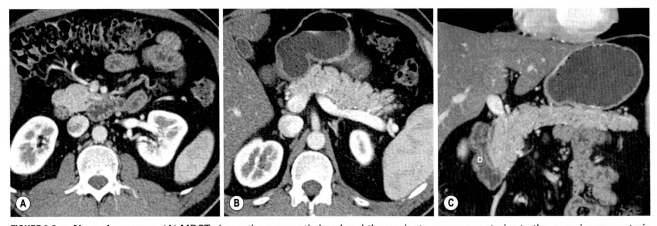

FIGURE 9-3 ■ **Normal pancreas.** (A) MDCT shows the pancreatic head and the uncinate process posterior to the superior mesenteric artery and vein. (B) The body and tail are demonstrated, lying anterior to the splenic vein. (C) The curved planar reformation along the pancreas shows the relationship between pancreas and duodenal *(D)* C-sweep.

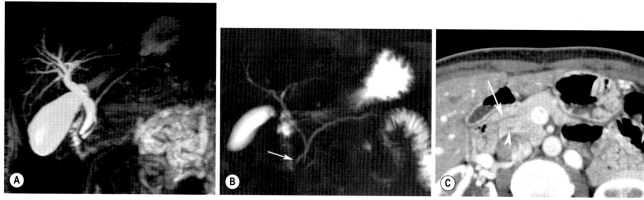

FIGURE 9-4 ■ **Duct morphology of normal pancreas and pancreas divisum.** (A) Normal anatomy as demonstrated on MRCP. (B) Dorsal (Santorini) duct drains into the minor papilla (arrow). Small ventral duct drains into the major papilla. (C) MDCT shows the typical configuration of pancreas divisum, with the dorsal duct (arrow) coursing anterior to the common bile duct (arrowhead).

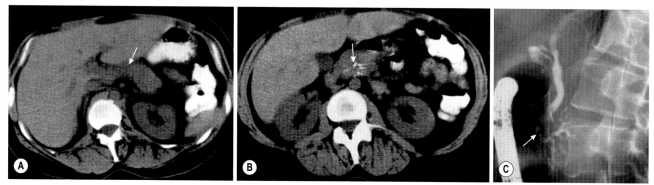

FIGURE 9-5 ■ **Pancreatitis in pancreas divisum.** (A) Normal unenhanced CT of the pancreatic body (white arrow). (B) Coarse calcifications in the pancreatic head (white arrow). (C) ERCP showing pancreas divisum with an abnormal separate ventral duct (white arrow) with dilatation and irregularity of side branches.

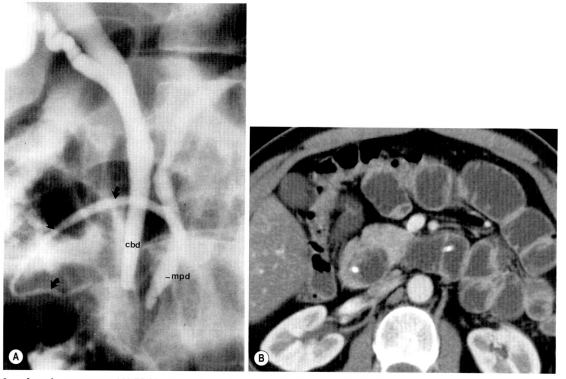

FIGURE 9-6 ■ **Annular pancreas.** (A) ERCP shows the main pancreatic duct (mpd) with the accessory duct surrounding the duodenum (arrows); cbd = common bile duct. (B) CT enteroclysis shows pancreatic parenchyma around the descending part of the duodenum, which is well distended by fluid. Note that there is a nasojejunal tube in place.

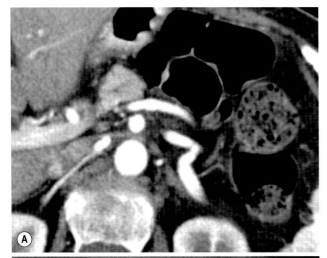

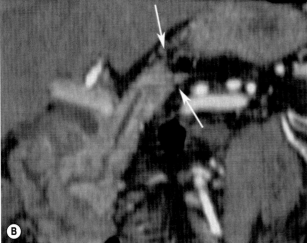

FIGURE 9-7 ▪ Aplasia of the dorsal pancreas. (A) CT demonstrates only the pancreatic head in a patient who had not undergone pancreatic surgery. (B) Coronal MPR shows the gland in its entirety, with the body and tail missing (arrows).

In these cases CT may show absence of the body and tail of the gland, with a corresponding short duct in the dorsal anlage (Fig. 9-7).

Ectopic islands of pancreatic tissue may be found remote from the gland, most commonly in the gastric or duodenal wall. The diagnosis is usually made incidentally during barium examination or upper gastrointestinal endoscopy when the ectopic pancreatic tissue is seen as a polypoid nodule, often with central umbilication representing a rudimentary pancreatic duct.

ACUTE PANCREATITIS

There are many causes of acute pancreatitis, including alcohol, cholelithiasis (Fig. 9-8), trauma, iatrogenic (e.g. post-ERCP) as well as metabolic disorders such as hyperlipidaemia and hypercalcaemia. Pancreatitis may also be associated with viral infections, examples being mumps and cytomegalovirus. Numerous drugs are known to cause acute pancreatitis. In 10–30% of cases there is no apparent cause, in which case it is classified as idiopathic

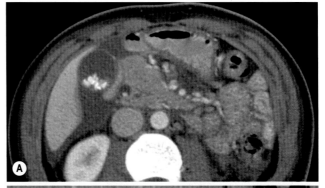

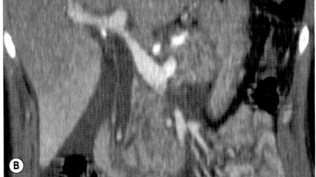

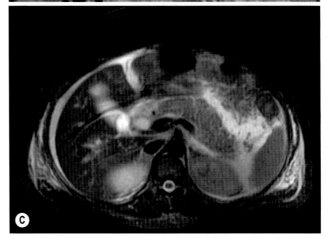

FIGURE 9-8 ▪ Pancreatitis secondary to cholelithiasis (biliary pancreatitis). (A) Axial CT shows dilated CBD with a hyperattenuating calculus. (B) Reformatted image of dilated duct with stone. (C) MRCP shows that the pancreas is swollen and oedematous with surrounding peripancreatic fluid. Appearances are consistent with acute pancreatitis.

pancreatitis, although there is evidence that some of these cases are associated with congenital duct anomalies.[3]

In many cases the diagnosis is a straightforward clinical one, for example in a patient with a history of heavy alcohol intake, upper abdominal pain and hyperamylasaemia or a raised plasma lipase. In 2008, an international group of experts in the field of pancreatitis, led by the Acute Pancreatitis Classification Group, gathered input using an iterative, web-based consultation process led by a working group, and revised the Atlanta classification system in an effort to improve clinical assessment and management of acute pancreatitis and to standardise terms for peripancreatic fluid collections, pancreatic and/

or peripancreatic necrosis and how these entities evolve over the time, as well as any complications that may arise.[5-7] The revised Atlanta classification (2012) of acute pancreatitis divides the condition into interstitial oedematous pancreatitis and necrotising pancreatitis, (formerly termed mild and severe acute pancreatitis).[5-7] This morphological classification system is based on findings on contrast-enhanced CT. Briefly, the imaging findings in interstitial oedematous pancreatitis include focal or diffuse enlargement of the gland, with normal homogeneous enhancement or slightly heterogeneous enhancement of the pancreatic parenchyma, which is attributable to oedema.[5] Necrotising pancreatitis is seen in fewer than 5% of patients and appears on contrast-enhanced CT images as lack of parenchymal enhancement.[5] In the 2012 classification, necrotising pancreatitis is further subdivided into parenchymal necrosis alone, peripancreatic necrosis alone and a combined type (areas of pancreatic parenchymal and peripancreatic necrosis) with and without infection.[5] Peripancreatic necrosis is seen as heterogeneous areas of non-enhancement that contain non-liquefied components.[5] Pancreatic parenchymal necrosis with peripancreatic necrosis is characterised on imaging by a combination of imaging features observed with pancreatic parenchymal necrosis alone and peripancreatic necrosis.[5]

In (mild) interstitial oedematous pancreatitis, proteolytic enzymes injure the acinar cell, causing oedema and swelling of the gland, but the inflammatory response is not strong enough to cause necrosis. In interstitial oedematous pancreatitis, which constitutes 70–80% of cases, the ultrasound (US) appearances may be entirely normal but common findings may include generalised (or less commonly, focal) enlargement of the gland with reduced reflectivity. The pancreatic margins may be difficult to define and peripancreatic fluid may be visualised. The presence of necrosis (necrotising pancreatitis) indicates that the inflammatory response has triggered cellular apoptosis.[7] The major determinant of morbidity and mortality in patients with acute pancreatitis is the development of pancreatic necrosis.[8] Conventional US cannot reliably detect this complication. Serum markers, such as C-reactive protein, have been identified for the diagnosis of pancreatic necrosis but their usefulness is limited by their specificity and/or availability. The clinical grading of severity has utilised a number of scoring systems such as Ranson's, APACHE-II, Marshall scoring system or BISAP score. There is an ongoing discussion about the use of imaging in the diagnosis of acute pancreatitis. Although in mild acute pancreatitis US may suffice to rule out complications and to assess for aetiologies such as gallstones, contrast-enhanced CT has emerged as the main diagnostic pillar in suspected or confirmed acute pancreatitis. Contrast-enhanced CT is the investigation of choice to assess the presence and extent of pancreatic necrosis, the extent of peripancreatic inflammation and necrosis and the presence of fluid collections.[9] The CT severity index (CTSI) for staging of acute pancreatitis has been developed,[10] considering the amount of fluid collections and the presence or absence of pancreatic necrosis (Table 9-1). The CTSI correlates with morbidity and mortality (Table 9-2). However, it has recently been

TABLE 9-1 Scoring System for Severity of Acute Pancreatitis: CT Severity Index (CTSI)

CT Features	Score
Grade	
Normal gland	0
Focal/diffuse enlargement	1
Peripancreatic inflammatory change	2
Single pancreatic fluid collection	3
Two or more fluid collections or abscess	4
Necrosis	
None	0
<30%	2
30–50%	4
>50%	6

TABLE 9-2 CT Severity Index (CTSI) vs Morbidity and Mortality

Score	Morbidity (%)	Mortality (%)
0–3	8	3
4–6	35	6
7–10	92	17

shown that CT scoring does not supersede clinical scoring systems (BISAP, Ranson's, APACHE-II) for identification of patients with severe pancreatitis.[11,12]

Imaging in Acute Pancreatitis

According to the revised Atlanta classification, contrast-enhanced CT is the primary tool for assessing and staging patients with acute pancreatitis, helping to assess for complications and assessing response to treatment.[5] Not all patients with acute pancreatitis require contrast-enhanced CT imaging. Recent UK guidelines suggest that immediate CT is indicated if the clinical and biochemical findings are inconclusive, especially if signs raise the possibility of an alternative abdominal emergency.[13] If carried out very early (in the first 24 h after clinical onset), it is also possible that CT may underestimate the degree of necrosis and in most patients it will not influence management in the first few days. The optimal time for performance of contrast-enhanced CT imaging is greater than 72 h after the onset of symptoms.[5] CT imaging should be repeated if clinical picture changes, such as development of fever or drop in haematocrit.[5] Also, patients with persisting or new organ failure and those with continuing pain or signs of sepsis will require a contrast-enhanced study as the presence of necrosis as detected on CT has a high correlation with the risk of local and systemic complications.[12] CT is the most reliable imaging technique for the staging of acute pancreatitis, if performed with IV contrast medium. Other than how CT is performed for pancreatic cancer detection and staging, a single venous phase CT image (100–150 mL at 4 mL/s with a fixed delay of 70 s) will be sufficient to stage acute pancreatitis, and unenhanced or arterial-phase imaging is not routinely necessary.[14] In the clinical context of acute pancreatitis, CT protocol design should consider radiation exposure, as many patients with severe acute pancreatitis are young and will require several sessions of CT imaging during the course of their disease.[14]

It has been shown that early removal of bile duct stones (by ERCP) may influence the prognosis in patients with biliary pancreatitis and obstructive jaundice.[15–17] Thus MRCP (or if available endosonography) should be used to detect choledocholithiasis and to aid in selection of candidates for ERCP, if performed without delay (Fig. 9-9).[18] MR imaging may also have a role in detecting non-liquefied material within a pancreatic or peripancreatic collection.[5]

Interstitial Oedematous Pancreatitis

As already discussed, the imaging findings in interstitial oedematous pancreatitis include focal or diffuse enlargement of the gland, with normal homogeneous enhancement (Figs. 9-10 and 9-11) or slightly heterogeneous enhancement of the pancreatic parenchyma, which is attributable to oedema.[5] It is important to highlight, however, that on a contrast-enhanced CT image obtained in the first few days after presentation with acute pancreatitis, the pancreas may demonstrate increased enhancement of the pancreatic parenchyma, which cannot be definitively characterised as either acute oedematous pancreatitis or necrotising pancreatitis.[5,6] In this situation, it is important for the radiologist to conclude

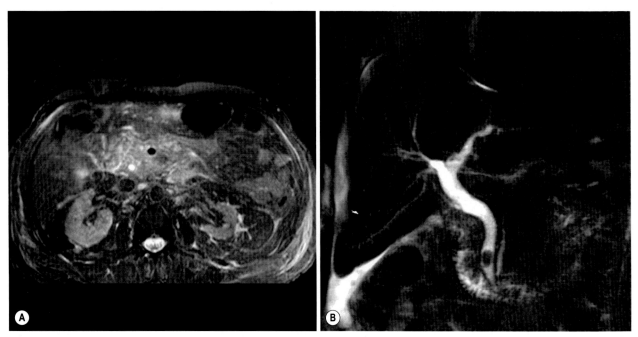

FIGURE 9-9 ■ **MRCP of biliary pancreatitis.** (A) Axial T2-weighted TSE image shows oedematous changes of the pancreas with oedema of the peripancreatic fat. (B) MRCP shows a large calculus in the CBD.

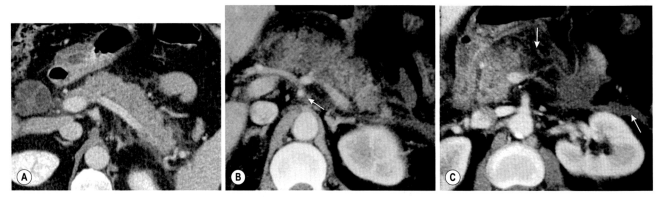

FIGURE 9-10 ■ **Mild acute (interstitial oedematous) pancreatitis.** (A) Minimal swelling of the tail of the pancreas with peripancreatic oedema. (B) Different patient: mild swelling of the gland that enhances uniformly but has indistinct margins because of peripancreatic oedema. There is inflammatory tissue around the coeliac axis (arrow). (C) Image at the level of the pancreatic head showing infiltration of the peripancreatic fat and fluid anterior to Gerota's fascia (arrows).

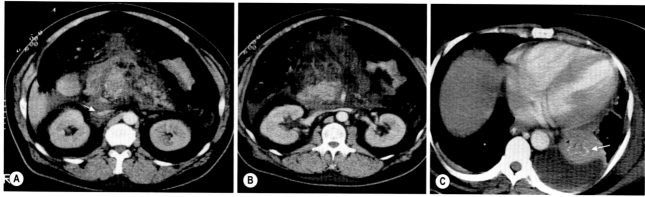

FIGURE 9-11 ■ **Moderately severe acute (interstitial oedematous) pancreatitis.** (A) Inflammatory fluid is seen surrounding the inferior vena cava (arrow). (B) Extensive exudation involving the mesentery. (C) There is a left basal pleural effusion and atelectasis in the left lower lobe (arrow).

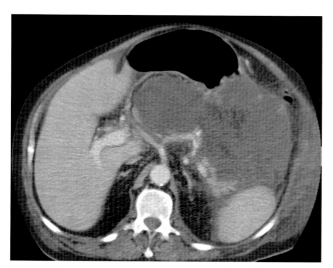

FIGURE 9-12 ■ **Acute necrotising pancreatitis.** Enhanced CT shows a largely necrotic non-enhancing body and tail of pancreas. There is a massive fluid collection surrounding the gland—an acute necrotic collection.

that the CT is indeterminate and that contrast-enhanced CT imaging should be repeated 5–7 days later, if the patient's clinical status is not improving.[5] Fluid collections may be seen around the pancreas, in the pararenal space along fascial planes, at the mesenteric root or in the bursa omentalis. For grading of acute pancreatitis, the CT severity index has been proposed, which takes into account the presence of gland swelling, peripancreatic fluid collections and the presence of necrosis as an indicator for the prognosis.[10]

Necrotising Pancreatitis

This is the hallmark of severe acute pancreatitis. The revised Atlanta classification distinguishes three forms of acute necrotising pancreatitis: pancreatic parenchymal necrosis alone, peripancreatic necrosis alone, and pancreatic necrosis with peripancreatic necrosis.[5,6] All three types can be sterile or infected. Necrotic glandular tissue is seen as an area of non-enhancement within the pancreatic parenchyma (Fig. 9-12). With time, non-viable or

necrotic tissue pancreatic parenchyma or peripancreatic fat liquefies.[5] The presence of peripancreatic necrosis alone carries a much better prognosis than parenchymal necrosis.[5] The extent of necrosis may be categorised into less than 30%, 30–50% or more than 50% of the gland. Patients with CT evidence of more than 30% necrosis have an overall reported mortality rate of 29%.[19] In the study of Heiss et al.[20] two CT features correlated with mortality: first, the presence of necrosis of more than one part (i.e. head, body or tail) of the pancreas and, secondly, the presence of distant fluid collections (in the posterior pararenal space and/or paracolic gutter).

Infected necrosis occurs in 20–70% of patients with necrotic pancreatic tissue[21] and is responsible for an estimated 80% of deaths from acute pancreatitis. The presence of gas bubbles within an area of necrotic tissue (in the absence of recent intervention in the region or existence of a communication between gastrointestinal tract and the pancreatic collection/area of necrosis) is highly suggestive of infection (Fig. 9-13). Confirmation of infection requires fine-needle aspiration. If infection is shown to be present within necrotic tissue, percutaneous drainage may not evacuate thick debris. Surgical intervention is the method of choice, although recent studies have shown that a conservative approach avoiding open necrosectomy lowers the mortality considerably (8.3 vs 45%).[22] Thus necrosectomy is nowadays reserved for patients with concomitant intra-abdominal complications not amenable to conservative therapy.[22]

Pancreatic and Peripancreatic Collections

Acute pancreatitis can be accompanied by pancreatic parenchymal or peripancreatic collections.[5,6] The acute collections are referred to as either acute peripancreatic fluid collections (APFCs) or as acute necrotic collections (ANCs), depending on the presence or absence of pancreatic necrosis.[5,6] Thus, in the acute period interstitial oedematous pancreatitis will be associated with APFCs and after a period of 4 weeks by a pseudocyst. Necrotising pancreatitis in its three forms is potentially associated with ANCs and after a period of 4 weeks by walled-off

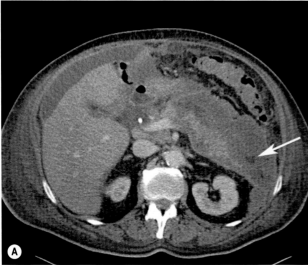

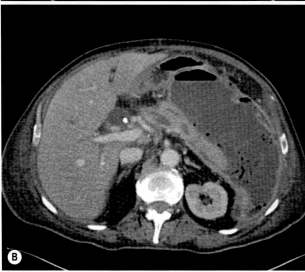

FIGURE 9-13 ■ **Infected pancreatic necrosis.** (A) MDCT shows heterogeneity of pancreatic parenchyma due to spotty necrosis. In addition there is a fluid collection containing chunks of fat attenuation (arrow) due to fat necrosis. (B) Follow-up CT 6 weeks later demonstrates a gas–fluid level (arrow) and multiple gas bubbles (arrowheads) indicative of secondary infection (an infected walled-off necrosis).

necrosis (WON). All of these collections can be sterile or infected.[5,6]

APFCs in general are self-limiting and are reabsorbed within the first few weeks, and usually do not become infected. These collections therefore rarely require any intervention unless they become infected.[5,6]

Pseudocyst

If an APFC is not resolved within 4 weeks after onset of acute pancreatitis, it transitions into a pancreatic pseudocyst. Pseudocysts develop as a complication of acute pancreatitis in 10–20% of cases.[5,6] The imaging characteristics of a pseudocyst, according to the 2012 classification, include a round or oval fluid collection surrounded by a well-defined enhancing wall or capsule. Pseudocysts

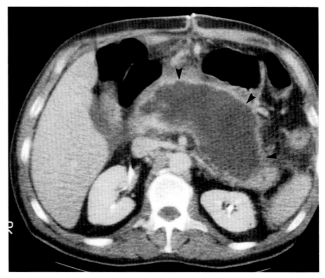

FIGURE 9-14 ■ **Walled-off necrosis containing necrotic debris.** The more solid necrotic tissue contained within the abscess will not be adequately drained by percutaneous catheter drainage. The collection was successfully drained surgically.

should not contain any non-liquefied components within the fluid collection.[5,6] In some cases, pseudocysts may communicate with the pancreatic duct, a feature which can have a bearing on management of these fluid collections. Pseudocysts can become infected and superinfection can be manifest as air within the collection on contrast-enhanced CT imaging.

Acute Necrotic Collection (ANC)

In the first 4 weeks after development of necrotising pancreatitis, a persistent collection is called an ANC.[5,6] This collection may contain variable amounts of debris and necrotic material. The natural history of ANC is progressive liquefaction over a 3- to 6-week period.[5,6] An important change with the new classification is that any collection in the pancreatic parenchyma should be called an ANC and not a pseudocyst. An ANC may have a communication to the pancreatic duct.[5,6]

Walled-Off Necrosis (WON)

Acute necrotic collection associated with NP, usually 4 weeks or later following first development of symptoms, develops a thickened non-epithelialised wall and is called a WON. Like ANC, WON can involve the pancreas, and/or the peripancreatic area.[5,6] Any fluid collection that occupies or replaces the pancreas should be called a WON after 4 weeks. Like APFC, ANC and pseudocyts, WON can be sterile or infected. Unlike pseudocyst, WON may contain varying amounts of non-liquefied material and therefore, if infected, is less easily treated by percutaneous catheter drainage when compared to a pseudocyst.[5,6] Infected WON has replaced the term 'pancreatic abscess', which was previously reported to occur in 3% of patients with severe pancreatitis[22] (Fig. 9-14). Gas bubbles are a helpful pointer to the presence of

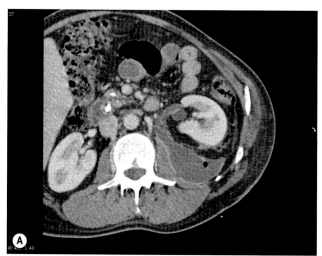

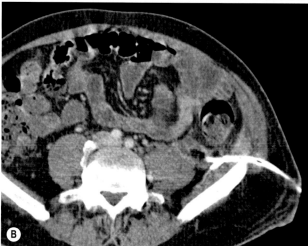

FIGURE 9-15 ■ Infected walled-off necrosis. (A) Contrast-enhanced MDCT shows an infected walled-off necrotic collection in the posterior pararenal space, (B) which is successfully drained percutaneously.

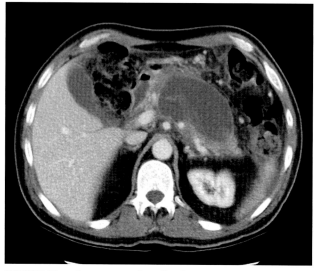

FIGURE 9-16 ■ Acute necrotic collection. Three weeks after the onset of acute pancreatitis, a fluid collection persists. This is developing a thin capsule. As this collection is located within the substance of the pancreas, it is called an acute necrotic collection.

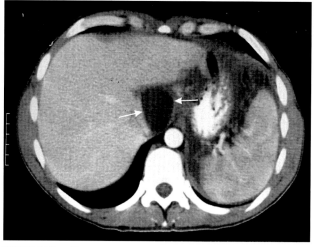

FIGURE 9-17 ■ Pancreatic pseudocyst. A well-defined fluid collection with a thin wall (arrows) lies superior to the pancreas.

infection, but most infected WONs appear as thick-walled fluid collections. It is also important to remember, that the presence of air bubbles within a WON is not always indicative of infection, as air bubbles can also be encountered when communication between WON and gastrointestinal tract exists. Imaging-based differentiation of sterile and infected fluid collections can be challenging. Thus, clinical signs and symptoms of infection should be correlated with laboratory indices of infection such as white cell count and C-reactive protein. If infection is confirmed by fine-needle aspiration and the collection is at least partially liquefied, percutaneous catheter drainage may be attempted but large catheters (up to 30Fr) may be required (Fig. 9-15).

Pseudocysts

As discussed previously, most APFCs resolve spontaneously without clinical sequelae.[5,6,23] In some cases, they persist and over several weeks develop into pseudocysts, which classically have a fibrous capsule

(Figs. 9-16–9-18). Pseudocysts may rarely even extend into the mediastinum.

More than 70% of pseudocysts resolve spontaneously or decrease in size. Thus a wait-and-see policy for more than 6 weeks is suggested for asymptomatic pseudocysts.[24] However, they may be associated with complications, including rupture, infection (Fig. 9-19), haemorrhage (Fig. 9-20), pain, biliary or pancreatic duct obstruction (Fig. 9-18), or gastrointestinal tract involvement. Effective treatment may be provided by percutaneous catheter drainage.

Vascular Complications

This is a not uncommon complication of pancreatitis. Intrapancreatic and peripancreatic arteries and veins may

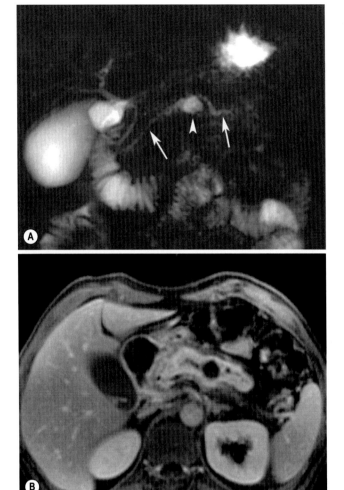

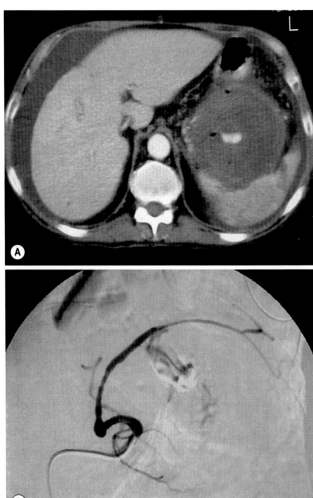

FIGURE 9-18 ■ **MRCP of walled-off necrosis.** (A) MRCP reveals signs of chronic pancreatitis: irregularities of the pancreatic duct with a stricture (arrows). There is a small intrapancreatic cyst (arrowhead). (B) Gadolinium-enhanced T1-weighted GRE images shows the non-enhancing cyst and subtle dilation of the pancreatic duct.

FIGURE 9-20 ■ **Haemorrhage into a pseudocyst.** (A) Contrast agent extravasation is seen within a well-defined pseudocyst. There are also small gas bubbles. (B) Selective DSA of the splenic artery shows displacement of the vessel by the pseudocyst and contrast extravasation. This was successfully treated by coil embolisation.

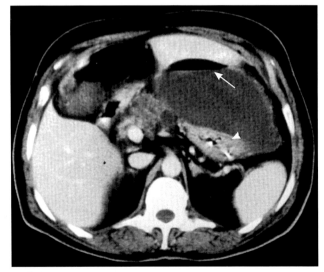

FIGURE 9-19 ■ **Infected pseudocyst.** A gas–fluid level is seen in the pseudocyst (arrow), which lies anterior to the stomach (arrowhead). This was successfully treated by percutaneous drainage.

be eroded or thrombosed by the digestive effect of pancreatic enzymes or as a result of compression by a pseudocyst. Vascular involvement may be manifested by thombosis of an artery or vein. The splenic artery and vein are especially at risk of being involved in acute pancreatitis, leading to splenic vein thrombosis with infarction or splenic haemorrhage.[25] Enzymatic damage to the splenic or gastroduodenal artery can cause development of a pseudoaneurysm, rupture of which may lead to life-threatening bleeding. Contrast-enhanced CT images reliably identify the site of vascular involvement. In cases of severe acute haemorrhage or pseudoaneurysm formation, angiography and vascular embolisation may be an alternative to surgery (Fig. 9-20).

Gastrointestinal Involvement

The gastrointestinal tract is frequently involved by direct extension of the inflammatory process from the inflamed

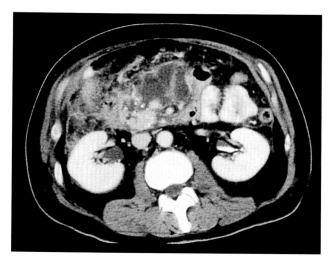

FIGURE 9-21 ■ **Acute-on-chronic pancreatitis.** Enhanced CT showing acute inflammatory changes in the pancreas with fluid collections superimposed on chronic pancreatitis with calcification.

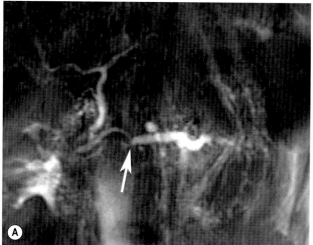

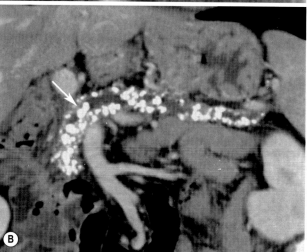

FIGURE 9-22 ■ **Chronic pancreatitis.** (A) MRCP shows typical stricture (arrow) with upstream duct dilatation, contour irregularities and dilated side branches. (B) Different patient: MDCT (curved planar reformation along the pancreatic duct) reveals extensive parenchymal calcification and an intraductal calculus (arrow) with duct dilatation.

pancreas and this can result in oedema, necrosis, or perforation of the wall of the stomach or duodenum. Patients are at higher risk if there is close contact between bowel loops and the inflammatory process. Secondary involvement of bowel may occur when pancreatic enzymes permeate through mesenteric attachments, or secondary to vascular complications resulting in bowel ischaemia.

CHRONIC PANCREATITIS

Chronic pancreatitis (CP) is an irreversible inflammatory disease of the pancreas, resulting in fibrosis. Patients often give a history of multiple prior attacks of acute pancreatitis (Fig. 9-21). Chronic pancreatitis produces abdominal pain and loss of exocrine and endocrine function, resulting in weight loss, steatorrhoea and diabetes. A variety of classification systems have been proposed, including the Marseille, the Manchester, the Cambridge and the Zurich classifications.[26] These classification systems are either based on histology or ductal morphology at ERCP, or a combination of ERCP morphology and clinical symptoms. For cross-sectional imaging, the diagnosis is based on ductal morphology and other findings. Plain abdominal radiographs may reveal pancreatic calcification with or without evidence of a mass. The presence of calcification is highly suggestive of a diagnosis of chronic alcohol-related pancreatitis. The size of the pancreas in chronic pancreatitis is very variable. Atrophy of the whole gland is a common consequence of chronic inflammation and fibrosis but enlargement of the gland may also be seen, either in a generalised or focal pattern. On US the internal echo texture may be heterogeneous. Dilatation of the side branches and of the main pancreatic duct (beyond its usual size of up to 2.5 mm) is, in the absence of an obstructing mass, a key feature of CP. Intraductal stones may seen with CT or MRCP (Fig. 9-22), with secondary dilatation of the common bile duct. Early CT diagnosis of CP is difficult, as no single imaging

feature is pathognomonic for CP. When a combination of at least three out of the four imaging features, i.e. parenchymal calcifications, intraductal calcifications, parenchymal atrophy and cystic lesions, is present, diagnosis of CP can be made with high specificity.[27]

When duct dilatation accompanies focal enlargement of the gland, the appearance may mimic that of pancreatic carcinoma. Indeed, pancreatitis and carcinoma may coexist, as patients with long-standing chronic pancreatitis have an up to 16-fold increased risk of developing pancreatic cancer.[28] On the other hand, chronic pancreatitis may present with a focal mass, thus mimicking ductal adenocarcinoma (Fig. 9-23). Differentiation of focal chronic pancreatitis and cancer can be extremely difficult,[29] requiring multiple imaging techniques (CT, MRI, EUS) and often multiple biopsies.[30] US and CT may also show cysts and vascular changes. Long-standing chronic pancreatitis is associated with a high incidence of vascular complications, including splenic, mesenteric or portal vein thrombosis. EUS assessment of the pancreas allows

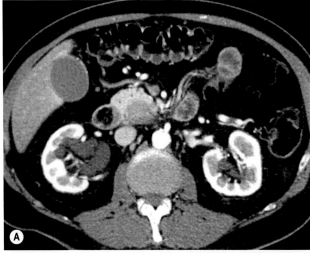

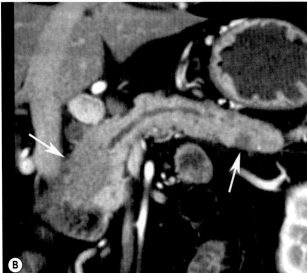

FIGURE 9-23 ■ **Focal pancreatitis mimicking pancreatic cancer.** (A) Axial MDCT shows a hypoattenuating mass in the uncinate process in a patient without clinical symptoms of acute pancreatitis. (B) Curved planar reformation better shows the mass (arrow) with pancreatic duct obstruction. There is another small hypoattenuating mass in the tail (arrow). Histopathological evaluation of the surgical specimen revealed only inflammation.

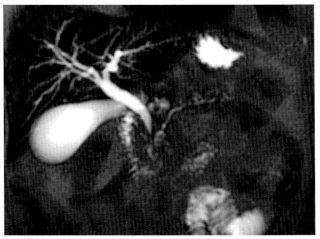

FIGURE 9-24 ■ **Mild chronic pancreatitis: MRCP features.** MRCP shows minimal dilatation and marginal irregularity of the main pancreatic duct and abnormal lateral side branches.

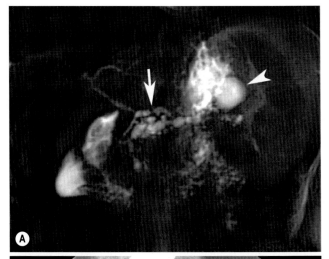

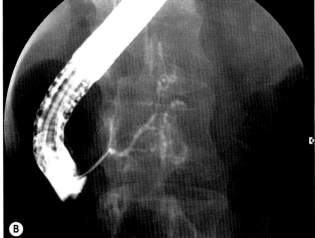

FIGURE 9-25 ■ **Severe chronic pancreatitis.** (A) MRCP shows a tight stricture with duct dilatation, contour irregularities, dilated side branches and a pseudocyst at the tail (arrowhead). (B) ERCP shows complete duct obstruction. The duct system upstream cannot be visualised.

high-resolution images to be obtained and may allow parenchymal changes to be detected early in the disease. It should be used when cross-sectional imaging is non-diagnostic.[31]

While CT may be used to make the diagnosis of chronic pancreatitis, specific imaging of the duct system with ERCP or MRCP has the advantage of providing detailed images of the duct system (Fig. 9-24), although ERCP often cannot visualise the entire pancreatic duct if pancreatic duct strictures are present (Fig. 9-25). Findings in chronic pancreatitis include dilatation or multifocal stenoses of the main pancreatic duct and its lateral side branches, intraductal filling defects representing protein plugs, areas of calcification and narrowing of the intrapancreatic segment of the common bile duct. The rapid development of MRCP and MRI has largely replaced the diagnostic use of ERCP for suspected

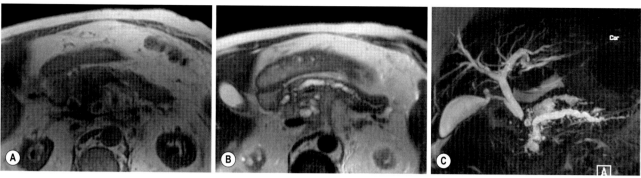

FIGURE 9-26 ■ **Chronic pancreatitis. MR images of the pancreas.** (A) T1-weighted GRE image reveals low signal intensity (due to fibrosis) and atrophy of the gland. (B) The T2-weighted HASTE image better demonstrates duct morphology. (C) MRCP shows severe duct changes. In addition, there is severe biliary duct dilatation, which is unusual for chronic pancreatitis.

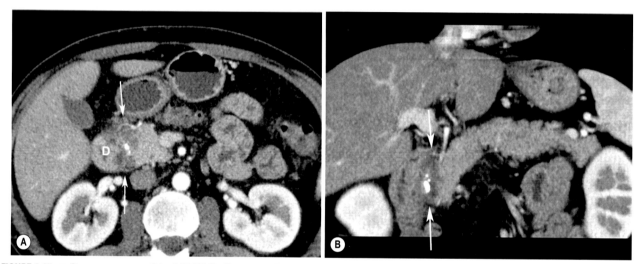

FIGURE 9-27 ■ **Groove pancreatitis: MDCT findings.** (A) There is a low-density mass (arrows) with some calcifications between the pancreatic head and duodenum (D). (B) Curved planar reformation shows the mass (arrows) and the largely unaffected pancreas.

chronic pancreatitis (Fig. 9-26) and has the major advantage of avoiding the complications of ERCP. These include acute pancreatitis, haemorrhage and cholangitis.

Groove Pancreatitis

Groove pancreatitis is a distinct form of CP, affecting the groove between the pancreatic head, duodenum and common bile duct.[32] It was formerly called 'cystic dystrophy of the duodenum', which refers to the presence of cystic changes of the duodenum, caused by heterotopic pancreatic tissue located in the duodenal wall. CT shows elegantly the imaging spectrum of groove pancreatitis, including a plate-like hypoattenuating (poorly enhancing) lesion located between the pancreatic head and the descending part of the duodenum (Fig. 9-27). This may lead to pancreatic and/or bile duct dilatation. MRCP is important in the diagnostic work-up, as it shows not only the hypovascular plate-like lesion but also pathognomonic cystic changes therein (Fig. 9-28). The differential diagnosis includes duodenal cancer, cholangiocarcinoma, pancreatic cancer or acute pancreatitis with inflammatory changes along the groove.[32,33]

Thus, EUS-guided biopsy is often helpful to corroborate the diagnosis.

Autoimmune Pancreatitis

Autoimmune pancreatitis (AIP) is another distinct form of CP, typically affecting patients without a history of alcohol abuse or biliary stone disease.[34] Although the pathogenesis remains unclear, an immune-mediated mechanism has been postulated: the gland shows infiltration by CD4-positive T lymphocytes and plasma cells. Serum levels of IgG4 are abnormally elevated. CT and MRI features are either diffuse or focal gland enlargement, narrowing of the pancreatic duct (without dilatation) and delayed contrast enhancement[34] (Fig. 9-29). Prognosis of AIP is fundamentally different from CP, as steroid therapy will lead to significant improvement or even resolution of symptoms. Focal AIP is difficult to differentiate from pancreatic cancer. Different diagnostic strategies have been proposed by Japanese and Korean pancreatologists with regard to the use of ERCP. It has been shown that typical CT findings (i.e. diffuse pancreatic enlargement with delayed enhancement with or

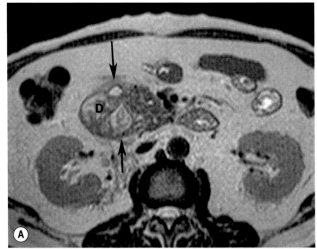

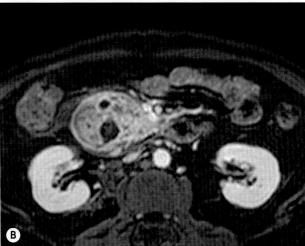

FIGURE 9-28 ■ **Groove pancreatitis: MRI findings.** (A) Axial T2-weighted TSE image shows typical cysts in such a mass located between the head and duodenum (D). (B) With a gadolinium-enhanced MRI, the cysts show no enhancement.

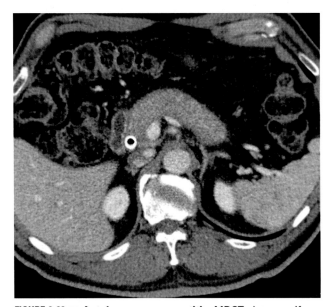

FIGURE 9-29 ■ **Autoimmune pancreatitis.** MDCT shows uniform swelling of the gland in a patient without risk factors for pancreatitis.

without capsule-like rim), together with positive serology, allow a confident diagnosis. However, in case of atypical CT findings, performance of ERCP has added benefit.[35] Whether tissue diagnosis is necessary is a matter of discussion. Histological confirmation is required if laboratory values are indeterminate or when there is incomplete resolution of the mass in response to steroid therapy.[33,36]

PANCREATIC NEOPLASMS

Tumours, both benign and malignant, may arise in the exocrine or endocrine tissue of the pancreas. By far the most common of these is ductal adenocarcinoma.

Ductal Adenocarcinoma

In Europe and the USA pancreatic cancer is the fourth most common cause of cancer death. It is an aggressive malignant disease with early advanced local or distant tumour spread. Adenocarcinoma tends to involve adjacent structures early by perivascular, perineural and lymphatic spread. There is also early metastatic spread to the liver and the peritoneum. As a result of these tumour characteristics, at the time of diagnosis, only approximately 10–20% of patients have surgically resectable disease and the overall 5-year survival rate is of the order of only 5%. Radical pancreaticoduodenectomy (Whipple's resection or pylorus-preserving pancreaticoduodenecetomy) has a significant associated morbidity and mortality. Thus, preoperative local staging should reliably identify patients with unresectable disease to avoid unnecessary laparotomies. The symptoms of pancreatic carcinoma vary, with weight loss and anorexia frequently being present, with or without abdominal pain. Tumours arising in the pancreatic head may obstruct the common bile duct early, resulting in obstructive jaundice, whereas adenocarcinoma arising in the uncinate process causes jaundice and pruritus significantly less often.[37] The tumour marker CA 19–9 is associated with pancreatic cancer but is neither sensitive nor specific enough to be used for screening or the differentiation of benign from malignant pancreatic masses.[38,39] The role of imaging is to detect the tumour, establish the diagnosis of cancer, and stage the disease with a view to determining resectability (Table 9-3).[40,41]

Imaging Techniques

US (transabdominal and endoscopic), MDCT, MRI and MRCP, and ECRP may, in different circumstances, each have a role in the diagnosis of ductal adenocarcinoma. In practice, because it is inexpensive and widely available, transabdominal US is frequently the first imaging investigation carried out in patients with pancreatic carcinoma, particularly in those who present with non-specific abdominal pain or jaundice. It is highly accurate in differentiating obstructive from non-obstructive causes of jaundice and with meticulous technique small pancreatic tumours in the head may be detected. However, negative transabdominal ultrasound neither excludes the presence

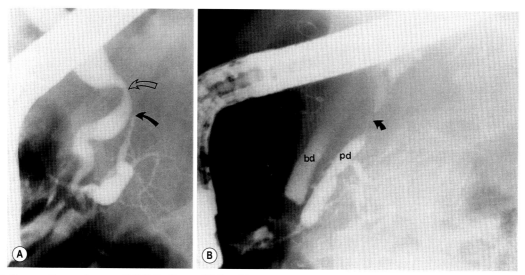

FIGURE 9-30 ■ **Pancreatic carcinoma: ERCP findings.** (A) Double duct sign. ERCP shows obstruction of the pancreatic duct (closed arrow) and focal encasement of the adjacent common bile duct (open arrow). (B) Pancreatic duct obstruction. ERCP shows focal narrowing (arrow) of the pancreatic duct (pd). The common bile duct (bd) is normal, although incompletely filled with contrast.

TABLE 9-3   TNM Staging of Pancreatic Cancer

TNM	Definitions
Tx	Primary tumour cannot be assessed
T0	No evidence of primary tumour
Tis	Carcinoma in situ
T1	Tumour limited to the pancreas, ≤ 2 cm in greatest dimension
T2	Tumour limited to pancreas, > 2 cm in greatest dimension
T3	Tumour extends beyond the pancreas, but without involvement of the coeliac axis or superior mesenteric artery
T4	Tumour involves the coeliac axis or the superior mesenteric artery
Nx	Regional lymph nodes cannot be assessed
N1	No regional lymph nodes
N2	Regional (peripancreatic) lymph node metastasis
M0	No distant metastasis
M1	Distant metastasis

of pancreatic tumour nor is it sufficient for staging pancreatic cancer. Contrast-enhanced MDCT with water as an oral contrast agent, in the pancreatic parenchymal and venous phases, is currently the most widely used technique for the diagnosis and staging of pancreatic cancer. MRI has potential theoretical advantages over CT for detection and characterisation of small tumours but most studies have failed to show a significant advantage over MDCT,[42,43] which is a more accessible and less costly investigation. ERCP is still used in many cases because of its ability to visualise the duodenum and ampulla of Vater directly and allow cytological sampling and access for stent insertion (Fig. 9-30), if required. However, endoscopic stent insertion and cholangitis seriously degrade the capability of subsequent MDCT or MRI studies for detection of small obstructing tumours and to define the longitudinal spread of tumour. Thus, 'exploratory' ERCP without appropriate prior cross-sectional imaging should be avoided. Endoscopic US, in particular, has a role in the

biopsy of equivocal, non-obstructing lesions, with an accuracy of 97.6% for diagnosing malignancy.[44] In addition, it is also a helpful in patients with potentially resectable disease, as it may define the anatomic relationship between tumour and peripancreatic vessels.[45] At present, [18]FDG-PET/CT has a limited role in the initial diagnosis of pancreatic carcinoma because of its inability to differentiate between malignant and inflammatory pancreatic masses and its low sensitivity for detection of liver metastases,[46] but it has been reported to have a high accuracy in the detection of local recurrence.

Imaging Appearances

Approximately 70% of adenocarcinomas arise in the head or uncinate process, with the remainder arising in the body or tail. On US the tumour typically has a lower echogenicity than adjacent pancreatic tissue. On CT the mass may not be visible on a preliminary unenhanced image but, because the tumour is typically less vascular than the surrounding normal pancreatic parenchyma, it will be seen as a poorly enhancing focal area within the densely enhancing normal pancreatic tissue on dynamic contrast-enhanced MDCT (Fig. 9-31). Tumours in the head of the pancreas may cause early dilatation of the common bile duct, although masses arising in the uncinate process are often quite large, encasing the superior mesenteric artery before bile duct obstruction occurs.[37] Upstream dilatation of the main pancreatic duct is a frequent finding in pancreatic carcinoma and is often associated with atrophy of the pancreatic tissue surrounding it.

For detection of pancreatic cancer, there are direct and indirect tumour signs. The classical direct tumour sign is the presence of a hypoattenuating/hypointense mass at contrast-enhanced MDCT or MRI. However, 11% of adenocarcinomas are isoattenuating at CT,[47] and in the category of tumours up to 2 cm in size, up to 27% are isoattenuating[48] and would not be seen, if only this imaging feature was used. There are also six indirect

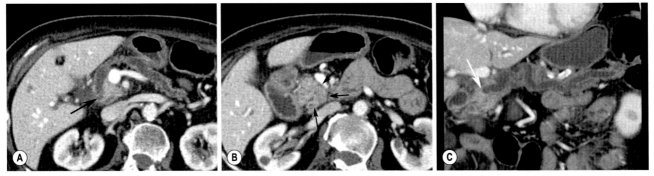

FIGURE 9-31 ■ **Isoattenuating pancreatic cancer: indirect tumour signs.** (A) MDCT shows duct dilatation with abrupt narrowing in the head (arrow). (B) At a slightly inferior level, the gland seems enlarged with convex contours (arrows), although no distinct mass is seen. (C) The curved planar reformation reveals to better advantage the duct dilatation with atrophy of the body and tail. There is a duct cut-off (arrow) due an isoattenuating mass in the head, which turned out to be ductal adenocarcinoma.

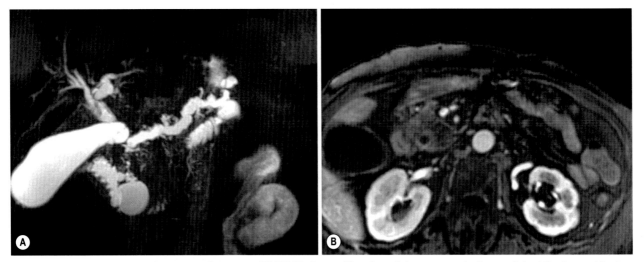

FIGURE 9-32 ■ **Double duct sign in pancreatic cancer.** (A) MRCP shows dilatation of the pancreatic duct and the bile duct, with abrupt cut-off at the pancreatic head. These findings are suggestive, although not pathognomonic for cancer. (B) Gadolinium-enhanced MRI shows the hypointense mass in the head.

tumour signs (Fig. 9-31), which should suggest the possibility of a pancreatic mass: the presence of (1) biliary duct dilatation, (2) pancreatic duct dilatation, or a (3) double duct sign, which may lead to (4) focal atrophy of the gland. If a mass is sufficiently large it will (5) distort the contour of the gland, and (6) loss of pancreatic lobulation is also a subtle, but often early sign.[49]

Pancreatic tissue enhances most intensely when a large volume of contrast medium (2 mL/kg b.w.) is given by rapid infusion (flow rate 4 mL/s) and MDCT is used in the parenchymal phase, with an imaging delay of aortic transit time plus 25 s. This is the optimum imaging for the detection of the primary pancreatic mass.[50] However, as it is necessary to evaluate not only the primary mass and the arterial vasculature but also the presence or absence of venous involvement and hepatic metastatic disease, biphasic imaging including the entire liver (or the entire abdomen) in the venous phase is likely to provide the maximum diagnostic information. Many also find that water provides a better (and cheaper) oral contrast

medium than positive contrast agents in these patients, as enhancement of the wall of the stomach and duodenum is more readily appreciated and this can help with assessment for invasion. On MRI the appearance of the primary mass will depend on the imaging sequence used. With MRCP the appearance of a double duct sign (i.e. dilatation of common bile duct and pancreatic duct) is quite typical in the case of pancreatic head tumours, although it is not pathognomonic (Fig. 9-32). On T2-weighted images the tumour is often hyperintense, but may be of variable signal intensity. At T1-weighted GRE images with spectral fat suppresssion the mass has low signal intensity relative to normal adjacent pancreatic parenchyma. Gadolinium enhancement of adenocarcinoma is typically less than that of normal pancreatic tissue (Figs. 9-32 and 9-33), whereas acinar carcinoma and neuroendocrine tumours tend to be hypervascular. It has been shown that dedicated pancreatic-protocol imaging leads to a significant improvement of preoperative staging.[51]

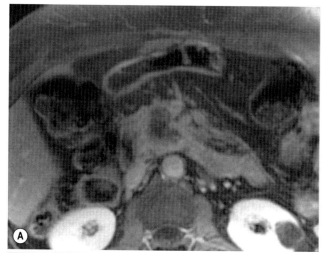

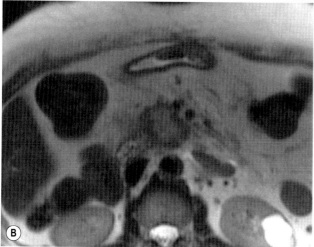

FIGURE 9-33 ▪ **MR signal intensity of pancreatic cancer.** (A) There is low signal intensity on gadolinium-enhanced T1-weighted GRE due to hypovascularity. (B) The mass is slightly hyperintense on T2-weighted TSE.

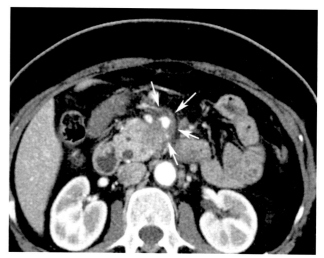

FIGURE 9-34 ▪ **Arterial invasion by pancreatic cancer.** MDCT shows a mass (arrows) in the uncinate process, which encases the superior mesenteric artery by more than 180° of vessel circumference.

Local Staging

This involves assessment of the degree of vascular involvement, and invasion of adjacent organs. In the absence of distant metastatic disease, perivascular invasion or vascular encasement are the most important criteria for unresectability. Pancreatic angiography formerly played an important role in the assessment of vascular involvement, but has been replaced by MDCT or MRI, which are capable of demonstrating even small pancreatic arteries. As well as being non-invasive, it is able to detect periarterial extension of disease, which precedes luminal narrowing. CT findings that indicate perivascular invasion of arteries include soft-tissue infiltration obscuring the vessel margin, calibre change, or contour deformity. Lu et al. assessed the presence of circumferential vessel contact with tumour to define vascular infiltration (either arterial or venous).[52] They found that a tumour-vessel contact of more than 180° circumference indicated vascular involvement (Fig. 9-34), whereas less than 90° vessel circumference having contact with tumour indicated low probability of vessel infiltration (Fig. 9-33).

With the adapted criteria defined by Li et al., different criteria apply for arterial and venous invasion.[53] Tumour surrounding more than 180° circumference of vessel or venous occlusion or deformation of vein contour due to adjacent tumour (so-called tear drop deformity) are highly suggestive of tumour involvement. For arterial invasion, arterial embedment in tumour or the presence of more than 180° circumference of vessel having contact with tumour *and* vessel irregularity or stenosis are indicative (Fig. 9-35). Arterial involvement of the coeliac trunk or SMA (stage T4) suggests unresectablility, whereas limited venous invasion (stage T3) may suggest resectability in specialised cancer centres, where vein resection and interposition is surgically feasible. Occlusion of major veins typically results in multiple venous collaterals (Fig. 9-35). Another quite specific sign for venous infiltration is the 'tear drop deformity sign' of the superior mesenteric vein or portal vein. As ductal adenocarcinoma is very fibrotic, tumour abutting the vein may lead to deformity of the venous contour, which is indicative of venous infiltration (Fig. 9-36). When normally enhancing pancreatic tissue is seen between the tumour and an adjacent vessel, vascular involvement is unlikely.

Invasion of adjacent structures, particularly the stomach and duodenum, will be shown by interruption of the normally enhancing wall. Duodenal involvement (stage T3) does not necessarily preclude curative surgery as the duodenum is removed as part of the Whipple's resection. Where MRI is used for staging, identical criteria are used to determine resectability.

Distant Metastases

US or CT may show evidence of metastatic disease in the liver (Fig. 9-37). Nodal staging has limitations in pancreatic carcinoma because nodes may be involved without enlargement; this represents a problem when assessing lymph nodes on cross-sectional imaging where enlargement is the main criterion for prediction of lymph node

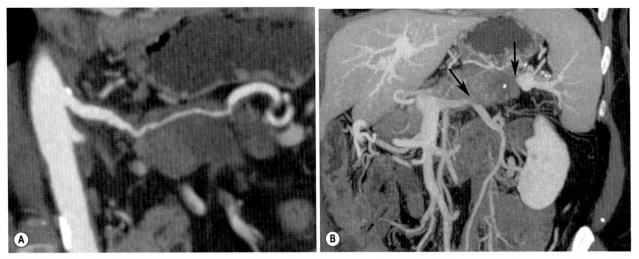

FIGURE 9-35 ■ **Vascular invasion by pancreatic cancer.** (A) The adapted criteria for arterial tumour invasion rely on the additional imaging feature of arterial stenosis or vessel irregularity. This tumour shows circumferential growth with a long irregular arterial stenosis (arrow). (B) Venous invasion: a large cancer in the tail occludes the splenic vein (arrows), as shown in this MIP image.

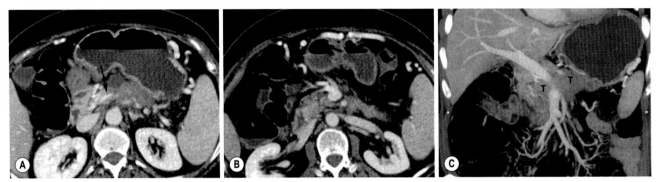

FIGURE 9-36 ■ **Tear drop sign as indicator for venous tumour invasion.** (A) A large cancer in the pancreatic body shows slit-like compression of the venous confluence (arrow). (B) At a slightly inferior level, the superior mesenteric vein has its normal ovoid shape, with some dilated venous tributaries. (C) The MIP image reveals obstruction of the venous confluence by circumferential tumour growth (T).

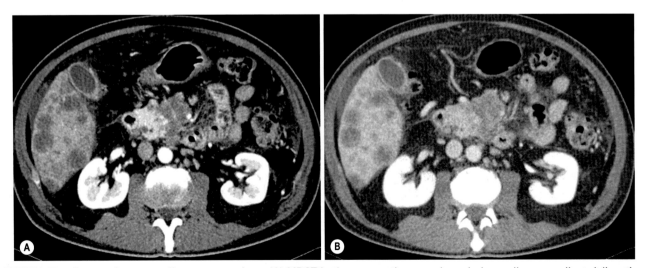

FIGURE 9-37 ■ **Pancreatic cancer: direct tumour signs.** (A) MDCT in the pancreatic parenchymal phase allows excellent delineation of the hypoattenuating mass in the uncinate process, encasing the mesenteric vessels. (B) In the venous phase the peripancreatic veins and the liver metastases are better visualised.

involvement. The lymph nodes initially involved are those adjacent to the pancreas, followed by the coeliac, common hepatic, mesenteric and para-aortic groups. Peritoneal spread from pancreatic adenocarcinoma is common but the lesions are typically small and difficult to detect. The presence of peritoneal involvement may be inferred if abdominal ascites is present.

Follow-Up

Very few imaging studies have focused on the detection of pancreatic cancer recurrence, because recurrence had a dismal prognosis and was not treated. However, radio-chemotherapy has been instituted as therapy for local or systemic recurrence. Normal postoperative appearance after Whipple's resection includes stranding or even a solid nodular component at the coeliac trunk or SMA, which, however, should not grow during follow-up. Knowledge of the resection status (R0, R1 or R2) is critical to interpret the imaging appearance. Tumour recurrence is most often found around the SMA, either as a localised tumour mass or as a cuff-like formation or in an area bordered by the coeliac trunk, the portal vein and the IVC.[54]

Neuroendocrine Pancreatic Tumours (NET)

Neuroendocrine tumours belong to a heterogeneous group of tumours, which share common histological, biological and clinical features.[55,56] NETs are divided into functioning or non-functioning tumours based on the presence or absence of hormonal hypersecretion. They were formerly known as 'islet cell tumours'. Functioning tumours are those in which a peptide hormone is produced by the tumour and results in a characteristic clinical syndrome; non-functioning tumours may have an appearance similar to pancreatic carcinoma but enjoy a much better prognosis.

Functioning Tumours

Five clinical syndromes have been described secondary to the presence of insulinoma, gastrinoma, glucagonoma, VIPoma (vasoactive intestinal polypeptide) and somatostatinoma. Of these, insulinoma and gastrinoma are the most common. Patients with insulinoma present with hypoglycaemic episodes and because the symptoms are non-specific there may be a delay in considering the diagnosis. The diagnosis is confirmed biochemically, with radiology having the task to localise the tumour. Insulinomas are usually solitary, benign, and in 78% of cases measure less than 2 cm in diameter.[57] Insulinomas are treated by surgical resection. Gastrinomas are the second most common islet cell tumours and cause the Zollinger–Ellison syndrome characterised by gastric hyperacidity and recurrent gastric and duodenal ulceration. These tumours are often multiple and 60% are malignant. Gastrinoma tend to be localised in the 'gastrinoma triangle', which is formed by the junction of the cystic and the common hepatic ducts superiorly, the second and third parts of the duodenum inferiorly, and the pancreatic neck

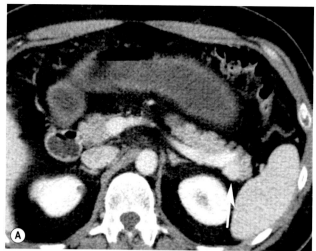

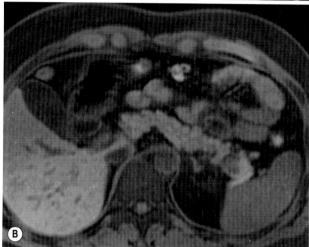

FIGURE 9-38 ■ **Insulinoma.** (A) Arterial-phase CT shows a small moderately hypervascular lesion adjacent to the splenic vessels, which could easily be missed (arrow). (B) The unenhanced T1-weighted GRE fat-suppressed sequence readily shows the hypointense mass in the tail.

medially. They are also frequently associated with multiple endocrine neoplasia type 1. The role of radiology in these functioning tumours, which may be very small, is to provide accurate preoperative localisation.[58] Transabdominal US is not indicated, because it will not allow assessment of the pancreatic body and tail. Other US techniques, including endoscopic US, have also been used.[59] CT is commonly used to localise these tumours, but because of their small size, fine cuts and meticulous technique must be used.[60] Neuroendocrine tumours typically show early but transient enhancement (Fig. 9-38), although better depiction on the portal phase images has also been described[38] and reported sensitivities for the technique range from 63 to 94%.[59–61] Fat-suppressed T1W GRE and dynamic gadolinium-enhanced MRI sequences are very helpful[62,63] (Fig. 9-38). There is also high potential for functional imaging in these tumours. ^{111}In-somatostatin receptor has largely been replaced by PET/CT using somatostatin receptor tracers (^{68}Ga-DOTATOC, ^{68}Ga-DOTANOC, ^{68}Ga-DOTATATE), which has the highest sensitivity and specificity for

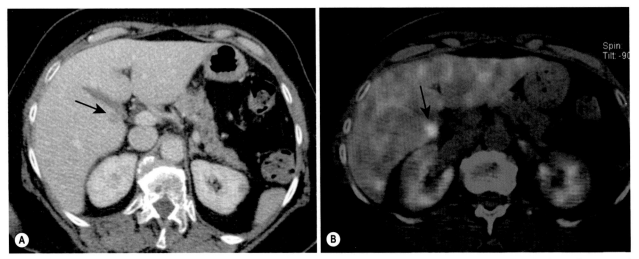

FIGURE 9-39 ■ **Value of Ga-DOTATOC-PET/CT for staging of NET.** (A) Enhanced CT shows a small focal liver lesion adjacent to the gall bladder (arrow), which cannot be characterised. (B) PET/CT clearly shows hypermetabolism, indicative of a metastasis (arrow).

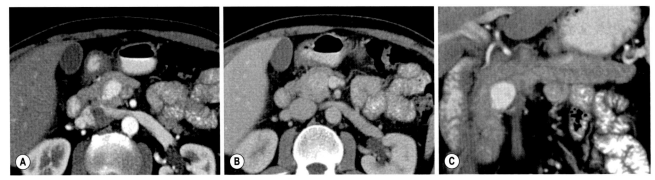

FIGURE 9-40 ■ **MDCT of non-functioning NET.** (A) Arterial-phase MDCT shows a hypervascular mass, (B) which is nearly isoattenuating in the venous phase. (C) The curved planar reformation shows the mass in the head, which is deeply embedded in the parenchyma.

localisation of pancreatic and extrapancreatic tumour load[64,65] (Fig. 9-39). More invasive techniques of localisation such as selective arterial calcium stimulation followed by venous sampling, have also been used and may successfully localise the tumour to the head, body, or tail of the gland.[66–68]

Non-functioning NETs

These may present with symptoms similar to pancreatic adenocarcinoma and are nearly always malignant. However, differentiation between ductal adenocarcinoma and non-functioning islet cell tumour is important, as the latter can often be curatively resected and may be successfully treated with chemotherapy. Two CT features of non-functioning endocrine tumours may be particularly helpful in suggesting the diagnosis. The first is the presence of calcification, which is seen in 22% of NETs and the second, tumour contrast enhancement. Strong enhancement is not a feature of ductal adenocarcinoma and an enhancing mass should suggest the possibility of a NET (Fig. 9-40).

Cystic Masses

The majority of cystic masses in the pancreas are post-inflammatory pseudocysts, although the reported proportion of 90% of cystic masses being pseudocysts is likely much too high.[69,70] However, cystic neoplasms are encountered in increasing frequency, which renders the characterisation of cystic pancreatic lesions important. Although a variety of histological types of cystic neoplasms have been reported, the most prevalent types are serous cystadenoma, mucinous cystadenoma and intraductal papillary mucinous neoplasm (IPMN), which account for approximately 90% of cystic neoplasms.[71] Characterisation of cystic masses should be based on clinical history, imaging features and, if necessary, aspiration or core biopsy. Mucinous cystic neoplasms are the most common. There is a spectrum from benign to malignant lesions, but ultimately most behave in a malignant fashion. A typical imaging feature of mucinous cystadenoma is a mass composed of a few, larger (> 2 cm) cysts (Fig. 9-41). If CT or MRI depicts solid, contrast-enhanced nodules, the presence of a mucinous

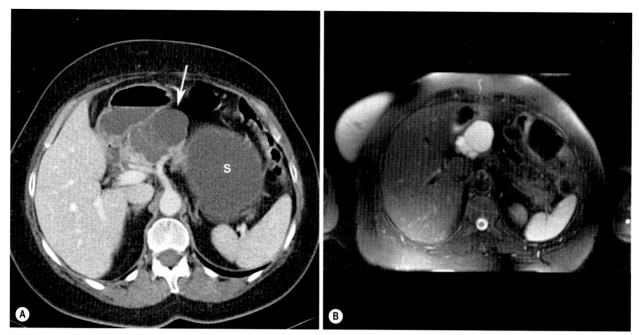

FIGURE 9-41 ▪ **Mucinous cystadenoma.** (A) Contrast-enhanced MDCT shows a macrocystic mass in the pancreas (arrow) with thin septations. Fluid-filled stomach (S). (B) The macrocystic structure and the septations are better demonstrated by a T2-weighted TSE image.

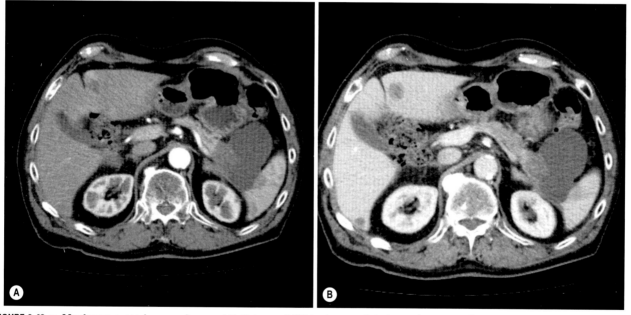

FIGURE 9-42 ▪ **Mucinous cystadenocarcinoma.** (A) Enhanced CT in the arterial phase shows a solid mass in the tail (arrow) with a large cystic component. Absence of history or signs of chronic pancreatitis makes a diagnosis of pseudocyst unlikely. (B) At venous-phase CT, liver metastases are shown with high conspicuity, which is in line with a diagnosis of cystadenocarcinoma.

cystadenocarcinoma should be suspected[72] (Fig. 9-42). Since mucinous cystadenomas may undergo malignant degeneration, they should be resected. Serous cystic tumours (formerly called 'microcystic cystadenomas') are generally benign. Serous cystadenomas are usually composed of numerous tiny cysts, generally more than six in number and less than 2 cm in diameter, which may have a central scar or central stellate calcification (Fig. 9-43).

If the cysts are too small to be resolved on CT, the mass may appear solid.[73] Treatment recommendations are based on size and the presence of symptoms.[73] In these cases, MRI may readily depict the true nature of the lesions, containing innumerable microcysts. Rarely a serous cystadenoma is macrocystic. In this case it cannot be differentiated from mucinous tumours by imaging. IPMNs originate from the epithelial cells of the main

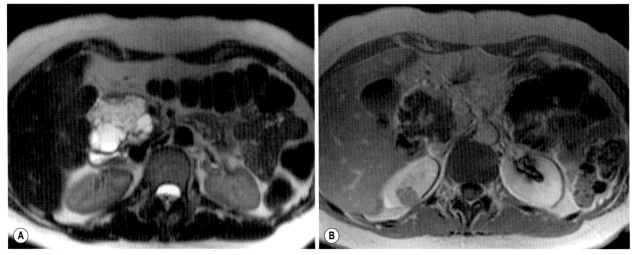

FIGURE 9-43 ■ **Serous cystadenoma.** (A) T2-weighted TSE MR image shows a microcystic mass in the pancreatic head. Only one of the innumerable cysts has a considerable size. (B) Gadolinium-enhanced T1-weighted GRE image demonstrates enhancement of the septations and of the central scar. No other solid components are seen.

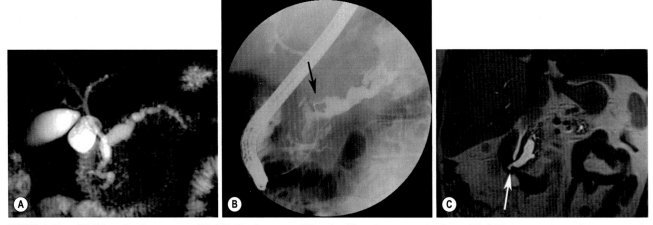

FIGURE 9-44 ■ **IPMN main duct type.** (A) MRCP shows a diffusely dilated pancreatic duct. (B) Different patient: the pancreatic duct is severely dilated. At ERCP there is a contrast material filling defect (arrow) in the main duct, which is traversed by the guide-wire. Imaging findings are suggestive of mucin filling the duct. At endoscopy mucin spilling out of the bulging papilla was seen. (C) Corresponding T2-weighted HASTE image shows the bulging papilla (arrow).

duct or the side branches, producing large amounts of mucin. Pathologically, a wide spectrum of benign to malignant lesions have been described, which is divided according to the WHO into four categories: adenoma, borderline, carcinoma in situ and IPMN with invasive cancer. According to the location, IPMNs are described as main duct type, branch duct type or mixed type (growing in the main duct and side branches).

Imaging findings include diffuse or segmental duct dilatation (Fig. 9-44). Branch duct type shows a sac-like dilatation, and is often difficult to differentiate from other cystic lesions (Fig. 9-45). Mixed-type IPMNs demonstrate dilatation of the main duct and side branches (Fig. 9-46). The presence of solid nodular protrusions is suspicious for malignancy.[74,75] In general, IPMNs affecting the main duct have a higher likelihood of undergoing malignant degeneration than branch duct types. Thus, management of main duct type IPMN is surgical, whereas

branch duct type IPMN < 3 cm in asymptomatic patients can be followed by serial imaging.[76,77]

The most reliable way of differentiating between pseudocyst, serous and mucinous cystic tumours is fine-needle aspiration of the fluid. If the fluid contains a high amylase level, this is likely to represent a pseudocyst rather than a cystic neoplasm. Mucinous neoplasms show elevated CEA levels in the fluid.[78,79] If the amylase level is low, cytological/histological examination of the specimen may characterise the nature of the cystic tumour.

What To Do With Small Incidental Cystic Lesions

Incidental, unsuspected pancreatic cysts are frequently encountered at MDCT or MRI (Fig. 9-47). Recent studies reported a prevalence of 2.6% at MDCT.[80] In liver-transplant patients MRI may reveal small cysts in up

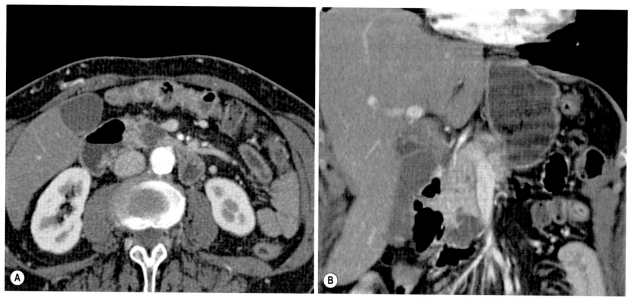

FIGURE 9-45 ■ **IPMN branch duct type.** (A) Axial MDCT shows a small cystic lesion in the uncinate process, which is difficult to characterise, unless a communication with the ductal system is seen. (B) Coronal MPR better demonstrates the cystic lesion to be a sac-like side branch variety.

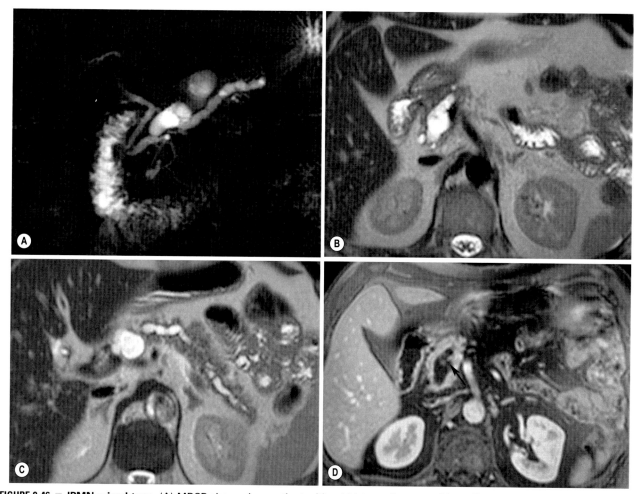

FIGURE 9-46 ■ **IPMN mixed type.** (A) MRCP shows, in a patient without history of pancreatitis, a dilated main duct with some cystic structures. (B, C) Axial T2-weighted HASTE images show the severe duct dilatation in the head. (D) Axial gadolinium-enhanced T1-weighted GRE image shows some solid nodular structures in the head (arrow), which are suspicious for malignancy.

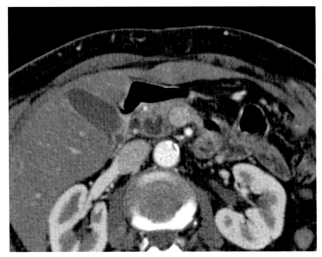

FIGURE 9-47 ■ **Incidentally found cystic lesion in the pancreatic head, which cannot be characterised with MDCT.**

to 59.6%.[81] The majority of these small cystic lesions are likely branch duct type IPMNs or simple cysts. It has been shown that follow-up of cystic lesions without a main duct dilatation or solid nodules seems to be safe.[82,83] However, they should not be ignored, as recent studies have demonstrated that patients with small cystic lesions tend to have a higher likelihood of developing pancreatic ductal adenocarcinoma in the future.[84]

Rare Pancreatic Neoplasms

There are a variety of rare pancreatic neoplasms that can be detected and, occasionally, diagnosed by imaging techniques. These include pancreatoblastoma, solid and papillary epithelial neoplasms, adenosquamous carcinoma, acinar cell carcinoma, haemangioma, lymphangioma and primary pancreatic lymphoma.

MULTISYSTEM DISEASES WITH INVOLVEMENT OF THE PANCREAS

Cystic Fibrosis

Cystic fibrosis is a condition with autosomal recessive inheritance in which there are defects of serous and mucous secretion involving multiple organs; 85% of patients have severe exocrine pancreatic insufficiency and steatorrhoea. Obstruction of the main pancreatic duct and side branches by inspissated secretions results in acinar and ductal dilatation and subsequent atrophy of the acinar tissue. US, CT or MR imaging may show marked fatty replacement of the pancreatic parenchyma (Fig. 9-48), dystrophic calcifications and pancreatic cysts resulting from ductal obstruction.

Von Hippel–Lindau Disease

Von Hippel–Lindau disease is inherited as an autosomal dominant condition characterised by renal cell carcinomas, phaeochromocytomas, retinal angiomatosis and

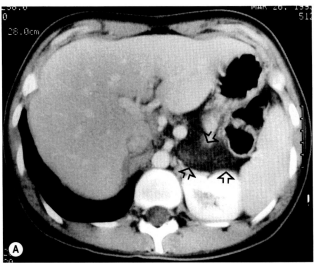

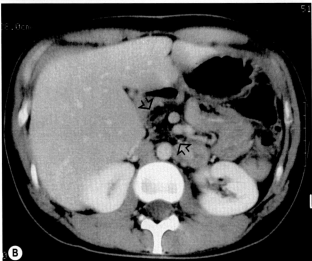

FIGURE 9-48 ■ **Cystic fibrosis.** (A) CT through the level of the body and tail of the pancreas (arrows) shows fatty replacement of the gland. (B) CT at the level of the pancreatic head (arrows) shows almost complete replacement of the pancreas by fat. Only a few strands of enhancing pancreatic parenchyma are identified.

haemangioblastomas of the cerebellum. The most common pancreatic lesions in this condition are simple pancreatic cysts, but serous cystic pancreatic neoplasms and pancreatic islet cell tumours may also occur[85] (Fig. 9-49).

Polycystic Kidney Disease

The hallmark of the autosomal dominant inherited form of polycystic renal disease is the presence of multiple renal cysts, but other organs may also be involved. Hepatic cysts may occur and in 10% of patients the pancreas also shows cystic change (Fig. 9-50).

Osler–Weber–Rendu Disease

Osler–Weber–Rendu disease is a vascular disorder characterised by telangiectasia of the skin, mucous

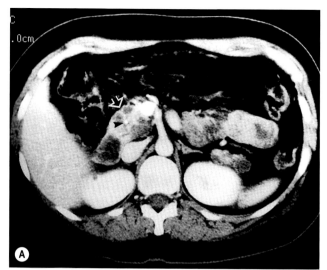

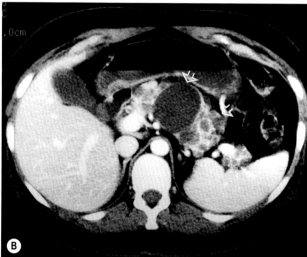

FIGURE 9-49 ■ von Hippel–Lindau disease. (A) CT through the level of the head of the pancreas (open arrow) shows multiple small cysts and a central area of calcification (arrowhead) sited in a small serous cystadenoma. (B) Image at the level of the body and tail of the pancreas (arrows) shows multiple cysts of different sizes. These were simple cysts, as distinct from the serous cystic neoplasm in the head of the pancreas.

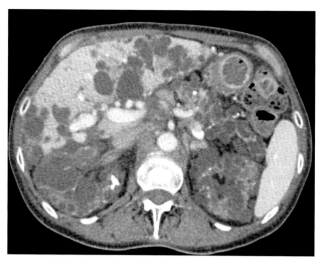

FIGURE 9-50 ■ Simple cysts in adult polycystic kidney disease. MDCT shows innumerable cysts in both kidneys, the liver and the pancreas.

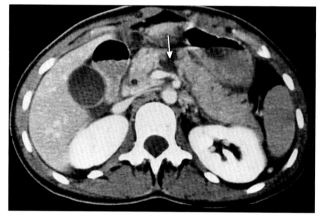

FIGURE 9-51 ■ Pancreatic trauma. Following direct blunt trauma to the abdomen, the pancreas is seen to be fractured (arrow). There was disruption of the main pancreatic duct.

membranes, gastrointestinal and urinary tracts, liver and pancreas. The angiographic findings of pancreatic involvement are characteristic and consist of dilated pancreatic arteries supplying a racemose collection of vessels with early draining veins.

TRAUMA

Pancreatic injury is relatively uncommon, being encountered in only around 3% of abdominal trauma cases that require surgical treatment.[86] The injuries are usually caused by severe direct impact or forceful deceleration injuries, such as those from a steering wheel or bicycle handlebar, which result in midline compression of the pancreas against the vertebral column. These injuries are often associated with other visceral injuries, especially of

the liver and duodenum. Blunt pancreatic injuries without ductal leakage usually resolve spontaneously without recourse to surgery. However, if there is leakage from the pancreatic duct, post-traumatic pancreatitis may result and main pancreatic duct disruption is an important indicator of severity. US may show peripancreatic fluid or discontinuity in the normal pancreatic contour, but CT is the most effective imaging technique for the diagnosis of pancreatic injury. Best results are obtained with thin-slice examinations. Findings may be very subtle and non-specific, such as thickening of the anterior renal fascia and fluid in the lesser sac. More specific features include fluid lying between the splenic vein and pancreas and increased attenuation of the peripancreatic fat. It may be possible to demonstrate a fracture line through the pancreas, with or without separation of the fracture fragments (Fig. 9-51), or focal enlargement of the pancreas,

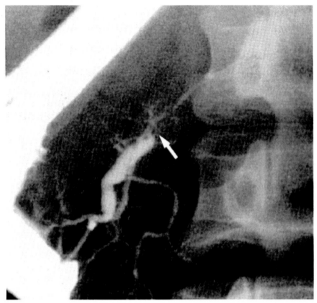

FIGURE 9-52 ■ **ERCP shows occlusion of the main pancreatic duct in the head of the pancreas (arrow) as a result of the laceration.**

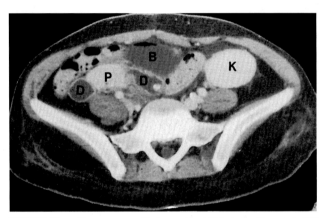

FIGURE 9-53 ■ **Post-pancreatic transplant CT study.** Dynamic CT at the level of the head of the pancreatic allograft (P) shows an apparently normal gland. The attached duodenum (D) has been anastomosed to the urinary bladder (B). Contrast excretion by the transplanted kidney (K) has not yet reached the urinary bladder.

with or without haematoma. When there is a high suspicion of ductal injury, ERCP or MRCP may be performed (Fig. 9-52).

PANCREATIC TRANSPLANT IMAGING

The increasing use of pancreatic transplantation for the treatment of diabetes has necessitated the use of imaging of the graft to determine the presence of complications, such as graft rejection, anastomotic leakage, perigraft fluid collections or abscesses and ischaemia (Fig. 9-53). Pancreatic graft rejection can be detected using US, MRI

and radionuclide imaging. The US findings in acute graft rejection include patchy or diffuse areas of decreased parenchymal echogenicity and enlargement of the graft, while in chronic rejection increased echogenicity and decreased graft size are seen. Radionuclide studies using ^{99m}Tc-DTPA blood-pool imaging can also detect rejection by demonstrating decreased graft perfusion, with a sensitivity of around 86%. MRI is the most sensitive and specific technique for detecting graft rejection. The findings of rejection include a decrease in signal intensity of the graft on T1-weighted sequences, such that the signal intensity becomes similar to that of skeletal muscle, and an increased signal on T2-weighted sequences, in which the signal intensity becomes equal to that of fluid.

Transplant pancreatitis and associated perigraft fluid collections are not uncommon complications following transplantation. These may be effectively treated with percutaneous catheter drainage, obviating the need for surgery in many cases. Disruption of the cystoduodenostomy and anastomosis with leakage of urine and pancreatic juice into the peritoneal cavity may be readily demonstrated by performing a CT cystogram (Fig. 9-54), with the instillation of dilute water-soluble contrast into the bladder.

INTERVENTIONAL RADIOLOGY

In addition to their ability to image the pancreas, radiologists are integral to the management of patients with pancreatic disease because of their ability to perform minimally invasive procedures, such as percutaneous biopsy of focal pancreatic masses and percutaneous drainage of pancreatic fluid collections.

Biopsy of Pancreatic Lesions

Some solid pancreatic lesions cannot be characterised fully by imaging methods alone. In order for clinicians to plan the appropriate treatment strategy, focal pancreatic masses should be biopsied. Almost all pancreatic masses can be biopsied under endosonography (EUS) or CT guidance. If available, EUS-guided biopsy is the method of choice, as it avoids transgression of the left lobe of the liver or the stomach with the biopsy needle. However, the use of small-calibre needles with EUS carries the risk of inadequate tissue sampling. CT guidance is usually reserved for lesions not successfully biopsied under EUS guidance. CT-guided biopsy may be performed from an anterior, posterior or even lateral approach (Fig. 9-55). Because of the location of the pancreas, it is usually necessary to pass the needle through normal abdominal tissue to reach it. Most structures (including stomach, small bowel, but not the spleen) can be traversed by 18G needles with little risk of morbidity.[87] Cutting needles (16–18G) are preferred for biopsy of pancreatic lesions, yielding a core of tissue for histological examination.[87] A fine-needle aspiration biopsy (FNAB) technique may be used to obtain a cytological aspirate.

The sensitivity of pancreatic biopsy is 78–99%.[87,88] Mild-to-moderate complications occur in up to 15% of cases, including post-procedural abdominal pain and

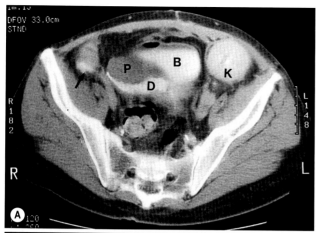
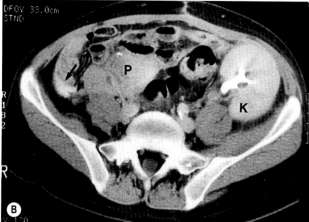

FIGURE 9-54 ■ **CT cystogram after pancreatic allograft transplant.** (A) Dilute contrast medium has been instilled into the urinary bladder (B) via a Foley catheter. Contrast medium fills the urinary bladder and the anastomosed duodenal loop (D) surrounding the head of the pancreatic allograft (P). Contrast medium extravasation is seen adjacent to the end of the duodenal loop (arrow). (B) CT at a slightly higher level shows free contrast medium extravasation from the CT cystogram (arrow). 12Fr K = renal allograft transplant.

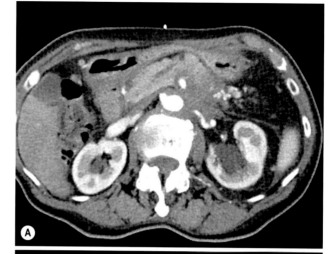
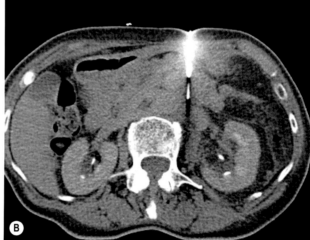

FIGURE 9-55 ■ **CT-guided biopsy of pancreatic cancer.** (A) A pancreatic tumour is present in the body, with extensive vascular infiltration. Histological evidence is sought prior to palliative chemotherapy. (B) The 17G coaxial needle (for an 18G cutting needle) is advanced in an anterior approach, traversing the stomach. The inner stylet is being pulled back to minimise the tip artefact, which may otherwise obscure the exact position of the needle tip.

pancreatitis, which occurs in 3%. Less common complications include severe haemorrhage and, very rarely, needle-track seeding.

Drainage of Pancreatic/Peripancreatic Fluid Collections

As with other abdominal fluid collections, pancreatic fluid collections are amenable to percutaneous drainage. Most pancreatic fluid collections requiring drainage are related to acute pancreatitis. The two main indications for percutaneous drainage in acute pancreatitis are to assess whether a fluid collection is infected and drainage of a known infected collection.[89]

Patients with acute pancreatitis with pancreatic or peripancreatic fluid collections are often febrile, and fine-needle aspiration under US or CT guidance of a few millilitres of fluid, followed by prompt microbiological analysis, may be necessary to confirm or exclude infection. If the fluid is infected, the collection can be drained by percutaneous insertion of a drainage catheter at the same time.

Infected ANC or WON should be drained by a catheter of the appropriate size. The contents of most infected collections are relatively viscous and large tubes are required (12Fr or more) to provide efficient drainage. The best results of percutaneous drainage of infected ANC or WON will be achieved with large catheters and it may be necessary to drain multiple collections; careful radiological follow-up is frequently needed (Fig. 9-56). Using these methods, successful cure rates of up to 86% for percutaneous drainage of infected pancreatic and peripancreatic fluid collections can be achieved.[90–92] Percutaneous drainage of liquefied walled-off necrosis has unpredictable success rates, as thick debris cannot be

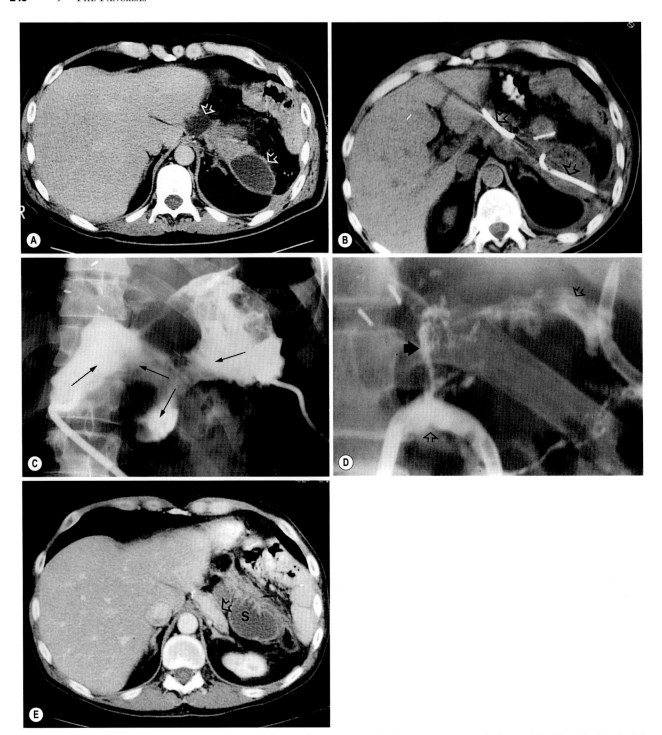

FIGURE 9-56 ■ **Postoperative pancreatitis with acute fluid collection treated with percutaneous drainage.** (A) CT at the level of the tail of the pancreas shows two fluid collections (arrows). Additional CT images (not shown) showed a larger fluid collection just inferior to the pancreas. (B) CT performed following percutaneous catheter drainage shows two 12Fr catheters (arrows) in place. (C) A contrast study through the two catheters shows communication (arrows) of the fluid collections around the pancreas. (D) Contrast study just before catheter removal shows only a small space remaining adjacent to both catheters (open arrows) and small sinus tracks between the two catheters (solid arrows). No GI or pancreatic duct communications were seen. (E) CT obtained 2 weeks after removal of catheter shows normal contrast enhancement of the tail of the pancreas (open arrow). No remaining fluid collections were identified. S = stomach.

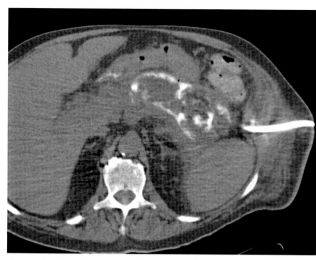

FIGURE 9-57 ■ **Unsuccessful CT-guided drainage of pancreatic necrosis.** CT sinogram shows extensive amount of necrotic debris in the collection, which precludes effective drainage.

drained even with large-calibre drains (Fig. 9-57). In these cases, a joint approach of radiology and surgery may be sought: percutaneous CT-guided puncture with insertion of a stiff guidewire may allow laparoscopic access via the tract with performance of a more minimally invasive necrosectomy.

REFERENCES

1. Morgan DE, Logan K, Baron TH, et al. Pancreas divisum: implications for diagnostic and therapeutic pancreatography. Am J Roentgenol 1999;173:193–8.
2. Gonoi W, Akai H, Hagiwara K, et al. Pancreas divisum as a predisposing factor for chronic and recurrent idiopathic pancreatitis: initial in vivo survey. Gut 2011;60:1103–8.
3. Kamisawa T, Yoshiike M, Egawa N, et al. Pancreatic tumor associated with pancreas divisum. J Gastroenterol Hepatol 2005;20:915–18.
4. Pasaoglu L, Vural M, Hatipglu HG, et al. Agenesis of the dorsal pancreas. World J Gastroenterol 2008;14:2915–16.
5. Thoeni RF. The revised Atlanta classification of acute pancreatitis: its importance for the radiologist and its effect on treatment. Radiology 2012;262:751–64.
6. Banks PA, Bollen TL, Dervenis C, et al. Classification of acute pancreatitis—2012: revision of the Atlanta classification and definitions by international consensus. Gut 2012;62:101–11.
7. Sheu Y, Furlan A, Almusa O, et al. The revised Atlanta classification for acute pancreatitis: a CT imaging guide for radiologists. Emerg Radiol 2012;19:237–41.
8. Beger HG, Rau B, Mayer J, Pralle U. Natural course of acute pancreatitis. World J Surg 1997;21:130–5.
9. Paulson EK, Vitellas KM, Keogan MT, et al. Acute pancreatitis complicated by gland necrosis: spectrum of findings on contrast-enhanced CT. Am J Roentgenol 1999;172:609–13.
10. Balthazar EJ. Staging of acute pancreatitis. Radiol Clin North Am 2002;40:1199–209.
11. Papachristou GI, Muddana V, Yadav D, et al. Comparison of BISAP, Ranson's, APACHE-II, and CTSI scores in predicting organ failure, complications, and mortality in acute pancreatitis. Am J Gastroenterol 2010;105:435–41; quiz 442.
12. Bollen TL, Singh VK, Maurer R, et al. A comparative evaluation of radiologic and clinical scoring systems in the early prediction of severity in acute pancreatitis. Am J Gastroenterol 2012;107:612–19.
13. UK guidelines for the management of acute pancreatitis. Gut 2005;54(Suppl. 3):iii, 1–9.
14. Kwon Y, Park HS, Kim YJ, et al. Multidetector row computed tomography of acute pancreatitis: Utility of single portal phase CT scan in short-term follow up. Eur J Radiol 2012;81(8):1728–34.
15. Neoptolemos JP, Carr-Locke DL, London N, et al. ERCP findings and the role of endoscopic sphincterotomy in acute gallstone pancreatitis. Br J Surg 1988;75:954–60.
16. Neoptolemos JP, Carr-Locke DL, London NJ, et al. Controlled trial of urgent endoscopic retrograde cholangiopancreatography and endoscopic sphincterotomy versus conservative treatment for acute pancreatitis due to gallstones. Lancet 1988;2:979–83.
17. Folsch UR, Nitsche R, Ludtke R, et al. Early ERCP and papillotomy compared with conservative treatment for acute biliary pancreatitis. The German Study Group on Acute Biliary Pancreatitis. N Engl J Med 1997;336:237–42.
18. Hallal AH, Amortegui JD, Jeroukhimov IM, et al. Magnetic resonance cholangiopancreatography accurately detects common bile duct stones in resolving gallstone pancreatitis. J Am Coll Surg 2005;200:869–75.
19. Balthazar EJ. Acute pancreatitis: assessment of severity with clinical and CT evaluation. Radiology 2002;223:603-13.
20. Heiss P, Bruennler T, Salzberger B, et al. Severe acute pancreatitis requiring drainage therapy: findings on computed tomography as predictor of patient outcome. Pancreatology 2010;10:726–33.
21. Beger HG, Bittner R, Block S, Buchler M. Bacterial contamination of pancreatic necrosis. A prospective clinical study. Gastroenterology 1986;91:433–8.
22. Alsfasser G, Schwandner F, Pertschy A, et al. Treatment of necrotizing pancreatitis: redefining the role of surgery. World J Surg 2012;36:1142–7.
23. Kourtesis G, Wilson SE, Williams RA. The clinical significance of fluid collections in acute pancreatitis. Am Surg 1990;56:796–9.
24. Kim KO, Kim TN. Acute pancreatic pseudocyst: incidence, risk factors, and clinical outcomes. Pancreas 2012;41:577–81.
25. Patil PV, Khalil A, Thaha MA. Splenic parenchymal complications in pancreatitis. JOP 2011;12:287–91.
26. Bagul A, Siriwardena AK. Evaluation of the Manchester classification system for chronic pancreatitis. JOP 2006;7:390–6.
27. Campisi A, Brancatelli G, Vullierme MP, et al. Are pancreatic calcifications specific for the diagnosis of chronic pancreatitis? A multidetector-row CT analysis. Clin Radiol 2009;64:903–11.
28. Lowenfels AB, Maisonneuve PM, Cavallini G, et al. Pancreatitis and the risk of pancreatic cancer. N Engl J Med 1993;328:1435–7.
29. Johnson PT, Outwater EK. Pancreatic carcinoma versus chronic pancreatitis: dynamic MR imaging. Radiology 1999;212:213–18.
30. Balthazar EJ. Pancreatitis associated with pancreatic carcinoma. Preoperative diagnosis: role of CT imaging in detection and evaluation. Pancreatology 2005;5:330–44.
31. Morris-Stiff G, Webster P, Frost B, et al. Endoscopic ultrasound reliably identifies chronic pancreatitis when other imaging modalities have been non-diagnostic. JOP 2009;10:280–3.
32. Triantopoulou C, Dervenis C, Giannakou N, et al. Groove pancreatitis: a diagnostic challenge. Eur Radiol 2009;19:1736–43.
33. Shanbhogue AK, Fasih N, Surabhi VR, et al. A clinical and radiologic review of uncommon types and causes of pancreatitis. Radiographics 2009;29:1003–26.
34. Manfredi R, Frulloni L, Mantovani W, et al. Autoimmune pancreatitis: pancreatic and extrapancreatic MR imaging-MR cholangiopancreatography findings at diagnosis, after steroid therapy, and at recurrence. Radiology 2011;260:428–36.
35. Kim JH, Kim MH, Byun JH, et al. Diagnostic strategy for differentiating autoimmune pancreatitis from pancreatic cancer: is an endoscopic retrograde pancreatography essential? Pancreas 2012. (epub ahead of print).
36. Toomey DP, Swan N, Torreggiani W, Conlon KC. Autoimmune pancreatitis: medical and surgical management. JOP 2007;8:335–43.
37. Padilla-Thornton AE, Willmann JK, Jeffrey RB. Adenocarcinoma of the uncinate process of the pancreas: MDCT patterns of local invasion and clinical features at presentation. Eur Radiol 2012;22:1067–74.
38. Ozkan H, Kaya M, Cengiz A. Comparison of tumor marker CA 242 with CA 19-9 and carcinoembryonic antigen (CEA) in pancreatic cancer. Hepatogastroenterology 2003;50:1669–74.
39. Markocka-Maczka K. [Ca 19-9 antigen in differentiation of pancreatic inflammatory and neoplastic tumours]. Wiad Lek 2003;56:537–40.

40. Schima W, Ba-Ssalamah A, Kolblinger C, et al. Pancreatic adeno-carcinoma. Eur Radiol 2007;17:638–49.

41. Schima W, Ba-Ssalamah A, Goetzinger P, et al. State-of-the-art magnetic resonance imaging of pancreatic cancer. Top Magn Reson Imaging 2007;18:421–9.

42. Koelblinger C, Ba-Ssalamah A, Goetzinger P, et al. Gadobenate dimeglumine-enhanced 3.0-T MR imaging versus multiphasic 64-detector row CT: prospective evaluation in patients suspected of having pancreatic cancer. Radiology 2011;259: 757–66.

43. Rao SX, Zeng MS, Cheng WZ, et al. Small solid tumours (< or = 2 cm) of the pancreas: relative accuracy and differentiation of CT and MR imaging. Hepato-gastroenterology 2011;58: 996–1001.

44. Krishna NB, LaBundy JL, Saripalli S, et al. Diagnostic value of EUS-FNA in patients suspected of having pancreatic cancer with a focal lesion on CT scan/MRI but without obstructive jaundice. Pancreas 2009;38:625–30.

45. Tellez-Avila FI, Chavez-Tapia NC, Lopez-Arce G, et al. Vascular invasion in pancreatic cancer: predictive values for endoscopic ultrasound and computed tomography imaging. Pancreas 2012;41: 636–8.

46. Maemura K, Takao S, Shinchi H, et al. Role of positron emission tomography in decisions on treatment strategies for pancreatic cancer. J Hepatobiliary Panc Surg 2006;13:435–41.

47. Prokesch R, Chow LC, Beaulieu CF, et al. Isoattenuating pancreatic carcinoma at multi-detector row CT: secondary signs. Radiology 2002;224:764–8.

48. Yoon SH, Lee JM, Cho JY, et al. Small (≤ 20 mm) pancreatic adenocarcinomas: analysis of enhancement patterns and secondary signs with multiphasic multidetector CT. Radiology 2011;259: 442–52.

49. Takeshita K, Kutomi K, Haruyama T, et al. Imaging of early pancreatic cancer on multidetector row helical computed tomography. Br J Radiol 2010;83:823-30.

50. Schueller G, Schima W, Schueller-Weidekamm C, et al. Multidetector CT of pancreas: effects of contrast material flow rate and individualized scan delay on enhancement of pancreas and tumor contrast. Radiology 2006;241:441–8.

51. Walters DM, Lapar DJ, de Lange EE, et al. Pancreas-protocol imaging at a high-volume center leads to improved preoperative staging of pancreatic ductal adenocarcinoma. Ann Surg Oncol 2011;18:2764–71.

52. Lu DSK, Reber HA, Krasny RM, et al. Local staging of pancreatic cancer: criteria for unresectability of major vessels as revealed by pancreatic-phase thin section helical CT. Am J Roentgenol 1997; 168:1439–43.

53. Li H, Zeng MS, Zhou KR, et al. Pancreatic adenocarcinoma. The different CT criteria for peripancreatic major arterial and venous invasion. J Comput Assist Tomogr 2005;29:170–5.

54. Heye T, Zausig N, Klauss M, et al. CT diagnosis of recurrence after pancreatic cancer: is there a pattern? World J Gastroenterol 2011;17:1126–34.

55. Chang S, Choi D, Lee SJ, et al. Neuroendocrine neoplasms of the gastrointestinal tract: classification, pathologic basis, and imaging features. Radiographics 2007;27:1667–79.

56. Rha SE, Jung SE, Lee KL, et al. CT and MR imaging findings of endocrine tumor acccording to WHO classification. Eur J Radiol 2007;62:371–7.

57. Zhao Y, Wang X, Yang B, et al. Pancreatic insulinomas: experience in 220 patients. Zhonghua wai ke za zhi [Chin J Surg] 2000;38: 10–13.

58. Reznek RH. CT/MRI of neuroendocrine tumours. Cancer Imaging 2006;6:S163–177.

59. Gouya H, Vignaux O, Augui J, et al. CT, endoscopic sonography, and a combined protocol for preoperative evaluation of pancreatic insulinomas. Am J Roentgenol 2003;181:987–92.

60. Rappeport ED, Hansen CP, Kjaer A, Knigge U. Multidetector computed tomography and neuroendocrine pancreaticoduodenal tumours. Acta Radiol 2006;47:248–56.

61. Fidler JL, Fletcher JG, Reading CC, et al. Preoperative detection of pancreatic insulinomas on multiphasic helical CT. Am J Roentgenol 2003;181:775–80.

62. Ichikawa T, Peterson MS, Federle MP, et al. Islet cell tumor of the pancreas: biphasic CT versus MR imaging in tumor detection. Radiology 2000;216:163–71.

63. Caramella C, Dromain C, De Baere T, et al. Endocrine pancreatic tumours: which are the most useful MRI sequences? Eur Radiol 2010;20:2618–27.

64. Frilling A, Sotiropoulos GC, Radtke A, et al. The impact of 68Ga-DOTATOC positron emission tomography/computed tomography on the multimodal management of patients with neuroendocrine tumours. Ann Surg 2010;252:850–6.

65. Kumar R, Sharma P, Garg P, et al. Role of (68)Ga-DOTATOC PET-CT in the diagnosis and staging of pancreatic neuroendocrine tumours. Eur Radiol 2011;21:2408–16.

66. Happel B, Niederle B, Puespoek A, et al. [Benign neuroendocrine and other rare benign tumours of the pancreas]. Radiologe 2008; 48:752–63.

67. Pereira PL, Roche AJ, Maier GW, et al. Insulinoma and islet cell hyperplasia: value of the calcium intraarterial stimulation test when findings of other preoperative studies are negative. Radiology 1998;206:703–9.

68. Wiesli P, Brandle M, Schmid C, et al. Selective arterial calcium stimulation and hepatic venous sampling in the evaluation of hyperinsulinaemic hypoglycaemia: potential and limitations. J Vasc Interv Radiol 2004;15:1251–6.

69. Sahani DV, Kadavigere R, Saokar A, et al. Cystic pancreatic lesions: a simple imaging-based classification system for guiding management. Radiographics 2005;25:1471–84.

70. Morana G, Guarise A. Cystic tumours of the pancreas. Cancer Imaging 2006;6:60–71.

71. Fernandez-del Castillo C, Warshaw AL. Cystic tumours of the pancreas. Surg Clin North Am 1995;75:1001–16.

72. Crippa S, Salvia R, Warshaw AL, et al. Mucinous cystic neoplasm of the pancreas is not an aggressive entity: lessons from 163 resected patients. Ann Surg 2008;247:571–9.

73. Kim HJ, Lee DH, Ko YT, et al. CT of serous cystadenoma of the pancreas and mimicking masses. Am J Roentgenol 2008;190: 406–12.

74. Ogawa H, Itoh S, Ikeda M, et al. Intraductal papillary mucinous neoplasm of the pancreas: assessment of the likelihood of invasiveness with multisection CT. Radiology 2008;248:876–86.

75. Sugiyama M, Hagi H, Atomi Y, Saito M. Diagnosis of portal venous invasion by pancreatobiliary carcinoma: value of endoscopic ultrasonography. Abdom Imaging 1997;22:434–8.

76. Tanaka M, Chari S, Adsay V, et al. International consensus guidelines for management of intraductal papillary mucinous neoplasms and mucinous cystic neoplasms of the pancreas. Pancreatology 2006;6:17–32.

77. Guarise A, Faccioli N, Ferrari M, et al. Evaluation of serial changes of pancreatic branch duct intraductal papillary mucinous neoplasms by follow-up with magnetic resonance imaging. Cancer Imaging 2008;8:220–8.

78. Linder JD, Geenen JE, Catalano MF. Cyst fluid analysis obtained by EUS-guided FNA in the evaluation of discrete cystic neoplasms of the pancreas: a prospective single-center experience. Gastrointest Endoscopy 2006;64:697–702.

79. Attasaranya S, Pais S, LeBlanc J, et al. Endoscopic ultrasound-guided fine needle aspiration and cyst fluid analysis for pancreatic cysts. JOP 2007;8:553–63.

80. Laffan TA, Horton KM, Klein AP, et al. Prevalence of unsuspected pancreatic cysts on MDCT. Am J Roentgenol 2008; 191:802–7.

81. Girometti R, Intini SG, Cereser L, et al. Incidental pancreatic cysts: a frequent finding in liver-transplanted patients as assessed by 3D T2-weighted turbo spin echo magnetic resonance cholangiopancreatography. JOP 2009;10:507–14.

82. Kirkpatrick ID, Desser TS, Nino-Murcia M, Jeffrey RB. Small cystic lesions of the pancreas: clinical significance and findings at follow-up. Abdom Imaging 2007;32:119–25.

83. Handrich SJ, Hough DM, Fletcher JG, Sarr MG. The natural history of the incidentally discovered small simple pancreatic cyst: long-term follow-up and clinical implications. Am J Roentgenol 2005;184:20–3.

84. Uehara H, Nakaizumi A, Ishikawa O, et al. Development of ductal carcinoma of the pancreas during follow-up of branch duct intraductal papillary mucinous neoplasm of the pancreas. Gut 2008; 57:1561–5.

85. Iwamuro M, Kawamoto H, Shiraha H, et al. Pancreatic involvement in 11 cases of von Hippel–Lindau disease. Hepatogastroenterology 2012;59:589–91.

86. Raptopoulos V. Abdominal trauma. Emphasis on computed tomography. Radiol Clin North Am 1994;32:969–87.

87. Xu K, Zhou L, Liang B, et al. Safety and accuracy of percutaneous core needle biopsy in examining pancreatic neoplasms. Pancreas 2012;41:649–51.

88. Zech CJ, Helmberger T, Wichmann MW, et al. Large core biopsy of the pancreas under CT fluoroscopy control: results and complications. J Comput Assist Tomogr 2002;26:743–9.

89. Koo BC, Chinogureyi A, Shaw AS. Imaging acute pancreatitis. Br J Radiol 2010;83:104–12.

90. Shankar S, van Sonnenberg E, Silverman SG, et al. Imaging and percutaneous management of acute complicated pancreatitis. Cardiovasc Intervent Radiol 2004;27:567–80.

91. Van Sonnenberg E, Wittich GR, Chon KS, et al. Percutaneous radiologic drainage of pancreatic abscesses. Am J Roentgenol 1997;168:979–84.

92. Mithofer K, Mueller PR, Warshaw AL. Interventional and surgical treatment of pancreatic abscess. World J Surgery 1997;21:162–8.

CHAPTER 10

COMMON URORADIOLOGICAL REFERRALS: HAEMATURIA, LOIN PAIN, RENAL FAILURE AND INFECTION

Owen J. O'Connor • Tarek El-Diasty • Mohamed Abou El-Ghar • Michael M. Maher

CHAPTER OUTLINE

HAEMATURIA

Haematuria refers to the presence of red blood cells in urine. Radiological referral of selected patients is often necessary as part of clinical management for this problem; however, the optimal method of patient selection and the best imaging algorithm are subject to debate.[1] In this chapter we will outline current opinion regarding best practices for such patients.

Haematuria visible to the naked eye is said to be macroscopic, but when a microscope is required for detection, the term *microscopic haematuria* is used. Macroscopic haematuria is a strong predictor of serious underlying urological pathology. In one large study, 21% of patients with macroscopic haematuria were found to have malignancy, and repeat assessment yielded malignant findings in 12 of 35 (17%) patients with persistent symptoms, though initial tests were negative.[2] Microscopic haematuria is often initially detected using a urine dipstick test: a simple inexpensive examination that is useful if positive but insufficient to exclude haematuria on its own, especially at a single time point. Screening for haematuria in asymptomatic patients is of dubious value, since less than 2% of young patients with a positive dipstick test have a serious treatable urinary tract disease and data are conflicting in older patients.[3] In one study, 75% of patients referred for consultation following a positive urine dipstick test did not have microscopic haematuria at microscopy.[4] Myoglobin and free haemoglobin in urine account for many of these false-positive results. Therefore, it is recommended by the American Urological Association that urological referral for asymptomatic patients should only be made if there are greater than three red blood cells per high power field in two of three urine analyses.[5]

It is also recommended that specialist referral should be initiated after a single positive urinalysis, if patients have symptomatic microscopic haematuria, gross haematuria or if they are considered to be at increased risk for urological malignancy; subgroups of patients which are at increased risk of urological malignancy include smokers, those with occupational exposure to benzene or aromatic amines, irritation on voiding, resistant urinary tract infections, pelvic irradiation and analgesic abuse.[6] Patients with haematuria of suspected glomerular or tubular origin, suggested by the presence of proteinuria, red blood cell casts, raised creatinine or hypertension, should be evaluated by a nephrologist.[7] The remaining patients, who are more likely to have an epithelial source of haematuria, should be reviewed by a urologist.[7] A large number of lesions can give rise to haematuria; individual causes are discussed in greater detail in relevant chapters of this book. The most common non-glomerular causes of haematuria include stone disease, malignancy and infection. This chapter will assess aspects relevant to the radiological assessment of non-glomerular causes of haematuria (Table 10-1).

Renal Tract Calcifications

Uroradiological referral for patients with haematuria due to stone disease is common. Approximately 95% of patients with acute renal colic have haematuria.[8] Pathological calcification can occur in the renal parenchyma or collecting system. Nephrocalcinosis refers to the presence of pathological calcification in the renal parenchyma; 95% of cases of nephrocalcinosis occur in the medulla and the remainder in the cortex. Medullary nephrocalcinosis is caused by hyperparathyroidism, medullary sponge kidney, renal tubular acidosis, hypervitaminosis D and primary hyperoxaluria.[9] Cortical nephrocalcinosis is caused by acute cortical necrosis, chronic glomerulonephritis and primary hyperoxaluria. Nephrocalcinosis can be seen on conventional radiography and

TABLE 10-1　**Non-glomerular Causes of Haematuria Divided on the Basis of Renal or Extrarenal Aetiology**

Renal	Extrarenal
Tumour (renal cell cancer, transitional cell cancer angiomyolipoma, oncocytoma)	Tumour (transitional cell and prostate cancer, benign prostatic hyperplasia)
Vascular (arteriovenous malformation, renal vein thrombosis, infarct, transplant rejection, malignant hypertension, sickle cell disease)	Renal or ureteric stones
Metabolic (hypercalciuria, hyperuricuria)	Infection (cystitis, prostatitis, urinary schistosomiasis, tuberculosis, condyloma acuminatum)
Familial (polycystic kidney disease, medullary sponge kidney)	Coagulopathy or bleeding diathesis
Infection (pyelonephritis, tuberculosis, cytomegalovirus, infectious mononucleosis)	Trauma (including catheterisation and radiation)
Papillary necrosis	Medications (heparin, warfarin, cyclophosphamide)

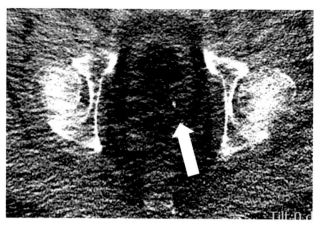

FIGURE 10-1 ■ **Low-dose renal stone protocol CT in a 34-year-old man with left vesicoureteric junction stone.** There is a 3-mm stone in the left vesicoureteric junction region (arrow). There is considerable noise in the image; however, with the application of adaptive statistical iterative reconstruction, this is acceptable since the stone is clearly visible. The effective dose was only 0.5 mSv, and therefore less than conventional radiography.

ultrasound. Stippled patterns of calcification are observed on conventional radiographs in the cortical and medullary regions of the kidneys due to cortical and medullary nephrocalcinosis, respectively. On ultrasound, increased echogenicity rather than discrete calcification may be perceived.

Nephrolithiasis refers to stone disease in the renal collecting system. The incidence of nephrolithiasis in patients with microscopic and macroscopic haematuria is 7.8 and 8.8%, respectively.[10] Calcium phosphate and calcium oxalate stones, which account for the majority of renal stones, are radio-opaque, as are struvite stones, which represent 15% of renal stones, and develop in the setting of infection and alkaline urine. Urate and xanthine stones represent 5% of renal stones and are radiolucent. Most renal stones are hyperattenuating on unenhanced computed tomography (CT) (150–1000 Hounsfield units (HU)). Crystalline stones are an exception; these are associated with use of protease inhibitors and are hypoattenuating. Calcification within tumours, haematoma, or fungal masses tends to have attenuation of less than 50 HU.[11]

Imaging of Renal and Ureteric Stones

Unenhanced CT or stone protocol CT is gradually becoming established as the one-stop imaging study of choice for renal and ureteric stone evaluation. Conventional radiography has a sensitivity of only 60% for renal stone detection, whereas ultrasound has a sensitivity and specificity for urolithiasis of 40 and 84%, respectively, compared with CT.[12,13] Ultrasound tends to overestimate stone size and has reduced sensitivity and specificity for small stones and those located in the ureters.[14]

Meta-analysis of unenhanced CT compared with intravenous urography (IVU) also confirms superiority of CT for acute urolithiasis.[15] CT radiation dose reduction techniques have dramatically reduced dose and strengthens the case in favour of CT as first-line imaging for urolithiasis. For example, adaptive statistical iterative reconstruction blended with filtered back projection can provide diagnostic imaging at approximately 20% of the normal radiation dose (Fig. 10-1).[16] This is possible since most renal stones are conspicuous relative to surrounding tissues and therefore less radiation dose is required for diagnosis since a greater degree of image noise may be tolerated. This of course comes at the cost of potentially missing other lesions that have soft-tissue attenuation. CT is not only excellent for stone detection but also helps clinical decision-making. The presence and severity of ureteric or renal obstruction can be estimated and the likelihood of spontaneous stone passage may also be determined (Fig. 10-2). Spontaneous passage occurs in 76% of calculi that measure 2–4 mm, 60% for calculi that measure 5–7 mm, 48% for calculi that measure 7–9 mm and less than 25% for stones greater than 9 mm.[17]

Imaging of Renal and Ureteric Tumours

CT is excellent for the detection and assessment of renal and urothelial tumours and is considered the imaging technique of choice for renal mass evaluation. CT imaging in this context is typically performed in the control, corticomedullary and nephrographic phases after intravenous contrast medium administration (Fig. 10-3). Unenhanced CT is useful for detection of calcification in renal tumours or fat in an angiomyolipoma (Fig. 10-4). Corticomedullary phase imaging is useful for cortical assessment, detection of angiogenesis in clear cell carcinoma, and recognition of pseudotumours, which may not be appreciated on later phase imaging. Most renal and urothelial tumours are maximally conspicuous during the

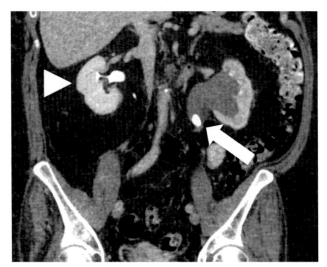

FIGURE 10-2 ■ **Obstructing left renal stone in a 61-year-old female patient.** There is a 7-mm stone in the upper left ureter (arrow), hydronephrosis and delayed left renal enhancement relative to the right kidney (arrowhead) on this CT urogram obtained in the nephropyelographic phase by split bolus intravenous contrast medium injection.

nephrographic phase. A difference of greater than 20 HU between unenhanced and nephrographic phase units is strongly predictive of enhancement and therefore renal neoplasm, as is a Hounsfield unit difference of greater than 10 between the corticomedullary and nephrographic phases (Fig. 10-5).[18] A difference of 10 HU between unenhanced and nephrographic phase CT is not indicative of enhancement, and a difference of 10–20 HU is equivocal. Increased attenuation can be observed in non-enhancing tissues after contrast administration due to a phenomenon known as pseudoenhancement, which is likely due to CT reconstruction algorithms. In addition, care must be taken when measuring enhancement, ensuring that the enhancing solid portion of a lesion is studied and not the cystic component (Fig. 10-6). The authors have a low threshold for biopsy in cases where imaging is equivocal and surgical management will be determined by whether a lesion is neoplastic.

Unfortunately, oncocytomas cannot be accurately distinguished from renal cell carcinoma using CT, although it is suggested that magnetic resonance imaging (MRI) may be helpful for making this important distinction (Fig. 10-7). Contrast medium-enhanced MRI is also very useful for renal lesion characterisation, especially for detection of fat within an angiomyolipoma and diffusion- and perfusion-weighted imaging has also improved lesion detection and characterisation.[19] CT assessment of haematuria can be performed using unenhanced CT and post-intravenous contrast medium-enhanced CT, including CT urography (CTU). CTU entails imaging the kidneys and collecting systems in the pyelographic phase. Normally, the collecting systems can also be examined in the control and nephrographic phases as part of a complete CTU protocol. The CTU technique is discussed in detail in Chapter 38. There is good evidence to indicate that traditional methods of haematuria assessment using IVU and ultrasound are improved upon by CTU. One

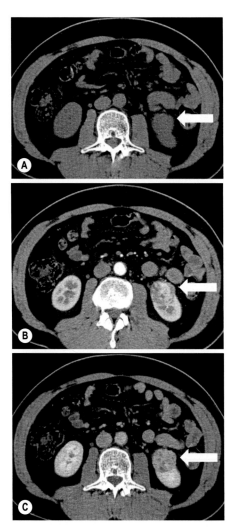

FIGURE 10-3 ■ **Renal mass protocol CT in a 75-year-old man with renal cell carcinoma.** (A) There is an exophytic mass (arrow) in the left kidney on unenhanced CT. (B) There is avid heterogeneous enhancement (arrow) in the corticomedullary phase. (C) The mass enhances to a lesser degree (arrow) than normal renal tissue in the nephrographic phase.

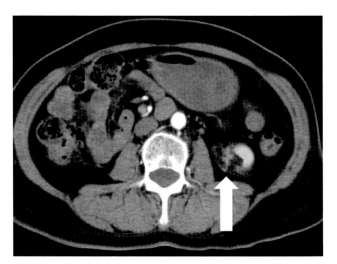

FIGURE 10-4 ■ **Non-contrast CT of 44-year-old woman with angiomyolipoma.** There is a left renal mass (arrow) that has hypoattenuating components consistent with fat, which is virtually diagnostic of angiomyolipoma.

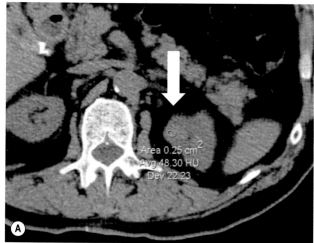

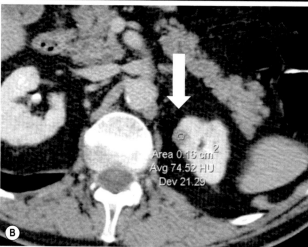

FIGURE 10-5 ■ **Renal cell carcinoma on CT in a 71-year-old man.** (A) There is a cortical-based left upper pole renal mass (arrow) which has attenuation of 48 HU on unenhanced CT within a region of interest placed over the lesion. This alone is suspicious for a solid lesion. (B) Following intravenous contrast administration, the lesion (arrow) measures 75 HU, indicating definitive enhancement and suggesting renal neoplasm.

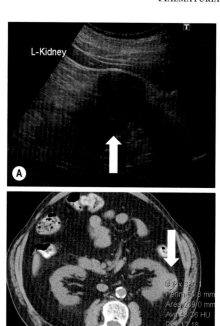

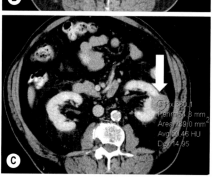

FIGURE 10-6 ■ **Renal cell carcinoma in a 72-year-old man.** (A) There is a mixed solid/cystic lesion (arrow) in the left kidney on ultrasound. (B) The attenuation within the region of interest (arrow) drawn over the lesion measured 43 HU. (C) The attenuation in the region of interest (arrow) was not considerably greater (50 HU) following intravenous contrast administration. The kidney was removed and the lesion confirmed to be a cystic renal cell carcinoma. The region of interest was probably drawn over cystic components of the lesion.

compelling study compared retrograde ureteropyelography (UP), the imaging gold standard for assessing the ureters and renal pelvis, with CTU.[20] A cohort of 106 patients who had initial assessment with IVU and cystoscopy underwent CTU and UP with a 3- to 5-year follow-up period and histological reference standard. The sensitivity, specificity, positive predictive value and negative predictive value of CTU for diagnosing transitional cell carcinoma of the upper urinary tract was 0.97, 0.93, 0.79 and 0.99, respectively. This was comparable to UP. Of note, the positive predictive value of CTU, 0.79, is not very strong. Patients should have histological confirmation prior to undergoing surgery for findings on CTU.

Risk Stratification of Patients with Haematuria for Triage to Computed Tomography

One would prefer to use CTU for legitimate indications and minimise wasted resources and radiation exposure.

A reasonable algorithm has been suggested to address this issue.[21] Patients with haematuria could be divided into low- and high-risk groups following exclusion of urinary tract infection. Low-risk patients include patients with either microscopic or macroscopic haematuria aged less than 40 years and patients with microscopic haematuria aged greater than 40 years. High-risk patients include those with macroscopic haematuria aged greater than 40 years. Low-risk patients would be imaged with ultrasound if aged less than 40 years for the assessment of medical renal disease and non-contrast CT would be used for patients aged less than 40 years with macroscopic haematuria or patients aged greater than 40 years with microscopic haematuria, since renal stone disease is the most common cause of haematuria in these patients. Patients in the high-risk group would be imaged with CTU. It has also been suggested that a risk stratification score could be incorporated into this algorithm to ensure

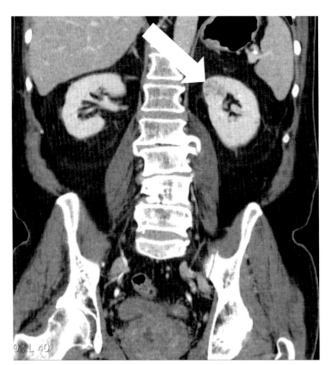

FIGURE 10-7 ■ **Oncocytoma in an elderly female patient.** There is a heterogeneously enhancing left upper pole renal mass (arrow) on coronal nephrographic phase CT. The lesion is indistinguishable from renal cell carcinoma based on imaging features alone.

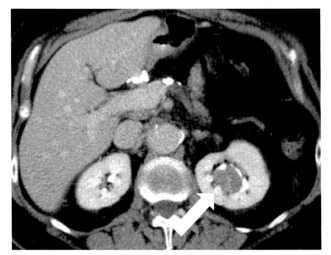

FIGURE 10-8 ■ **Transitional cell carcinoma on split bolus CT urogram.** There is a filling defect in the interpolar region of the left kidney (arrow) due to transitional cell carcinoma.

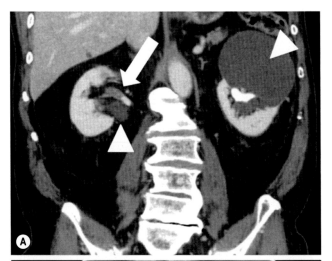

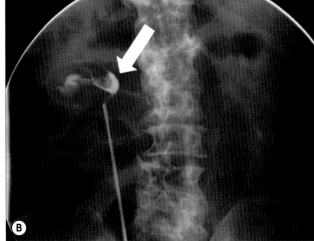

FIGURE 10-9 ■ **Transitional cell carcinoma of renal collecting system.** (A) There is a hypoenhancing mass (arrow) in the upper pole collecting system of the right kidney on CT urography obtained in the nephropyelographic phase by split bolus technique. There are parapelvic cysts in both kidneys (arrowheads). (B) There is a smooth filling defect (arrow) in the upper pole collecting system producing a phantom calyx appearance on retrograde pyelography.

optimal patient selection for CTU. Similarly, CTU can be used as a triage tool for intravesical transitional cell carcinoma assessment in the setting of haematuria. Based on a large study of 778 patients with visible haematuria aged >40 years, it was suggested that, rather than investigating all patients initially with flexible cystoscopy, patients should first undergo CTU. If a bladder lesion is detected by CTU, patients should undergo rigid cystoscopy, whereas a normal CTU should be followed with flexible cystoscopy. The authors suggested that following this strategy would reduce the number of flexible cystoscopies by 17% without reducing detection rates.[22] Urine cytology has had a poor sensitivity and some suggest that it no longer has a role at a rapid diagnosis clinic where CTU and cystoscopy are available.

Imaging Features of Urothelial Tumours on Computed Tomography

Although CT has superseded IVU and ultrasound for detection of urothelial cancers, many of the imaging signs sought on CT imaging have been previously described using IVU.[23] Early urothelial neoplasms appear as subtle filling defects or focal mural thickening on IVU and CT (Fig. 10-8). Transitional cell cancers (TCC) can appear as fixed smooth or irregular, single or multiple filling defects within the renal collecting systems. Renal TCC can obstruct an infundibulum, creating a phantom calyx that may or may not fill with contrast (Fig. 10-9). Pelviureteric junction obstruction can produce a delayed nephrogram or ureteric involvement can cause acute hydronephrosis. Signs of ureteric TCC include absent

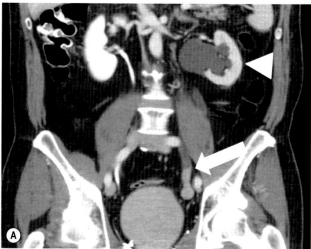

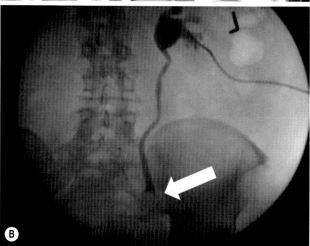

FIGURE 10-10 ■ **Transitional cell carcinoma of the ureter.** (A) There is an enhancing mass in the distal ureter (arrow) at CT urography. There is proximal hydronephrosis and delayed nephrogram of the left renal collecting system and kidney (arrowhead) relative to the right. (B) There is an abrupt filling defect of the ureter (arrow) on antegrade pyelography due to the mass in the left ureter.

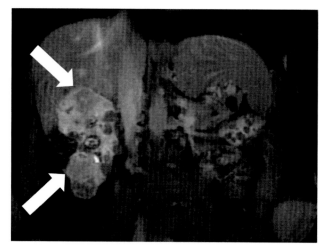

FIGURE 10-11 ■ **MRI in a patient with two right renal cell carcinomas.** Coronal T1 fat-saturated post-contrast imaging depicts masses in the upper and lower poles of the right kidney (arrows). These were renal cell carcinomas. The patient had prior left nephrectomy for renal cell carcinoma.

renal function, eccentric or circumferential fixed wall thickening, filling defects, hydronephrosis with or without hydroureter and irregular ureteric narrowing with proximal shouldering termed the *goblet sign* (Fig. 10-10). Filling detects may also be produced by metastases, calculi, blood clots, infection, a vascular impression or congenital abnormality such as pyelourethritis cystica. The ultrasonic characteristics of urothelial tumours are variable. Transitional cell cancer is often slightly hyperechoic, but may be difficult to differentiate from renal sinus fat, and further imaging is always needed for confirmation.

There are many other causes of haematuria. Infection will be discussed later in this chapter. Many causes are diagnosed early in life using ultrasound, based on family history, or clinical findings, such as von Hippel–Lindau syndrome, tuberous sclerosis, polycystic kidney disease and medullary sponge kidney. Repeated imaging plays an essential role in screening for renal tumour development in many of these cases. It is preferable in many cases that this be done using MRI if possible since contrast

resolution will be superior to unenhanced CT in patients with renal insufficiency, and, even in the absence of renal insufficiency, the use of MRI will limit the number of CT studies performed over a patient's lifetime and lifetime cumulative radiation exposure (Fig. 10-11).

Haematuria as a result of trauma requires imaging to determine whether there is renal parenchymal injury, involvement of perirenal or periureteric tissues, bladder rupture and/or presence of pseudoaneurysm. Unenhanced imaging as part of CT evaluation in the setting of suspected trauma is essential. When performing angiography in the setting of iatrogenic haematuria following percutaneous nephrostomy drain insertion, an angiographic run may need to be performed while the nephrostomy drain is removed over a guidewire, to detect active bleeding or pseudoaneurysm formation, when not seen on initial angiographic sequences (Fig. 10-12).

LOIN PAIN

The loin or *flank* is an anatomical area between the ribs and pelvis lateral to the spine. The kidneys and ureters receive visceral nerve supply from T10–L1 and T11–L1, respectively. Renal or ureteric pathology causes referred painful stimuli transmitted by the somatic fibres to be perceived over the dermatomes at the loin. Acute flank pain is a common clinical entity which may be secondary to urinary or extraurinary causes.[24] Urinary obstruction secondary to urinary tract calculi is the most common cause. Urinary tract calculi are very common, affecting 3–5% of the population,[25] men more than women, and the incidence increases with age up to 60 years.[23] Caucasian patients are more likely to develop urinary tract calculi than patients of African origin and calculi are much less common in children than adults.[23] Calculi typically become lodged in specific anatomic areas along the course of the ureter: the ureteropelvic junction, where the ureter crosses the iliac vessels, and at the vesicoureteric junction.[26] It is important to remember that the

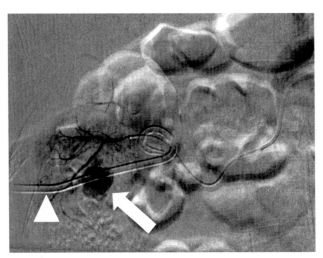

FIGURE 10-12 ■ **Renal pseudoaneurysm on angiography in a male patient with haematuria post percutaneous nephrostomy.** There is a pseudoaneurysm (arrow) in the lower pole of the right kidney on digital subtraction angiography. The patient's percutaneous nephrostomy is seen (arrowhead). Sometimes it is necessary to withdraw the catheter over a wire at angiography for optimal assessment so that the tamponade effect is removed and the pseudoaneurym is seen. If there is abrupt haemorrhage, the nephrostomy catheter should be promptly replaced until definitive treatment can be completed.

probability of spontaneous passage of small calculi (less than or equal to 5 mm) is very high but that larger stones (over 10 mm) are unlikely to pass spontaneously.[25] Therefore, determination of the size of a ureteric calculus is fundamental to deciding the appropriate management.

Imaging of Patients with Loin Pain

An ideal imaging investigation for patients with acute flank pain should be a single imaging test that provides accurate information not only about the present or absence of urinary tract stones but also about the size and position of the calculus and the presence of related complications, such as obstruction. One of the major clinical challenges managing patients with urinary tract calculi is that symptoms are frequently non-specific and also that urinary tract calculi tend to be recurrent. In addition, there are many other potential causes of acute loin pain. Other urological causes of loin pain include blood clots or tumour in the collecting systems, obstruction of the pelviureteric junction and infection such as acute pyelonephritis or pyonephrosis. There are several non-urological causes of acute loin pain including gallbladder problems such as biliary colic or acute cholecystitis, abdominal aortic aneurysm leakage, pneumonia, myocardial infarction, ovarian or testicular torsion, ectopic pregnancy, appendicitis, omental infarction, epiploic appendigitis, inflammatory bowel disease, acute diverticulitis or even intervertebral disc prolapse. Chronic loin pain can be caused by urological neoplasms including renal cell carcinoma, transitional cell carcinoma, renal and ureteric stones, tuberculosis, pelvic ureteric junction obstruction, testicular cancer, gastrointestinal neoplasms and spinal disease. Therefore, evaluation with imaging is recommended at initial presentation.

Radiography

The evaluation of acute flank pain commonly includes urinalysis, plain radiography of the kidneys, ureter and bladder (KUB), intravenous urography, ultrasound, or unenhanced CT (known as stone protocol CT or CT KUB) used alone or in combination.[25] The role of MR urography in this setting is still being studied, but limited sensitivity for calcification remains a major limitation. Plain radiography is still often the first imaging study performed for a patient with loin pain. The sensitivity of plain radiography for detection of urinary tract calculi has been reported in the range 58–62%. Using CT as a reference standard, Levine et al. reported sensitivities of only 59% for detecting urinary tract calculi on KUB.[27] Currently the role of KUB is limited when performed alone, but may be very useful when used in combination with ultrasound for detection of urinary tract calculi. However, even when KUB is used in combination with ultrasound, their combined sensitivities are well below unenhanced CT.[25]

Ultrasound

Ultrasound in the setting of acute flank pain may be very useful. First, exposure to ionising radiation is avoided, which is especially important in children and pregnant patients. Ultrasound is capable of determining whether there is obstruction of urinary tract by assessing for direct signs of obstruction such as hydronephrosis and hydroureter. Early ultrasound in this setting, however, can miss acute obstruction in up to 30% of patients since it can take several hours for hydronephrosis and hydroureter to develop following stone impaction.[25] Ultrasound suffers further disadvantages in pregnant patients due to the phenomenon of physiological hydronephrosis, which is observed in up to 80% of patients. This occurs in the absence of urinary stones and affects the right side more often than the left. Neither ultrasound, IVU or MR urography is as sensitive or specific as CT for determining the cause of obstruction. Combined imaging using ultrasound to determine the presence or absence of hydronephrosis and hydroureter in conjunction with KUB to examine for urinary tract calculi is a common imaging strategy in the setting of acute loin pain. This remains less sensitive for urinary tract calculus detection compared with IVU and is much less sensitive than unenhanced CT (stone protocol).

MR Urography

MR urography in the evaluation of patients with acute flank pain is limited by poor access in the acute setting at many centres, increased study duration compared with unenhanced CT, and most importantly, by substantially reduced sensitivity for urinary tract stones and, therefore, for definitive direct stone identification.[28] Differentiation of a urinary stone from other intraluminal filling defects such as blood clot or tumour is difficult on MR urography. MR urography is frequently used in pregnant patients with loin pain and suspected obstructing urinary tract calculi. This is often performed following ultrasound of the kidneys. MR urography in this setting is useful for confirming the presence of true hydronephrosis and determining the level of apparent obstruction. As with MR urography in the non-pregnant patient, definitive detection of renal and ureteric calculi is difficult because of the limited sensitivity for calcification. Recent advances in low-dose CT have shown good sensitivity and specificity for stone diagnosis in pregnant patients, but the use of low-dose CT in this setting remains unproven and still very controversial.

Computed Tomography

Since Smith et al. first described the use of unenhanced CT or *stone protocol* CT in evaluation of the patients with loin pain, multiple studies have confirmed impressive sensitivities of 95–96% and specificities of 98% for detection of urinary tract calculi.[29] Not only is unenhanced CT good for determining the presence of calculi but also it can detect associated obstruction and also immediately determines the level of obstruction and the size of the obstructing stone. Obstruction is suggested by identifying hydronephrosis and hydroureter above the level of the obstructing calculus and also by the presence of secondary signs of obstruction such as perirenal and periureteric fat stranding. Indeed, the degree of perinephric fat stranding in the obstructed kidney has been reported in some studies to correlate inversely with the likelihood of stone passage. Unenhanced CT also enjoys the advantage of contrast medium avoidance over IVU. CT is rapid and does not require repeated imaging (compared with IVU) to determine the site of obstruction. The major concern associated with the use of unenhanced CT, however, is associated exposure to ionising radiation. In recent years, unenhanced CT protocols which can provide comprehensive evaluation of the urinary tract for the presence of calculi with effective doses reported in a range comparable to IVU or even lower have been described. A meta-analysis of studies assessing diagnostic accuracy of low-dose unenhanced CT for evaluation of patients with suspected urinary tract calculi in the sub 3-mSv range found sensitivities of 97% and specificity of 95% for detection of urinary tract calculi.[25,30] Recently, there has been increasing interest in the use of dual-energy CT as a means of characterising urinary tract calculi composition. Some studies have suggested that dual-energy CT imaging can be used to differentiate various subtypes of urinary tract calculi such as uric acid stones, cysteine stones and struvite stones.[31]

Intravenous Urography

Before the development of unenhanced CT protocols for suspected urinary stones, IVU was the investigation of choice in this setting.[25] There are several reasons why IVU has been replaced by CT: avoidance of the requirement for intravenous contrast medium administration with CT, avoidance of repeated studies up to 24 hours after commencing IVU, and better determination of the site of ureteric obstruction using CT. Another major advantage of CT is the ability to detect alternative causes of flank pain such as acute appendicitis, acute diverticulitis, epiploic appendagitis and others which can be difficult to diagnose with ultrasound and are almost never identified de novo on IVU and plain radiography.

Useful Signs on Unenhanced CT and Potential Pitfalls

The most important imaging finding on CT in acute ureteral obstruction secondary to urinary stone disease is direct visualisation of a calculus in the ureteric lumen. The certainty of diagnosis is strengthened by finding a dilated ureter above the stone. Definitive characterisation of a calcification as a calculus is supported by the identification of a *soft-tissue rim sign*.[23] This is a soft-tissue attenuation surrounding the calcification and indicates that the calcification is in the ureter. Pelvic phleboliths do not have surrounding soft tissue and therefore this sign is crucial for distinction. The presence of increased perinephric or pereuretericfat stranding also represents a secondary sign suggestive of downstream ureteric obstruction.

There are also a number of potential pitfalls on unenhanced CT in the detection of urinary tract calculi and in the characterisation of an abdominal or pelvic calcification as a urinary tract calculus. Calcifications of iliac vessels and their branches can be difficult to differentiate from an adjacent ureteric calculus.[23] When it is difficult to definitively conclude that an abdominal or pelvic calcification lies in the lumen of the left ureter, intravenous contrast medium administration and pyelographic phase CT imaging can help make the distinction between ureteric calculi and extraluminal calcifications.[23] Currently, this strategy carries a disadvantage of increased exposure to ionising radiation and potential nephrotoxicity from iodinated contrast media. Other problems for radiologists on unenhanced CT include parapelvic cysts or an extrarenal pelvis which can mimic hydronephrosis;[23] the distinction of these entities can be made by ultrasound or on pyelographic phase enhanced CT. A large adnexal cyst can simulate a distended bladder. Following the entire ureteric course on unenhanced CT in a thin patient with paucity of peritoneal and retroperitoneal fat can be very difficult and this situation can be exacerbated by the present of multiple phleboliths in the pelvis.

RENAL FAILURE

Imaging of the kidneys in the setting of renal failure has two principal aims: to demonstrate or exclude obstruction and to show renal size, since small kidneys indicate irreversible chronic renal failure. Ultrasound is generally the first imaging investigation performed in this clinical setting, since it assesses renal size and collecting system appearances. Underlying causes of renal impairment such as autosomal dominant polycystic kidney disease or collecting system stones can also be identified during the course of this examination.

Renal obstruction is demonstrated on ultrasound in an indirect manner by showing pelvicalyceal and/or ureteric dilatation proximal to the level of obstruction, with a change in calibre of the collecting system and/or ureter at the level of obstruction which is often not well seen using ultrasound alone. Obstructive appearances can be difficult to distinguish from non-obstructive lesions such as an extrarenal pelvis or parapelvic cyst. The Doppler resistive index ((peak systolic − end diastolic velocity)/

peak systolic velocity) measure is a useful means of differentiating acute renal collecting system obstruction from non-obstructive causes of collecting system dilatation. The resistive index is greater than normal (0.7) in the setting of acute obstruction. Ultrasound can help differentiate between the two most common causes of acute renal failure. An increased resistive index is observed in non-obstructive renal failure due to acute tubular necrosis but not in the setting of prerenal azotaemia.[32] Unenhanced CT is indicated to assess the pelvicalyceal system if ultrasound is inconclusive, to detect stones or as part of a multiphase study. Unenhanced MRI may be used as an alternative to CT and provides similar anatomical information, with coronal T2-weighted sequences providing detailed imaging of the collecting system. Dynamic radionuclide renography is the simplest and safest way to assess renal perfusion in patients with renal failure, helping to differentiate reversible causes such as acute tubular necrosis from other conditions with a poorer prognosis such as renal cortical necrosis.

Ultrasound is also a practical means of image guidance for non-focal biopsy in the setting of renal dysfunction. Imaging-guided renal biopsy is indicated for patients with unexplained acute renal failure. Haemorrhage is one of the potentially serious complications of renal biopsy. Renal biopsy is considered a high-risk procedure in terms of bleeding risk since bleeding can be hard to detect and control.[33] Asymptomatic perinephric haematoma is demonstrated in up to 90% of patients on CT and 44% on ultrasound following renal biopsy. Asymptomatic arteriovenous fistulae also occur but these often spontaneously close.[34] Symptomatic bleeding, macroscopic haematuria or perinephric haematoma occur in less than 10% of patients after biopsy and less than 5% of these patients require transfusion or surgery. Mortality rate of renal biopsy is approximately 1 per 1000. Small kidneys with a parenchymal thickness of 1 cm or less are not usually biopsied because histological samples have a greater chance of being non-diagnostic and biopsy has an increased associated complication rate in these cases.

Renal size and parenchymal thickness are used to categorize non-obstructive renal failure as acute or chronic; chronic renal failure is characterised by small kidneys with thin parenchyma. Ultrasound provides accurate measurements of renal length, although this is normally less than the corresponding urographic measurement, with 9 cm representing the lower limit of normal adult kidney length, equivalent to a urographic measurement of 11.5 cm. Renal parenchymal thinning occurs before renal length decreases.

Chronic Renal Failure

Chronic kidney disease is divided into five stages:

Stage 1: normal (glomerular filtration rate > 90 mL/min/1.73 m^2).

Stage 2: mild impairment (glomerular filtration rate 60–89 mL/min/1.73 m^2).

Stage 3: moderate (glomerular filtration rate 31–59 mL/min/1.73 m^2).

Stages 4 and 5: severe (glomerular filtration rate 15–29 and < 15 mL/min/1.73 m^2, respectively).[35]

In non-obstructive chronic renal failure, ultrasound demonstrates small kidneys with diffuse or focally reduced parenchymal thickness. As in acute renal failure, parenchymal reflectivity may be normal or increased, and increased reflectivity does not point towards a specific diagnosis. Although an increased resistive index (RI) may be detected in the intrarenal arteries on Doppler interrogation, this is often insufficient alone to identify the cause of renal failure. Ultrasound elastography for renal assessment is currently being investigated as a means of quantifying renal fibrosis. The most common cause of chronic kidney disease is diabetes. Non-diabetic causes are divided into glomerular, vascular, tubulointerstitial and cystic aetiologies. Notable causes of renal failure relevant to imaging include the following conditions.

Autosomal Dominant Polycystic Kidney Disease (Adult Polycystic Kidney Disease)

Autosomal dominant polycystic kidney disease is responsible for renal failure in 10–15% of patients who receive dialysis.

Tuberous Sclerosis

Between 5 and 15% of patients with tuberous sclerosis develop renal failure and have multiple cysts with an appearance indistinguishable from autosomal dominant polycystic kidney disease. Differentiation depends on detecting the other typical clinical features of tuberous sclerosis (e.g. central nervous system features).

Acquired Cystic Kidney Disease (ACKD)

Acquired cystic kidney disease is observed in up to 13% of patients with chronic renal disease before commencing dialysis.[36] It also occurs in patients on long-term haemo- or peritoneal dialysis and depends on the duration of dialysis, occurring in over 90% of patients after 5 years of dialysis. The majority of patients are asymptomatic but in some patients cysts bleed and cause pain or haematuria. ACKD can usually be distinguished from autosomal dominant polycystic kidney disease because the kidneys are small or normal in size and cysts are less numerous. Patients with ACKD have an increased incidence of renal cell carcinoma, including low-grade papillary tumours. Following renal transplantation, ACKD persists and the risk of haemorrhage and development of renal cell cancer also continues.

Renovascular Disease

Renovascular disease is an important cause of chronic renal failure, responsible for renal failure in 14% of patients over the age of 50 years old accepted for renal replacement therapy and, more importantly, it represents one of the few treatable causes. Doppler resistive index is increased in patients with non-obstructive causes of renal failure. A decreased resistive index can be observed in patients with flow-limiting renal artery stenosis and can cause a parvus tardus wave pattern due to reduced arterial flow, and a resistive index difference of more than 0.05 between kidneys helps in the identification of renal artery stenosis. Overall, resistive index measurements are not specific for renal artery stenosis detection, since the index can also be increased by renal vein thrombosis and renal obstruction. Cross-sectional imaging by CT or MR angiography should be considered for confirmation in these cases.

Contrast Medium-Induced Nephrotoxicity

Contrast medium nephrotoxicity is defined as a serum creatinine increase of more than 25% or 44 µmol/L within 3 days of intravascular contrast medium administration, for which there is no other explanation.[37,38] The causality link between intravenous contrast medium administration and nephropathy has received renewed interest recently. This is based on the observation that many assumptions have been made when extrapolating results from invasive angiographic studies which lacked control arms and that 13 control studies showed that patients who received contrast medium were less likely to suffer acute kidney injury.[39] A large single-centre retrospective case-control study of 15,7140 CT examinations which stratified patients into low-, medium- and high-risk subgroups demonstrated no increased risk of nephropathy following intravenous contrast medium administration.[40] Until this issue has been resolved through prospective study one would suggest continued caution regarding intravenous contrast medium administration to patients with renal impairment. Alternative imaging methods, without iodinated contrast media, should be chosen in patients with considerably impaired renal function (CKD 4 or 5) where possible. When it is essential to give contrast media to patients with moderate renal impairment (low or moderate impairment; CKD 3), precautionary administration of *N*-acetylcysteine and normal saline are associated with a low incidence of contrast medium-induced nephropathy.[41]

Nephrogenic Systemic Fibrosis

Gadolinium-enhanced MRI was once the default cross-sectional imaging method for patients with marked renal impairment and was also sometimes used instead of iodine-based contrast media for conventional angiography. This has had deleterious consequences for some patients. Gadolinium administration can result in a debilitating condition known as nephrogenic systemic fibrosis. Nephrogenic systemic fibrosis is a systemic condition that primarily affects the skin of patients with renal impairment. Increased numbers of fibrocytes result in skin thickening and plaque formation which evolves to cause flexion contractures, paraesthesia and pruritus.[42] Gadolinium administration should therefore be judiciously used in patients in chronic renal impairment depending on the severity of disease and the type of gadolinium agent.[43] Although the mechanism by which gadolinium induces nephrogenic systemic fibrosis is not known, adoption of precautionary measures has reduced the number of cases reported.[44]

INFECTION

Urinary tract infection is the most common human infection, responsible for seven million physician visits and 100,000 hospitalisations annually in the Unites States.[45] Urinary tract infections (UTIs) account for the greatest proportion (31%) of nosocomial infections in American medical intensive care units, while they represent the second most common nosocomial infection in Europe after respiratory infection.[46,47] Healthy adults with a UTI who exhibit a prompt response to medical treatment do not require diagnostic imaging. A first UTI in a man should be imaged, whereas female patients should be imaged if 2–3 UTIs occur within a 12-month period.[48] Complicated UTIs require imaging to assess for predisposing factors and to direct medical or interventional management. Complicated UTIs entail infection with an uncommon organism, severe symptoms, findings suggestive of renal obstruction such as renal colic, or failure to respond within 72 hours after appropriate antibiotic therapy.[47] Early imaging is indicated for suspected pyonephrosis, renal infarction or where urinalysis and symptomatology are incongruent.[49] A lower threshold exists for imaging high-risk patients; diabetics, elderly, transplant recipients, those receiving chemotherapy, human immunodeficiency virus (HIV) sufferers and other immunocompromised groups.[50] Many radiological imaging techniques have been used to image UTIs, including ultrasound, IVU, CT, MRI, renal cortical scintigraphy and positron emission tomography (PET).[51]

Acute Pyelonephritis

Acute pyelonephritis (APN) is an acute infection of the renal parenchyma and collecting system. It is a clinical syndrome characterized by *upper tract signs* including high-grade fever (>38.5°C), rigors, nausea/vomiting and costovertebral angle tenderness. Symptoms include flank or suprapubic pain, dysuria, frequency or urgency.[50] Tubulointerstitial inflammation causes parenchymal swelling and renal enlargement. Inflammation can affect the perinephric fat, Gerota's fascia, and, very rarely the extrarenal space.[52] Extrarenal extension usually occurs in untreated cases, uncontrolled diabetics or immunocompromised patients. Microabscesses can coalesce to form a renal abscess, which may rupture into the perirenal space or extend to adjacent organs such as the liver. Usually infection ascends through the collecting system; occasionally it seeds haematogenously, or rarely enters through lymphatics. Ascending infection from the urethra to bladder causes cystitis; this extends to the upper tract in half of cases.[53] Major risk factors include long-term catheterisation, faecal soiling in chronic ill patients or vesicoureteric reflux (VUR).[54] Ureteric peristalsis is hindered by Gram-negative endotoxins and anatomic obstruction to urinary flow; therefore, VUR is not essential for infection ascent.[55] Bacteria enter the renal parenchyma through collecting ducts at renal papillae, causing an infectious-inflammatory response extending from the collecting tubules into the renal interstitium.[56] Leucocytes and debris tend to occlude renal tubules and patchy or lobar vasoconstriction of intrarenal arteries and arterioles also occurs.[51]

Haematogenous seeding tends to occur among intravenous drug abusers, those with extrarenal infection (dental, cutaneous, or coronary valves), immuno-compromised or paediatric patients.[51] Urinary tract obstruction may precipitate haematogenous seeding through reduced urinary clearance of the responsible organisms.[57] In contradistinction to ascending infection, haematogenous seeding begins in the cortex and involves the medulla 24–48 hours after bacterial inoculation. Initially, haematogenous infection causes multiple, small, peripheral round lesions without a lobar distribution. Once the medulla is involved, differentiation between ascending and haematogenous infection is not easily made with imaging.[51] Lymphatic spread of infection to the kidney is rare, occurring with severe retroperitoneal infection or abscess, bowel perforation or infection. Lymphatics may permit lower urinary tract infections to ascend to the kidney.[51,58]

Imaging of Acute Pyelonephritis

In general, acute pyelonephritis is diagnosed clinically and does not require imaging. The indications for imaging of suspected APN are the same as for any UTI. The type of imaging is determined by the indication, suspected abnormality, patient background, availability, and personal preference. The Society of Uroradiology recommends that imaging should document if APN is unilateral or bilateral, diffuse or focal, and if renal enlargement is present.[59]

Intravenous Urography. IVU was once commonly used to diagnose APN but currently only plays a minor role to screen for urinary tract obstruction, which is now better performed by other imaging investigations, if available.[60] IVU depicts abnormalities in approximately 25% of patient with APN. This is determined by the degree and extent to which parenchymal involvement disturbs renal excretion.[61] IVU findings include diffuse renal enlargement, delayed contrast excretion with dense persistent striated nephrogram, delayed faint filling of the calyces and effacement or dilation of the collecting system. Caliectasis may be due to either urinary obstruction or impaired peristaltic activity secondary to released endotoxins.[60] The sensitivity of IVU is insufficient to reliably diagnose APN, characterise the type of parenchymal involvement or demonstrate complications. Intravenous contrast medium administration for IVU is not possible in patients with severe renal impairment and is not recommended in the routine assessment of acute pyelonephritis.[62,63]

Ultrasound. Ultrasound is the optimal imaging investigation of the urinary tract evaluation for suspected acute pyelonephritis. Ultrasound has a low sensitivity, is operator dependent and has limited diagnostic accuracy in obese patients. Ultrasound does not demonstrate renal abnormalities in 75–80% of patients with uncomplicated infection and often underestimates the infection severity, particularly with multifocal disease or perinephric extension.[64,65] Nevertheless, ultrasound is the technique of choice for APN assessment during pregnancy due to lack of ionising radiation.[62] Features of APN on ultrasound include renal enlargement caused by generalised renal oedema from inflammation and congestion. Renal length exceeding 15 cm or increase in length of greater than

1.5 cm compared with the unaffected kidney can be attributed to APN on ultrasound.[66] Oedema can also efface renal sinus fat. Renal parenchymal echogenicity may be normal, hyperechoic from haemorrhage or hypoechoic due to oedema. Loss of corticomedullary differentiation may be observed. This is suggestive of but not diagnostic for APN on ultrasound.[67] Hydronephrosis, either as a cause for infection or secondary to pyelonephritis, can be seen on ultrasound and internal echoes in a dilated pelvicalyceal system should raise concern for pyonephrosis. In children where infection can easily extend to the pelvis there may be relatively increased renal sinus echogenicity. Ultrasound can diagnose underlying congenital anomalies that predispose to infection such as pelviureteral junction obstruction or duplicated pelvicalyceal system.[61]

Doppler ultrasound increases the sensitivity for detection of renal parenchymal abnormalities due to APN.[68] Power Doppler US can help demonstrate areas of parenchymal hypoperfusion due to arteriolar vasoconstriction and interstitial edema.[66] It is suggested that contrast-enhanced ultrasonography (CEUS) better demonstrates hypoperfusion from APN and has comparable sensitivity and specificity with intravenous contrast medium-enhanced CT.[69,70] CEUS does not demonstrate a striated nephrogram or delayed persistent enhancement from tubular obstruction since it is a purely intravascular contrast agent.[71] The main advantage of CEUS for APN assessment is for abscess detection. Careful analysis of all phases of enhancement is important to differentiate pure APN from abscess.[70] CEUS can differentiate infarction from APN; although both may have wedge-shaped appearances, APN usually shows some degree of enhancement, whereas infarction does not enhance. Infarction usually does not produce cortical deformity, whereas pyelonephritis usually causes deformity when it reaches sufficient size. Infarction may show penumbral enhancement due to collateral blood supply.[72] Ultrasound of the urinary bladder should be performed in cases of suspected acute pyelonephritis. Measurement of bladder wall thickness and calculation of postmicturition residual urine volume can support a diagnosis of bladder outflow obstruction, as can an enlarged prostate in male patients.[61]

Computed Tomography. The sensitivity and specificity of CT for APN is 86.8 and 87.5%, compared with 74.3 and 56.7% for US, respectively.[64] CT is considered the imaging technique of choice for diagnosis or follow-up of acute pyelonephritis despite radiation exposure, use of iodinated contrast media and the relatively high cost. CT is readily available and sensitive and can also assess for complications or extrarenal involvement.[73] CT for pyelonephritis should include an unenhanced phase, an early nephrographic phase and a pyelographic phase. Occasionally, CT 3 hours after intravenous contrast medium administration may demonstrate retention of contrast medium and help differentiate APN from tumour or infarction. Unenhanced CT evaluates renal size, areas of increased attenuation due to haemorrhage, calcification or perinephric stranding and areas of hypoattenuation due to gas, mass or fluid. Unenhanced

CT detects causes of renal obstruction such as stones or soft-tissue masses. APN is typically hypoattenuating due to oedema or necrosis; rarely, hyperattenuation is observed due to haemorrhagic bacterial nephritis.[61] A normal unenhanced CT does not exclude APN and intravenous contrast medium-enhanced imaging is required.

Nephrographic-phase imaging allows accurate detection and assessment of APN. Loss of corticomedullary differentiation with one or more wedge-shaped zones or streaky areas of reduced enhancement extending from the papilla through the medulla to the renal capsule are observed (Fig. 10-13). APN causes homogeneous or heterogeneous reduced parenchymal enhancement due to tubular obstruction by inflammatory debris, interstitial oedema and vasospasm.[58] Increased time-to-peak enhancement results in delayed persistent enhancement 3–6 hours after contrast medium administration.[74] A striated nephrogram may be observed; however, this may occur in normal subjects when low-osmolar iodinated contrast is used in a dehydrated patient.[51] Peripherally located rounded hypoattenuating renal lesions with clinical features supportive of APN favour haematogenous aetiology (Fig. 10-14) since ascending infection usually creates wedge-shaped abnormalities. When the entire kidney is involved, differentiation between haematogenous and ascending infection is difficult.[75] Early enhanced CT is highly sensitive for pelvicalyceal involvement. Thickened enhancing walls may be the only sign of ascending infection. Later, extrarenal extension or involvement of Gerota's fascia may also be seen. The presence of non-enhancing fluid locules within an area of APN suggests fluid liquefaction and abscess formation (Fig. 10-15). Diffuse renal involvement with APN causes impaired contrast medium excretion proportional to the severity of infection.[48] Pelvicalyceal filling defects at the excretory-phase CT can be due to sloughed papillae, blood clots or fungus balls.

CT is important for differentiating pyelonephritis from tumour or infarction. Imaging features of APN should show improvement after medical treatment but tumour or infarction will not. Occasionally, CT features of APN lag behind clinical resolution. This can create clinical uncertainty and precipitate biopsy for histopathologic reassurance (Fig. 10-14).[76] Extrarenal manifestations of APN that are observed on CT include gallbladder wall thickening, periportal oedema and renal vein or inferior vena cava thrombosis (Fig. 10-15).[77]

Magnetic Resonance Imaging. MRI has gained wide acceptance in the diagnosis of APN. MRI is recommended when CT cannot be performed (pregnancy, previous reactions to contrast medium, children, etc.). MRI features of APN resemble those observed at CT: renal enlargement, alterations of signal intensity due to haemorrhage or oedema, striated nephrograms, parenchymal or perinephric fluid collection (Fig. 10-16). Signal void in the urinary tract on MRI may be due to either stone or gas. With MRI, APN demonstrates heterogeneous low signal on T1-weighted sequences and high-signal intensity on T2-weighted sequences.[78] MRI has excellent soft-tissue contrast resolution

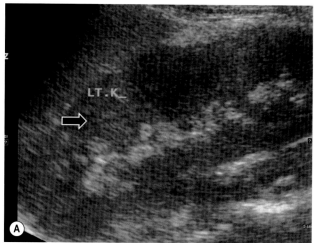
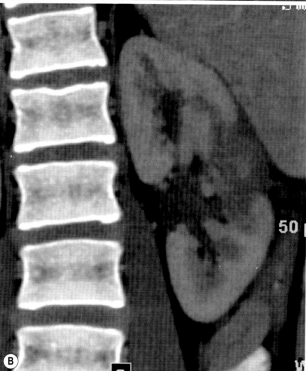

FIGURE 10-13 ■ **Acute focal nephritis.** (A) Ultrasound of left kidney shows a focal area of increased echogenicity (arrow) adjacent to an ill-defined relatively hypoechogenic lesion at the anterior parenchyma of the left mid pole (arrow). (B) Coronal reformatted post-contrast CT image identifies a subcapsular cortical lesion extending to the medulla with thickened perinephric fascia and distorted perinephric fat.

which provides accurate information regarding APN, helping to differentiate APN from renal scar, and detection of the extrarenal extension at least as well as CT (Fig. 10-17).[79]

MRI with intravenous gadolinium helps depict areas of renal parenchymal involvement. Gadolinium-enhanced inversion recovery imaging can help detect intrarenal APN. This method emphasises negative enhancement in diseased areas compared with normal perfused kidney, which becomes hypointense after the administration of contrast agent.[78] MRI using a gadolinium-enhanced

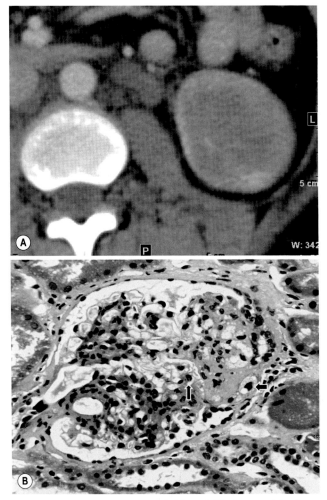

FIGURE 10-14 ■ **Acute pyelonephritis.** (A) Nephrographic-phase CT shows an ill-defined upper pole hypoenhancing abnormality. (B) Cytopathology slide demonstrates multiple neutrophils in the glomerular capillaries (arrows).

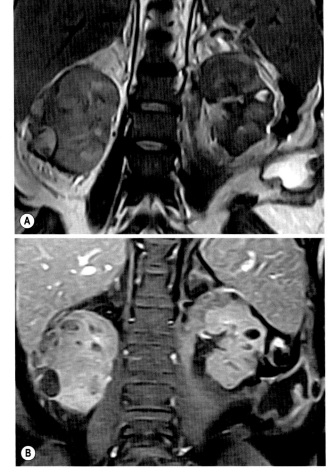

FIGURE 10-16 ■ **Bilateral acute pyelonephritis on MRI.** (A) Coronal T2-weighted MRI shows irregular outline of both kidneys with bilateral subcapsular fluid locules and laterally located fluid collection. (B) Gd-enhanced GRE T1-weighted coronal MRI identifies linear streaks of non-enhancing tubules with small subcapsular fluid locules and marginally enhancing infected laterally located fluid collection.

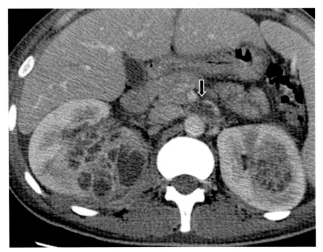

FIGURE 10-15 ■ **Bilateral pyelonephritis with bilateral renal vein thrombosis.** Axial post-intravenous contrast medium CT image shows evidence of bilateral pyelonephritis with areas of lique-faction and bilateral renal vein thrombosis extending to the left renal vein (arrow).

short-tau inversion recovery (STIR) sequence can diagnose APN accurately in children compared with DMSA scintigraphy.[80] MR urography using heavily T2-weighted sequences (such as half-Fourier acquisition single-shot turbo spin echo (HASTE) can detect urinary tract dilatation in cases of obstruction and perinephric inflammatory extension, especially when fat suppression is used. Diffusion-weighted (DW) MRI (or DWI) helps characterise tissues without ionising radiation or contrast medium injection. On diffusion-weighted imaging, APN is typically seen as areas of restricted diffusion which are hyperintense on high b value MRI > 600 (Fig. 10-18),[63] and hypointense at $b = 0$ and on apparent diffusion coefficient (ADC) mapping. Quantitative assessment of affected areas shows low ADC values in comparison with the cortex and medulla, but this is not specific and can be also seen in tumours and ischaemia.

Renal Scintigraphy. Renal scintigraphy using ^{99m}Tc-dimercaptosuccinic acid (DMSA) is commonly used to

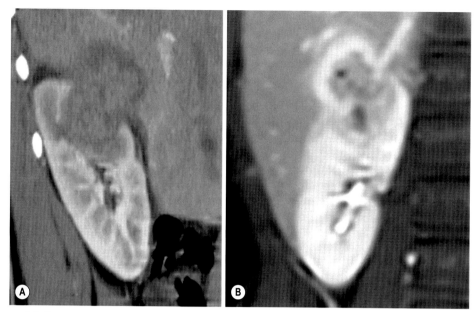

FIGURE 10-17 ■ **Right renal inflammatory mass extending to the liver.** (A) Sagittal post-intravenous contrast medium CT shows a right upper polar mass extending to the liver with hypodense margin at the liver interface. (B) Gd-enhanced GRE T1-weighted coronal MRI shows marginal marked enhancement with non-enhancing central component due to liquefaction.

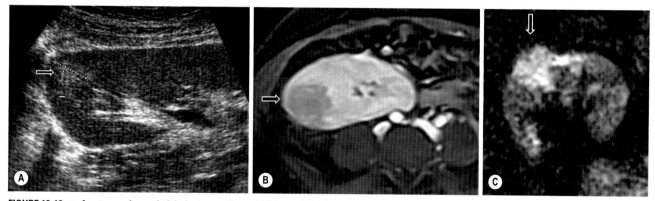

FIGURE 10-18 ■ **Acute pyelonephritis in transplanted kidney.** (A) Ultrasound of the kidney shows a right renal upper pole hyperechoic lesion (arrow). (B) The lesion is hypoenhancing on post- contrast GRE T1-weighted axial MR image. (C) There is diffusion restriction in the lesion on a coronal DW image (*b* = 800).

assess for renal scarring as part of APN evaluation. Approximately 60% of the administered dose of ^{99m}Tc-DMSA is taken up by the proximal tubular cells, mainly through peritubular arterioles and some through filtration and tubular reabsorption.[81] The remaining DMSA is filtered and excreted at low concentrations in the urine. Tracer accumulates in the cortical tubules within 1 hour and remains for 24 hours. Homogeneous distribution of tracer throughout the cortex on anterior and posterior high-spatial resolution imaging 2–3 hours after DMSA administration can confirm that the cortex is normal. In the early phase of APN, there is reduced tracer uptake due to ischemia. In later stages, there is associated tubular obstruction with impairment of the kidney function and isotope accumulation.[82] Renal scarring, on the other hand, appears photopenic.

DMSA should ideally be performed at least 6 months after APN to allow the reversible changes to resolve.[83] Photopenia can occur due to renal abscess, hydronephrosis, cysts, or duplex morphology. Scintigraphy should be performed with ultrasound for diagnostic purposes.[51] Assessment of left and right renal DMSA uptake relative to one another is generally performed on the posterior view. The lower limit of normal for renal uptake is approximately 45%. Less than 45% uptake during APN is predictive of permanent damage.[84,85] DMSA scintigraphy is 92% sensitive for the diagnosis of experimentally induced APN in an animal model.[22] DMSA is superior to IVU for renal scar detection and more or less equal to US, but MRI is superior for diagnosis of APN. In children, it is arguable if cortical imaging should be performed to determine parenchymal involvement before voiding cystourethrography (VCUG). Some authors have suggested that the diagnosis of parenchymal scar at DMSA scintigraphy is an indication for VCUG.[84]

Renal and Perirenal Abscess

Abscess formation affects the renal parenchyma more often than the perinephric space, usually as a complication of APN but occasionally due to haematogenous or direct spread from acute diverticulitis or pancreatitis. Inflammation from APN causes vasospasm, which can cause liquefactive necrosis and microabscess formation. Coalescence of small microabscesses leads to abscess formation.[51] Absent clinical response to medical management should raise concern for abscess formation.[61] Patients receiving renal replacement therapy, intravenous drug abusers and diabetic patients (75% of cases) are particularly at risk for renal abscess formation. Most abscesses are unilateral and solitary; multifocal lesions suggest haematogenous dissemination.[51] A perirenal abscess may rupture through Gerota's fascia to become a paranephric abscess.[86] Urine culture is negative in 20–25%, usually when an abscess is isolated from the pelvicalyceal system.[87]

Imaging of Renal and Perirenal Abscess

IVU is limited for renal abscess detection; at best it can demonstrate some of the findings of APN, including renal enlargement, delayed contrast excretion with dense persistent striated nephrogram and delayed faint filling of the calyces. A large abscess may compress and displace adjacent calyces, the kidney itself and mask the renal contour or a peripheral lesion may deform the renal contour. Ultrasound can be used for initial evaluation of suspected renal or perirenal abscess and it has an important role in follow-up to assess treatment response (Fig. 10-19). At US, a renal abscess appears as a hypoechoic thick-walled lesion containing internal echoes, which tend to disappear as the abscess matures and the thickened walls become more distinct. The kidney may be displaced or rotated and is usually enlarged with distorted contour. The perirenal abscess appears as a cystic mass of variable echogenicity adjacent to the kidney.[88] The presence of gas inside the abscess causes 'dirty' acoustic shadowing. There is usually no flow inside an abscess on power Doppler US and the mobile debris inside the abscess shouldn't be misinterpreted as colour flow.[55] CEUS will show no enhancement by an abscess but 50% of mature abscesses will have mural enhancement and diagnosis of a cystic neoplasm should also be considered.[51]

CT is the imaging study of choice for the diagnosis of renal and perirenal abscess. At contrast medium-enhanced CT, the contents of an evolving abscess may be dense but a mature abscess will contain hypoattenuating non-enhancing fluid. An enhancing rim, due to a pseudocapsule may be observed, and a halo of hypoenhancement may occur at nephrographic-phase CT.[61] Renal fascial thickening, fat stranding, septal thickening and perinephric fat obliteration are commonly found (Fig. 10-19).

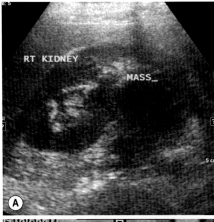

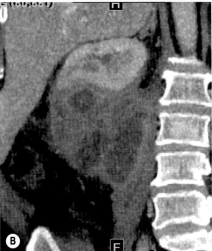

FIGURE 10-19 ■ **Perirenal and psoas abscess.** (A) Ultrasound shows a hypoechoic lesion which appears to lie within and posterior to the lower pole of the right kidney. (B) Contrast medium-enhanced coronal CT demonstrates a multilocular cystic lesion with marginal and septal enhancement extending to the right psoas muscle.

Gas is occasionally seen on CT, as can extension into the psoas muscle, perirenal, anterior or posterior pararenal spaces, and the pelvis.[87] Ultrasound or CT can guide diagnostic aspiration or drainage.

Contrast medium-enhanced and diffusion-weighted (DW) MRI have important roles in renal disease assessment, particularly during pregnancy, in children and if CT is contraindicated. MRI can help differentiate an abscess from a renal mass and when serum creatinine is raised conventional MRI with DWI can help accurately diagnose renal and perirenal abscesses. An intrarenal abscess generally appears as an ovoid or rounded thick-walled lesion with low signal intensity on T1-weighted images and increased signal intensity on T2-weighted images, depending on the presence of protein, fluid and cellular debris (Fig. 10-20).[89] Fluid–fluid levels or irregular septations, perinephric oedema can be observed. Gadolinium-enhanced MRI can help detect extrarenal extension.[51] Cytotoxic oedema and increased fluid viscosity restrict diffusion and help differentiate collections from parenchyma (Fig. 10-21).[90]

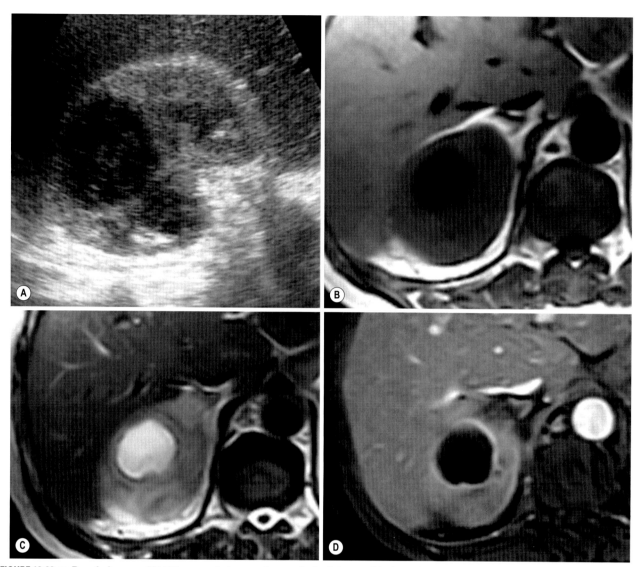

FIGURE 10-20 ■ **Renal abscess.** (A) Ultrasound shows a hypoechoic right renal lesion with internal echoes. (B) Axial T1-weighted MRI shows a hypointense parenchymal lesion. (C) Axial T2-weighted MRI demonstrates hyperintensity relative to the surrounding renal parenchyma with a thick margin. (D) There is marginal enhancement on Gd-enhanced GRE T1-weighted axial image.

Emphysematous Pyelonephritis

Emphysematous pyelonephritis is a life-threatening, fulminant, necrotising upper urinary tract infection associated with gas within or surrounding the kidney, acute flank pain, rapid-onset fever and chills and occasionally shock. Gas confined to the renal pelvis is called emphysematous pyelitis, but in the perinephric space, the term perinephric emphysema is more appropriate.[91] Uncontrolled diabetes is a major predisposing condition (90%), and to a lesser extent immunocompromise or urinary obstruction due to tumour, stone or sloughed papillae from papillary necrosis. *Escherichia coli*, *Klebsiella pneumoniae* and *Proteus mirabilis* are typically responsible.[67]

Imaging of Emphysematous Pyelonephritis

Abnormal gas collections can be detected in 70% of patients with emphysematous pyelonephritis on plain

abdominal radiography (Fig. 10-22).[92] At US, multiple non-dependent echogenic foci with low-level reverberations are seen in an enlarged kidney.[91] Adjacent bowel gas or renal stones create diagnostic difficulty. Ultrasound is inferior to CT for this indication. CT is the most reliable and sensitive technique for evaluating and characterising patients with emphysematous pyelonephritis. Findings include parenchymal enlargement and destruction, small bubbly or linear streaks of gas radiating from the papillae, gas–fluid levels, and focal tissue necrosis with or without renal and perirenal abscess (Fig. 10-23).[93] CT differentiates type 1 emphysematous pyelonephritis (parenchymal destruction with loculated gas without perinephric fluid or collection) from type 2 (parenchymal loculated gas with renal or perirenal fluid or collection). Type 2 emphysematous pyelonephritis has a better prognosis, likely due to better immune response.[91] CT-guided drainage in addition to antibiotics can be used for management of

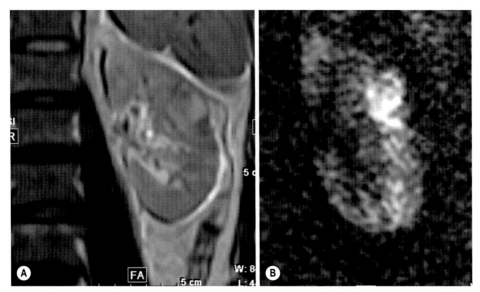

FIGURE 10-21 ■ **MRI of renal abscess.** MRI was carried out to evaluate left acute pyelonephritis with possible abscess formation on ultrasound of diabetic patient who was allergic to iodinated contrast medium. (A) There is a hyperintense left renal midpole lesion on coronal T2-weighted imaging. (B) Coronal DWI MRI demonstrates fluid restriction at the lesion.

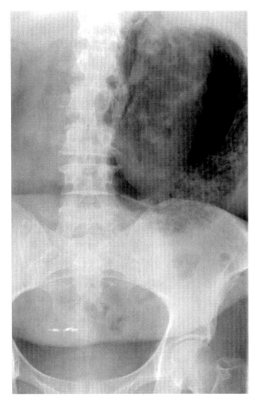

FIGURE 10-22 ■ **Emphysematous pyelonephritis.** A 38-year-old female patient with uncontrolled diabetes. Plain radiograph shows abnormal soft-tissue opacity and air lucencies projected over the left hypochondrium, lumbar and iliac regions.

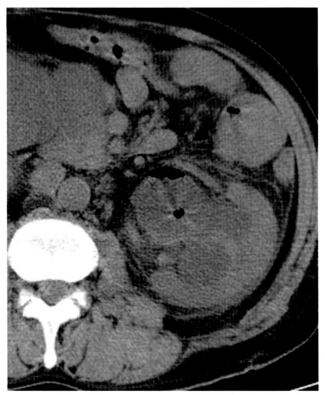

FIGURE 10-23 ■ **Emphysematous pyelitis.** Axial unenhanced CT image shows an air locule inside a dilated left renal pelvis with peripelvic and perinephric fat stranding and thickening of perinephric fascial planes.

emphysematous pyelonephritis, particularly in patients with a solitary kidney. Emphysematous pyelitis without parenchymal involvement can be depicted easily at CT, but MRI is reserved for cases where CT is contraindicated since signal-void due to gas on T1- and T2-weighted images simulates calculi or fluid movement. Perinephric and intraparenchymal fluid collections are accurately delineated on MRI.[94] Emphysematous pyelonephritis should be differentiated from other causes of air inside the kidney such as air reflux from the bladder, air within a renal abscess, renal fistulae or retroperitoneal air from perforated viscus.

Xanthogranulomatous Pyelonephritis (XGP)

XGP is a chronic granulomatous inflammatory process caused by abnormal host response to bacterial infection often associated with renal pelvic stones, which results in parenchymal destruction, replacement with lipid-laden macrophages and renal impairment.[91] The renal pelvis is initially affected; later the corticomedullary territories become involved and eventually extension into the perinephric space or retroperitoneum occurs.[59] It is commonest in middle-aged women and diabetic patients (approximately 10%); *P. mirabilis* and *E. coli* are most often cultured, and occasionally transitional cell carcinoma, haematuria, retroperitoneal haemorrhage or renal vein thrombosis occur.[95] Patients have non-specific symptoms such as loin pain, low-grade fever, chills, dysuria and weight loss.

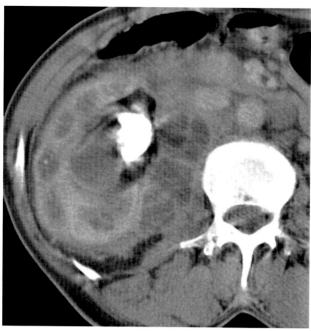

FIGURE 10-24 ■ **Xanthogranulomatous pyelonephritis.** Contrast-enhanced axial CT shows hydronephrotic changes in the right kidney due to a staghorn calculus and with multiple renal parenchymal collections. There is a multilocular fluid collection/abscess medial to the kidney which is displacing the kidney laterally.

Imaging of XGP

Staghorn stones are often seen on plain abdominal radiography and affected kidneys are usually enlarged and non-functioning, or partially enhance and excrete on IVU. Inflammatory extension to the perirenal space will obscure the kidney margins. Ultrasound typically demonstrates renal enlargement and a staghorn calculus. Loss of corticomedullary differentiation, stenosis of the renal pelvis and replacement of the renal parenchyma by hypoechoic masses with internal echos may be observed. CT is indicated and essential for preoperative assessment, in particular for documenting extrarenal disease. A non-functioning enlarged kidney, containing a central calculus within a contracted renal pelvis, expansion of the calyces, and inflammatory changes in the perinephric fat are strongly suggestive of xanthogranulomatous pyelonephritis (Fig. 10-24). Although hypoattenuating branching patterns (due to its lipid content) extending from the contracted renal pelvis may suggest hydronephrosis, the low attenuation corresponds to an extensive inflammatory infiltrate rather than fluid in almost all cases (Fig. 10-25). Xanthomatous material does not enhance and approximately 10% of cases are acalculous.[96] Psoas abscess and fistula formation (which is often cutaneous or colonic) are among the more clinically significant patterns of disease progression.[97] The disease may be focal in 10% of cases, presenting as a mass in an otherwise functioning kidney; the mass is usually hypoattenuating and only rim enhancement may be seen. Focal disease may occur in

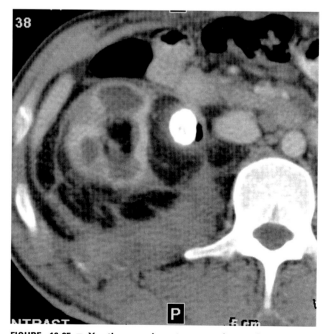

FIGURE 10-25 ■ **Xanthogranulomatous and emphysematous pyelonephritis.** Contrast-enhanced axial CT image reveals multiple parenchymal hypodense areas, thickened perinephric fascia and distorted perinephric fat with staghorn calculus.

one moiety of a duplex kidney or the kidney may be atrophic.[98] MRI accurately depicts extrarenal extension of XGP, and can differentiate focal XGP from renal tumour. On T1-weighted MR images, the solid component of the lesion may be isointense or hyperintense, due to the xanthine and fatty component. On T2-weighted images, the signal intensity of the solid component is isointense to slightly hypointense relative to the normal kidney. The parenchymal cavities filled with fluid and pus show high signal intensity on T2-weighted images and low signal intensity on T1-weighted images, varying according to the protein concentration in the cavity.[99] Restricted water movement may be observed due to increased viscosity at DW MRI.

Pyonephrosis

Pyonephrosis refers to an obstructed infected kidney. Pyonephrosis represents an emergency; the kidney is usually enlarged, and if not drained immediately permanent parenchymal damage and septicaemia will ensue.[72] In the adult, pyonephrosis occurs from acute or chronic obstruction secondary to calculus, tumour, stricture or congenital anomaly with superimposed UTI and extensive parenchymal involvement.[54] Patients are asymptomatic in 15% of cases, or present with fever, chills, loin pain or septicaemia.

Imaging of Pyonephrosis

Plain abdominal radiography can show renal enlargement or an opaque stone. IVU is not recommended for assessment of suspected pyonephrosis. Ultrasound can detect pelvicalyceal dilatation with echogenic debris or fluid–fluid levels.[100] Echogenic debris in a dilated pelvicalyceal system is the most reliable sign of pyonephrosis, with a sensitivity of 90%, specificity of 97% and accuracy of 96%. US is important for diagnostic aspiration and drainage catheter insertion. CT is the investigation of choice; it delineates hydronephrosis, its cause, severity, and information regarding renal function. Typical findings include hydronephrosis with high-density fluid, perirenal inflammation (Fig. 10-26) and thickening of the renal pelvis (> 2 mm). Excretory-phase CT demonstrates contrast-debris layering. MRI provides little additional information over CT but MRI may be preferred to avoid intravenous contrast medium; on T1-weighted images the signal intensity of the infected fluid will be hypointense or slightly increased and on T2-weighted images it will be intermediate to low. MRI may demonstrate fluid–fluid layering and renal pelvis thickening (Fig. 10-27). DW MRI can differentiate between hydronephrosis and pyonephrosis since thick infected fluid in pyonephrosis will lead to restricted diffusion.[101]

Chronic Pyelonephritis

Chronic pyelonephritis is characterised by chronic renal inflammatory and fibrotic change induced by recurrent or continuous infection, vesicoureteral reflux (VUR), or urinary tract obstruction.[102] Renal damage and scarring from childhood VUR is termed reflux nephropathy.[78]

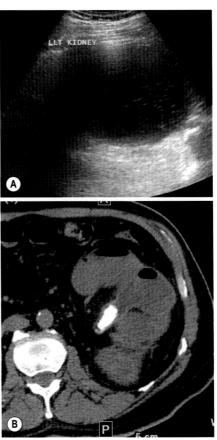

FIGURE 10-26 ■ **Pyonephrosis.** (A) Ultrasound shows marked left hydronephrosis with multiple internal echoes. (B) Axial unenhanced CT shows multiple stones in the renal pelvis and lower pole calyces with marked hydronephrosis. Air–fluid levels are identified within the calyces. The fluid is of increased density relative to the clear urine.

Progressive renal scarring can lead to end-stage renal disease, although scarring may occur without VUR.[64]

Imaging of Chronic Pyelonephritis

Chronic pyelonephritis (reflux nephropathy) is characterised by renal scarring, atrophy and cortical thinning, hypertrophy of residual normal tissue (which may mimic a mass lesion), calyceal clubbing secondary to retraction of the papilla from overlying scar, thickening and dilatation of the calyceal system and overall renal asymmetry.[61] IVU is less sensitive than CT and US and requires a functioning kidney to demonstrate calyceal and contour irregularities. IVU in many cases cannot differentiate between renal scar secondary to pyelonephritis and focal contour changes in cases of renal infarction, papillary necrosis and fetal lobulation.[61] On US, chronically pyelonephritic kidneys are usually small with focal contour irregularities and areas of fibrosis may also be seen.[103] DMSA demonstrates photopenia in scarred areas of kidney (Fig. 10-28). CT with intravenous contrast medium differentiates non-enhancing areas of infarction from the scar tissue; it also can differentiate pseudotumours of hypertrophied parenchyma from neoplasia.

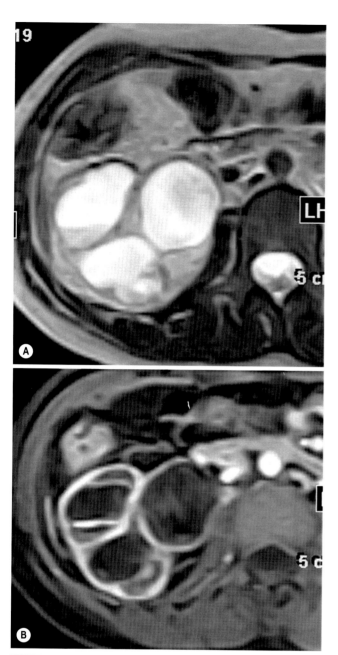

FIGURE 10-27 ■ **Pyonephrosis on MRI.** (A) Axial T2-weighted MRI shows fluid–fluid levels inside dilated right renal calyces. (B) Axial contrast-enhanced GRE T1-weighted MRI demonstrates thickened renal pelvis with mural enhancement.

MRI provides information equivalent to CT without intravenous contrast medium. A rare chronic severe form of renal and bladder infection and inflammation is called alkaline-encrusted pyelitis and cystitis. It is characterised by encrustations and calcifications of the urothelium due to Gram-positive urea-splitting organisms. On unenhanced CT, linear hyperdense calcifications occur along the thickened urothelium (Fig. 10-29).

Renal Tuberculosis

The urinary system is the most common extrapulmonary site of TB, normally seeded haematogenously in

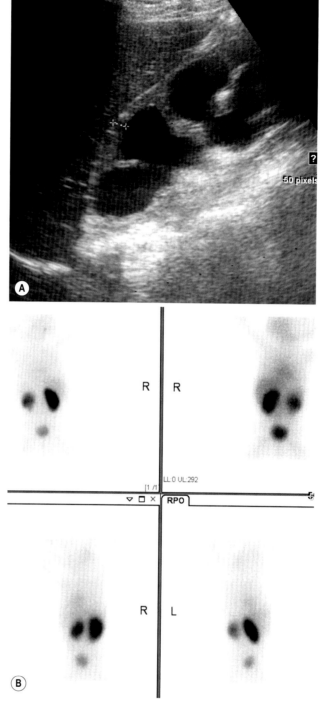

FIGURE 10-28 ■ **Chronic pyelonephritis.** (A) Ultrasound shows hydronephrotic changes with generalised atrophy of the left renal parenchyma. (B) ^{99m}Tc-DMSA demonstrates reduced tracer uptake with photopenic area at the left renal lower pole due to scarring.

periglomerular or peritubular regions from active or quiescent pulmonary TB. It has an incidence of 4–8% in patients with pulmonary TB but only 50% of patients with renal TB have concomitant pulmonary manifestations.[104] Renal TB has an insidious onset characterised by non-specific symptoms including flank pain, dysuria, low-grade fever, malaise or weakness due to parenchymal

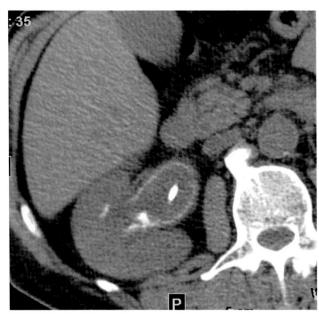

FIGURE 10-29 ■ **Alkaline-encrusted pyelitis.** Axial CT of the right kidney demonstrates marginal calcification at the renal pelvis and middle calyx. A stent is noted inside the dilated renal pelvis.

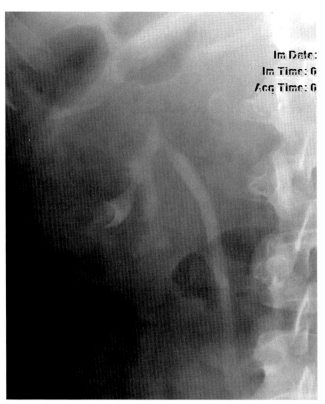

FIGURE 10-30 ■ **Renal TB.** IVU shows no contrast excretion by the upper calyces of the right kidney due to an amputated or *phantom* calyx.

destruction, impaired function and renal calcification (autonephrectomy).[105] Presentation is frequently late: activated infection has spread from the cortex into the medulla, papillae and the collecting system with haematuria and culture-negative pyuria on urinalysis.[67] Extrarenal spread can involve perinephric and retroperitoneal tissues and adjacent organs including the gastrointestinal tract or skin.[56]

Imaging of Renal Tuberculosis

Imaging appearances of renal TB are non-specific and rely on detection of features of papillary necrosis and parenchymal destruction. The presence of three or more of the following features is highly suggestive of TB: pelvicalyceal thickening; ulceration; and fibrosis with or without stricture. Infindibular strictures obstruct renal segments creating a *phantom calyx* against background of normal renal tissue. Strictures distort the collecting system, create cavities and contour deformities.[61] Later calcification can create a thin rim surrounding a necrotic area or completely replace renal parenchyma (autonephrectomy). Calcification occurs in 40–70% of renal TB cases.[106]

IVU can detect parenchymal calcification, cavitary lesions, infundibular stenosis with amputated calyces (Fig. 10-30), or pelviceal stenosis with hydronephrosis.[59] Focal hyper- or hypoechoic renal masses, diffuse parenchymal hyperechogenicity from calcification or renal abscess formation can be observed on ultrasound.[107] Reactivated disease causes inflammation and vasoconstriction, which causes hypoperfusion and a striated nephrogram at contrast medium-enhanced CT. CT can also detect papillary necrosis, which gives calyces a moth-eaten appearance and CT examines for extrarenal spread.[108] CT can detect parenchymal thinning and

scarring and is optimal for detection of calcification[109] (Fig. 10-31). Fibrotic strictures of infindibula, renal pelvis and ureters are highly suggestive of tuberculosis. TB granulomas contain caseous material or calcification on CT. CT is not as sensitive as excretory urography for detecting early urothelial changes. MRI is good at depicting TB cavities (Fig. 10-32), sinus tracts, fistulous communications and extrarenal spread. MRI features of renal macronodular tuberculoma include hypointensity on T1-weighted images, and a thick, irregular, hypointense peripheral wall with intralesional fluid-debris level on T2-weighted images.[110] TB granulomas appear as mildly enhancing soft-tissue masses on CT or MRI (Fig. 10-33). Putty kidney represents end-stage renal TB; dystrophic calcifications involve the entire non-functioning kidney (Fig. 10-34).

Cystitis

Cystitis refers to bladder inflammation. Symptoms include urgency, frequency, dysuria, haematuria, or suprapubic pain. Sources include infection (bacteria, TB, schistosomiasis), medications (cyclophosphamide) or radiation. Cystitis affects both sexes and all ages without racial predisposition. Women younger than 50 years are predisposed due to short urethral length and urethral proximity to the anus.[111] Imaging and urine cultures are unnecessary in uncomplicated cystitis but recurrent cystitis merits urine culture.[112]

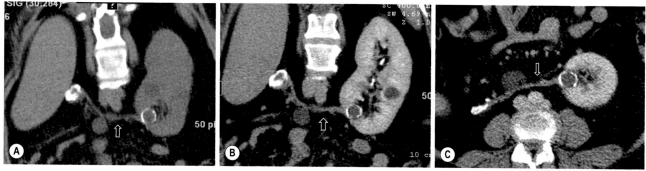

FIGURE 10-31 ■ **Bilateral renal TB in horseshoe kidney.** Coronal reformatted CT of the abdomen. (A) Unenhanced and (B) intravenous contrast medium-enhanced CTs show small atrophic calcified right kidney (autonephrectomy) with marginally calcified non-enhancing cystic lesion at the medial aspect of the lower pole of the left kidney, with a fibrous isthmus connecting the lower pole of both compartments (arrows) crossing the midline. (C) Contrast-enhanced axial CT of the kidney clearly delineates the isthmus (arrow) anterior to the aorta and IVC.

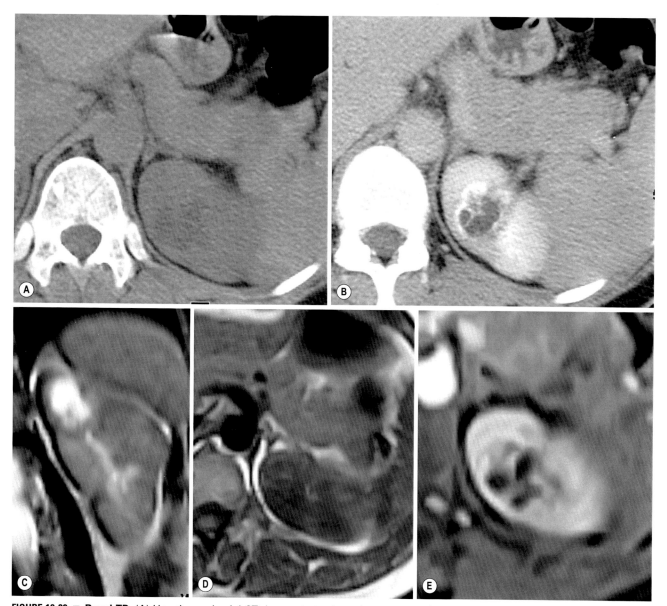

FIGURE 10-32 ■ **Renal TB.** (A) Unenhanced axial CT demonstrates hypodense area at the upper pole of the left kidney medially with marginal enhancement at contrast-enhanced axial CT (B). (C) Coronal T2-weighted MRI of the left kidney shows the lesion with high signal intensity. (D) T1-weighted MR image identifies the lesion as isointense to the renal parenchyma. (E) Contrast-enhanced T1-weighted GRE MRI shows rim enhancement and further subtle enhancement of the internal septations.

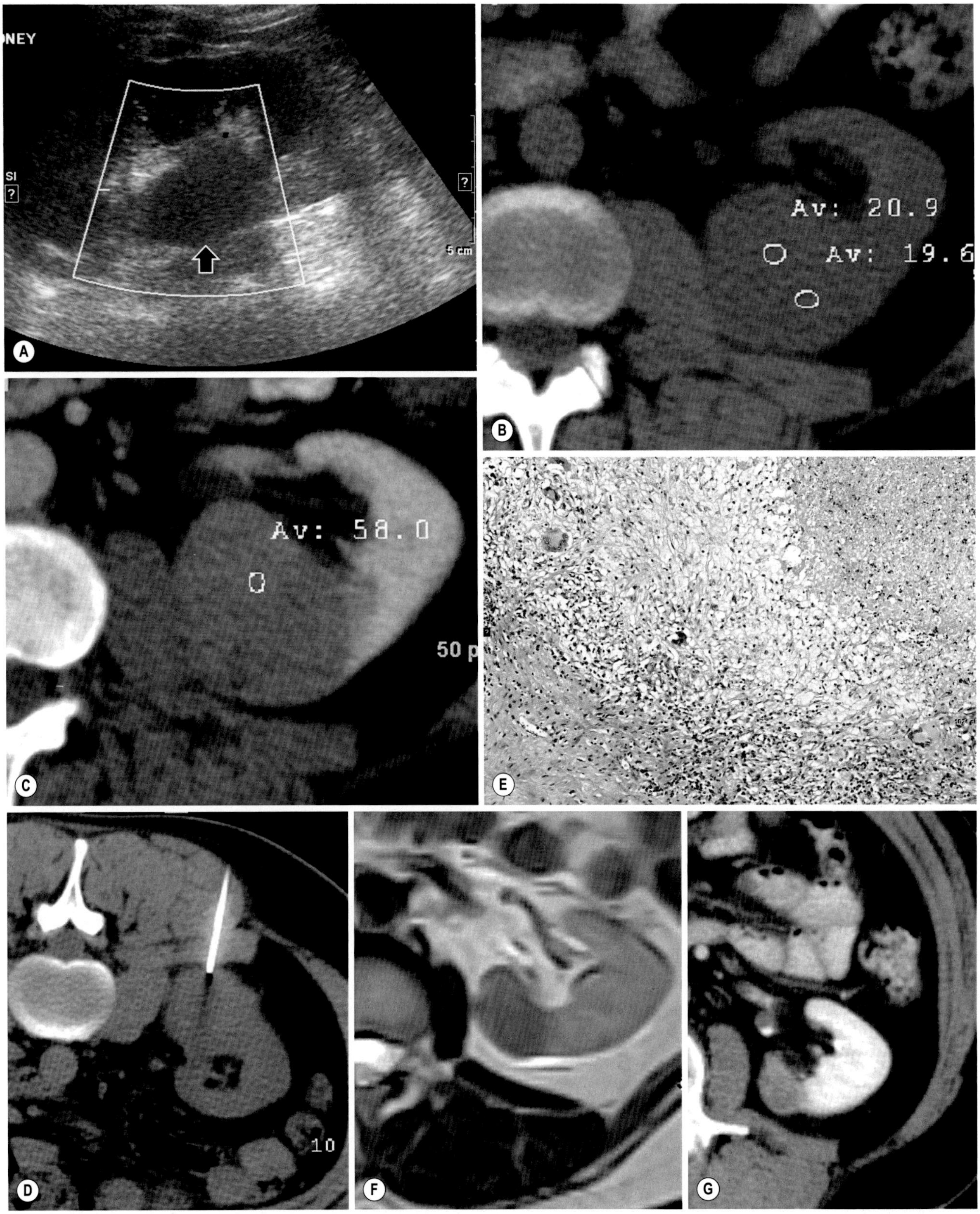

FIGURE 10-33 ■ **Renal tuberculoma.** (A) Colour Doppler ultrasound in axial plane at the midzone of left kidney shows a mildly hypoechoic lesion posteriorly with no internal color flow (arrow). (B) Unenhanced axial CT of the left kidney shows an isodense lesion at the posteromedial aspect of the kidney that demonstrates contour bulge and mild enhancement on the contrast medium-enhanced axial CT (C). (D) CT-guided needle biopsy of the mass. (E) Histological analysis of the needle biopsy shows dense lymphocytic infiltrates and multinucleated giant cells surrounded by some epithelial cells, lymphocytes and macrophages. There are wide areas of caseating necrosis. (F, G) Follow-up axial T2-weighted MRI and intravenous contrast medium-enhanced axial CT of the kidney after medical treatment shows significant reduction in the size of lesion. The lesion is seen as an area of low signal intensity on T2-weighted MRI.

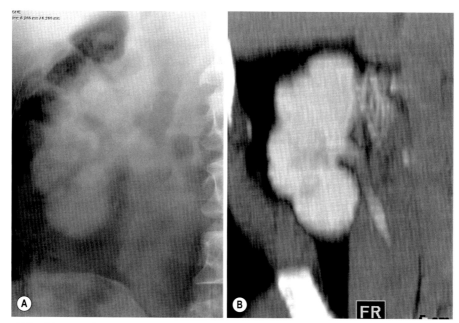

FIGURE 10-34 ■ **Urinary TB with putty kidney.** (A) Plain radiograph shows reniform-shaped radiopaque calcified mass. (B) Unenhanced coronal CT image shows hyperdense calcific material filling dilated calyces and upper ureter.

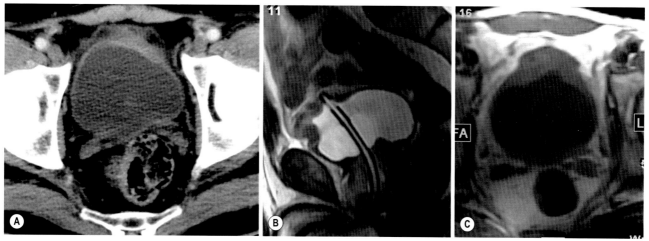

FIGURE 10-35 ■ **Chronic non-specific cystitis.** (A) Mildly dense thickened anterior bladder wall is identified on intravenous contrast medium-enhanced axial CT. (B) Sagittal T2-weighted MR image shows irregular thickening of the anterior bladder wall. (C) Thickened enhancing anterior bladder wall on axial T1-weighted MRI, taken early after intravenous contrast medium administration.

Imaging of Cystitis

Imaging is indicated for complicated cystitis and to differentiate pyelonephritis from cystitis, especially in children. IVU is generally normal in mild cystitis, but moderate-to-severe cases demonstrate focal mucosal oedema with a cobblestoned mucosa on full bladder or post-voiding images and progressive luminal contraction if severe. Ultrasound can assess mucosal thickness (normal mucosa < 2 mm with full bladder and < 5 mm with empty bladder), post-voiding residual urine, polyps or masses. VCUG can detect associated vesicoureteric reflux, bladder or urethral diverticula.

CT cystography is helpful for assessing wall thickness, detecting localised and diffuse mural hypertrophy, polyps or intraluminal masses. CT identifies calculi, diverticula, and complications including fistula or abscess. Blood within the bladder is used to diagnose haemorrhagic cystitis. Mural air due to emphysematous cystitis can occasionally be diagnosed at plain radiography or CT. MRI findings are non-specific; there may be focal or diffuse mural thickening. Gadolinium-enhanced MRI of the bladder shows differential enhancement proportional to the severity of inflammation but generally less than that of a tumour (Figs. 10-35 and 10-36). Cystoscopic

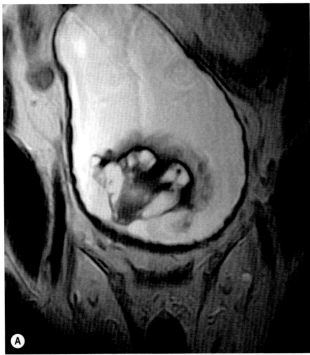

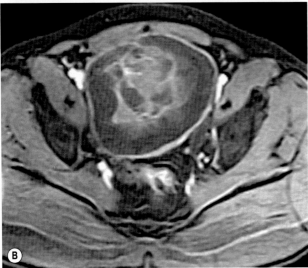

FIGURE 10-36 ■ **Polypoidal cystitis.** (A) Coronal T2-weighted MRI shows a multilocular cystic lesion with mixed high and low signal intensity in the anterior wall of the bladder. (B) Gd-enhanced GRE T1-weighted axial MR image shows mildly enhancing septa with other non-enhancing parts.

assessment and biopsy should be considered for focal mural thickening, polyps or masses.

Prostatitis

Prostatitis is a common urological diagnosis in men less than 50 years and the third most common urological diagnosis in men over 50 years after benign prostatic hyperplasia and prostate cancer. In 1999 The National Institutes of Health (NIH) classified prostatitis into four types:

1. Acute bacterial prostatitis.
2. Chronic bacterial prostatitis.

3. Chronic prostatitis/chronic pelvic pain syndrome (CPPS) (inflammatory (IIIA) and non-inflammatory (IIIB).
4. Asymptomatic inflammatory prostatitis.[113]

Acute Bacterial Prostatitis and Prostatic Abscess

Acute prostatitis presents with fever, chills, dysuria and pelvic pain (as per UTI) in men, which generally makes diagnosis straightforward. *Escherichia coli* and *Pseudomonas* are most commonly responsible. Approximately 10% of cases of acute bacterial prostatitis progress to chronic bacterial prostatitis and a further 10% progress to chronic pelvic pain syndrome.[114] Risk factors for acute bacterial prostatitis include prostate biopsy, urethral catheterisation and instrumentation, especially in immunocompromised and diabetic patients.

Imaging of Acute Prostatitis and Prostatic Abscess. Transrectal ultrasound (TRUS) is indicated for patients who fail initial therapy and especially for abscess detection. Acute prostatitis causes symmetrically reduced periurethral echogenicity and increased periprostatic adipose tissue blood flow. Loss of capsular definition can occur, and appearances may overlap with invasive carcinoma. Occasionally, multiple hypoechoic areas, particularly in the peripheral zone, are seen. Abscesses are generally a late complication of acute prostatitis and can spontaneously decompress into the urethra, rectum or periprostatic adipose tissues.[115]

An early abscess on TRUS appears heterogeneous or anechoic with fine internal echoes. Margins become progressively irregular over time and, in refractory or untreated cases, can extend throughout the gland and beyond the capsule. TRUS also guides abscess drainage and provides sample for microbiological culture.[114] CT has no role in acute prostatitis, but it can diagnose an abscess or extracapsular extension. Although MRI can depict the diffuse asymmetric prostate swelling, it is usually performed for suspected prostatic abscess, which appears as a cystic lesion with thickened walls, septations, or heterogeneous contents. Signal intensity is usually iso- to hyperintense on T1, and iso- to hypointense on T2-weighted images due to pus and debris. Thick-walled fluid collections due to abscess formation are well-depicted at contrast medium-enhanced images. Excellent soft-tissue resolution provided by MRI is useful for assessing the extent of a prostatic abscess and involvement of adjacent structures (Figs. 10-37 and 10-38). Extracapsular extension is important to detect, as this influences treatment. DW MRI will define the abscess as an area of restricted diffusion that correlates with T2-weighted abnormality.

Chronic Prostatitis

Bacterial or non-bacterial forms of chronic prostatitis are usually characterised by irritative urinary symptoms, occasionally haematuria and rarely urinary obstruction due to recurrent urinary tract infections. Chronic bacterial prostatitis cannot be differentiated from chronic

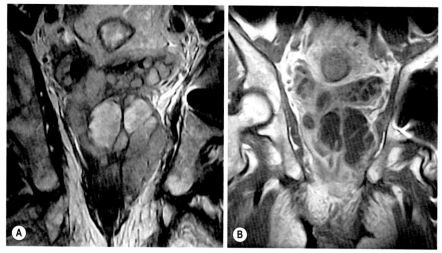

FIGURE 10-37 ■ **Prostatic abscess.** (A) Coronal T2-weighted MRI shows a multilocular cystic lesion replacing most of the left lobe of prostate with extension to the left pelvic wall. (B) Coronal Gd-enhanced GRE T1-weighted MRI demonstrates marginal and septal enhancement with irregular enhancement of the seminal vesicles suggesting involvement.

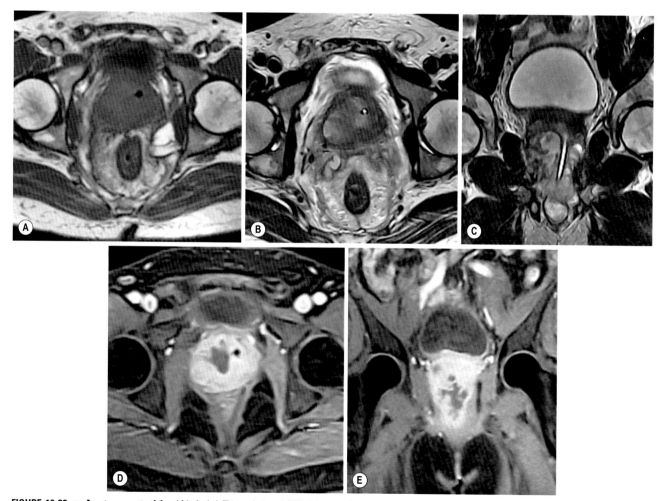

FIGURE 10-38 ■ **Acute prostatitis.** (A) Axial T1-weighted MR image shows asymmetric enlargement of the prostate with distorted periprostatic fat. (B, C) Axial and coronal T2-weighted MRI depict asymmetric enlargement of the prostate with hyperintense fluid locules and periprostatic fat distortion. (D, E) Axial and coronal GRE T1-weighted MRI show diffuse heterogeneous enhancement with central liquefaction.

pelvic pain syndrome, based on clinical findings alone. Quantitative sequential bacteriological localisation cultures are essential for diagnosis. *Escherichia coli* is most often the causative organism in cases of chronic bacterial prostatitis.[116] Non-specific granulomatous prostatitis is a variety of chronic prostatitis which has eosinophilic and non-eosinophilic variants. This presents as palpable mass on digital rectal examination and increased prostate specific antigen (PSA), which can be mistaken for prostate cancer.[114] Chronic prostatitis may be associated with calculosis, especially in young subjects, inflammation of the ductus deferens and seminal vesicles or purely mechanical obstruction of one or both ejaculatory ducts due to scarring and retraction or compression from adjacent calculi, with consequent sterility.[114]

Imaging of Chronic Prostatitis. TRUS is normal in most cases of chronic prostatitis; there may be areas of hypo-, iso- or hyperechogenicity in one or both lobes. Calcification is not specific for chronic prostatitis. Granulomatous prostatitis can appear similar to carcinoma on ultrasound; focal hypoechoic areas, which may disrupt the capsule due to extension, can be seen. Where there is a palpable mass, TRUS-guided biopsy is indicated. Overlapping features between prostate cancer and chronic prostatitis are also seen on MRI.[117] DW MRI shows restricted diffusion in both cancer and prostatitis, but ADC values less than 1.2×10^{-3} mm^2/s increase its sensitivity and specificity for prostatitis detection.[118]

REFERENCES

1. Rodgers M, Nixon J, Hempel S, et al. Diagnostic tests and algorithms used in the investigation of haematuria: systematic reviews and economic evaluation. Health Technol Assess 2006;10(18):iii–iv, xi–259.
2. Mishrike SF, Vint R, Somani BK. Half of visible and half of recurrent visible hematuria cases have underlying pathology: prospective large cohort study with long-term follow-up. J Urol 2012; 187(5):1561–5.
3. Woolhandler S, Pels RJ, Bor DH, et al. Dipstick urinalysis screening of asymptomatic adults for urinary tract disorders. I. Hematuria and proteinuria. JAMA 1989;262(9):1214–19.
4. Rao PK, Gao T, Pohl M, Jones JS. Dipstick pseudohematuria: unnecessary consultation and evaluation. J Urol 2010;183(2): 560–4.
5. Grossfeld GD, Litwin MS, Wolf JS, et al. Evaluation of asymptomatic microscopic hematuria in adults: The American Urological Association best practice policy. Part 1: definition, detection, prevalence, and etiology. Urology 2001;57:599–603.
6. Burger M, Catto JW, Dalbagni G, et al. Epidemiology and risk factors of urothelial bladder cancer. Eur Urol 2013;63(2): 234–41.
7. O'Connor OJ, McSweeney SE, Maher MM. Imaging of haematuria. Radiol Clin North Am 2008;46:113–32.
8. Argyropoules A, Farmakis A, Doumas K, Lykourinas M. The presence of microscopic haematuria detected by urine dipstick test in the evaluation of patients with renal colic. Urol Res 2004;32: 294–7.
9. Pressler CA, Heinzinger J, Jeck N, et al. Late-onset manifestation of antenatal Bartter syndrome as a result of residual function of the mutated renal Na1-K1-2Cl-co-transporter. J Am Soc Nephrol 2006;17(8):2136–42.
10. Edwards TJ, Dickinson AJ, Natale S, et al. A prospective analysis of the diagnostic yield resulting from the attendance of 4020 patients at a protocol-driven haematuria clinic. BJU Int 2006; 97(2):301–5.
11. McNamara MM, Lockhart ME. In: Canon C, editor. Speciality Board Review Radiology. New York: McGraw-Hill; 2010. 56: pp. 441–8.
12. Caoli EM, Cohan RH, Korobkin M, et al. Urinary tract abnormalities: initial experience with multi-detector row CT urography. Radiology 2002;222:353–60.
13. Viprakasit DP, Sawyer MD, Herrell SD, Miller NL. Limitations of ultrasonography in the evaluation of urolithiasis: a correlation with computed tomography. J Endourol 2012;26(3): 209–13.
14. Ray AA, Ghiculete D, Pace KT, Honey RJ. Limitation to ultrasound in the detection and measurement of urinary tract calculi. Urology 2010;76(2):295–300.
15. Worster A, Preyra I, Weaver B, Haines T. The accuracy of non-contrast helical computed tomography versus intravenous pyelography in the diagnosis of suspected acute urolithiasis: a meta-analysis. Ann Emerg Med 2002;40(3):280–6.
16. Kulkarni NM, Uppot RN, Eisner BH, Sahani DV. Radiation dose reduction at multidetector CT with adaptive statistical iterative reconstruction for evaluation of urolithiasis: how low can we go? Radiology 2012;265(1):158–66.
17. Coll DM, Varanelli MJ, Smith RC. Relationship of spontaneous passage of ureteral calculi to stone size and location as revealed by unenhanced helical CT. Am J Roentgenol 2002;178(1): 101–3.
18. Zagoria RJ, Gasser T, Leydendecker JR, et al. Differentiation of renal neoplasms from high-density cysts: use of attenuation changes between the corticomedullary and nephrographic phases of computed tomography. J Comput Assist Tomogr 2007;31(1): 37–41.
19. Taouli B, Thakur RK, Mannelli L, et al. Renal lesions: characterization with diffusion-weighted imaging versus contrast-enhanced MR imaging. Radiology 2009;251:398–407.
20. Cowan NC, Turney BW, Taylor NJ, et al. Multidetector computed tomography urography (MDCTU) for diagnosing upper urinary tract tumour. BJU Int 2007;99:1363–70.
21. Cowan NC. CT urography for haematuria. Nat Rev Urol 2012;9(4):218–26.
22. Blick CG, Nazir SA, Mallett S, et al. Evaluation of diagnostic strategies for bladder cancer using computed tomography (CT) urography, flexible cystoscopy and voided urine cytology: results for 778 patients from a hospital haematuria clinic. BJU Int 2012;110(1):84–94.
23. O'Connor OJ, Maher MM. CT urography. Am J Roentgenol 2010;195(5):W320–4.
24. Turkbey B, Akpinar E, Ozer C, et al. Multidetector CT technique and imaging findings of urinary stone disease: an expanded review. Diagn Interv Radiol 2010;16:134–44.
25. Hiatt RA, Dales LG, Friedman GD, Hunkeler EM. Frequency of urolithiasis in a prepaid medical care program. Am J Epidemiol 1982;115:255–65.
26. Coursey CA, Casalino DD, Remer EM, et al. ACR Appropriateness Criteria: acute onset flank pain—suspicion of stone disease. Ultrasound Q 2012;28(3):227–33.
27. Levine JA, Neitlich JD, Verga M, et al. Identification of ureteral calculi on plain radiographs in patients with flank pain: correlation with helical CT. Radiology 1997;204:27–31.
28. Regan F, Bohlman ME, Khazan R, et al. MR urography using HASTE imaging in the assessment of ureteric obstruction. Am J Roentgenol 1996;167:1115–20.
29. Smith RC, Rosenfield AT, Choe KA, et al. Acute flank pain: comparison of non-contrast-enhanced CT and intravenous urography. Radiology 1995;194:789–94.
30. Jin DH. Effect of reduced radiation CT protocols on the detection of renal calculi. Radiology 2010;255(1):100–7.
31. Eliahou R, Hidas G, Duvdevani M, Sosna J. Determination of renal stone composition with dual-energy computed tomography: an emerging application. Semin Ultrasound CT MR 2010;31: 315–20.
32. Platt JF. Duplex Doppler evaluation of native kidney dysfunction: obstructive and nonobstructive disease. Am J Roentgenol 1992; 158(5):1035–42.
33. Malloy PC, Grassi CJ, Kundu S, et al; Standards of Practice Committee with Cardiovascular and Interventional Radiological Society of Europe (CIRSE). Endorsement. Consensus guidelines for periprocedural management of coagulation status and hemostasis risk in percutaneous image-guided interventions. J Vasc Interv Radiol 2009;207(Suppl):S240–9.

34. Sateriale M, Cronan JJ, Savadier LD. A five-year experience with 307 CT-guided renal biopsies: results and complications. J Vasc Interv Radiol 1991;2:401–7.

35. Fink HA, Ishani A, Taylor BC, et al. Screening for, monitoring, and treatment of chronic kidney disease stages 1 to 3: a systematic review for the U.S. Preventive Services Task Force and for an American College of Physicians Clinical Practice Guideline. Ann Intern Med 2012;156(8):570–81.

36. Levine E. Acquired cystic kidney disease. Radiol Clin North Am 1996;34:947–64.

37. Brigouri C, Colombo A, Airoldi F, et al. Nephrotoxicity of low-osmolality versus iso-osmolality contrast agents: impact of N-acetyl cysteine. Kidney Int 2005;68:2250–5.

38. Thomsen HS, Morcos SK. Contrast media and the kidney: European Society of Urogenital Radiology (ESUR) guidelines. Br J Radiol 2003;76:513–18.

39. McDonald JS, McDonald RJ, Comin J, et al. Frequency of acute kidney injury following intravenous contrast administration: a systematic review and meta-analysis. Radiology 2013;267(1):119–28.

40. McDonald RJ, McDonald JS, Bida JP, et al. Intravenous contrast material-induced nephropathy: causal or coincident phenomenon? Radiology 2013;267(1):106–18.

41. Kim SM, Cha RH, Lee JP, et al. Incidence and outcomes of contrast-induced nephropathy after computed tomography in patients with CKD: a quality improvement report. Am J Kidney Dis 2010;55(6):1018–25.

42. Sadowski EA, Bennett LK, Chan MR, et al. Nephrogenic systemic fibrosis: risk factors and incidence estimation. Radiology 2007;243(1):148–57.

43. Stacul F, van der Molen AJ, Reimer P, et al; Contrast Media Safety Committee of European Society of Urogenital Radiology (ESUR). Contrast induced nephropathy: updated ESUR Contrast Media Safety Committee guidelines. Eur Radiol 2011;21(12):2527–41.

44. Wang Y, Alkasab TK, Narin O, et al. Incidence of nephrogenic systemic fibrosis after adoption of restrictive gadolinium-based contrast agent guidelines. Radiology 2011;260(1):105–11.

45. Foxman B, Brown P. Epidemiology of urinary tract infections: transmission and risk factors, incidence, and costs. Infect Dis Clin North Am 2003;17(2):227–41.

46. Richards MJ, Edwards JR, Culver DH, Gaynes RP. Nosocomial infections in medical intensive care units in the United States. National Nosocomial Infections Surveillance System. Crit Care Med 1999;27(5):887–92.

47. Vincent JL, Bihari DJ, Suter PM, et al. The prevalence of nosocomial infection in intensive care units in Europe. Results of the European Prevalence of Infection in Intensive Care (EPIC) Study. EPIC International Advisory Committee. JAMA 1995;274(8):639–43.

48. Hooton T, Stamm W. Acute pyelonephritis: symptoms; diagnosis; and treatment. In: Rose BD, editor. 2006 UpToDate. Waltham, MA: UpToDate; 2006.

49. Webb JAW. The role of imaging in adult acute urinary tract infection. Eur Radiol 1997;7:837–43.

50. Stunell H, Buckley O, Feeney J, et al. Imaging of acute pyelonephritis in the adult. Eur Radiol 2007;17(7):1820–8.

51. Schaeffer AJ, Schaeffer MD. Infections of the urinary tract. In: Vein AJ, Kavoussi LR, Novick AC, et al, editors. Campbell-Walsh Urology. 9th ed. Philadelphia: Saunders; 2007. pp. 135–98.

52. Blandino A, Mazziotti S, Ascenti G, Gaeta M. Acute renal infections. In: Quaia A, editor. Radiologic Imaging of the Kidney. Berlin: Springer-Verlag; 2011. pp. 417–44.

53. Sobel JD. Pathogenesis of urinary tract infection. Role of host defenses. Infect Dis Clin North Am 1997;11(3):531–49.

54. Hooton TM, Johnson C, Winter C, et al. Single-dose and three-day regimens of ofloxacin versus trimethoprim-sulfamethoxazole for acute cystitis in women. Antimicrob Agents Chemother 1991;35(7):1479–83.

55. Thulesius O, Araj G. The effect of uropathogenic bacteria on ureteral motility. Urol Res 1987;15(5):273–6.

56. Kawashima A, Sandler CM, Goldman SM. Imaging in acute renal infection. BJU Int 2000;86:70–9.

57. Measley RE Jr, Levison ME. Host defense mechanisms in the pathogenesis of urinary tract infection. Med Clin North Am 1991;75(2):275–86.

58. Bechtold RE, Dyer RB, Zagoria RJ, Chen MY. The perirenal space: relationship of pathologic processes to normal retroperitoneal anatomy. Radiographics 1996;16(4):841–54.

59. Talner LB, Davidson AJ, Lebowitz RL, et al. Acute pyelonephritis: can we agree on terminology? Radiology 1994;192(2):297–305.

60. Baumgarten DA, Baumgartner BR. Imaging and radiologic management of upper urinary tract infection. Urol Clin North Am 1997;24:545–69.

61. Dunnick NR, Sandler CM, Newhouse JH, et al. Textbook of Uroradiology. 3rd ed. Philadelphia: Lippincott Williams & Wilkins; 2001. pp. 150–77.

62. Craig WD, Wagner BF, Travis MD. Pyelonephritis: radiologic-pathologic review. Radiographics 2008;28:255–76.

63. Stunel H, Bucley O, Feeney J, et al. Imaging of acute pyelonephritis in adult. Eur Radiol 2007;17:1820–8.

64. Browne RFJ, Zwirewich C, Torreggiani WC. Imaging of urinary tract infection in the adult. Eur Radiol 2004;14:168–83.

65. Majd M, Nussbaum Blask AM, Markle BM, et al. Acute pyelonephritis: comparison of diagnosis with 99mTc-DMSA SPECT, spiral CT, MR imaging, and power Doppler US in an experimental pig model. Radiology 2001;218:101–8.

66. Vourganti S, Agarwal PK, Bodner DR, et al. Ultrasonographic evaluation of renal infections. Radiol Clin North Am 2006;44:763–75.

67. Rigsby CM, Rosenfield AT, Glickman MG, Hodson J. Hemorrhagic focal bacterial nephritis: findings on gray-scale sonography and CT. Am J Roentgenol 1986;146:1173–7.

68. Morehouse H, Darwish M, Ginsberg M, et al. Comparison of contrast CT with duplex ultrasonography in the evaluation of patients with acute severe pyelonephritis. Am J Roentgenol 1995;165:217.

69. Mitterberger M, Pinggera GM, Colleselli D, et al. Acute pyelonephritis: comparison of diagnosis with computed tomography and contrast-enhanced ultrasonography. BJU Int 2007;101:341–4.

70. Iványi B, Thoenes W. Microvascular injury and repair in acute human bacterial pyelonephritis. Virchows Arch A 1987;411(3):257–65.

71. Fontanilla T, Minaya J, Cortés C, et al. Acute complicated pyelonephritis: contrast-enhanced ultrasound. Abdom Imaging 2011;37(4):639–46.

72. Bertolotto M, Martegani A, Aiani L, et al. Value of contrast-enhanced ultrasonography for detecting renal infarcts proven by contrast enhanced CT—a feasibility study. Eur Radiol 2008;18(2):376–83.

73. Demertzis J, Menias CO. State of the art: imaging of renal infections. Emerg Radiol 2007;14(1):13–22.

74. Dalla-Palma L, Pozzi-Mucelli F, Pozzi-Mucelli RS. Delayed CT findings in acute renal infection. Clin Radiol 1995;50:364–70.

75. Lee JK, McClennan BL, Melson GL, et al. Acute focal bacterial nephritis: emphasis on gray scale sonography and computed tomography. Am J Roentgenol 1980;135:87–92.

76. Kawashima A, Sandler CM, Goldman SM, et al. CT of renal inflammatory disease. Radiographics 1997;17(4):851–66.

77. Zissin R, Osadchy A, Gayer G, Kitay-Cohen Y. Extrarenal manifestations of severe acute pyelonephritis: CT findings in 21 cases. Emerg Radiol 2006;13(2):73–7.

78. Piccoli GB, Consiglio V, Deagostini MC, et al. The clinical and imaging presentation of acute 'non complicated' pyelonephritis: a new profile for an ancient disease. BMC Nephrol 2011;12:68.

79. Poustchi-Amin M, Leonidas JC, Palestro C, et al. Magnetic resonance imaging in acute pyelonephritis. Pediatr Nephrol 1998;12:579–80.

80. Lonergan GJ, Pennington DJ, Morrison JC, et al. Childhood pyelonephritis: comparison of gadolinium enhanced MR imaging and renal cortical scintigraphy for diagnosis. Radiology 1998;207:377–84.

81. De Lange MJ, Piers DA, Kosterink JGW, et al. Renal handling of technetium-99m DMSA: evidence for glomerular filtration and peritubular uptake. J Nucl Med 1989;30:1219–23.

82. Majd M, Rushton HG. Renal cortical scintigraphy in the diagnosis of acute pyelonephritis. Semin Nucl Med 1992;22:98–111.

83. Stokland E, Hellstrom M, Jakobsson B, et al. Imaging of renal scarring. Acta Paediatr Suppl 1999;88:13–21.

84. De Sadeleer C, De Boe V, Keuppens F, et al. Can the outcome of renal abnormalities be predicted on the basis of the initial Tc-99m DMSA scintigraphy? Eur J Nucl Med 1993;20:867.

85. Hansson S, Dhamey M, Sigstrom O, et al. Dimercaptosuccinic acid scintigraphy instead of voiding cystourethrography for infants with urinary tract infection. J Urol 2004;172:1071–3.

86. Dembry L-M, Andriole VT. Renal and perirenal abscesses. Infect Dis Clin North Am 1997;11:663–80.

87. Thornbury JR. Acute renal infections. Urol Radiol 1991;12: 209–13.

88. Cho JY. Renal infection. In: Kim SH, editor. Radiology Illustrated—Uroradiology. Berlin: Springer-Verlag; 2012. pp. 393–424.

89. Puvaneswary M, Bisits A, Hosken B. Renal abscess with paranephric extension in a gravid woman: ultrasound and magnetic resonance imaging findings. Australas Radiol 2005;49: 230–2.

90. Verswijvel G, Vandecaveye V, Gelin G. Diffusion-weighted MR imaging in the evaluation of renal infection: preliminary results. Br J Radiol 2002;85:100–3.

91. Shokeir AA, El-Azab M, Mohsen T, El-Diasty T. Emphysematous pyelonephritis: a 15-year experience with 20 cases. Urology 1997;49(3):343–6.

92. Wan YL, Lee TY, Bullard MJ, Tsai CC. Acute gas-producing bacterial renal infection: correlation between imaging findings and clinical outcome. Radiology 1996;198:433–8.

93. Grayson DE, Abbott RM, Levy AD, Sherman PM. Emphysematous infections of the abdomen and pelvis: a pictorial review. Radiographics 2002;22:543–61.

94. Huang JJ, Tseng CC. Emphysematous pyelonephritis: clinicoradiological classification, management, prognosis, and pathogenesis. Arch Intern Med 2000;160:797–805.

95. Hayes WS, Hartman DS, Sesterbenn IA. Xanthogranulomatous pyelonephritis. Radiographics 1991;11:485–98.

96. Kenney PJ. Imaging of chronic renal infections. Am J Roentgenol 1990;155:485–94.

97. Matsuoka Y, Arai G, Ishimaru H, et al. Xanthogranulomatous pyelonephritis with a renocolic fistula caused by a parapelvic cyst. Int J Urol 2006;13:433–5.

98. Loffroy R, Guiu B, Watfa J, et al. Xanthogranulomatous pyelonephritis in adults: clinical and radiological findings in diffuse and focal forms. Clin Radiol 2007;62:884–90.

99. Cakmakci H, Tasdelen N, Obuz F, et al. Pediatric focal xanthogranulomatous pyelonephritis: dynamic contrast enhanced MRI findings. Clin Imaging 2002;26:183–6.

100. Subramanyam BR, Raghavendra BN, Bosniak MA, et al. Sonography of pyonephrosis: a prospective study. Am J Roentgenol 1983;140:991–3.

101. Chan J, Tsui E, Luk S, et al. MR diffusion-weighted imaging of kidney: Differentiation between hydronephrosis and pyonephrosis. J Clin Imaging 2001;25:110–13.

102. Guarino N, Casamassima MG, Tadini B, et al. Natural history of vesicoureteral reflux associated with kidney anomalies. Urology 2005;65(6):1208–11.

103. Goldman SM, Fishman EK. Upper urinary tract infection: the current role of CT, ultrasound, and MRI. Semin Ultrasound CT MR 1991;12:335–60.

104. Becker J. Renal tuberculosis. Urol Radiol 1988;10:25–30.

105. Sharma A, Rattan KN, Kumar S. Renal tuberculosis in children. Trop Doctor 2000;30:183–4.

106. Muttarak M, ChiangMai WN, Lojanapiwat B. Tuberculosis of the genitourinary tract: imaging features with pathological correlation. Singapore Med J 2005;46:568–74.

107. Das KM, Vaidyanathan S, Rajwanshi A, Indudhara R. Renal tuberculosis: diagnosis with sonographically guided aspiration cytology. Am J Roentgenol 1992;158:571–3.

108. Hammond N, Nikolaidis P, Miller F. Infectious and inflammatory diseases of the kidney. Radiol Clin N Am 2012;50:259–70.

109. Leder RA, Low VH. Tuberculosis of the abdomen. Radiol Clin North Am 1995;33:691–705.

110. Verswijvel G, Janssens F, Vandevenne J, et al. Renal macronodular tuberculoma: CT and MR findings in an asymptomatic patient. JBR-BTR 2002;85(4):203–5.

111. Hanno P, Nordling J, van Ophoven A. What is new in bladder pain syndrome/interstitial cystitis? Curr Opin Urol 2008;18(4): 353–8.

112. Bjerklund-Johansen TE. Diagnosis and imaging in urinary tract infections. Curr Opin Urol 2002;12:39–43.

113. Krieger JN, Nyberg L Jr, Nickel JC. NIH consensus definition and classification of prostatitis. JAMA 1999;282:236–7.

114. Yoon BI, Kim S, Han DS, et al. Acute bacterial prostatitis: how to prevent and manage chronic infection? J Infect Chemother 2012;18(4):444–50.

115. Olivetti L, Grazioli L. Diagnostic imaging of the prostate. In: Olivetti L, Grazioli L, editors. Imaging of Urogenital Diseases. Springer-Verlag Italia; 2009.

116. Meares EM, Stamey TA. Bacteriologic localization patterns in bacterial prostatitis and urethritis. Invest Urol 1968;5(5): 492–518.

117. Shukla-Dave A, Hricak H, Eberhardt SC, et al. Chronic prostatitis: MR imaging and 1H MR spectroscopic imaging findings—initial observations. Radiology 2004;23:717–24.

118. Ibrahiem EI, Mohsen T, Nabeeh AM, et al. DWI-MRI: single, informative, and noninvasive technique for prostate cancer diagnosis. ScientificWorldJournal 2012;973450.

CHAPTER 11

THE URINARY TRACT: OVERVIEW OF ANATOMY, TECHNIQUES AND RADIATION ISSUES

Owen J. O'Connor • Michael M. Maher

CHAPTER OUTLINE

INTRODUCTION

ANATOMY OF THE URINARY TRACT

TECHNIQUES

RADIATION ISSUES

CONCLUSION

INTRODUCTION

This chapter describes clinically important aspects of urinary tract imaging with specific reference to anatomy, techniques and radiation. We begin with an outline of urinary tract embryology in order to place urinary tract anatomy and many anatomic variations into context. We describe long-established techniques of urinary tract imaging and the principles used to guide development of newer techniques. Imaging of the urinary tract is an evolving process, which has seen the introduction of CT urography in recent years and also in recent efforts aimed at radiation dose reduction. Current low-dose imaging practices are described.

ANATOMY OF THE URINARY TRACT

Embryology

An understanding of urinary tract development helps foster better appreciation of urinary tract anatomy and the anatomical variation and anomalies that are encountered. Congenital urinary tract anomalies have a prevalence of approximately 10%. Due to complex inter-relationships during development, once one anomaly occurs, there is a 75% chance of another congenital anomaly either in the urinary tract, genital, musculoskeletal, gastrointestinal or cardiovascular system.

The kidneys develop from primitive excretory organs, which emerge in a craniocaudal sequence beginning in the cervical region of the fetus at three weeks' gestation. Renal development begins with a transient precursor organ called the pronephros, which is later replaced by the mesonephros at four to eight weeks' gestation. Although most of the mesonephros degenerates, a portion develops into the mesonephric or Wolffian duct, which

gives rise to the ureteric bud and male genital development. The ureteric bud emerges from mesonephric duct close to its insertion with the cloaca.[1] The segment of the mesonephric duct between the cloaca and ureteric bud origin is known as the common excretory duct.[2] The proximal ureteric bud enlarges into an ampulla, which undergoes dichotomous division to form the renal pelvis, calyces and collecting tubules of the renal medulla.[3] This results in the development of 10 to 14 minor calyces. Since the interpolar calyces are initially formed, the polar calyces are more likely to have fewer calyces or have incomplete divisions. The kidney itself develops from the metanephros, which is initially located in the sacral region of the fetus. The metanephric blastema forms the renal excretory ducts (proximal and distal convoluted tubules, loop of Henle), interstitium of the renal parenchyma, as well as Bowman's capsule, once contact is made with the ureteric bud.[4]

The bladder develops following craniocaudal division of the cloaca into the urogenital sinus anteriorly and the anorectal portion posteriorly by the urorectal septum at 3–7 weeks' gestation.[5] The caudal aspect of the urorectal septum forms the perineal body. The urogenital triangle lies anterior to the perineal body and the anal triangle posterior. The cranial portion of the urogenital sinus forms the bladder, the middle portion helps form anterior pelvic structures and the inferior portion the urogenital membrane. The common excretory duct is incorporated into the inferior portion of the bladder and proximal urethra during development. The ureteric ostia migrate laterally and cranially during bladder development while the distal portion of the metanephric duct remains medial and continues to communicate with the urethra forming ejaculatory ducts and seminal vesicles. Tissues between the developing distal ureter and the ejaculatory duct orifice form the superficial muscular layer of the trigone. The deep muscular layer of the trigone is contiguous with the detrusor muscle of the bladder. The genital ridges fuse to form the urethra in males or remain separate to form major and minor labia in females. The urachus develops from the urogenital diaphragm and connects the dome of bladder with the fetal allantoic duct within the space of Retzius anterior to the peritoneum and posterior to the abdominal wall musculature. Normally the urachus fibroses during the second trimester and forms the median umbilical ligament.

Normal Urinary Tract Anatomy

The upper urinary tract consists of paired kidneys and ureters, while the bladder and urethra constitute the lower urinary tract. The developing kidney gradually rotates medially and undergoes cranial migration relative to the spine due to lengthening of the lumbar and sacral spine during development, so that the normal final position is in the upper lumbar region. Arterial supply during development is from progressively more cranial aortic branches beginning initially at the lateral sacral artery. Final arterial supply is from the aorta at the level of the second lumbar vertebral body, by which time arteries that arose earlier in development should have involuted.[6] Accessory unilateral renal arteries occur in approximately 30% of the population and bilaterally in 10%.[7] The prevalence is higher when abnormal renal ascent occurs.[6] The left renal vein generally drains anterior to the aorta into the IVC. Involution anomalies of the embryonic circumaortic venous ring lead to retroaortic and circumaortic left renal drainages which are not normally associated with other renal deformities.[6] In this configuration, the ipsilateral adrenal and gonadal veins drain into the anterior and posterior renal veins, respectively. The renal veins lie anterior to the renal arteries, which lie anterior to the renal pelvices.

The kidneys are contained within the perirenal space, one of four retroperitoneal spaces which also include the anterior and posterior pararenal spaces, and the retroperitoneal vascular compartment. The perirenal space is bounded by a thin layer of connective tissue called Gerota's fascia (sometimes subdivided into a posterior fascia of Zuckerkandl and lateroconal fascia). Superiorly Gerota's fascia is closely related to the adrenal glands; it also envelops the renal pedicle consisting of the renal artery, vein, lymphatics and the urinary collecting system. The perirenal space contains thin septations called Kumin's septa that may thicken in response to renal disease, an appearance termed *perinephric stranding*. The perirenal space communicates with the bare area of the liver or spleen superiorly, the periureteric tissues inferiorly and the renal sinus fat medially. The perirenal spaces may communicate across the midline and with the retroperitoneal vascular space. The pararenal spaces communicate caudally and with the extraperitoneal spaces, including the prevesical space.

The renal collecting system consists of 10–14 concave-shaped minor calyces bounded laterally by forniceal angles. The minor calyces coalesce to form upper, mid and lower major calyces, or infundibula, and then the renal pelvis is either enveloped entirely in the renal sinus, or partially outside the kidney, termed an *extrarenal pelvis*.

Exuberant adipose proliferation termed *renal sinus lipomatosis* may occur in the renal sinus with increasing age, renal atrophy or steroid administration.[4] The normal kidney contains 14 lobes, each consisting of a calyx, collecting duct and cortex. The external contour of the kidney demonstrates lobulation at the intersection of lobes, evident up to five years of age as the kidneys mature and cells multiply. Beyond this age, external lobulation disappears and glomeruli may respond to injury such as partial or complete nephrectomy by hypertrophy. The normal kidney should be 12–14 cm in length and there should be less than 1cm difference in lengths between the kidneys. Renal length tends to be underestimated by ultrasound and overestimated by intravenous urography.

The ureters have three normal constrictions at points of temporary peristaltic arrest; at the pelvic inlet, crossing the iliac vessels, and at the ureteropelvic junctions. The normal ureter courses along the anterior psoas muscle within 1cm of the lateral margin of the vertebral transverse processes and outside the line of the pedicles to the level of L3 on an abdominal radiograph, sometimes with a short horizontal course as it crosses the lateral edge of the psoas at L3 (Fig. 11-1). The transverse distance between the ureters at this level should normally be greater than 5 cm.

The bladder has a superior surface with a peritoneal reflection, two inferolateral surfaces, a neck, which contains the ureteric ostia, a base which contains the trigone, and continues into the urethra from the apical region as the medial umbilical ligament. The trigone is bounded by the ureteric orifices posterolaterally and the urethral orifice anteroinferiorly. The muscular layer of the bladder is known as the detrusor muscle and the bladder is lined by transitional cell epithelial. The anterior division of the internal iliac artery supplies the bladder via the superior, middle, and inferior vesicle arteries. Many collateral arteries exist, including the obturator and inferior gluteal arteries. Venous drainage from the bladder is into the

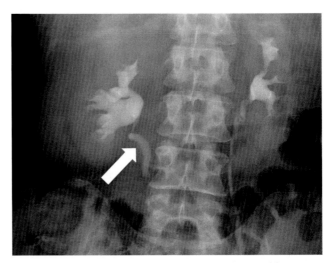

FIGURE 11-1 ■ **Intravenous urography in a 61-year-old woman.** Twenty-minute radiograph following release of compression demonstrates short horizontal course of right ureter as it traverses the lateral margin of the psoas muscle (arrow).

internal iliac vein, and lymphatic drainage occurs into internal, external, and common iliac nodal basins.

The male urethra consists of prostatic, membranous, bulbous, and penile divisions. The prostatic portion is lined by transitional cell epithelium, and the remainder by columnar epithelium. The prostatic and membranous portions constitute the posterior urethra. The prostatic portion has a posterior indentation as it traverses the transitional zone of the prostate called the verumontanum, which serves as a landmark for prostatic gland drainage lateral to this structure. The prostatic utricle is a vestigial remnant of the Müllerian duct located just inferior to the verumontanum and is the site of ejaculatory duct drainage. The membranous portion of the urethra has a thick outer circular rim of muscle, which forms the external urethral sphincter. This is the narrowest and shortest portion of the urethra, and is followed by the widest urethral segment, the bulbous urethra within the corpus spongiosum of the penis, from the level of the urogenital diaphragm which separates the posterior and anterior urethra (Fig. 11-2). The paired Cowper's glands drain into the proximal bulbous portion. The remainder of the anterior urethra is termed the penile portion from the level of the penoscrotal junction. The female urethra is widest at its origin and narrowest at the meatus adjacent to the external vagina. Skene's

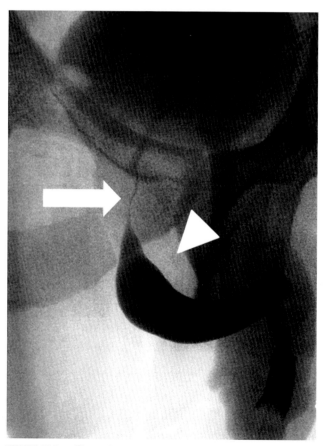

FIGURE 11-2 ■ **Normal retrograde urethrogram in a 35-year-old man.** Normal constriction at the membranous urethra (arrow) and dilation at the bulbous urethra (arrowhead) are depicted.

glands drain along the course of the urethra. The female urethra is approximately 4 cm in length and the external urethral sphincter is in the region of the mid urethra.

Congenital Abnormalities of the Urinary Tract

Renal

Renal abnormalities may be subclassified into those of number, position, fusion, vasculature, and ureteropelvic junction anomalies.[8] Failure of the ureteric bud to join the metanephric blastema causes renal agenesis. This is observed in 1 in 1000 live births and is associated with absence of the ipsilateral ureter or the presence of a ureteric stump.[6] Absent ipsilateral epididymis, vas deferens, seminal vesicle or presence of a seminal vesicle cyst is observed in up to 70% of patients with renal agenesis.[1] Interestingly, anomalies of the urinary tract are almost twice as common among men compared with women; however, congenital anomalies of the genital tract are much more common in women.[1] Woman patients with renal agenesis have a 70% incidence of Müllerian anomalies such as vaginal and uterine agenesis, or unicornuate uterus, which are part of Mayer–Rokitansky–Küster–Hauser syndrome. Absent ipsilateral adrenal gland is observed in 10%. Agenesis of the left kidney can be recognised on an abdominal radiograph if the splenic flexure is located medial to the lesser curve of stomach. Bilateral renal agenesis results in Potter's syndrome (1 in 3000 live births) consisting of oligohydramnios, pulmonary hypoplasia and facial anomalies such as low set ears, broad flat nose and prominent infraorbital skin folds. *Supernumerary kidney* on the other hand refers to the presence of an additional kidney. A supernumerary kidney is uncommon but normally occurs on the left, probably due to duplication of the ureteric bud. The supernumerary kidney is located caudal to the normal kidney drained by either a separate ureter or a branch of a bifid ureter.

An abnormal amount of renal rotation around its long axis can position the ureteropelvic junction anterior, or less commonly, posterior to the kidney. Abnormal caudocranial renal ascent during development results in an ectopic renal location (Fig. 11-3). An ectopic kidney is more commonly inferior to the normal anatomical position, or rarely, in the upper abdomen where it is referred to as a *thoracic kidney*. Ectopic kidneys can be located in the pelvis, in the iliac fossa or can cross the midline. There is an increased incidence of renal anomalies in both the ectopic kidney and its contralateral counterpart. A *pancake kidney* is produced when bilateral pelvic kidneys fuse (Fig. 11-4). Pelvic kidneys are more prone to decreased function, ureteropelvic junction obstruction, vesicoureteric reflux, stone formation and trauma (Fig. 11-5).

Fusion anomalies of several types and severity occur in the kidneys. A horseshoe kidney deformity consists of medial facing lower renal poles connected by an isthmus containing parenchyma or a relatively avascular fibrous tissue, which rotates the renal axis (Fig. 11-6). This

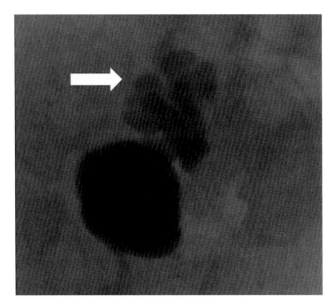

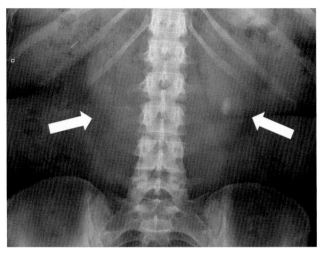

FIGURE 11-6 ■ Abdominal radiograph in a 28-year-old woman with horseshoe kidney containing two stones (arrows)

FIGURE 11-3 ■ Voiding cystourethrogram in a 3-month-old boy. There is a right-sided pelvic kidney present with reflux from the bladder into the renal pelvis and dilated calyces (arrow).

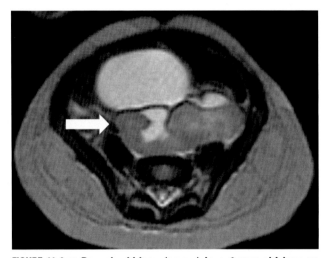

FIGURE 11-4 ■ Pancake kidney (arrow) in a 1-year-old boy on MRI.

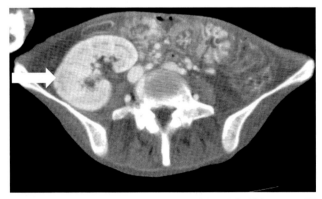

FIGURE 11-5 ■ A 61-year-old woman with pelvic kidney on CT (arrow).

anomaly occurs following metanephric contact and fusion during development. The incidence of horseshoe kidney is approximately 1 in 400 live births and has a 2-to-1 male-to-female preponderance.[4] The isthmus lies anterior to the inferior vena cava and aorta but posterior to the inferior mesenteric artery. As a result, renal assent is arrested at this level. Horseshoe kidney is associated with a 30% incidence of ureteropelvic junction obstruction, stone formation in 30%, and 10% chance of ureteric duplication. There is an increased incidence of genital, cardiovascular and anorectal abnormalities. Patients with horseshoe kidneys also have increased risk of renal tumours including Wilms' tumour, traumatic injury or infection.

Occasionally, one kidney crosses the midline and fuses with the contralateral kidney, a configuration known as *crossed fused ectopia* (Fig. 11-7). Unlike horseshoe kidney, both kidneys lie on one side of the spine (Fig. 11-8). Generally, the ureters drain in an orthopic manner into the bladder when crossed fused ectopia exists. This fusion pattern is more common in men and the left kidney is more commonly ectopically located (Fig. 11-9).

Overall, abnormalities of the renal vasculature occur in almost 25% of the population. Ectopic kidneys have a higher incidence of anomalous blood supply. Renal artery duplication is the most common vascular abnormality. The accessory artery normally supplies the lower pole renal territory. Accessory veins are much less common than accessory arteries. Vessels crossing the ureteropelvic junction can cause complete segmental renal obstruction, which can simulate duplication (pseudoduplication). Anomalous vessels generally cause few symptoms; however, inadvertent injury during open aortic and renal surgery, or ureteroscopic procedures can occur. The tissues anterior to the ureteropelvic junction, in particular, should be examined carefully on pre-procedure imaging, since anomalous vessels traverse anterior more frequently than posterior to the ureteropelvic junction.

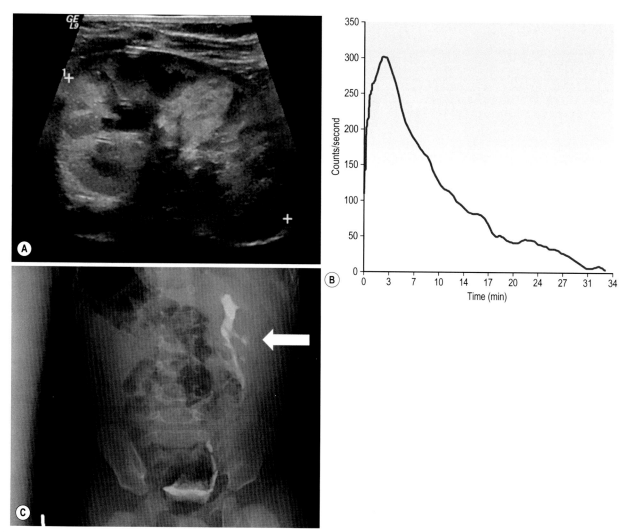

FIGURE 11-7 ■ **Ultrasound, MAG-3 renogram and IVU in a 4-month-old boy with crossed fused ectopia.** (A) Both kidneys are fused and located to the right of midline on ultrasound. The kidneys cannot be easily distinguished from one another. (B) Normal excretion seen on MAG-3 renogram. (C) Fused kidneys seen on IVU following intravenous contrast medium administration (arrow).

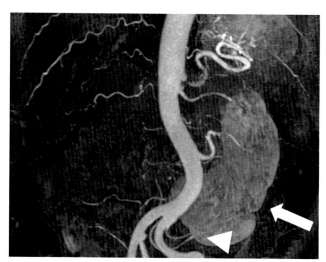

FIGURE 11-8 ■ **Reformatted images from a CT angiogram in a 36-year-old man with cross fused renal ectopia.** The ectopic kidney (arrow) receives blood supply from the contralateral iliac artery (arrowhead).

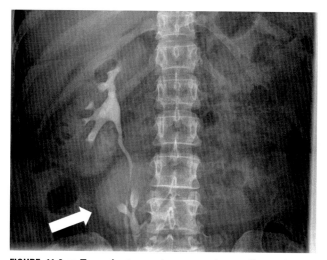

FIGURE 11-9 ■ **Ten-minute post-compression radiograph performed as part of an intravenous urogram in a 55-year-old man with ectopic left kidney.** The ectopic kidney has crossed to the right of midline (arrow) but has not fused with the contralateral kidney.

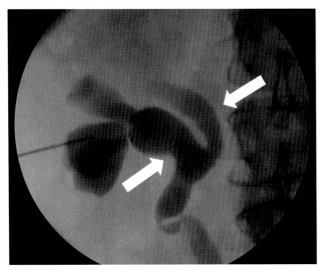

FIGURE 11-10 ■ Antegrade urogram in a 70-year-old female patient with hydronephrosis and bifid right renal collecting system (arrows).

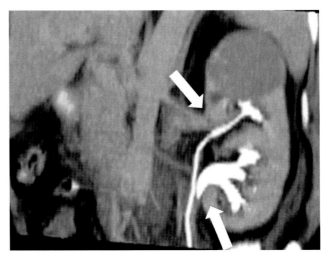

FIGURE 11-11 ■ **Partial duplication of the left renal collecting system on CT in a 61-year-old woman.** Coronal CT reformation shows separate drainage systems for the upper and lower moieties of the left kidney (arrows).

Ureter and Pelvis

Congenital ureteric anomalies can be generally subdivided into those of ureteric number, direction, diameter and filling defects.[8] The most common ureteric anomaly is that of ureteric number, which was observed in 0.7% of autopsies in one series.[9] The renal parenchyma may be divided into upper and lower components by a septum of Bertin. This anomaly is associated with a bifid collecting system consisting of two pelvices joined proximal to the ureteropelvic junction (Fig. 11-10). The upper calyces drain into the upper pelvis, while the mid and lower calyces drain into the lower pelvis. The ureters may also join distal to the ureteropelvic junction (Fig. 11-11) with a Y-configuration. This is normally asymptomatic unless urine refluxes from one ureter up the other causing ureteroureteric reflux, also termed *yo-yo reflux*, which should be considered if one ureteric segment is disproportionately enlarged.[10] This anomaly can precipitate recurrent infections and obstruction of a ureteric segment.

When there is complete duplication of the renal collecting system, the ureter draining the upper moiety tends to insert ectopically below and medial to the normal ureteric orifice or sometimes outside the bladder (extravesical). The ureter draining the upper moiety tends to drain ectopically due to delayed separation of the ureteric bud from its parent Wolffian duct, which migrates in a caudal direction during development.[11] For this reason it is suggested that if the upper urinary tract is normal, the ureter is likely to have an orthopic insertion; however, a dysplastic or malfunctioning upper tract is likely associated with an ectopic insertion. The ectopic ureter often has a strictured distal element which causes proximal dilatation in the bladder wall and ureterocele formation in 75% of affected patients and is eight times more common in women than men (Fig. 11-12).[10] A ureterocele contains layers of ureteric and bladder epithelium

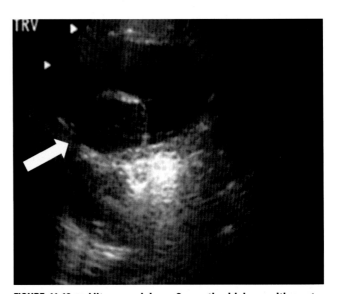

FIGURE 11-12 ■ **Ultrasound in a 6-month-old boy with ureterocele.** The ureterocele (arrow) is depicted as a circular filling defect within the bladder.

which are optimally appreciated on early imaging on a voiding cystourethrogram (VCUG) but can be obscured by contrast medium, effaced or everted similar to a diverticulum when the bladder is full (Fig. 11-13).[12] A *cobra-neck* appearance is observed at intravenous urography (IVU) consisting of a dilated contrast-filled ureter surrounded by thin rim of ureteric wall and bladder mucosa measuring less than 2 mm in diameter (Fig. 11-14). Ectopic ureteroceles often project into the bladder and are associated with recurrent infection, stone formation, complete ipsilateral or bilateral ureteric obstruction. Orthopic ureteric insertion in the setting of ureteric duplication is generally asymptomatic unless larger than

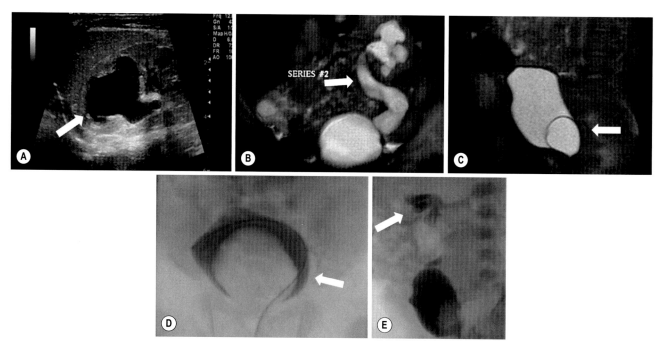

FIGURE 11-13 ■ **Ultrasound, MRI and micturating cystourethrogram in a 4-month-old girl with duplication of the left renal collecting system, upper pole obstruction, lower pole reflux and ureterocele formation.** (A) There is hydronephrosis of only the upper pole collecting system on ultrasound (arrow). (B) There is left- sided hydroureter (arrow) and upper pole hydronephrosis on MRI. (C) A crisp-walled ureterocele (arrow) is seen in the bladder on MRI. (D) Filling defect due to ureterocele at micturating cystourethrogram (arrow). (E) There is reflux into the lower moiety at micturating cystourethrogram. This has a 'drooping lilly' appearance (arrow).

2 cm. An ectopic ureter with extravesical insertion below the bladder neck, into the urethra or vagina, can cause urinary incontinence, infection and ureteric obstruction from fibrotic stricture formation. The ectopic ureter generally inserts above the external sphincter in men, thereby inhibiting incontinence but in about 50% of women this does not occur and patients present with dribbling incontinence but are able to void normally.

The ureter draining the lower moiety of a duplicated collecting system inserts orthopically but tends to reflux. In fact, reflux is the most common association of ureteric duplication. Lower pole hydronephrosis in the setting of duplication is mainly due to reflux rather than an obstructing ureterocele or stricture. In duplicated systems the dilated upper pole ureter can impinge and displace the lower pole ureter, which can be appreciated on voiding cystourethrogram. Conformity of a duplicated collecting system with this pattern of ureteric insertion is known as the *Weigert–Meyer Rule*.[10] Approximately one-third of patients with complete ureteric duplication have an additional congenital anomaly such as horseshoe kidney and multicystic dysplastic kidney.

Anomalies of ureteric course generally occur due to extrinsic processes, which push or pull complete or segmental portions of the ureter in medial or lateral directions. Potential causes of medial ureteric deviation include retrocaval ureter (Fig. 11-15), laterally based renal, retroperitoneal, lymph node, central pelvic or psoas masses, pelvic lipomatosis, vascular aneurysms or haematoma, retroperitoneal fibrosis and surgical resection of pelvic

organs such as the entire rectum. Lateral ureteric deviation is caused by retroperitoneal and central pelvic masses such as lymphadenopathy (testicular metastases), aortic aneurysm, psoas enlargement (young men) and abnormal renal position (malrotated or horseshoe kidney). Cross-sectional imaging is usually required to confirm aetiology. Acute medial deviation of the right ureter medial to corresponding vertebral pedicles on an abdominal radiograph is virtually diagnostic of retrocaval ureter. Pelvic lipomatosis pushes the distal ureters medially. This condition is more common in African-American men and can induce bilateral hydronephrosis. A characteristic pear-shaped bladder may be observed and cystitis glandularis of the bladder is an associated premalignant condition. Retroperitoneal fibrosis pulls one or both ureters medially in about half of cases. Psoas muscle hypertrophy can be recognised as the cause of lateral ureteric deviation if the lateral psoas border exceeds 8 cm from the lateral edge of the corresponding vertebral body at the level of the iliac crest.

Other congenital ureteric anomalies of note include ureteric stricture, megaureter and vesicoureteric reflux. Ureteric strictures are the most common of these anomalies. The ureteropelvic junction, in particular, and the ureterovesical junction to a lesser extent, are predisposed to stricture formation. Ischaemia during development is thought to incite fibrosis and stricture formation in these regions. There is consequent dilatation of the proximal ureter and possibly the renal pelvis, which may be detected by screening or as an incidental finding in

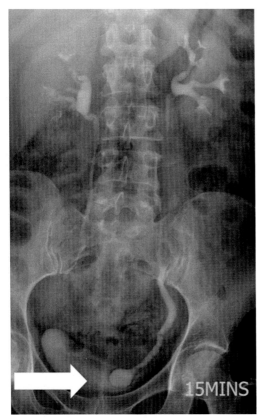

FIGURE 11-14 ■ Orthopic ureterocele in a 43-year-old man on intravenous urography. A cobra-neck appearance is seen at the distal left ureter on the 15-min radiograph at intravenous urography (arrow).

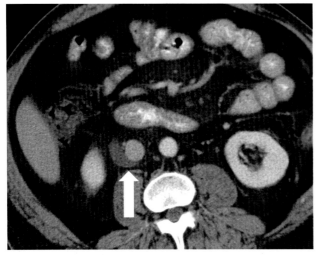

FIGURE 11-15 ■ Retrocaval ureter in a 52-year-old man on CT. Axial CT demonstrated retrocaval ureter (arrow).

asymptomatic patients, or associated with flank pain, recurrent infection, haematuria or stone formation, anywhere from in utero to adulthood (Fig. 11-16). Ureteric strictures may also be caused by a vessel crossing from medial to lateral with a convex lateral margin in about

1 in 20 cases of ureteropelvic junction obstruction (Fig. 11-17).

Ureteric diameter exceeding 7 mm is termed megaureter.[13] Megaureter may be a congenital phenomenon or secondary to a process in the bladder or urethra (Fig. 11-18). Primary megaureter is due to deficient ureteric musculature, which limits peristalsis and leads to upstream dilatation. Three forms are described: obstructing primary megaureter, refluxing primary megaureter, and non-obstructing non-refluxing primary megaureter. Primary refluxing megaureter is due to inadequate one-way valve mechanism at the vesicoureteric junction. In non-obstructing non-refluxing primary megaureter the calyces should maintain a crisp outline and not be blunted as with primary obstructing megaureter and there should be normal excretion (Fig. 11-19). Three-quarters of cases are unilateral; there is left-sided a male predominance.

Vesicoureteric reflux is caused by maldevelopment of the distal ureter characterised by a shortened intramucosal bladder tract with a deficient valve-like mechanism. Reflux increases the risks of renal infection, scarring and reflux nephropathy. Vesicoureteric reflux represents the most common cause of antenatal hydronephrosis, responsible for 40% of cases.[14] Grading is between 1 and 5 according to the International Reflux Study Committee as determined by the most severe degree of reflux at voiding cystourethrography: reflux into the ureter only (I), to the renal pelvis without calyceal dilatation (II), with mild or moderate ureteric and calyceal dilatation but preserves fornices (III), and severe ureteric and calyceal dilatation with obliteration of forniceal angles but maintained greater calyceal papillary impressions (IV), and finally gross dilatation with effacement of the papillary impressions (V).[15]

Bladder and Urethra

The term cloaca is derived from the Latin term for sewer. Cloacal malformation is believed to occur when the urorectal septum fails to separate the cloaca and results in a shared orifice for the genital, urinary and lower gastrointestinal tracts in a phenotypic female. A urogenital sinus anomaly occurs at a later stage in development and results in a common drainage tract for the genital and urinary systems. Extrophy of the cloaca occurs in males and females when there is failed closure of the infra-umbilical anterior abdominal wall, creating a defect larger than that observed with bladder extrophy.

Several anomalies of bladder development may occur, including agenesis, duplication, diverticula, prune-belly syndrome and anomalies of the cloaca. Agenesis of the bladder is very rare and its origin is uncertain, but since the hindgut often develops normally, maldevelopment of the anterior cloaca is usually responsible. The ureters insert ectopically in this situation and further urinary tract anomalies are common. Rarely, there may be duplication of the bladder and urethra created by a septum containing detrusor muscle. This occurs more commonly in a sagittal rather than in a coronal plane. This anomaly is associated with uni- or bilateral renal obstruction,

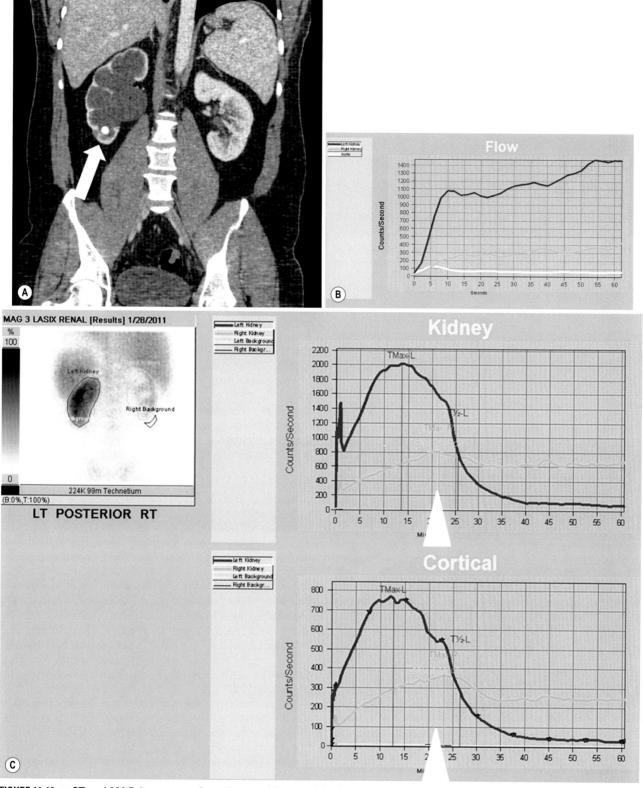

FIGURE 11-16 ■ **CT and MAG-3 renogram in a 40-year-old man with left ureteropelvic junction obstruction.** (A) Coronal reformation of CT shows severe right-sided hydronephrosis and a stone in a dilated lower pole calyx (arrow). (B) MAG-3 renogram shows reduced accumulation of radiotracer in the right kidney (green line). (C) MAG-3 renogram shows normal left renal excretion (red) response to furosemide injection (arrowheads) but no significant response in the right kidney (green).

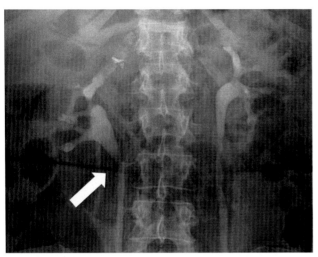

FIGURE 11-17 ■ **Crossing vessel on intravenous urogram in a 62-year-old man.** Radiograph 20 min following intravenous contrast medium injection shows a slight indentation of the ureteropelvic junction (arrow) due to a crossing vessel but no hydronephrosis.

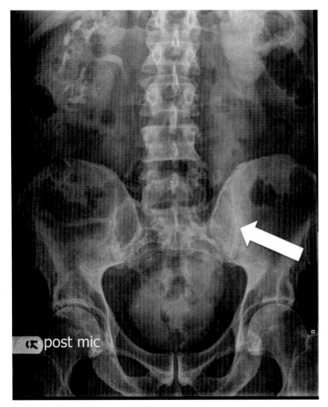

FIGURE 11-18 ■ **Primary megaureter on intravenous urogram in a 68-year-old man.** There is extensive dilatation of the left ureter (arrow) diagnosed in a delayed manner. The left ureter is less well opacified than the right ureter due to contrast medium dilution.

single or duplicated urethras, genital or lower gastrointestinal tract duplication.

Bladder diverticula in children in the absence of obstruction have an incidence of 1.7%.[16] A diverticulum at the vesicoureteric junction is known as a *Hutch diverticulum* and is associated with vesicoureteric reflux

(Fig. 11-20). The term *bladder ear*, on the other hand, refers to a diverticulum which descends into the internal inguinal ring (Fig. 11-21). Congenital diverticula are often asymptomatic; however, infection, stone formation and possibly cancer can occur, so surgical repair is sometimes necessary. Prune-belly syndrome, also known as Eagle–Barrett syndrome, is a rare constellation of findings consisting of absent rectus abdominis muscles with lax abdominal wall skin, bilateral undescended testes, dilated ureters and prostatic urethra and abnormal kidneys.[2] Vesicoureteric reflux is a common association and affected neonates generally die early. The bladder wall is characteristically thickened and the bladder enlarged though not trabeculated, owing to increased mural connective tissue. Associated anomalies are common, including those of the musculoskeletal, cardiorespiratory or gastrointestinal systems. The urachus is often patent in the setting of prune-belly syndrome.

Failure of the urachus to fibrose and obliterate causes a constellation of anomalies. Patent urachus presents with urine draining from the umbilicus at birth. Urachal cysts occur when the umbilical and vesical portions are occluded but a central segment remains patent. A urachal sinus forms when there is a blind-ending tract within the urachus contiguous with the umbilical opening, or a urachal diverticulum is observed when a segment of urachus remains in continuity with the bladder.[17] Infection is the most common complication affecting urachal remnants. Adenocarcinoma of urachal remnant is a rare cancer that often produces mucin and may contain calcification. Prognosis is typically worse compared with bladder malignancies.

Posterior urethral valves are the most common malformation of the urethra. The valve is created from a remnant of the Wolffian duct and consists of a raised mucosal fold which courses obliquely from the verumontanum to the inferior aspect of the prostatic urethra (Fig. 11-22). Diagnosis is often made after bilateral hydronephrosis is detected. Bladder outflow obstruction raises intravesical pressure, causes bladder wall thickening, trabeculation, and vesicoureteric reflux in approximately half of affected patients (Fig. 11-23). On a voiding cystourethrogram (VCUG), the valve itself may not be appreciated but the posterior urethra is both dilated and lengthened. VCUG may also diagnose anterior urethral valves, which represent an uncommon cause of urinary obstruction anywhere from the bulbar urethra to the penile urethra.

Other causes of abnormal urethral dilatation include megalourethra and urethral diverticulum and stricture. Megalourethra occurs due to abnormalities in the development of the corpus spongiosum and/or corpus cavernosum. The more common deformity occurs when only the corpus spongiosum is maldeveloped, which produces a scaphoid appearance during voiding. If the corpus cavernosum is also maldeveloped, a fusiform dilatation of the penile urethra is observed.[18] Focal stenosis or obstruction of the anterior urethra due to a ventrally located diverticulum is the second most common cause of urethral obstruction in men. A posteriorly located diverticulum can occur at the site of the prostatic utricle, a remnant of the Müllerian duct, on the verumontanum. Cowper's

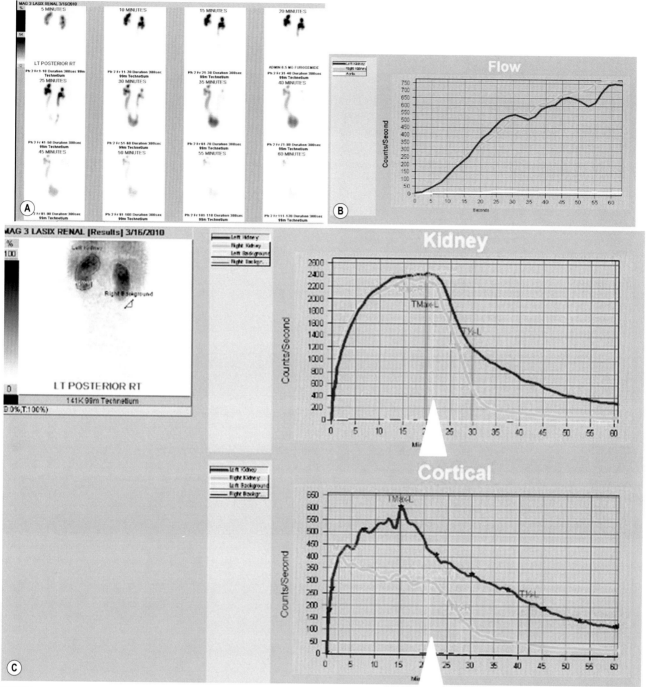

FIGURE 11-19 ■ **MAG-3 renogram in a 2-month-old girl with left-sided megaureter.** (A) Imaging every 5 min following radioisotope injection demonstrates increased accumulation in a dilated right ureter. (B) Normal radioisotope accumulation seen. (C) There is normal response to furosemide injection (arrowheads) bilaterally.

glands may be seen parallel to the urethra on a normal VCUG but occasionally they can enlarge, obstruct or fistulate into the bulbous urethra. A congenital stricture of the urethra may also be identified at VCUG. This anomaly usually occurs at the confluence of the anterior and posterior urethral segments. Stenosis of the orthopic urethra is among the associations of urethral duplication. Urethral duplication more commonly occurs in the coronal (one in front of the other) plane and usually the ventral urethra is more normal in calibre.[19] This anomaly

produces a Y-configuration with the accessory urethra originating from the prostatic portion of the normal tract. If the accessory urethra has its own origin from the bladder, incontinence ensues.

TECHNIQUES

The urinary tract may be evaluated using a wide variety of imaging techniques. The following pages provide an

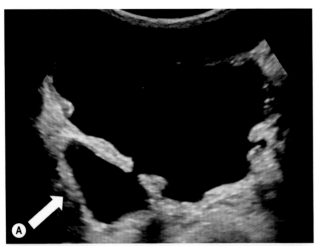

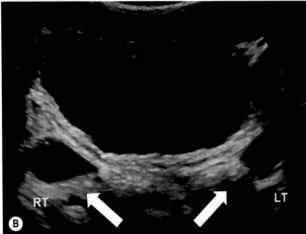

FIGURE 11-20 ■ **Hutch diverticulum on ultrasound in a 17-year-old woman with Hutch diverticulum and bilateral hydroureter.** (A) The bladder wall is trabeculated and there is a diverticulum close to the right ureteric orifice. (B) There is bilateral hydroureter (arrows).

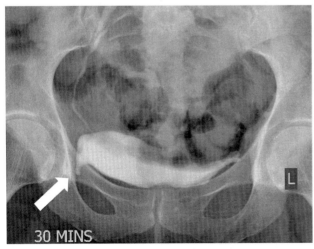

FIGURE 11-21 ■ **Bladder ear at intravenous urogram in a 61-year-old woman.** Pelvic radiograph 30 min following intravenous contrast medium administration demonstrates a bladder ear (arrow).

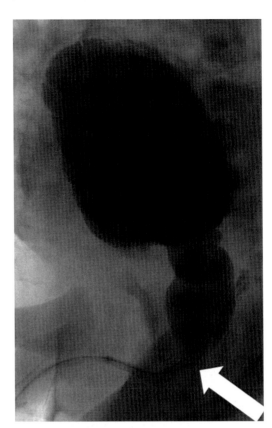

FIGURE 11-22 ■ **Posterior urethral valves in a 13-day-old boy on voiding cystourethrogram.** There is gross dilatation of the posterior urethra and a fine line is seen across the point of obstruction (arrow).

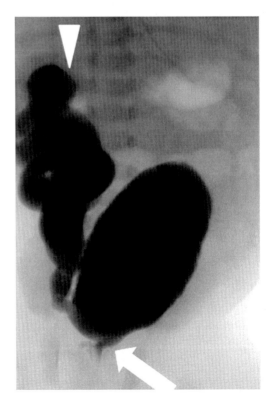

FIGURE 11-23 ■ **Posterior urethral valve in a 9-day-old boy causing grade 4 right-sided vesicoureteric reflux on voiding cystourethrogram.** There is dilatation of the posterior urethra (arrow) and severe reflux with pelvicalyceal dilatation.

overview of the techniques concerned. The optimal strategy for imaging the urinary tract is a matter of debate, particularly with recent developments in cross-sectional urography, and must be tailored to the patient's symptomatology and clinical context.[20,21] Intravenous/excretory urography (IVU) and retrograde urography are primarily used to image the upper urinary tract, whereas voiding cystourethrography and retrograde urethrography (RUG) primarily image the lower urinary tract. Ultrasound (US), nuclear scintigraphy, computed tomography (CT) and magnetic resonance imaging (MRI) are used to image the upper and lower urinary tracts.

Conventional Radiography

Conventional radiography has a low-cost, relatively open accessibility and appearances with which referring physicians are familiar. Unfortunately conventional radiography compares unfavourably with CT for the assessment of renal stone disease but cost, access and radiation dose concerns hamper the more widespread use of CT. The sensitivity of conventional radiography for the assessment of renal and ureteric stones is approximately 60% since it mainly relies on stone calcification for visualisation.[22] Conventional radiography also has a poor sensitivity for urinary malignancy since the incidence of calcification in transitional cell carcinoma (TCC) is approximately 7% and approximately 8–18% for renal cell carcinoma (RCC).[23,24] Conventional radiography therefore has little merit for urinary imaging as part of assessment for TCC and RCC, and is not indicated in high-risk patients with microscopic haematuria according to the American Urological Association Best Practice criteria. Such patients, which include those with history of smoking, pelvic radiation, analgesic abuse, certain occupational exposures and those older than 40 years,

will require upper urinary tract imaging irrespective of appearances on conventional radiography.[25]

Intravenous Urography (IVU)/Excretory Urography

Intravenous urography (IVU) can take one of two main forms: bolus infusion or drip infusion urography. Rapid instillation of 70–100 mL of 300 mmol/L non-ionic contrast medium for bolus urography achieves greater renal opacification than drip infusion, although the collecting system is visible for a shorter period of time. Drip infusion generally requires greater contrast medium volumes (100–130 mL) and fewer images need be acquired. Many variations of IVU technique exist. One suggested bolus infusion technique consists of a non-contrast medium *control* KUB and cross kidney tomogram, immediate and 1-min renal tomograms, 5-min cross kidney radiograph followed by application of compression, 10- and 20-min full-length radiographs, and coned images of the bladder before and after voiding (Fig. 11-24). The technique should be modified based upon findings as each radiograph is reviewed. For example, delayed images may be necessary if a kidney fails to excrete contrast medium, so that the degree of obstruction may be assessed. Placing the patient prone after the 10-minute image or having the patient mobilise may assist lower ureteric filling. Subsequent imaging of the patient in the supine position reduces distance from image intensifier and reduces artefacts. Patients with a single kidney should receive reduced contrast medium volumes. Pelvic compression enhances ureteric filling and may assist identification of small tumours or papillary necrosis. Contraindications to compression include suspicion of obstruction, ongoing abdominal pain, abdominal stoma or tender hernia, recent surgery, severe hypertension or abdominal aortic aneurysm.

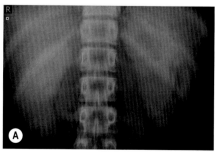 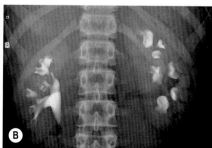 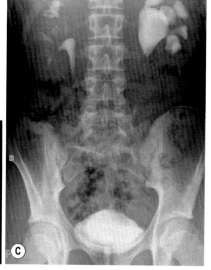

FIGURE 11-24 ■ **Intravenous urogram in an 18-year-old man with mild left hydronephrosis due to ureteropelvic junction obstruction.** (A) Bilateral symmetrical nephrotomograms. (B) Blunted calyces and preserved forniceal angles are seen on delayed phase imaging. (C) Normal excretion from the right renal collecting system noted with persistent and delayed opacification of the left renal pelvis with absent filling of the left ureter.

IVU can be time intensive, requires intravenous contrast medium and sometimes entails delayed imaging at 24 hours to localise obstruction.[20,26] In patients with impaired renal function (serum creatinine above 3.5 mg/dL) contrast medium excretion and therefore renal and ureteric visualisation are limited. The risk of contrast-induced nephropathy is increased if serum creatinine is greater than 1.5 mg/dL. The most common reasons for absent renal opacification include nephrectomy, agenesis and ectopia. Less common reasons include renal artery or vein occlusion, ureteric obstruction, pyonephrosis, pyelonephritis, xanthogranulomatous pyelonephritis, multicystic dysplastic kidney or tumour infiltration.

There has been a steady decline in the use of IVU for urinary imaging in recent decades which has raised concerns regarding reduction in skills among technologists and radiologists.[26] A 15-fold reduction in the number of IVUs performed in the United States between 1975 and 1995 has been observed.[27] CT has surpassed IVU for urinary stone assessment, with a sensitivity of 100% compared with 52–69% for IVU.[27] The superior diagnostic performance of CT versus IVU, increased patient acceptability, and equivalent or even lower radiation exposure using low-dose techniques were reasons for recommendation of CT over IVU in one evidence-based review.[28] The adoption of CT in favour of IVU is not a panacea. Even though CT is generally fast to perform and requires minimal preparation for the assessment of renal stone disease, limited CT access overnight in some hospitals can result in delayed time to imaging for patients presenting to the emergency department with renal colic, and delayed discharge.[29] A meta-analysis published in 2010 has shown that CT is superior to IVU for urinary tract tumour detection, with pooled sensitivity and specificity of 96% (95% CI: 88–100%) and 99% (95% CI: 98–100%), respectively.[30] IVU also compares unfavourably with US and CT for renal mass detection, with sensitivities of only 21, 52 and 85% for masses less than 2, 2–3 and greater than 3 cm, respectively.[31] In addition, masses detected by IVU inevitably require further imaging for lesion confirmation and characterisation by either US, CT or MRI.

The development of radiography suites capable of digital tomosynthesis may provide a lifeline for IVU. Digital tomosynthesis is being extensively evaluated in mammography, but a recent paper has shown potential for urinary imaging.[32,33] Digital tomosynthesis acquires a set of low-dose images at regular intervals for a limited degree of rotation in an arc-like pattern around a body part, which can be subsequently reconstructed to provide better resolution than conventional radiography.[32] A feasibility study of the adequacy of IVU using digital tomosynthesis compared with conventional IVU, has shown a significant improvement in the adequacy of renal and urinary imaging from 46.5% for conventional IVU to 95.5% for IVU with digital tomosynthesis.[33] There was also a reduction in length of procedure and a 56% radiation dose reduction. This facility may be most beneficial in situations where optimal renal parenchyma imaging is not required, obviating the need for cross-sectional imaging, such as for residual stone assessment after percutaneous lithotripsy.

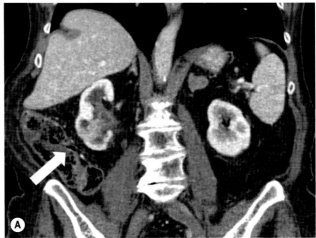

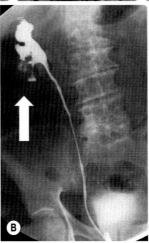

FIGURE 11-25 ■ **Transitional cell carcinoma in a 78-year-old female patient.** (A) There is right renal collecting system infiltrative mass on CT (arrow). (B) Findings confirmed on retrograde pyelogram (arrow).

Retrograde Urography

Retrograde urography is performed by gentle instillation of contrast medium devoid of air bubbles into a ureteric catheter placed by cystoscopy. The role for retrograde urography has been diminished due to isotropic CT imaging and multiplanar reconstruction. Retrograde urography can still be useful as a problem-solving tool when filling defects are detected in the upper urinary tracts on imaging and where diagnostic uncertainty exists, after negative endoscopic examination and cytology analysis, and for assessment of stone disease after renal and ureteric lithotripsy (Figs. 11-25 and 11-26).[34] There is little scientific evidence to substantiate the superiority of CT over retrograde urography. Limited studies comparing CTU with retrograde urography have shown increased sensitivity and specificity for CT detection of urothelial tumours.[34–36]

Retrograde Urethrography and Voiding Cystourethrogram

The male urethra may be imaged by retrograde urethrography (RUG) and voiding cystourethrogram

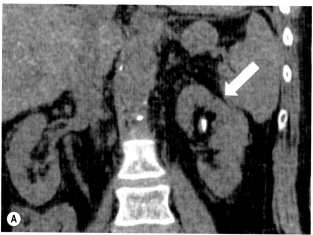

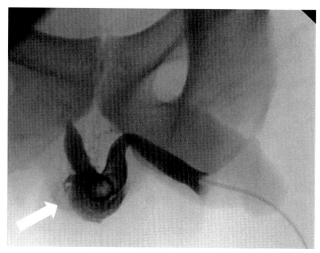

FIGURE 11-27 ■ **Urethral injury on retrograde urethrogram in a 28-year-old man after pelvic trauma.** There is extravasation of contrast medium from the bulbar urethra (arrow).

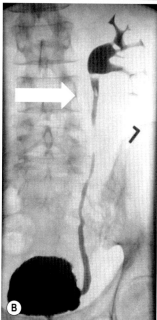

FIGURE 11-26 ■ **Patient with right renal stone, which displaced into the right ureter.** (A) CT demonstrates stone in left renal upper pole (arrow). (B) Retrograde pyelogram demonstrates the stone in the upper ureter without hydronephrosis (arrow).

(VCUG) using fluoroscopy and spot films, or overhead radiographs following cleansing of the glans penis, catheter insertion and contrast medium instillation. RUG is usually used to image the anterior urethra by placing a flushed catheter devoid of air bubbles with a 5-mm balloon in the fossa navicularis, inflating a retention balloon and then gently instilling up to 50 cc of iodinated contrast medium into a stretched penis with the patient positioned at a 45° left or right anterior oblique position and the dependent thigh flexed (Fig. 11-27). RUG performed with an external clamp just proximal to the glans penis after placement of a catheter which has no retention balloon is an alternative method of urethral imaging that causes less patient discomfort and hence allows more successful imaging than the traditional approach. RUG is also often performed after blunt perineal trauma to assess for urethral disruption.

The posterior urethra is usually imaged in an antegrade manner by VCUG after the bladder is initially drained of urine and later filled with contrast medium using a 14–18Fr Foley catheter or sometimes 18- to 20-gauge percutaneous suprapubic needle, which has been inserted directly into the bladder.[37] Radiographs of the bladder and renal fossae should be performed before contrast medium instillation. In the setting of ureteric duplication, early filling images of the bladder with the patient supine are important for the detection of ureterocele. Anteroposterior and oblique bladder imaging should be performed using intermittent fluoroscopy with spot images of abnormal findings. Lateral imaging is necessary to identify thin tracts or congenital deformities that may not otherwise be seen. Once the bladder is filled to capacity, the urethra is imaged in profile using an oblique projection after catheter removal and during micturition.

VCUG is particularly important for imaging of the urinary tract in paediatric patients. VCUG is indicated following urinary tract infection in male children or females less than 3 years old and a febrile urinary tract infection in females less than 5 years old. The presence and severity of vesicoureteric reflux should be sought and it should be noted whether reflux occurs during filling or micturition. Although nuclear cystography can also be used to diagnose vesicoureteric reflux, it lacks sufficient spatial resolution to provide accurate anatomical information regarding the bladder or urethra. Echo-enhanced voiding cystosonography and MR voiding cystography may also be used for screening or follow-up in patients with known or suspected vesicoureteric reflux, with promising initial experience. These modalities allow serial imaging, and so repeated stress testing of the bladder antireflux mechanism is feasible.

Ultrasound

Ultrasound (US) is inferior to CT for stone detection, even when combined with IVU.[38] In addition, the sensitivity of US for renal lesions smaller than 1 cm is only 26%. According to European Society of Urologic Radiology (ESUR), low- and medium-risk patients with painless haematuria should have ultrasound and cystoscopy, but high-risk patients require CT urography and cystoscopy for complete urinary tract imaging. US is up to 95% sensitive for bladder TCC; however, cystoscopy is required for assessment and biopsy to exclude mimics of TCC, including cystitis, bladder outlet obstruction, haematoma, postoperative change, prostate carcinoma, lymphoma, neurofibromatosis and endometriosis.[23] US is excellent for examination of cystic renal lesion architecture such as wall thickening, internal septations, calcification and solid components in order to prescribe a Bosniak grade. Grade 1 and 2 lesions have simple septations but no focal thickening and are considered benign, whereas lesions with focal wall or septal thickening or solid components are categorised at 3 or 4. US is also useful to assess a hyperattenuating renal lesion detected at CT, which could represent a hyperdense cyst (Bosniak 2) or solid mass. One potential pitfall is that internal echoes can sometimes give cystic lesions a solid appearance at US. In this scenario, correlation with CT or MRI can be helpful.

US is a safe method of examining the urinary tract, particularly in paediatric patients, where high-resolution imaging is normally feasible and radiation can be avoided.[39,40] US is most often performed for assessment of congenital abnormalities and infection. Postnatal US is recommended for urinary tract evaluation following documented prenatal fetal hydronephrosis. This should be performed within a week of birth, but not usually within the first 48 hours due to reduced urine output. Transient and physiologic hydronephrosis should resolve, but approximately 35% of patients with prenatal hydronephrosis will persist. The renal parenchyma should be assessed for scarring, the renal pelvis and ureter for confirmation of hydronephrosis and hydroureter, or for the presence of ureteric wall thickening and failure of peristaltic propagation. Dilatation may be primary or secondary to megaureter, vesicoureteric reflux or posterior urethral valves. VCUG is recommended if continued urinary tract dilatation is confirmed on ultrasound after birth.

If causes of megaureter such as vesicoureteric reflux and posterior urethral valves are excluded, diuresis renography should be performed next in order to differentiate primary obstructive megaureter, which requires intervention from non-obstructive non-refluxing megaureter, which is often treated conservatively (Fig. 11-18). Ultrasound is also indicated for assessment of suspected ureteric duplication in a paediatric patient. Ultrasound can be used to assess for upper moiety atrophy, ectopic ureter insertion and ureterocele formation. IVU, VCUG and nuclear scintigraphy are commonly performed for complete assessment, although MRI is showing utility in this setting and is being used to a limited extent instead of IVU (Fig. 11-13). Detection of hydronephrosis on US in an adult is an indication for CT for accurate determination of the level of obstruction (Fig. 11-16). Ultrasound can be performed for the assessment of acute pyelonephritis. A triangular zone of reduced flow can be observed

and the sensitivity of ultrasound for this purpose is comparable with that of cortical scintigraphy. Ultrasound is inferior to scintigraphy for renal scar detection.

Nuclear Medicine

Nuclear medicine provides data pertaining to renal function, perfusion and urinary tract dynamics which complements that of IVU, US, CT and MRI. ^{99m}Tc-dimercaptosuccinic acid (DMSA) is used to image the renal cortex when investigating suspected upper urinary tract infection. The merits of DMSA for imaging acute pyelonephritis are debated due to the inability to distinguish acute pyelonephritis from scarring is a limitation. It is acknowledged that DMSA is very sensitive for renal cortical scar detection. Imaging for the detection of renal scars can also be performed during assessment of urinary tract dilatation during the first few minutes after tracer injection; however, the isotopes used for this purpose are less sensitive than DMSA.

Vesicoureteric reflux is an indication for DMSA. Even though approximately 50% of patients with vesicoureteric reflux will resolve, complications such as scarring, hypertension and insufficiency can ensue. Diagnosis of vesicoureteric reflux may be made using direct of indirect radionucleotide cystography. Radiation doses are less than VCUG and continuous imaging is possible. The tracer is instilled into the bladder through a catheter (direct) or allowed to accumulate after ^{99m}Tc-mercaptoacetyltriglycine (MAG3) injection (indirect) (Figs. 11-16 and 11-18). Scintigraphy provides limited anatomic information when performed for assessment of vesicoureteric reflux and the grade of reflux cannot be assessed. The indirect method is less sensitive than either direct scintigraphy or VCUG; however, it is an appealing follow-up examination and is easy to perform as part of diuresis renography.

Diuresis renography is particularly important for the investigation of urinary tract dilatation. MAG-3 and ^{123}I-orthoiodohippurate are extracted and cleared by the renal tubules faster than the glomerular agent ^{99m}Tc-diethylenetriaminepentaacetate (DTPA) and so preferred for collecting system imaging in paediatric patients. Concentration of tubular agents in the kidneys should peak within 3 minutes after concomitant radiotracer and furosemide administration. Furosemide may be injected at differing phases of the examination depending on preference. Furosemide at a dose of 1 mg/kg for infants (max 20 mg), 0.5 mg/kg for children and 40 mg for adults may be injected when maximal renal distension is observed, 15 min prior to, at the time of, or 20 min after radiopharmaceutical injection.[41] Diuresis should begin 1–2 min after injection. Images should be taken after micturition, since a full bladder can affect urinary dynamics. Since hydration status affects furosemide response, patients are hydrated with 15 mL/kg within 30 min of examination. GFR less than 15 mL/min will reduce the renal response to furosemide.[42] Diuresis is often quantified in terms of time to peak and time or 50% of tracer washout. The extraction of radiotracer is used to calculate renal function. Function should be relatively evenly split between kidneys, with a range of 45 to 55%. Renal function less than 40 or 5% reduction compared with prior imaging is indicative of deterioration. These indices should be assessed in the context of other clinical data, and it should be remembered that renal failure, bilateral obstruction or single kidney limit sensitivity.

CT

Unenhanced CT is used to evaluate urinary tract stones, haematoma, and to obtain baseline attenuation of renal masses. Unenhanced CT is faster and more accurate than IVU for stone detection, and can identify extraurinary lesions that may mimic stone disease in clinical presentation, and avoids potential nephrotoxicity.[20,43] It is preferable to perform stone protocol CT without oral contrast medium in order to optimise stone detection. Some stones have soft-tissue attenuation on CT, including stones caused by protease inhibitors, such as indinavir sulfate, or mucoid matrix stones, which limits detection. Signs indicative of an obstructing stone include hydronephrosis, hydroureter, ipsilateral renal enlargement, perinephric and periureteral fat stranding, perinephric fluid, *ureter rim sign* and ureterovesical oedema. Combined hydronephrosis, hydroureter and perinephric stranding has a positive predictive value of 90% for an obstructing urinary tract stone (4). Alternatively, a *comet-tail* sign consisting of a linear or curvilinear soft-tissue structure extending from an abdominal or pelvic calcification indicates that a calcification represents a phlebolith rather than a stone.[44] Spontaneous passage occurs in 76% for 2–4 mm calculi, 60% for 5–7 mm calculi, 48% for 7- to 9-mm stones and less than 25% for stones greater than 9 mm.[45] Intravenous contrast medium administration is potentially indicated if doubt exists as to whether a stone lies in the collecting system or to distinguish parapelvic cysts from hydronephrosis. Renal masses are frequently detected on non-contrast CT performed for other purposes, such as CT colonography. Non-contrast CT of the bladder is important not only for stone detection but also to detect focal areas of mural calcification which can be associated with transitional cell or squamous cell carcinoma of the bladder, cyclophosphamide-induced cystitis, prior radiation treatment, schistosomiasis or urinary tract TB.

In addition to unenhanced urinary tract imaging, CT for renal parenchymal tumour detection requires arterial (15- to 30-s delay) and nephrographic post-intravenous contrast medium (80- to 100-s delay) acquisitions for renal mass detection, staging and characterisation.[46] A lesion which enhances by more than 10 HU following intravenous contrast medium is likely solid, and enhancement of 20 HU or more is considered highly suspicious of malignant lesion. In one study, the presence of an incidentally detected renal mass on non-contrast CT with attenuation between 20 and 70 HU was 100% sensitive and 89% specific for carcinoma.[47] Clear cell carcinomas are characterised by avid heterogeneous enhancement. Papillary cell carcinoma is characterised by homogeneous less avid enhancement. Homogeneous peripheral enhancement is a feature of chromophobe renal cell carcinoma which arises in the collecting duct epithelium as does an oncoctyoma (Fig. 11-28). These entities not only share

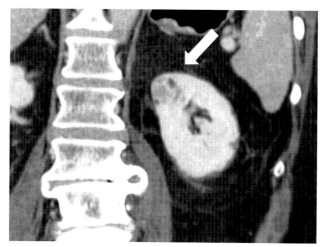

FIGURE 11-28 ■ **Oncocytoma in an 83-year-old man on CT.** There is a heterogeneously enhancing left upper pole renal mass (arrow). Biopsy confirmed an oncocytoma.

imaging features but can also be difficult to discriminate histopathologically. Multiplanar reformations are particularly important for optimal lesion detection in urinary tract imaging. Reformations help appreciate a mass at the corticomedullary junction or renal sinus fat displacement from a urothelial tumour. Wide window settings should be liberally used to evaluate pyelographic phase images to detect intraluminal filling defects surrounded by excessively dense endoluminal contrast medium.

Multiphase imaging of the urinary tract analogous to that of IVU is the method of choice for *one-stop* urinary tract imaging patients with high risk for upper urinary tract urothelial malignancy. CT urography (CTU) is defined by the European Society of Urogential Radiology as a CT optimised for renal, ureteric and bladder examination using thin–slice, excretory-phase imaging after intravenous contrast medium administration.[48] CTU typically consists of three imaging phases. Following unenhanced imaging, thin-section (2.5 mm) nephrographic phase imaging of the kidneys is acquired using non-ionic contrast medium (100–150 mL of 300 mg/mL iodine at 2–4 mL/s) after an 80- to 100-s delay.[49] Nephrographic phase imaging has the highest sensitivity for the detection of renal parenchymal masses. Correlation with unenhanced images confirms unequivocal enhancement. The excretory or pyelographic phase is imaged 5–15 min after injection and covers the upper urinary tract and bladder.

CTU protocols require continual refinement to optimise radiation exposure and urothelial imaging.[49] The number of imaging phases can be reduced using the *split-bolus* technique, by administering intravenous contrast medium in two quotients (Fig. 11-29). A 30- to 50-mL bolus of intravenous contrast medium is administered first, and 8–10 min later, after a period of mobilisation, 80–100 mL are administered prior to imaging with 80- to 100-s delay (Fig. 11-29). Thus, a hybrid *nephropyelographic phase* is acquired, in which the renal parenchyma (nephrographic phase) and the urinary collecting systems (pyelographic phase) are simultaneously imaged. One potential disadvantage of the split-bolus technique is that

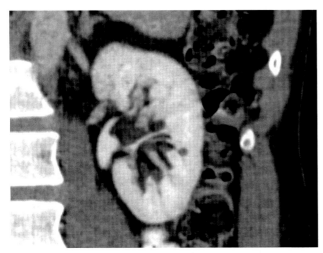

FIGURE 11-29 ■ **Parapelvic renal cysts on 51-year-old man on split-bolus CT.** Simultaneous nephrographic and pyelographic phase imaging demonstrated.

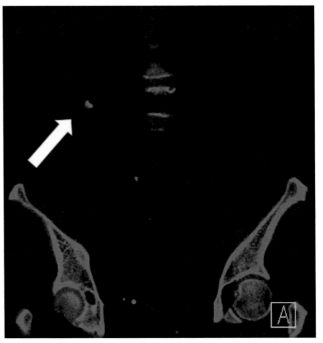

FIGURE 11-30 ■ **Calcium-containing stone on dual-energy CT in a 43-year-old female patient.** A colour overlay has been placed on the image; blue in this case indicates calcium composition (arrow).

the presence of contrast medium within the ureter at the time of imaging may obscure subtle isoattenuating tumours which are not seen on the low-dose non-contrast phase of imaging. This weakness may be potentially countered by diuretic administration, which dilutes collecting system contrast medium.

Imaging phases can potentially be reduced using dual-energy CT (DECT) which foregoes an unenhanced CT since a *virtual unenhanced CT* can be post-processed from a contrast-enhanced study acquired with two different tube voltages (usually 80 and 140 kV).[50] Three systems with this capability currently exist. Platforms use two energy sources, fast kV switching of a single source or two layers of detectors. Dual-source systems allow kV and mA to be altered separately in both tubes. A thin layer of tin allows better spectral separation and the lower kV to be set at 100 kV, which is beneficial in larger patients. The size of the gantry is increased compared with conventional single-source systems and this decreases the diameter of the bore 33 cm, which is too small for some large patients.[51] Fast kV switching uses a single-source detector platform, which reduces beam hardening artefacts, but rapid switching inhibits the use of automatic tube current modulation. Spectral filtration and separation of photon detection are limited by the use of only one tube. Dual-layer technology allows standard field-of-view imaging. Lower-energy photons from a 140-kV fan beam deposit energy in the inner detectors, and higher-energy photons are detected by the outer detectors. Spectral separation can be compromised by overlapping detection, which can limit assessment of material composition. Low- and high-energy data sets can be displayed separately. Low-energy images have high noise but good contrast resolution (closer to k edge of iodine), in counter-distinction to images obtained with higher energies.

In practice, a single composite image data set, comparable with a standard 120-kV scan, is created using non-linear blending, for optimal contrast resolution.[52] Material specific images can be created based on differential beam attenuation. This can be used to subtract base materials, including calcium, iodine and water, from an image, to quantify the amount of fat in an organ, or to discriminate uric acid from non-urate stones. This is important for characterising urinary tract calculi; for example, identification of uric acid stones which generally respond to medical treatment. Several types of calculi can be differentiated from one another on DECT, although many stones have mixed composition, which can be difficult to assess and characterise, and a dilemma to treat. Reconstructed DECT data sets can create iodine and water images for CT urography. Water images are referred to as a virtual non-contrast examination and can be created from a post-contrast study by the subtraction of iodine-containing tissues, obviating the need for an unenhanced acquisition. A colour can be assigned to stones of a particular composition or to iodine-containing structures using an overlay function for ease of interpretation or for facilitating communication of findings to referring physicians (Fig. 11-30). A colour overlay function is useful for depicting contrast enhancement in a renal mass or a nodule in a cystic lesion as part of assessment for malignancy. These data can vividly depict iodine-containing tissues, and so function as a subtraction-type study. This application adequately identifies stones over 3 mm in size lying in dilute contrast medium, but is less effective if stones are small or abut dense contrast medium.

Imaging of the urinary tract in the pyelographic phase is performed to assess for transitional cell carcinoma, the degree of obstruction due to a stone, or to identify a collecting system leak. Many variations of CT urography (CTU) protocol aim to optimise urinary tract distension to optimise tumour detection. Oral hydration, saline or diuretic infusion, compression, and prone imaging have all been assessed. One litre of water ingested 20 to 60 min before CT urography can enhance ureteric visualisation. European Society of Urogenital Radiology guidelines do not advocate routine use of saline infusion for ureteric distension.[49] Saline can stimulate peristalsis, causing temporary segmental ureteric contraction. Our group found that 100 mL saline, administered for ureteric distension and opacification in the split-bolus two-phase technique, had no effect. Furosemide (0.1 mg/kg up to 10 mg) is used to provoke diuresis for CTU when administered 1-min prior to imaging. Diuresis dilutes ureteric contrast medium, but improves mid and distal ureteric opacification and distension, compared with saline infusion alone.[53] A study has shown that dual-phase imaging with furosemide administration provided ureteric distension comparable with that of three-phase study, but benefitted from reduced artefact due to dilation of contrast medium in the collecting system.[54] Prone imaging arguably improves ureteric distension, and can help differentiate an impacted stone at the vesicoureteric junction from a mobile stone in the bladder. Although compression techniques increase proximal ureteric distension, more than one pyelographic phase scan is required, and effaced ureteric segments are observed just as often without compression. Complete ureteric distension is likely not an absolute requirement for adequate urinary tract imaging since urothelial neoplasms generally produce filling defects and obstruction. An unopacified ureter has a negative predictive value of 100% for the presence of tumour.[36]

Detection and characterisation of both intrinsic and extrinsic causes of ureteric obstruction such as mural thickening, benign and malignant strictures, retroperitoneal masses, lymphadenopathy, retroperitoneal fibrosis, and iatrogenic injury are all better assessed with CTU than IVU. CTU is superior to IVU for detection of upper urinary tract urothelial malignancies.[55] The sensitivity, specificity, positive predictive and negative predictive values of CTU for diagnosing upper urinary tract urothelial tumour are 0.97, 0.93, 0.79 and 0.99, respectively.[56] CTU is comparable with retrograde urography for diagnosis of upper urinary tract urothelial tumours. CTU has only a moderate positive predictive value for tumour detection, and for now at least, suspicious findings should be histologically confirmed before definitive surgery.[57] It is a reasonable policy to use CTU for first-line investigation of patient with haematuria and retrograde pyleography for patients in which CTU is equivocal. Enhancing focal bladder wall thickening is suggestive of lower urinary tract carcinoma, whereas diffuse or uniform bladder wall thickening is usually secondary to cystitis or changes related to obstructive uropathy. Cystoscopy is the gold standard for bladder assessment; however, good examination of the bladder is desirable due to high rates of synchronous tumours in the urinary tract. Good bladder distension is important and delayed-phase imaging a necessity for assessment.

MRI

MR urography (MRU) is capable of complete urinary tract medium imaging. Contrast resolution exceeds

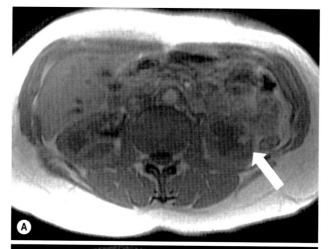
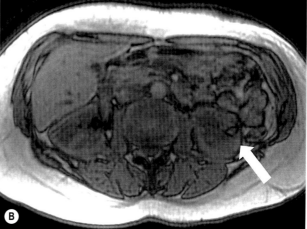

FIGURE 11-31 ■ Renal MRI in a 41-year-old female patient with angiomyelolipoma. (A) In-phase MRI demonstrates a T1 hyperintense lesion in the left kidney (arrow). (B) The lesion drops signal on out-of-phase imaging (arrow).

CTU, no ionising radiation is required, and no intravenous contrast medium need be administered. This is beneficial in pregnant females, and patients with renal insufficiency. MRU is also very effective for imaging most paediatric lesions and anomalies. Serial ureteric imaging can overcome the potential pitfalls associated with ureteric peristalsis and help characterise lesions, quantifying renal function, or assess for vascular invasion.[58]

Urinary tract imaging should commence with precontrast fat-suppressed T1- and T2-weighted sequences, and in- and out-of-phase gradient-echo sequences for intracytoplasmic lipid detection within lesions, such as angiomyolipoma or clear cell renal cell carcinoma (RCC) (Fig. 11-31). Some angiomyolipomas are lipid-poor and both lipid-poor angiomyolipomas and papillary carcinomas are of low signal on T2-weighted imaging. Clear cell RCCs are generally iso- or hyperintense to normal renal parenchyma on T2-weighted images.[59,60] Another complicating issue is that some RCC lesions may contain fat and extensive tumours may invade renal sinus or perinephric fat.[61,62] MRI for evaluation of RCC is most useful for assessment of vascular invasion, recurrence following ablative techniques, and for those in whom intravenous iodinated contrast medium is contraindicated.[63]

The collecting system is examined with static-fluid urography using heavily T2-weighted sequences such as half-Fourier acquisition single-shot turbo spin-echo (HASTE), or excretory urography with breath-hold fat-suppressed T1-weighted 3D gradient-echo sequences following intravenous contrast medium. Intravenous hydration, diuretics (0.1 mg/kg furosemide) and oral restriction may all be used to optimise contrast from urine. Intravenous contrast medium usually needs to be supplemented by one of these measures in order to avoid T2* effects due to high concentrations of gadolinium. Excretory T1-weighted sequences can image the kidneys in the corticomedullary, nephrographic and excretory phases as for CTU. Fat-poor angiomyolipomas and clear cell carcinoma tend to avidly enhance, whereas papillary carcinomas tend to poorly enhance, reflecting the diminished vascularity of the latter compared with the former.[64,65] A wide spectrum of enhancement exists and biopsy is often advised for definitive diagnosis.[66] Combined static fluid and excretory MRU can provide useful information in obstructive uropathy, since T2-weighted sequences demonstrate collecting system dilatation and excretory images help estimate the degree of obstruction. Imaging is usually performed in the coronal and axial planes, with excretory imaging approximately 5 min following intravenous gadolinium.[67] Imaging resolution is 2–3 mm, which is inferior to that of CTU. Signal-to-noise ratio is optimised by using phased-array surface coins and segmental imaging of the upper and lower urinary tract; however, this is not normally necessary.

Calcified lesions create signal drop-out or filling defects. Stones less than 5 mm are not well visualised and appearances can be simulated by blood clots, surgical clips or small tumours.[68] In pregnant patients, HASTE imaging appears useful for the assessment of hydronephrosis related to pregnancy and for stone detection.[69] Spin-echo MRI helps differentiate blood clots and stones from tumour by demonstrating contrast enhancement on post-contrast T1-weighted imaging.[70] Stone detection is improved by using gadolinium-DTPA (sensitivity between 94 and 100%) as for conventional excretory urography.[71] Furosemide administration enhances the ability of MRU to evaluate the non-dilated urinary systems by increasing glomerular filtration.[72] However, static MRU sequences can demonstrate secondary signs of obstruction such as renal oedema better than CTU by detecting hyperintense urine within renal tubules.[73] T1-weighted imaging is advantageous in the setting of incomplete obstruction because with the aid of contrast medium, the ureteric tract can be demonstrated above and below the site of obstruction and can provide an estimation of the degree of ureteric stenosis.[73] T2-weighted imaging is likely sufficient in the setting of high grade or complete obstruction. MRI is showing increasing utility for examining the urinary tract for urothelial tumours and to exclude synchronous and metachronous lesions.[73] Limited access and difficulties detecting calcification or air are among the principal obstacles to increased use for urinary tract imaging. MRU provides a comprehensive and non-invasive diagnostic tool for urinary tract imaging that is showing increasing utility as experience grows and limitations are better understood.

RADIATION ISSUES

An increased awareness of the importance of radiation exposure reduction and optimisation in medical imaging has become apparent over the past decade. The optimal strategy for minimising radiation exposure in urinary tract imaging requires collaboration, including educational initiatives and modification of referral practices. Radiologists must ensure that all studies with ionising radiation are indicated and integrate low-dose CT protocols into routine practice and use alternative imaging such as ultrasound and MRI where feasible.

Mean annual exposures due to ionising radiation from medical sources are 1.5 and 0.48 mSv among patients in the United States and the Netherlands, respectively.[74,75] The ill effects of X-rays can be either deterministic or stochastic. Deterministic effects, including skin erythema, become worse with increasing exposure, have thresholds but fortunately rarely occur[76] as a result of exposure to ionising radiation from diagnostic studies. The probability of a stochastic effect occurring is variable and has no threshold. Increasing radiation exposure increases the likelihood of a stochastic effect but no safe lower limit exists. Cancer is a stochastic effect, which may occur years following exposure. Young age, large exposure and possibly frequent exposures increase risks.[77]

Radiation Exposure from Medical Imaging

Conventional Radiography

Conventional radiography (CR) is only moderately sensitive for detecting renal and urinary tract stones. Low-dose CT (0.5 mSv in men and 0.7 mSv in women) with doses equivalent to that of CR has a sensitivity and specificity for stone detection of 97 and 95%, respectively.[78] Factors which limit the abandonment of conventional radiography and replacement with CT include expense, limited accessibility and, importantly, the increased radiation dose associated with standard-dose CT (3.63 mSv) compared with plain radiography (0.7 mSv) at most centres.[79,80] A study of cumulative effective doses from CT examinations in 176 patients with chronic nephrolithiasis showed that patients had 3–18 CT images, each with effective doses of 6–17 mSv.[81] For reassessment of patients with urinary tract calculi diagnosed by CT, conventional radiography and scout films from CT studies can potentially be used.[82] Correlating CT scout images with conventional radiographs can help localise stones for the purposes of follow-up. At our institution, we favour low-dose CT protocols, where feasible, for follow-up.

IVU

CTU has largely replaced IVU for the assessment of the urinary tracts in many centres.[83] CT can impart much higher radiation doses compared with IVU, depending on the protocol used. An average IVU including nephrotomograms can result in a total of 12 images and an effective dose between 5 and 15 mSv.[84] In another study, 9.3 radiographs were used for an average IVU, and the mean effective dose was 3 mSv.[85] A three-phase CT can have a mean effective dose of 15 ± 9 mSv (155–200 mAs at 120 kV, 1–2.5 mm collimation), and has a radiation dose 1.5 times higher than IVU.[86] Interestingly, the mean skin dose of IVU has been noted to be 2.7 times than that of CT, which has a more uniform dose distribution. Skin doses with IVU are higher than CT due to exponential decrease in radiation dose between entrance and exit sites.

CT

CT examinations represent approximately 10% of all studies that use ionising radiation, yet they are responsible for two-thirds of radiation dose related to medical imaging.[86] Radiation dose is a major concern due to replacement of CR and IVU by CTU. Although modern CT provides excellent spatial resolution and isotropic reformations, 4% of patients with urinary stones, for example, require repeated CT imaging, which is an increasing cause of concern.[82] Four-phase CTU can have an effective dose of 25–35 mSv.[87] A CTU protocol can have a radiation dose between 6 and 18 mSv; the wide range in radiation exposure is explained by variation in scan parameters.[88] Radiation dose can be reduced by carefully monitoring scanning parameters for each phase, reducing the number of phases, and optimising reconstruction methods.

Radiation dose reduction for *stone-protocol* CT is feasible since increased image noise does not significantly limit discrimination of stones from surrounding soft tissue. This single-phase protocol is sufficient in many patients requiring urinary tract imaging, particularly for stone assessment in a patient with ureteric colic. Radiation doses in CTU can also be reduced by limiting the number of imaging phases. Benign conditions such as a suspected congenital anomaly or ureteric trauma may only require a single excretory phase CT.[89] In high-grade ureteric obstruction, where asymmetric contrast excretion is anticipated, a longer delay of the excretory phase can be performed, rather than scanning multiple times.[89] The *split-bolus* technique is a practical alternative to three-phase imaging.[90] The European Society of Urologic Radiology has recommended that the split-bolus technique be used for CTU in younger patients (<40) to minimise radiation dose and that three-phase protocols be reserved for older patients or those at high risk of malignant disease, albeit with close adherence to the ALARA principle.[89] The split-bolus technique has been shown to decrease radiation dose by 65% compared with the three-phase technique.[54]

There is a linear relationship between tube current and radiation dose. A 43–66% dose reduction with *stone-protocol* CT is feasible using automatic tube current modulation (ATM), which automatically adjusts tube current depending on body attenuation relative to a user-prescribed image quality range.[91] Detection of urinary tract stones with ATM is feasible even with high noise indices of 14 to 20 without compromising stone depiction.[92] At present ATM cannot be used in conjunction with fast-kV switching single source dual-energy CT systems.[92] Using an animal model, a current–time product of 70 mAs has been reported to be sufficient for CTU with effective doses of between 3 and 5 mSv.[93,94] A current–time product equalling the value of a patient's weight in kilograms is another suggested method for low-dose examinations, which can reduce radiation doses to 50%.[95] It has been noted that effective CTU radiation exposures increase by a factor of 2 when patient thickness doubles.[84] This observation supports the suggestion that technical settings could be tailored to patients' body habitus in order to reduce doses. Tube voltage reduction at CTU from 120 to 90 kV in an experimental model reduces radiation dose by 60%.[96] A tube voltage of 80 kV combined with noise reduction filters is equivalent to 120 kV imaging according to one study, but only for upper urinary tract assessment.[97] Contrast material in the urinary tract absorbs a greater proportion of X-rays relative to biological tissues at 80 kV as energy approaches the k edge of iodine, which helps maintain sensitivity for stones or contrast.[98] A potential disadvantage of this approach for CTU is that low-contrast lesions can potentially be missed, which may result in failure to detect urothelial tumours. Noise reduction filters can be applied to low-dose data sets in order to improve image acceptability and have shown a 25% dose saving.[99]

Radiation dose reductions of 30–40% are achievable in practice using adaptive statistical iterative reconstruction (ASIR).[100] Further dose reductions should be feasible using full iterative reconstruction techniques which have recently been made available on CT platforms. A study of 50 patients with Crohn's disease that compared low-dose and conventional-dose CT images reconstructed using ASIR[101] showed that low-dose CTs had a mean dose of 0.98 mSv and a dose reduction of 72% compared with conventional dose images, which had a mean dose of 3.5 mSv. Even though there was some sacrifice of image quality using low-dose imaging, this was not at the cost of reduced imaging accuracy. No clinically significant diagnostic findings were missed on the low-dose CT images. Importantly, low-dose CT accurately excluded clinically significant pathology such as perforation or abscess in the remaining 50 patients, which, in some cases allowed safe consideration of immunosuppressive therapy. It is important to note, however, that solid organ imaging is currently suboptimal at doses approaching 1 mSv and caution is advised in extrapolating these results to all clinical settings, without due consideration.

CONCLUSION

The anatomy of the urinary tract is subject to great variation, which often influences the subsequent development of pathology. The urinary tract may be imaged using many techniques. The optimal method for imaging frequently depends upon the clinical concerns, patient circumstances and available techniques. A collaborative approach between referring physicians and radiologists is important for good patient outcome. Referring physicians and radiologists also share responsibility for the justification of radiation exposure and an onus exists to minimise exposures. Based on current data, there is cause for optimism that increased availability and integration of dose reduction techniques will achieve significant radiation dose reduction and acceptable image quality for urinary tract imaging in the near future.

REFERENCES

1. Kenney PJ, Spirt BA, Leeson MD. Genitourinary anomalies: radiologic-anatomic correlations. Radiographics 1984;4(2): 233–60.
2. Berrocal T, López-Pereira P, Arjonilla A, Gutiérrez J. Anomalies of the distal ureter, bladder, and urethra in children: embryologic, radiologic, and pathologic features. Radiographics 2002;22(5): 1139–64.
3. Moore KL. The urogenital system. In: Moore KL, editor. The Developing Human: Clinically Oriented Embryology. 3rd ed. Philadelphia: Saunders; 1982. pp. 255–97.
4. Zagoria RJ. The kidney and retroperitoneum: anatomy and congenital abnormalities. In: Zagoria RJ, editor. Requisites Genitourinary Radiology. 2nd ed. Philadelphia: Mosby; 2004. pp. 51–79.
5. Zagoria RJ. The lower urinary tract. In: Zagoria RJ, editor. Requisites Genitourinary Radiology. 2nd ed. Philadelphia: Mosby; 2004. pp. 201–55.
6. Gay SB, Armistead JP, Weber ME, Williamson BR. Left infrarenal region: anatomic variants, pathologic conditions, and diagnostic pitfalls. Radiographics 1991;11(4):549–70.
7. Kadir S. Angiography of the kidneys. In: Kadir S, editor. Diagnostic Angiography. Philadelphia: Saunders; 1986. pp. 445–95.
8. Zagoria RJ. The renal sinus, pelvicaliceal system and ureter. In: Zagoria R, editor. Requisites Genitourinary Radiology. 2nd ed. Philadelphia: Mosby; 2004. pp. 158–200.
9. Hartman GW, Hodson CJ. The duplex kidney and related abnormalities. Clin Radiol 1969;20:387–400.
10. Fernbach SK, Feinstein KA, Spencer K, Lindstrom CA. Ureteral duplication and its complications. Radiographics 1997;17(1): 109–27.
11. Mackie GG, Stephens FD. Duplex kidneys: a correlation of renal dysplasia with position of the ureteral orifice. J Urol 1975; 1(14):274–80.
12. Fenelon MJ, Alton DJ. Prolapsing ectopic ureteroceles in boys. Radiology 1981;140:373–6.
13. Kass EJ. Megaureter. In: Kelalis PP, King LR, Belman AB, editors. Clinical Pediatric Urology. 3rd ed. Philadelphia: Saunders; 1992. pp. 781–821.
14. Zerin JM. Hydronephrosis in the neonate and young infant: current concepts. Semin Ultrasound CT MR 1994;15: 306–16.
15. Lebowitz RL, Olbing H, Parkkulainen KV, et al. International system of radiographic grading of vesicoureteric reflux. Pediatr Radiol 1985;15:105–9.
16. Blane CE, Zerin JM, Bloom DA. Bladder diverticula in children. Radiology 1994;190:695–7.
17. Suita S, Nagasaki A. Urachal remnants. Semin Pediatr Surg 1996;5:107–15.
18. Kester RR, Woopan UM, Ohm HK, Kim H. Congenital megalourethra. J Urol 1990;4:1213–15.
19. Effman EL, Lebowitz RL, Colodny AH. Duplication of the urethra. Radiology 1976;119:179–85.
20. Maher MM, Kalra MK, Rizzo S, et al. Multidetector CT urography in imaging of the urinary tract in patients with hematuria. Kor J Radiol 2004;5:1–10.
21. Nolte-Ernsting C, Cowan N. Understanding multislice CT urography techniques: many roads lead to Rome. Eur Radiol 2006;16: 2670–86.
22. Caoli EM, Cohan RH, Korobkin M, et al. Urinary tract abnormalities: initial experience with multi-detector row CT urography. Radiology 2002;222:353–60.
23. Thurston W, Wilson SR. The urinary tract. In: Rumack CM, Wilson SR, Charboneau JW, editors. Diagnostic Ultrasound. 3rd ed. St. Louis: Elsevier Mosby; 2005. pp. 321–93.

24. Wong-You-Cheong JJ, Wagner BJ, Davis CJ Jr. Transitional cell carcinoma of the urinary tract: radiologic-pathologic correlation. Radiographics 1998;18(1):123–42.
25. Grossfeld GD, Litwin MS, Wolf JS, et al. Evaluation of asymptomatic microscopic hematuria in adults: the American Urological Association best practice policy—part I: definition, detection, prevalence, and etiology. Urology 2001;57(4):599–603.
26. Vrtiska TJ. Quantitation of stone burden: imaging advances. Urol Res 2005;33:398–402.
27. Dalla Palma L. What is left of i.v. urography? Eur Radiol 2001;11(6):931–9.
28. Shine S. Urinary calculus: IVU vs CT renal stone? A critically appraised topic. Abdom Imaging 2008;33(1):41–3.
29. Quirke M, Divilly F, O'Kelly P, et al. Imaging patients with renal colic: a comparative analysis of the impact of non-contrast helical computed tomography versus intravenous urography on the speed of patient processing in the Emergency Department. Emerg Med J 2011;28(3):197–200.
30. Chlapoutakis K, Theocharopoulos N, Yarmenitis S, Damilakis J. Performance of computed tomographic urography in diagnosis of upper urinary tract urothelial carcinoma, in patients presenting with hematuria: Systematic review and meta-analysis. Eur J Radiol 2010;73(2):334–8.
31. Warshauer DM, McCarthy SM, Street L, et al. Detection of renal masses: sensitivities and specificities of excretory urography/ linear tomography, US, and CT. Radiology 1988;169(2): 363–5.
32. Wells IT, Raju VM, Rowberry BK, et al. Digital tomosynthesis—a new lease of life for the intravenous urogram? Br J Radiol 2011;84(1001):464–8.
33. Wallis MG, Moa E, Zanca F, et al. Two-view and single-view tomosynthesis versus full-field digital mammography: high-resolution X-ray imaging observer study. Radiology 2012;262(3): 788–96.
34. Cowan NC, Turney BW, Taylor NJ, et al. Multidetector computed tomography urography for diagnosing upper urinary tract urothelial tumour. BJU Int 2007;99:1363–70.
35. Caoili EM, Cohan RH, Inampudi P, et al. MDCT urography of upper tract urothelial neoplasms. Am J Roentgenol 2005;184(6): 1873–81.
36. Tsili AC, Efremidis SC, Kalef-Ezra J, et al. Multi-detector row CT urography on a 16-row CT scanner in the evaluation of urothelial tumors. Eur Radiol 2007;17(4):1046–54.
37. Kawashima A, Sandler CM, Wasserman NF, et al. Imaging of urethral disease: a pictorial review. Radiographics 2004; 24(suppl 1):S195–216.
38. Levine JA, Neitlich J, Verga M, et al. Ureteral calculi in patients with flank pain: correlation of plain film radiography with unenhanced helical CT. Radiology 1997;204:27–31.
39. Greenfield SP, Williot P, Kaplan D. Gross hematuria in children: a ten-year review. Urology 2007;69(1):166–9.
40. Hulton SA. Evaluation of urinary tract calculi in children. Arch Dis Child 2001;84(4):320–3.
41. O'Reilly PH. Standardization of the renogram technique for investigating the dilated upper urinary tract and assessing the results of surgery. BJU Int 2003;91:239–43.
42. Boubaker A, Prior JO, Meuwly JY, Bischof-Delaloye A. Radionuclide investigations of the urinary tract in the era of multimodality imaging. J Nucl Med 2006;47(11):1819–36.
43. Sourtzis S, Thibeau JF, Damry N, et al. Radiologic investigation of renal colic: Unenhanced helical CT compared with excretory urography. Am J Roentgenol 1999;172:1491–4.
44. Guest AR, Cohan RH, Korobkin M, et al. Assessment of the clinical utility of the rim and comet-tail signs in differentiating ureteral stones from phleboliths. Am J Roentgenol 2001;177(6): 1285–91.
45. Coll DM, Varanelli MJ, Smith RC. Relationship of spontaneous passage of ureteral calculi to stone size and location as revealed by unenhanced helical CT. Am J Roentgenol 2002;178(1): 101–3.
46. Ng CS, Wood CG, Silverman PM, et al. Renal cell carcinoma: diagnosis, staging, and surveillance. Am J Roentgenol 2008;191(4): 1220–32.
47. O'Connor SD, Pickhardt PJ, Kim DH, et al. Incidental finding of renal masses at unenhanced CT: prevalence and analysis of

REFERENCES **303**

48. Van der Molen AJ, Cowan NC, Mueller-Lisse UG, et al; CT Urography Working Group of the European Society of Urogenital Radiology (ESUR). CT urography: definition, indications and techniques. A guideline for clinical practice. Eur Radiol 2008; 18:4–17.

49. O'Connor OJ, McSweeney SE, Maher MM. Imaging of hematuria. Radiol Clin N Am 2008;46:113–32.

50. Graser A, Johnson TR, Chandarana H, Macari M. Dual energy CT: preliminary observations and potential clinical applications in the abdomen. Eur Radiol 2009;19(1):13–23.

51. Hartman R, Kawashima A, Takahashi N, et al. Applications of dual-energy CT in urologic imaging: an update. Radiol Clin N Am 2012;50:191–205.

52. Yu L, Primak AN, Liu X, et al. Image quality optimization and evaluation of linearly mixed images in dual source, dual-energy CT. Med Phys 2009;36(3):1019–24.

53. Silverman SG, Leyendecker JR, Amis ES Jr. What is the current role of CT urography and MR urography in the evaluation of the urinary tract? Radiology 2009;250(2):309–23.

54. Portnoy O, Guranda L, Apter S, et al. Optimization of 64-MDCT urography: effect of dual-phase imaging with furosemide on collecting system opacification and radiation dose. Am J Roentgenol 2011;197(5):W882–86.

55. Wang LJ, Wong YC, Huang CC, et al. Multidetector computerized tomography urography is more accurate than excretory urography for diagnosing transitional cell carcinoma of the upper urinary tract in adults with hematuria. J Urol 2010;183(1): 48–55.

56. Blick CG, Nazir SA, Mallett S, et al. Evaluation of diagnostic strategies for bladder cancer using computed tomography (CT) urography, flexible cystoscopy and voided urine cytology: results for 778 patients from a hospital haematuria clinic. BJU Int 2011;110(1):84–94.

57. Cowan NC. CT urography for hematuria. Nat Rev Urol 2012; 9(4):218–26.

58. Vivier PH, Dolores M, Taylor M, Dacher JN. MR urography in children. Part 2: how to use ImageJ MR urography processing software. Pediatr Radiol 2010;40(5):739–46.

59. Jinzaki M, Tanimoto A, Narimatsu Y, et al. Angiomyolipoma: imaging findings in lesions with minimal fat. Radiology 1997;205: 497–502.

60. Shinmoto H, Yuasa Y, Tanimoto A, et al. Small renal cell carcinoma: MRI with pathologic correlation. J Magn Reson Imaging 1998;8:690–4.

61. Lesavre A, Correas J, Merran S, et al. CT of papillary renal cell carcinomas with cholesterol necrosis mimicking angiomyolipomas. Am J Roentgenol 2003;181:143–5.

62. Prando A. Intratumoral fat in a renal cell carcinoma. Am J Roentgenol 1991;156:871.

63. Kabala JE, Gillatt DA, Persad RA, et al. Magnetic resonance imaging in the staging of renal cell carcinoma. Br J Radiol 1991; 64(764):683–9.

64. Yamashita Y, Takahashi M, Watanabe O, et al. Small renal cell carcinoma: pathologic and radiologic correlation. Radiology 1992; 184:493–8.

65. Kim JK, Park S, Shon J, Cho K. Angiomyolipoma with minimal fat: differentiation from renal cell carcinoma at biphasic helical CT. Radiology 2004;230:677–84.

66. Silverman SG, Mortele KJ, Tuncali K, et al. Hyperattenuating renal masses: etiologies, pathogenesis, and imaging evaluation. Radiographics 2007;27(4):1131–43.

67. Silverman S, Leyendecker J, Amis S. What is the current role of CT urography and MR urography in the evaluation of the urinary tract? Radiology 2009;250:309–23.

68. Kawashima A, Glockner JF, King BFJ. CT urography and MR urography. Radiol Clin North Am 2003;41:945–54.

69. Mullins JK, Semins MJ, Hyams ES, et al. Half Fourier single-shot turbo spin-echo magnetic resonance urography for the evaluation of suspected renal colic in pregnancy. Urology 2012;79(6): 1252–5.

70. Catalano C, Pavone P, Laghi A, et al. MR urography and conventional MR imaging in urinary tract obstruction. Acta Radiol 1999;40:198–202.

71. Sudah M, Vanninen R, Partanen K, et al. Patients with acute flank pain: comparison of MR urography with unenhanced helical CT. Radiology 2002;223:98–105.

72. Nolte-Ernsting CCA, Bucker A, Adam GB, et al. Gadolinium-enhanced excretory MR urography after low-dose diuretic injection: comparison with conventional excretory urography. Radiology 1998;209:147–57.

73. Blandino A, Minutoli F, Scribano E, et al. Combined magnetic resonance urography and targeted helical CT in patients with renal colic: a new approach to reduce delivered dose. J Mag Reson Imag 2004;20:264–71.

74. United States Medical Regulatory Commission. Fact Sheet on Biological Effects of Radiation. Available at <http://www.nrc.gov/reading-rm/doc-collections/fact-sheets/bio-effects-radiation.html>; 2012.

75. Aroua A, Olerud HM, et al. Collective doses from medical exposures: an intercomparison of the 'Top 20' radiological examinations based on the EC guidelines RP 154. Proceedings of the Third European IRPA Congress, Helsinki, Finland. Available at <http://www.irpa2010europe.com/pdfs/Proceedings_-_Third_European_IRPA_Congress_2010.pdf>; 2010.

76. Koenig TR, Wolff D, Mettler FA, Wagner LK. Skin injuries from fluoroscopically guided procedures: part 1, characteristics of radiation injury. Am J Roentgenol 2001;177:3–11.

77. Brenner D, Elliston C, Hall E, Berdon W. Estimated risks of radiation-induced fatal cancer from pediatric CT. Am J Roentgenol 2001;176(2):289–96.

78. Kluner C, Hein PA, Gralla O, et al. Does ultra-low-dose CT with a radiation dose equivalent to that of KUB suffice to detect renal and ureteral calculi? J Comput Assist Tomogr 2006;30(1):44–50.

79. Eikefjord EN, Thorsen F, Rorvik J. Comparison of effective radiation doses in patients undergoing unenhanced MDCT and excretory urography for acute flank pain. Am J Roentgenol 2007; 188(4):934–9.

80. Wall BF, Hart D. Revised radiation doses for typical X-ray examinations. Report on a recent review of doses to patients from medical X-ray examinations in the UK by NRPB. National Radiological Protection Board. Br J Radiol 1997;70:437–9.

81. Katz SI, Saluja S, Brink JA, Forman HP. Radiation dose associated with unenhanced CT for suspected renal colic: impact of repetitive studies. Am J Roentgenol 2006;186(4):1120–4.

82. Jackman SV, Potter SR, Regan F, Jarrett TW. Plain abdominal X-ray versus computerized tomography screening: sensitivity for stone localization after nonenhanced spiral computerized tomography. J Urol 2000;164(2):308–10.

83. Mueller-Lisse UL, Coppenrath EM, Meindl T, et al. Delineation of upper urinary tract segments at MDCT urography in patients with extra-urinary mass lesions: retrospective comparison of standard and low-dose protocols for the excretory phase of imaging. Eur Radiol 2011;21(2):378–84.

84. Nawfel RD, Judy PF, Schleipman AR, Silverman SG. Patient radiation dose at CT urography and conventional urography. Radiology 2004;232:126–32.

85. Yakoumakis E, Tsalafoutas IA, Nikolaou D, et al. Differences in effective dose estimation from dose are product and entrance surface dose measurements in intravenous urography. Br J Radiol 2001;74:727–34.

86. Mettler FA, Wiest PW, Locken JA, Kelsey CA. CT scanning: patterns of use and dose. J Radiol Prot 2000;20:353–9.

87. Caoili EM, Inampudi P, Cohan RH, Ellis JH. Optimization of multi-detector row CT urography: effect of compression, saline administration, and prolongation of acquisition delay. Radiology 2005;235:116–23.

88. Martingano P, Stacul F, Cavallaro MF, et al. 64-Slice CT urography: optimisation of radiation dose. Radiol Med 2011;116(3): 417–31.

89. Van der Molen AJ, Cowan NC, Mueller-Lisse UG, et al; CT Urography Working Group of the European Society of Urogenital Radiology (ESUR). CT urography: definition, indications and techniques. A guideline for clinical practice. Eur Radiol 2008; 18:4–17.

90. Takeyama N, Ohgiya Y, Hayashi T, et al. CT urography in the urinary bladder: to compare excretory phase images using a low noise index and a high noise index with adaptive noise reduction filter. Acta Radiol 2011;52(6):692–8.

features for guiding management. Am J Roentgenol 2011;197(1): 139–45.

91. Kalra MK, Maher MM, D'Souza RV, et al. Detection of urinary tract stones at low-radiation-dose CT with z-axis automatic tube current modulation: phantom and clinical studies. Radiology 2005;235(2):523–9.

92. Silva AC, Morse BG, Hara AK, et al. Dual-energy (spectral) CT: applications in abdominal imaging. Radiographics 2011;31(4): 1031–46.

93. Kemper J, Bergmann PGC, Regier M, et al. Multislice-CT-urography: experimental evaluation of low-dose protocols. Eur Radiol 2005;15(Suppl 1):273.

94. Stamm G, Nagel HD. CT-expo-a novel program for dose evaluation in CT. Fortschr Rontgenstr 2002;174:1570–6.

95. Nolte-Ernsting C, Cowan N. Understanding multislice CT urography techniques: many roads lead to Rome. Eur Radiol 2006;16: 2670–86.

96. Coppenrath E, Meindl T, Herzog P, et al. Dose reduction in multidetector CT of the urinary tract. Studies in a phantom model. Eur Radiol 2006;16:1982–9.

97. Yanaga Y, Awai K, Funama Y, et al. Low-dose MDCT urography: feasibility study of low-tube-voltage technique and adaptive noise reduction filter. Am J Roentgenol 2009;193:W220–9.

98. Seltzer SM. Calculation of photo mass energy-transfer and mass energy absorption coefficients. Radiat Res 1993;136:147–70.

99. Sung MK, Singh S, Kalra MK. Current status of low dose multi-detector CT in the urinary tract. World J Radiol 2011;3(11): 256–65.

100. Singh S, Kalra MK, Shenoy-Bhangle AS, et al. Radiation dose reduction with hybrid iterative reconstruction for pediatric CT. Radiology 2012;263(2):537–46.

101. Craig O, O'Neill S, O'Neill F, et al. Diagnostic accuracy of computed tomography using lower doses of radiation for patients with Crohn's disease. Clin Gastroenterol Hepatol 2012; 10(8):886–92.

CHAPTER 12

RENAL MASSES: IMAGING AND BIOPSY

Giles Rottenberg • Zaid Viney

METHODS OF ANALYSIS

Plain Abdominal Radiography

The plain abdominal radiograph (KUB—kidneys, ureters, bladder) is rarely used to diagnose a renal mass. Loss of the psoas margin or displacement of retroperitoneal fat may suggest the presence of one, as may an opacity projected over the renal outline, or a loss of the renal outline. Central calcification within a renal mass is more suggestive of malignancy than peripheral calcification (87 vs 20–30%).

Intravenous Urography

Intravenous urography (IVU) is a relatively insensitive method for detecting renal masses, particularly if they occur centrally rather than peripherally; cross-sectional techniques are a more appropriate method for investigating a patient with a suspected renal mass.

Radionuclide Imaging

Differentiation between a definite mass and an anatomical variant that simulates a mass (pseudotumour) can be made using radionuclide imaging, although this is rarely useful in practice.

Ultrasound

Ultrasound (US) is usually the first method for evaluating a patient for a renal mass and is the most appropriate technique for evaluating an abnormal IVU. Ultrasound is ideally suited for children, pregnant women and patients with renal impairment. Ultrasound can reliably differentiate solid masses from simple cysts, which are the most common space-occupying lesions in the kidney. A lesion that appears solid on ultrasound, or demonstrates any suspicious features, merits further analysis with CT or MRI.

Ultrasound is less accurate in staging renal cell carcinoma than computed tomography (CT) or MRI. It is poor at demonstrating lymph node disease, skeletal or lung metastases.

Computed Tomography

Computed tomography (CT) is still the Investigation of choice for evaluating and characterising solid renal masses. It can accurately assess 'pseudomasses' (see Fig. 12-1) and other anatomical variants and can provide attenuation values that can confirm the presence of fluid in cysts or fat in angiomyolipomas. As CT can delineate accurately the perinephric space and the retroperitoneum, it is useful in the diagnosis of complicated renal sepsis and the assessment of the extent of haemorrhage; it can also identify tumour recurrence after radical nephrectomy. Accurate analysis of renal masses requires the use of intravenous contrast medium.

The continued development of multislice CT has improved the detection, characterisation and staging of renal tumours and allows high-quality multiplanar imaging of the kidneys, which is useful for evaluating small areas of enhancement and for presurgical planning. With the increased use of laparoscopic, robotic and nephron-sparing surgery, it is vitally important to be able to review the coronal and sagittal images with surgical colleagues to decide upon appropriate management.

Unenhanced CT images are essential for identifying calcification and allow true evaluation of enhancement following IV contrast. Corticomedullary phase (25–40 s post-IV contrast administration) imaging is helpful in demonstrating normal variants, pseudotumours, tumour vascularity and the renal vein. The nephrographic phase (90–100 s post-IV contrast administration) is best for the detection of central renal masses, as the medulla is optimally enhanced and small medullary lesions are better visualised.[1,2] For optimal lesion detection and characterisation, images should be obtained in both phases; however, if only one phase is to be used, to reduce radiation dose, it should be the nephrographic phase. If surveillance imaging of a lesion is to be undertaken, the single optimal phase for detection of the mass can be used rather than repeating a three-phase examination.

MRI

The ability of MRI to characterise renal masses has improved with the development of phased-array multicoils, fast breath-hold imaging and the use of Gd-DTPA contrast enhancement. Protocols vary widely but usually

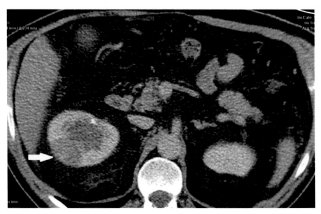

FIGURE 12-1 ■ **Pseudomass of the kidney secondary to renal obstruction.** Post-contrast CT performed in a patient with an obstructed kidney reveals an apparent soft-tissue mass in the upper pole of the kidney which was initially misinterpreted as a probable incidental renal cell carcinoma (see arrow). Follow-up imaging demonstrated near-complete resolution of these changes with the development of a small focal scar.

include pre- and post-contrast T1-weighted images with and without fat suppression. The coronal and sagittal planes are helpful for evaluating the extent of lesions. MR angiography can demonstrate the renal arteries and veins, and the inferior vena cava. MRI can be used as an alternative to CT for detection and surveillance of masses, although this depends upon local resources, and availability of equipment. Many radiologists prefer to use CT for the initial evaluation of renal masses as it is such a reliable technique, and easier to interpret than MRI. There has been recent interest in the use of diffusion-weighted imaging for the characterisation of renal masses. Malignant tumours are associated with a significantly reduced analog-to-digital converter (ADC) value[3,4] compared to benign lesions, although the utility of this technique is not definitively confirmed at present and not widely practised outside the research setting.

Simple renal cysts and angiomyolipomas have characteristic appearances, but the signal from most other masses is nonspecific.

MRI is an alternative to CT in patients with renal insufficiency or severe previous reactions to contrast medium. MRI is superior to CT in differentiating benign thrombus from tumour thrombus and in identifying its extent. MRI is ideally suited for monitoring patients who have a genetically increased risk of renal malignancy, such as von Hippel–Lindau disease, who require repeated imaging for surveillance.

MRI is no more specific than CT at differentiating malignant from reactive lymphadenopathy, although the development of tissue-specific agents might alter this in the future. MRI is a more lengthy and complex investigation than CT. The role of MRI has reduced with the development of multislice CT, which allows the production of reliable and high-quality multiplanar reconstructions.

Renal Arteriography

Renal arteriography is seldom used to diagnose or characterise a renal mass as the necessary information is usually provided by cross-sectional imaging. Angiography can play a role in preoperative embolisation of very vascular tumours immediately before partial nephrectomy. CT or MR angiography is usually sufficient to provide a road map for surgery, and to identify the size, number and position of renal vessels.

Needle Aspiration and Biopsy

Percutaneous aspiration of renal cysts is indicated in the investigation of an indeterminate cystic renal mass to diagnose an abscess or an infected cyst.

Fluid obtained at aspiration should be sent for cytological examination, although negative cytology does not exclude malignancy; this applies particularly in some cystic renal cell carcinomas, in which malignant disease is confined to the wall of the lesion. If the fluid is found to be turbid, microbiological examination should also be performed. Needle biopsy of a cyst wall can be performed to improve the diagnostic yield although there are small but potential risks in this setting including seeding of tumour and false-negative diagnosis.[5]

Biopsy is used to confirm the histology of a renal mass in patients with underlying non-renal malignancy or radiological features suggestive of lymphoma. Biopsy is also used to confirm the presence of malignancy before radiofrequency or cryoablation of a renal mass. Histological techniques have improved over the past 10 years and are more reliable at classifying a renal mass and differentiating between oncocytoma and renal cell carcinoma. In patients with significant other comorbidity, this may significantly alter the management of an asymptomatic renal mass. Biopsy should also be considered in bilateral masses to characterise whether the lesions represent multifocal oncocytoma or papillary tumour. This information may make such lesions suitable for attempted nephron-sparing surgery even if potentially suboptimal for this approach.

NON-NEOPLASTIC RENAL MASSES

A number of non-neoplastic tumours must be differentiated from renal cell carcinoma. Fetal lobulation occurs as a result of incomplete fusion of the fetal lobules, which results in a lobulated contour to the lateral border of the kidney occurring between the underlying calices. Dromedary humps are bulges occurring on the lateral side of the left kidney. Many of these pseudomasses can be identified with ultrasound but occasionally further imaging is required. This is usually achieved with CT or MRI, although scintigraphic techniques can be used.

PATHOLOGICAL RENAL MASSES

Renal Cysts

Serous Renal Cyst

This is the commonest form of cystic disease and is seen with increasing frequency with advancing age. Autopsy studies have demonstrated a prevalence of almost 50%.

The cysts are frequently multiple and occur in various sizes. On ultrasound examination renal cysts appear as anechoic, well-defined masses, with thin walls and good through transmission of sound. On CT, a simple cyst usually appears as a well-defined rounded mass with an attenuation value of 0–20 HU, with an imperceptible wall and no enhancement after injection of contrast medium. The MRI appearance of a simple renal cyst is characterised by a sharply demarcated, homogeneous, hypointense mass on T1-weighted images, which becomes uniformly hyperintense on T2-weighted images and shows no enhancement following contrast medium administration on T1-weighted images.

'Complicated Cysts'[6,7]

A classification of cystic lesions was suggested in 1986 by Bosniak, based upon CT characteristics, and is used to guide management.[7] Class I is a simple benign cyst. Class II cysts have one or more thin septa running through them (<1 mm), thin areas of mural calcification or fluid contents of increased attenuation; they do not enhance following injection of contrast medium and are benign (see Figs. 12-2–12-4). These two categories of cysts are benign, and do not require surgery or radiological follow-up.

Class III cysts are more complicated and contain thickened septa, nodular areas of calcification or solid non-enhancing areas. Mural enhancement can be seen in class III lesions, which are indeterminate for malignancy and should be biopsied or surgically explored. Less than 50% of these will turn out to be malignant, although there can be significant interobserver variation in how such cysts are classified.

Class IV cystic masses are clearly malignant, with solid enhancing nodules and should be treated accordingly.

A subcategory, IIF, has been suggested for lesions with multiple class II features, and these require follow-up for up to 5 years to exclude malignancy (see Fig. 12-5). Surveillance of these lesions may demonstrate growth or

change in calcification, but it is the development of enhancing soft tissue that should upgrade the cystic lesion and result in surgical treatment. Category IIF lesions are large (>3 cm) hyperdense cysts or hyperdense cysts that are totally intrarenal.

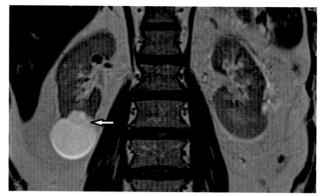

FIGURE 12-3 ■ **MRI of a Bosniak II cyst.** Coronal T2 MRI demonstrates a large right lower pole renal cyst with internal septation, categorised as a Bosniak II cyst (see arrow). MRI usually shows greater detail of internal cyst architecture than CT.

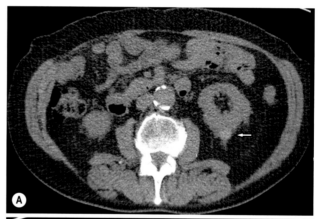

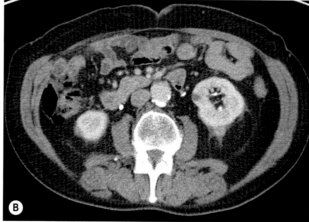

FIGURE 12-4 ■ **Haemorrhagic cyst of the kidney.** Pre-contrast (A) image reveals high-density, round, smooth mass in the right kidney (see arrow). There is minor inflammatory change surrounding the lesion which may be due to recent trauma, or infection. (B) Following contrast medium there is no significant change in the appearance or density of the mass. It is easy to misdiagnose a haemorrhagic cyst as a solid renal mass, and review of a non-contrast CT is vital to evaluate the presence of enhancement.

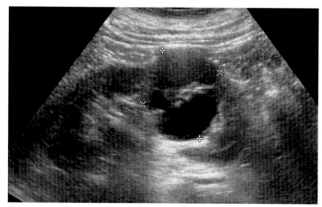

FIGURE 12-2 ■ **US of a Bosniak II cyst.** Ultrasound demonstrates a large cyst in the mid pole of the kidney with thick internal septation. No abnormal colour flow was seen on US, and CT confirmed the absence of solid enhancement. The lesion was classified as a IIF cyst and did not demonstrate significant change over the subsequent 5 years.

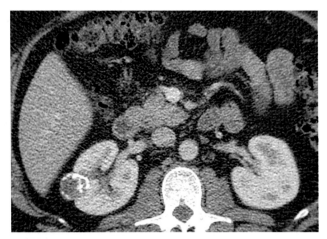

FIGURE 12-5 ■ **Bosniak IIF renal cyst.** CT demonstrates heavy calcification in a small cyst which was difficult to evaluate at US. Despite the absence of enhancement on CT, the lesion was considered too atypical to be a Bosniak II lesion, and was classified as a 2F cyst for observation.

A simple benign cyst on ultrasound or CT requires no further investigation or follow-up. If there is wall thickening or the contents of the cyst are not of water density, the lesion is indeterminate. Haemorrhage or infection may result in cyst fluid of high attenuation but, unlike tumours, such lesions do not enhance following the administration of contrast medium. It is usually necessary to obtain a pre-contrast CT to adequately assess a rounded homogeneous lesion on a post-contrast CT that is not of water density to exclude low-grade enhancement signifying a renal mass, e.g. papillary tumour, rather than a benign cyst. Ultrasound is helpful if the hyperdense mass satisfies the sonographic criteria of a benign simple cyst.

Thick and irregular mural calcification can be seen with both cystic renal cell carcinomas and complicated renal cysts.[8] CT attenuation values in both lesions may be identical. Cystic renal cell carcinomas (especially papillary cystadenocarcinomas) may have fluid-range densities, while benign haemorrhagic cysts may have attenuation values much higher than those acceptable for benign cysts.

Parapelvic and Peripelvic Cysts

These occur in the renal sinus and frequently cause distortion, but rarely obstruction, of the renal collecting system. Peripelvic cysts are of lymphatic origin, whereas parapelvic cysts are renal serous cysts arising from the renal parenchyma that is present in the sinus. Although parapelvic cysts may be evaluated satisfactorily using ultrasound, peripelvic cysts can occasionally lead to confusion with hydronephrosis, as they track along the renal infundibula. Careful examination should demonstrate that the apparently dilated infundibula do not connect to a dilated renal pelvis. If necessary, urography or CT in the pyelographic phase is usually confirmatory.

Adult Polycystic Kidney Disease (ADPKD)

This is an autosomal dominant hereditary condition which affects many organs in addition to the kidneys.

Although it has 100% penetrance, it has variable expression and does not generally produce symptoms until adult life. Renal cysts are seen in addition to cysts within the liver, pancreas and spleen, although hepatic failure does not tend to occur despite extensive infiltration. Coexisting aneurysms of the circle of Willis are seen in 10–16% of patients in autopsy series and as many as 41% of patients undergoing cerebral angiography.

The imaging appearances vary with the severity of the disease. Ultrasound demonstrates cysts in the adolescent or young adult, who is usually not yet clinically symptomatic. CT and MRI are more sensitive and frequently show more cysts than US. Adults presenting with ADPKD usually have enlarged kidneys with numerous cysts of varying sizes.

Occasionally, an infected cyst, a hyperdense cyst and, less commonly, a renal neoplasm may coexist with adult polycystic renal disease and the diagnosis becomes somewhat difficult in these cases. MRI may prove to be a useful technique in differentiating between simple cysts, haemorrhagic cysts and neoplasms when the findings on CT and ultrasound are equivocal. Infected cysts can be difficult to diagnose, and aspiration of a dominant or hyperdense cyst may be required for definitive evaluation. Fluorodeoxyglucose positron emission tomography (FDG PET) can be helpful in evaluating for the presence of an infected cyst, and has logistical advantages over white cell scintigraphy in such cases.

Multicystic Renal Dysplasia

This is a non-hereditary, congenital, usually unilateral form of renal cystic disease and is one of the commonest causes of an abdominal mass in the newborn.

Localised Cystic Disease of the Kidney

Localised cystic disease is characterised by the presence of multiple cysts seen throughout part, or all, of one kidney (see Fig. 12-6). The aetiology of this disorder is not known. Normal cortex is seen between the individual cysts, which helps distinguish the disease from multicystic dysplastic kidney. The contralateral kidney is usually entirely normal or contains several small cysts, which can help distinguish it from ADPKD, in which multiple cysts of varying size are seen in enlarged kidneys bilaterally. It is equally important to distinguish localised cystic disease of the kidney from multilocular cystic nephroma, which is achieved by the demonstration of normal parenchyma between the cysts.

Hydatid (Echinococcal) Cysts of the Kidney

These are rare in most parts of the world and uncommon even in endemic areas. They are thick-walled, mainly intrarenal, and sometimes calcified. Hydatid cysts may present as flank or perinephric masses, which rupture into the collecting system, giving rise to acute flank pain followed by the voiding of hydatid scolices, with or without haematuria. Ultrasound demonstrates a multicystic lesion of mixed reflectivity.

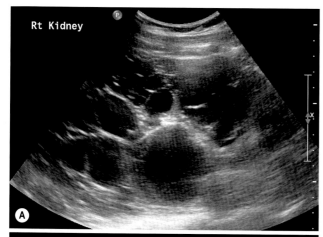

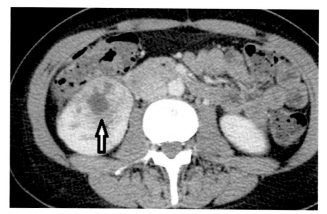

FIGURE 12-7 ■ **Renal abscess.** A 30-year-old woman presents with symptoms of urinary infection with loin pain. CT demonstrates a thick-walled cystic lesion in the right kidney (see arrow) in keeping with an abscess. CT is particularly helpful for infections that involve the perinephric space which are not well demonstrated with US.

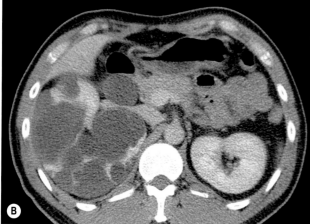

FIGURE 12-6 ■ **Localised cystic kidney disease.** Ultrasound (A) and CT (B) demonstrate multiple cysts throughout both kidneys with no solid elements. The initial US was interpreted as a probable multicystic dysplastic kidney (contralateral kidney was normal), although the CT demonstrates the presence of some normal renal parenchyma surrounding the kidney in keeping with localised cystic kidney disease.

Inflammatory Masses

Renal Abscesses

Renal abscesses are increasingly uncommon, as urinary tract infection is usually treated early. Most abscesses are due to ascending infection, commonly by *Escherichia coli* (see Fig. 12-7). Immunocompromised and diabetic patients, as well as those with infected renal stones, are at a higher risk of developing renal infection. Haematogenous infection is usually secondary to *Staphylococcus*. Although renal abscess formation is generally associated with symptomatic urinary tract infection, it can present with vague symptoms such as flank pain and weight loss. Rupture of a renal abscess can lead to spread of infection into the perinephric space.

CT is the best technique for the diagnosis and staging of renal and perinephric abscesses. The central portion of an abscess is of near-fluid density and does not demonstrate contrast enhancement, making it more obvious following contrast administration. There is often a thick irregular wall, which enhances together with inflammatory changes in the perinephric space. The presence of

gas within a lesion is diagnostic of an abscess but is very rarely seen. The differential diagnosis of these appearances includes renal lymphoma, metastatic disease, renal infarction and complicated cystic disease.

Acute Focal Pyelonephritis

A renal mass may be caused by acute focal pyelonephritis with localised swelling of the kidney but without liquefaction. Focal pyelonephritis appears as a round or wedge-shaped focal mass without a defined wall, which tends to extend from the papilla to the outer cortex. Contrast administration demonstrates heterogeneous enhancement of the affected area, which can often be greater than that of the normal parenchyma on delayed images. Perinephric inflammation is frequently seen. CT may demonstrate persistent renal abnormality for several weeks after infection and a focal mass may persist for several months.

Malacoplakia

This is a rare disease of the renal parenchyma caused by granulomatous inflammation. Malacoplakia is most commonly seen in middle-aged women and is more prevalent in individuals who are immunosuppressed. Renal involvement is usually associated with disease in the lower urinary tract. Focal hypoechoic renal masses may simulate renal abscesses, and heterogeneous masses that undergo calcification may be mistaken for renal carcinoma. Renal malacoplakia can extend outside the kidney into the perinephric space and can also undergo spontaneous haemorrhage.

Vascular Masses

Haematomas

These may present as masses following trauma or as a result of spontaneous intrarenal bleeding. It may be difficult to determine whether there is underlying renal pathology, such as a tumour that has bled because of anticoagulation, or whether the kidney is otherwise healthy. Follow-up examination will be required to clarify whether there is an underlying mass.

The ultrasound appearance of a haematoma varies according to its age. Fresh haematomas behave primarily as fluid collections, whereas organised haematomas may be highly reflective because they contain fragments of clot. CT during the acute phase will demonstrate an area of high attenuation, which is diagnostic of haematoma.

Intrarenal Vascular Masses

Two uncommon vascular lesions that may present as intrarenal masses are aneurysms and arteriovenous malformations (or fistulas). Aneurysms are usually caused by atherosclerosis, but may be congenital, post-traumatic or secondary to vasculitis. Rim calcification is common. Arteriovenous communications are usually congenital, but may be caused by trauma (particularly renal biopsy) or atherosclerosis.

Angiomyolipomas[9]

Angiomyolipomas are benign lesions composed of variable amounts of fat, smooth muscle and abnormal blood vessels (see Figs. 12-8–12-10). They occur spontaneously in the general population, mainly in women during their fifth decade; they occur at a much younger age and are frequently multiple in patients with tuberous sclerosis, with an incidence of 50–80%. They are rarely seen in neurofibromatosis and in autosomal dominant polycystic kidney disease. Angiomyolipomas are composed of thick-walled, inelastic blood vessels. The risk of haemorrhage is related to the size of the tumour, and is significantly higher in lesions greater than 4 cm in diameter.

The appearance on ultrasound depends on the proportions of fat, smooth muscle and vascular elements, and on the presence of haemorrhage. Typically, angiomyolipoma appears as a circumscribed, highly reflective mass, more echogenic than the central sinus fat. Because of this high reflectivity, very tiny lesions can be detected with ultrasound. Tumours with a greater proportion of muscle, and those which have undergone haemorrhage or necrosis, may not be echogenic. Recent work has indicated that 32% of renal carcinomas smaller than 3 cm in diameter are also highly reflective, although there will often be other suspicious features, such as a hyporeflective rim or small focal spotty areas of reduced central reflectivity.[8] A further feature that may be of help in distinguishing an angiomyolipoma from a small renal cell carcinoma is

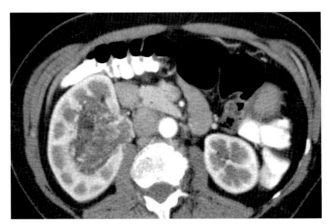

FIGURE 12-9 ■ **Central angiomyolipoma of the kidney.** There is a large predominantly fat-containing lesion in the right mid pole of the kidney involving the renal pelvis in keeping with an AML. The presence of macroscopic fat is strongly suggestive of the diagnosis. Large renal cancers can engulf perinephric fat, and mimic an AML. The patient in this case actually had a tumour extending into the vena cava, which was confirmed as benign AML at surgery.

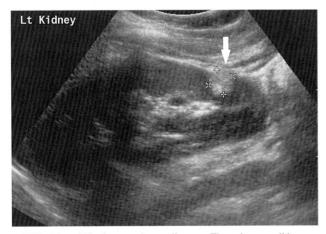

FIGURE 12-8 ■ **US of an angiomyolipoma.** There is a small hyperechoic mass in the lower pole of the kidney characteristic of an AML (see arrow). Confirmation of the diagnosis can be made with CT or MRI as small renal cell cancers may occasionally mimic the hyperechoic appearance of an AML.

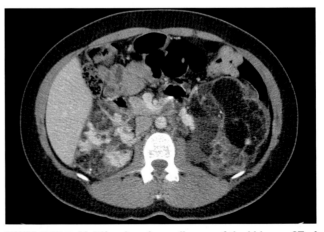

FIGURE 12-10 ■ **Multifocal angiomyolipoma of the kidneys.** CT of the kidneys demonstrates extensive infiltration of both kidneys with multiple fat-containing lesions in a patient with tuberous sclerosis. Angiography should be considered in patients with such large tumours with a view to prophylactic embolisation as the risk of bleeding is high.

posterior shadowing, which is seen in approximately 30% of angiomyolipomas but not seen in the small hyper-reflective renal carcinoma.

CT usually demonstrates a fatty mass intermixed with areas of increased tissue density, although the amount of fat present is variable and it can even be absent.[9] Generally, the detection by CT of even a small amount of fat within a renal mass establishes the diagnosis of angiomyolipoma. An attenuation value of –15 HU is considered diagnostic of fat, although some authors specify a lower level, such as –20 HU. If there is coexistent haemorrhage, CT and other techniques may not provide an accurate preoperative diagnosis.[9] It is important to assess the relationship of the fat to the remainder of the tumour to be certain that the fat is intratumoral, and not perirenal fat that has been engulfed by an expanding renal cell carcinoma.

Angiography can demonstrate multiple aneurysms and an 'onion layer' appearance. Embolisation can control bleeding tumours, and can also be used to treat enlarging tumours to reduce the risk of haemorrhage.

Focal Hydronephrosis

Hydronephrosis confined to one part of the kidney can simulate a mass on urography. This most commonly occurs in patients with an obstructed upper segment of a duplex system. Obstruction to an infundibulum may be caused by a variety of conditions, such as tuberculosis and tumour.

Renal Sinus Lipomatosis

Sinus lipomatosis is an overabundance of normal renal sinus fat, which may produce stretching of the infundibula and compression of the renal pelvis, simulating a parapelvic cyst or other hilar renal mass. The diagnosis is generally clarified by CT or ultrasound. On ultrasound examination the area in question is usually echogenic.

Non-Renal Masses

Occasionally an extrarenal mass may extend into the kidney and appear to be intrarenal, e.g. pancreatic pseudocysts, tumours of the colon, spleen and adrenal gland.

NEOPLASTIC RENAL MASSES

Benign

Adenoma and Oncocytoma

Small renal tumours (<3 cm) have been regarded in the past as adenomas rather than carcinomas. Unfortunately the size of a renal mass is not a valid criterion for differentiating a benign from a malignant mass. There are reports of tumours that have produced metastases when less than 3 cm, although this is uncommon.

Oncocytomas are tubular adenomas with a specific histological appearance characterised by the oncocyte.[10] They have previously been considered benign, but it is now recognised that they can metastasise. Oncocytomas can occur at any age and are often asymptomatic at presentation. They can vary in size from 1 to 20 cm in diameter, but tend to be large. Although they are usually solitary and unilateral, they can be multiple (5%) and bilateral (3%). Ultrasound demonstrates a solid mass with internal echoes, which occasionally has a stellate hypoechoic centre. However, the echogenicity of the mass can be variable. Contrast-enhanced CT demonstrates a well-defined solid mass which, when large, can contain a low-attenuation central scar. Large lesions can extend into and engulf the perinephric fat, and can be mistaken for angiomyolipomas. There are no features on MRI that will differentiate an oncocytoma from renal carcinoma. Arteriography is also of limited value in discriminating between an oncocytoma and renal cell carcinoma.

Haemangioma

Haemangiomas of the kidney are rare lesions, which are generally cavernous rather than capillary. The most common symptom is haematuria. They are most commonly symptomatic in the middle years and are equally distributed between the sexes.

Excretory urography may demonstrate a renal mass, or more commonly pyelocalyceal distortion or a filling defect, attributable to the haemangioma or associated clot. Selective arteriography is often unhelpful, although occasionally will suggest the diagnosis.

Multilocular Cystic Nephroma

This is a rare benign neoplasm which presents as a unilateral septated encysted mass. It usually presents in young children but can be seen in adulthood, particularly in women. There are frequently septae which demonstrate enhancement. The cystic portion is usually of water density or slightly higher density with no enhancement. The best clue to the diagnosis is the presence of herniation of the mass into the renal hilum.

Malignant

Parenchymal

Renal Cell Carcinoma. Most cases arise spontaneously in the fifth to seventh decade, although an increasing number of cases are discovered in younger patients, some of whom have hereditary cancer syndromes.[11]

There are several main types of renal cancer, as well as a larger number of rarer subtypes. It occurs bilaterally in 3–5% of cases, and is the eighth most common malignancy, accounting for 3% of newly diagnosed neoplasms.

Clear cell carcinoma is the commonest renal malignancy, comprising 85% of all malignant renal tumours (see Figs. 12-11–12-13). Clear cell carcinoma is seen in about 36% of patients with von Hippel–Lindau disease[12] and is characterised by significant enhancement following contrast administration (see Fig. 12-14).

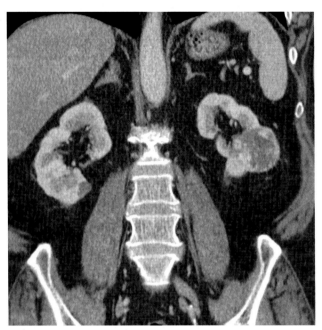

FIGURE 12-11 ■ **Clear cell carcinoma of the kidney.** Post-contrast CT demonstrates an enhancing soft-tissue mass in the lower pole of the left kidney, histologically confirmed as a clear cell cancer. Coronal reconstructions are critical in planning surgery and deciding upon the feasibility of nephron-sparing surgery.

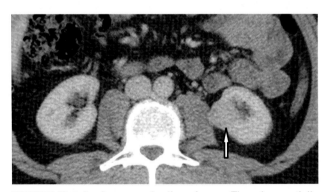

FIGURE 12-12 ■ **Isodense renal cell carcinoma.** There is a partially exophytic mass on the medial aspect of the mid pole of the left kidney (see arrow) which demonstrates isoenhancement compared with the rest of the renal parenchyma. Partial nephrectomy confirmed a T1 renal cell carcinoma.

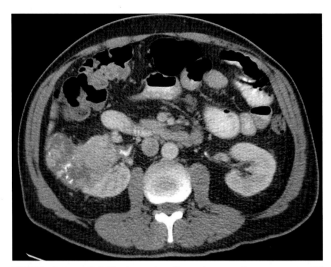

FIGURE 12-13 ■ **Calcified renal cell carcinoma.** Post-contrast CT demonstrates a large soft-tissue mass in the right kidney with central calcification. Whilst peripheral calcification is commonly seen in cysts and benign lesions, central calcification is usually seen with malignant lesions.

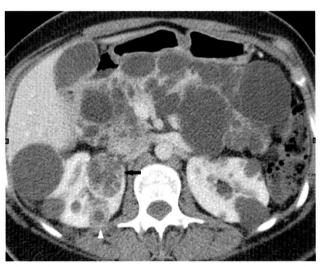

FIGURE 12-14 ■ **Von Hippel–Lindau and renal tumours.** Single-phase post-contrast CT demonstrates multiple renal and pancreatic cysts in a patient with known von Hippel–Lindau. There is a cystic RCC in the mid pole of the right kidney (see arrow), which was subsequently removed at open partial nephrectomy. There is a further smaller mass in the posterior aspect of the right kidney (see arrowhead).

Papillary tumours are the next most common subtype of tumour, occurring in 10–15% of cancers (see Figs. 12-15 and 12-16) These tumours are commonly seen in failing kidneys, and in some hereditary syndromes, and are not infrequently multiple. They have a characteristic appearance on CT and are associated with minimal contrast enhancement. They can be easily misinterpreted as a hyperdense cyst on CT if an unenhanced examination has not been performed.

There are two types of papillary tumour—type 1 and 2, the latter of which is less common and associated with a worse prognosis.

Chromophobe tumours (see Fig. 12-17) are the third most common tumour (5%). They have a similar appearance to oncocytomas with homogeneous enhancement and presence of a central scar. Ultrasound frequently demonstrates a hyperechoic mass.

Less common pathological subtypes include collecting duct tumours, which are associated with a poor prognosis.

Renal cancers can appear hyperechoic, hypoechoic or isoechoic on ultrasound. Most small renal carcinomas are hyperechoic compared with normal parenchyma, whereas up to 86% of large tumours are isoechoic. Central necrosis can produce a central hypoechoic region that is associated with posterior acoustic enhancement. Cystic tumours may have thick or irregular walls, together with small or large intracystic nodules of tumour. Ultrasound with colour Doppler is useful for detecting inferior vena cava thrombus and extension of tumour thrombus into the intrahepatic vena cava.

Renal cell carcinomas are often heterogeneous on unenhanced CT, with one or more low-density central areas. An extensively necrotic tumour may have a pseudocapsule. Unusually high- or low-density tumours have been described. CT is the most sensitive technique for the depiction of parenchymal calcification associated with renal malignancy. Most renal cell cancers are solid, with attenuation values of more than 20 HU on pre-contrast

CT. An increase in attenuation of more than 10 HU after IV contrast administration suggests a solid mass, and enhancement of more than 20 HU indicates malignancy. Tumours occurring in non-functioning kidneys may show little enhancement due to papillary subtype or poor renal arterial blood flow (see Fig. 12-18).

Attention should always be made when fully evaluating the contralateral kidney for a renal mass, as bilateral tumours are not infrequently seen. When tumours are seen bilaterally, they can have similar histological subtypes, although if the morphology is different, there may be two different pathological renal masses present (see Fig. 12-19).

MRI can be used to detect and stage renal cell carcinoma, with a sensitivity similar to that of CT. However, CT is better at detecting small foci of calcification. The signal characteristics of renal carcinoma are variable, with tumours appearing isointense or hypointense compared with the renal cortex on T1-weighted sequences, and slightly hyperintense on T2W sequences. Following administration of gadolinium intravenously, heterogeneous enhancement occurs immediately, decreasing on delayed images. Homogeneous enhancement is more likely in small, low-grade tumours. MRI is not significantly better at detecting lymph node disease. Although in most institutions CT is the technique of choice for the diagnosis and staging of renal cell cancer, MRI can play a role when contrast-enhanced CT is contraindicated, or if frequent follow-up is required in high-risk patients.

Angiography is no longer required for the diagnosis of renal cell carcinoma but is occasionally performed for embolisation of large tumours before surgery in order to reduce the risk of perioperative haemorrhage.

Staging of Renal Cancer. The TNM staging system is the most widely used system and is shown in Table 12-1. CT is the most frequently used staging technique, with accuracy ranging between 72 and 90%. CT is not very accurate in differentiating T2 from early T3a disease; however, this is not particularly important clinically, except in the context of nephron-sparing surgery. The

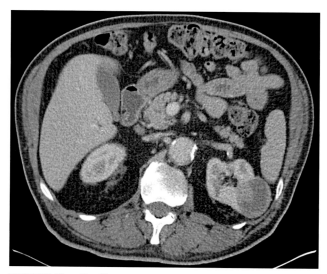

FIGURE 12-15 ■ **Papillary tumour of the kidney.** Post-contrast CT demonstrates a partially cystic, and partially solid, left renal mass, with a histologically proven papillary cell carcinoma type 1. These tumours often have characteristic appearances at CT or MRI, as they are often homogeneous in density and demonstrate minor enhancement only (see Fig. 12-16). Some lesions, as seen in this example, have a partially cystic component.

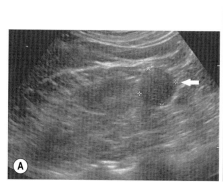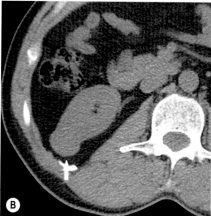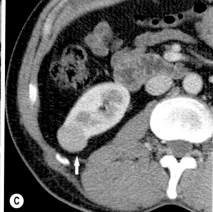

FIGURE 12-16 ■ **Papillary carcinoma of the kidney.** (A) US and (B) pre- and (C) post-contrast CT demonstrate an incidental solid mass detected on US which demonstrates low-grade enhancement (25 HU) post-contrast (see arrow). This appearance is typical for a papillary tumour. These can be multifocal, and close scrutiny of the ipsi- and contralateral kidney is recommended.

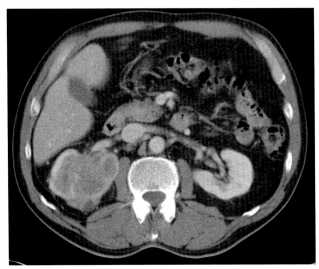

FIGURE 12-17 ■ **Chromophobe tumour.** Post-contrast CT demonstrates a large enhancing right renal mass which was confirmed following nephrectomy as a chromophobe renal cancer. The appearances are indistinguishable from that of a clear cell cancer. Chromophobe tumours have a better prognosis than clear cell carcinoma.

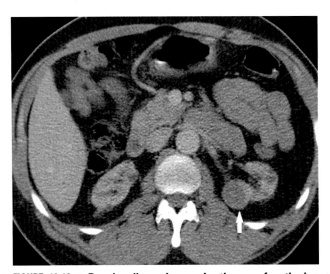

FIGURE 12-18 ■ **Renal cell carcinoma in the non-functioning kidney.** Single-phase post-contrast CT through the native kidneys in a patient with a renal transplant demonstrates a small left-sided renal mass which was confirmed as a solid lesion on US and subsequently resected and confirmed as a renal cell carcinoma. Native non-functioning kidneys demonstrate poor enhancement post-contrast and it can be difficult to differentiate a complex cyst from a poorly enhancing tumour.

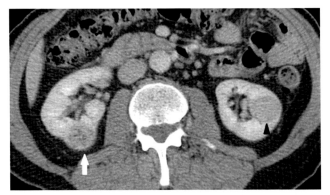

FIGURE 12-19 ■ **Bilateral renal tumours.** Post-contrast CT demonstrates a typical small right renal cell carcinoma (see arrow). The contralateral kidney contains a mass with different morphology (see arrowhead), which is more in keeping with a papillary tumour, although a haemorrhagic cyst could cause a similar appearance, and comparison with a pre-contrast image would be required to confirm that there is enhancement. Partial nephrectomy was performed bilaterally as a staged procedure.

TABLE 12-1   Staging of Renal Cell Carcinoma: TNM System 2010 Modification

Tumour confined to kidney, small <4 cm	T1a
Tumour confined to kidney >4 cm, <7 cm	T1b
Tumour confined to kidney >7 cm, <10 cm	T2a
Tumour confined to kidney >10 cm	T2b
Tumour spread to perinephric fat, or renal vein	T3a
Tumour spread to cava below diaphragm	T3b
Tumour spread to cava above diaphragm, or invades the wall of the cava	T3c
Tumour spread outside Gerota's fascia, or ipsilateral adrenal gland	T4
Metastasis in single lymph node	N1
Metastasis in more than one lymph node	N2
Distant metastasis	M1

presence of a discrete soft-tissue tumour mass in the perinephric space is a specific sign of T3a disease (98%) but has a sensitivity of only 46%. Perinephric stranding is found in most patients with T3 disease but is also detected in a significant number of patients with T1 or T2 disease, when it is caused not by tumour but by oedema, vascular engorgement or fibrosis.

CT has a limited ability to identify lymph node involvement, which is based entirely on size. Using 1 cm as the upper limit of normal, nodal micro-metastases will be missed in 4% of patients. There is also a variable false-positive rate due to nodal enlargement caused by reactive hyperplasia. This is more common when tumour necrosis or tumour thrombus is present. The overall accuracy for lymph node staging is reported to be between 83 and 89%.

Accurate identification of involvement of the renal vein and inferior vena cava is very important for correct patient management (see Figs. 12-20 and 12-21). The reported accuracy for detecting renal vein involvement using CT is approximately 96%. Optimal enhancement of the renal vein is seen during the corticomedullary phase of enhancement. Thrombus is seen as a filling defect within the vein. Isolated renal vein enlargement is an unreliable sign because it can be caused by increased blood flow secondary to tumour hypervascularity. It is usually difficult to differentiate tumour thrombus from bland thrombus unless enhancement can be seen within the thrombus. CT is a sensitive method for detecting lung metastases but is often reserved for patients with extensive regional disease or an abnormal chest radiograph. MRI has been reported as being the best technique for defining the extent of venous invasion. MRI is superior to CT in differentiating benign from malignant

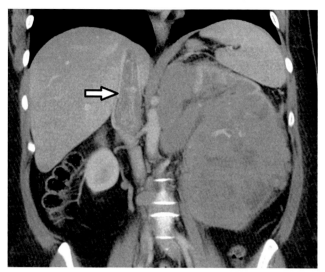

FIGURE 12-20 ■ **T3b Renal cell carcinoma.** Coronal post-contrast CT demonstrates tumour thrombus extending into the right renal vein and the cava (see arrow) (radiological stage T3b).

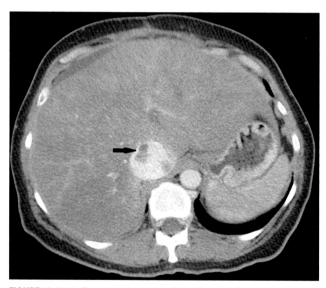

FIGURE 12-21 ■ **Recurrent renal cell carcinoma in the vena cava.** Post-contrast CT performed during follow-up for a previously resected renal cell carcinoma demonstrates a soft-tissue mass in the vena cava (see arrow) consistent with recurrent tumour.

thrombus, but offers no advantage in staging nodal disease.

Wilms' Tumour in the Adolescent and Adult. Approximately 90% of Wilms' tumours are diagnosed before 7 years of age. Presentation in adolescence is uncommon and it is very occasionally seen in adulthood. In adults, it generally presents as a palpable abdominal mass, although hypertension, abdominal pain and, less frequently, gross haematuria may be seen. Wilms' tumours are usually large at presentation and can occasionally be identified on plain abdominal radiographs.

As with renal cell carcinoma, invasion and obstruction of the renal vein or inferior vena cava may occur, as well as invasion of the renal pelvis and ureter.

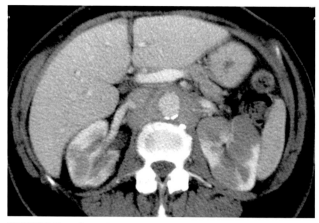

FIGURE 12-22 ■ **Lymphoma of the kidney.** Post-contrast CT demonstrates multifocal solid masses in both kidneys with para-aortic nodal disease highly suggestive of lymphoma. Biopsy of the renal mass is required to confirm and characterise before treatment, which will not be surgical.

Sarcoma. Sarcomas of the kidney are rare, solid, malignant tumours which develop from mesenchymal cells. Many of these tumours arise in close proximity to the renal capsule, making it difficult to distinguish whether they originate in the renal or perinephric tissues. Others arise from the wall of intrarenal blood vessels within the kidney, or close to the renal pelvis. The imaging characteristics are non-specific, making it difficult to distinguish a renal sarcoma from a renal cell carcinoma. The tumours are frequently large at presentation and tend to present with abdominal pain and discomfort. Renal vein and inferior vena cava invasion is seen, and metastases are common at initial diagnosis.

Lymphoma and Leukaemia.[13] Primary lymphoma of the kidney is very rare, as there is no lymphatic tissue within the kidneys. Renal involvement may be due to haematogenous spread or contiguous invasion from adjacent retroperitoneal lymphadenopathy (see Figs. 12-22 and 12-23). The kidneys are much more frequently involved in patients with non-Hodgkin's lymphoma, particularly when the disease has relapsed. Although clinically apparent renal involvement is seen in 5% of patients, and autopsy post mortem studies have shown that 30–50% of patients have involvement of the urinary tract.

CT may demonstrate sheet-like diffuse infiltration of the perirenal tissues or multiple focal nodules. Following intravenous injection of contrast medium, focal lesions are usually of low attenuation. Contrast enhancement may also be useful in demonstrating the presence of discrete focal abnormalities in diffusely enlarged kidneys. Lymph node enlargement is often seen surrounding the vessels and can lead to bilateral hydronephrosis.

[67]Ga citrate radionuclide imaging may also identify lymphomatous involvement of the kidney. CT- or ultrasound-guided biopsy may be helpful if lymphoma is suspected. Leukaemic renal infiltration is frequently seen at postmortem examination and can be associated with renal impairment. CT can demonstrate unilateral or bilateral renal enlargement or the presence of a focal mass or masses.

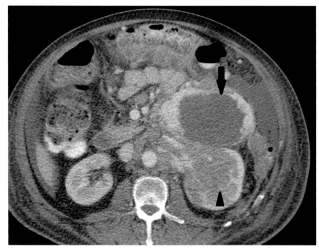

FIGURE 12-23 ■ **RCC and lymphoma.** Post-contrast CT demonstrates a complex left renal mass. There is an irregular hypervascular mass in the upper pole of the left kidney (see arrow), as well as a poorly enhancing soft-tissue mass in the lower pole (see arrowhead). Incidental para-aortic nodes were seen. Biopsy of both components was performed, confirming the presence of a clear cell carcinoma in the upper pole and a lymphoma of the lower pole. There was no previous history of lymphoma. Following chemotherapy, the lower pole renal mass responded, as did the nodal disease. Nephrectomy was performed for the clear cell carcinoma of the upper pole.

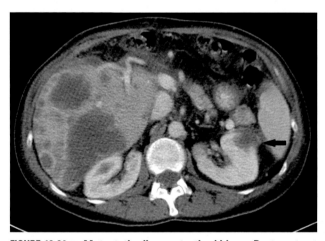

FIGURE 12-24 ■ **Metastatic disease to the kidney.** Post-contrast CT in a patient with advanced metastatic cholangiocarcinoma demonstrates multiple metastases to the liver with a similar metastatic deposit in the left kidney (see arrow). Renal metastases in advanced metastatic disease are not uncommon, but are rarely clinically significant.

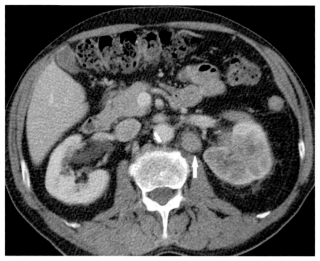

FIGURE 12-25 ■ **Transitional cell carcinoma of the kidney presenting as a solid renal mass.** CT performed with contrast demonstrates a large centrally placed and poorly vascular mass in the middle of the left kidney confirmed histologically as a TCC. There is an enlarged left para-aortic lymph node (see arrow), which is also metastatic.

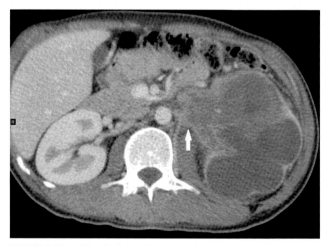

FIGURE 12-26 ■ **Urothelial cell cancer of the kidney.** Post-contrast CT performed in a 22-year-old with haematuria demonstrates a large central soft-tissue mass invading the renal pelvis, and causing hydronephrosis (see arrow). Resection was performed, confirming a transitional cell tumour. These can sometimes be difficult to differentiate from an RCC, and should always be considered in a poorly enhancing central endophytic mass. Surgical treatment for TCC includes ureterectomy, so preoperative differentiation is important.

Tumours Metastatic to the Kidney.[14] These tumours rarely cause symptoms during life but are frequently found in autopsy studies. They are increasingly detected as a result of the widespread use of CT in monitoring the response of extrarenal tumours to chemotherapy (see Fig. 12-24). Most renal metastases are haematogenous, although a few occur by direct invasion or from lymphatic spread. The commonest primary tumours are bronchial, colorectal, breast, testicular and gynaecological malignancies and malignant melanoma. Haematogenous metastases are usually small (<3 cm), multiple and confined to the cortex. They tend to present late in the

course of the disease and are associated with other evidence of metastatic disease. They are usually hypovascular on CT and do not tend to demonstrate calcification or renal vein invasion. Most metastases are more infiltrative and less exophytic than renal cell carcinoma. Fine-needle aspiration can confirm malignant disease if there is clinical doubt.

Non-Parenchymal

Urothelial Tumours

Transitional Cell Carcinoma (see Figs. 12-25 and 12-26). Transitional cell carcinoma of the renal pelvis

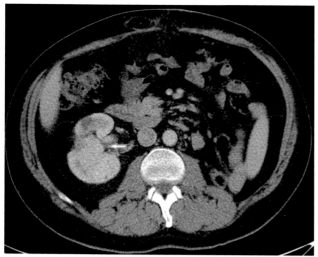

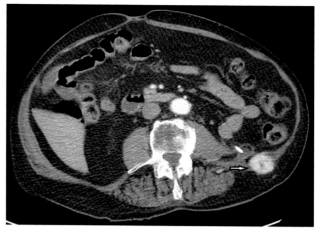

FIGURE 12-27 ■ **Local recurrence of renal cell carcinoma following cryotherapy.** Dynamic post-contrast CT demonstrates a soft-tissue mass in the mid pole of the right kidney (see arrow) with overlying cortical atrophy. The patient had received previous cryotherapy to a 3-cm mass, but follow-up imaging demonstrated a progressive mass. Biopsy confirmed recurrence, and under intraoperative US guidance, a successful open partial nephrectomy was performed.

FIGURE 12-29 ■ **Local recurrence of renal cell carcinoma.** Post-contrast axial CT performed 5 years after radical nephrectomy demonstrates a focal enhancing mass (see arrow) in the posterior abdominal wall. No other metastatic disease was evident. Originally the tumour had been treated with focal percutaneous therapy and the local recurrence was considered to be secondary to this. In view of the solitary nature of the lesion, and absence of metastatic disease, local excision was performed.

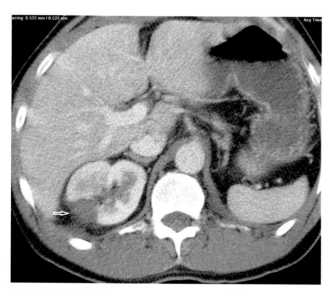

FIGURE 12-28 ■ **Post-treatment appearances following radiofrequency ablation of the kidney.** Recent radiofrequency (RF) treatment to a small right renal mass (see arrow) is seen as a wedge-shaped area of reduced attenuation. Increased use of local ablation with RF or cryotherapy produces a cohort of patients requiring follow-up for assessment of local disease, as well as detecting metachronous lesions in the same or contralateral kidney.

Squamous Cell Carcinoma. Squamous cell carcinoma of the renal pelvis is a relatively rare tumour, representing only a few per cent of all renal neoplasms. It is a highly aggressive tumour and carries a poor clinical prognosis. Chronic infection and calculi play an important aetiological role in this malignancy, with stones being present in 57% of patients. It often involves the renal parenchyma and perinephric tissues, and may present with metastases.

There has been an increased use of localised or minimally invasive treatments with radiofrequency and cryotherapy for small renal masses over the past 10 years. Although local treatment is an attractive approach, it requires a relatively higher intensity of follow-up to ensure treatment is adequate and that there is no local recurrence (Figs. 12-27 and 12-28).

A soft-tissue mass is usually seen around the site of local treatment which demonstrates involution over time, often leaving some residual soft tissue (Fig. 12-29). The development of new enhancing tissue on the lateral or medial surface of the kidney suggests local recurrence. It is important to scrutinise both these areas for disease, as well as for metachronous tumours or metastatic nodes.

REFERENCES

1. Cohan RH, Sherman LS, Korbkin M, et al. Renal masses: assessment of corticomedullary-phase and nephrographic-phase CT scans. Radiology 1995;196:445–51.
2. Szolar DH, Kammerhuber F, Altziebler S, et al. Multiphasic helical CT of the kidney: increased conspicuity for detection and characterization of small (<3 cm) renal masses. Radiology 1997;202: 211–17.
3. Paudyal B, Paudyal P, Tsushima Y, et al. The role of the ADC value in the characterisation of renal carcinoma by diffusion-weighted MRI. Br J Radiol 2010;83:336–43.
4. Faemi S, Knoll AN, Bendavid OJ, et al. Characterization of genitourinary lesions with diffusion-weighted imaging. Radiographics 2009;29:1295–317.

and calyceal system presents as a renal mass when it infiltrates into the renal substance, although most urothelial tumours present as filling defects within the renal pelvis or ureter. The infiltrative form may be mistaken for a primary renal cell carcinoma that has breached the renal pelvis. Renal cell carcinoma may, on occasion, invade the calyceal system.

5. Bosniak MA. Should we biopsy complex cystic renal masses (Bosniak category III)? Am J Roentgenol 2003;181:1425–6.
6. Bosniak MA. Diagnosis and management of patients with complicated cystic lesions of the kidney. Am J Roentgenol 1997;169: 819–22.
7. Bosniak MA. The current radiological approach to renal cysts. Radiology 1986;158:1–10.
8. Jinzaki M, Tanimoto A, Narimatsu Y, et al. Angiomyolipoma: imaging findings in lesions with minimal fat. Radiology 1997; 205:497–502.
9. Lemaitre L, Claudon M, Dubrulle F, Mazeman E. Imaging of angiomyolipoma. Semin Ultrasound CT MRI 1997;18:100–14.

10. Licht MR, Novick AC, Tubbs RR, et al. Renal oncocytoma: clinical and biological correlates. J Urol 1993;150:1380–3.
11. Choyke PL, Glenn GM, McClellan MW, et al. Hereditary renal cancers. Radiology 2003;226:33–46.
12. Choyke PL, Glenn GM, Walther MM, et al. von Hippel–Lindau disease: genetic, clinical and imaging features. Radiology 1995; 194:629–42.
13. Semelka RC, Kelekis NL, Burdeny DA, et al. Renal lymphoma: demonstration by MR imaging. Am J Roentgenol 1996;166: 823–7.
14. Ferrozzi F, Bova D, Campodonico F. Computed tomography of renal metastases. Semin Ultrasound CT MRI 1997;18:115–21.

CHAPTER 13

RENAL TRANSPLANTATION: IMAGING

Giles Rottenberg • Allan C. Andi

HISTORY OF TRANSPLANT

Renal transplantation was first performed in 1950 in the USA but with limited success due to the lack of immunosuppression. Initial success was experienced between identical twins where immunosuppression was not required. Cadaveric transplantation was only performed later when immunosuppression had been developed. There has been a recent increase in living donors—almost 50% in the USA and 30% in UK—due to the lack of availability of cadaveric kidneys. Recent development has seen the use of paired schemes or even more complicated pooled groups of donors sharing kidneys. ABO incompatibility is no longer a contraindication.

SURGICAL TECHNIQUE

Technique will vary amongst surgeons and is dependent upon the recipient's vascular anatomy and presence of previous renal transplants. The transplant is usually sited in the right or left iliac fossa. The artery is anastomosed end to side onto the common or external iliac artery. If there are multiple arteries, the anastomosis may be onto a patch, although this is only possible from a cadaveric donor. The venous anatomy is usually performed as an end-to-side anastomosis onto the external iliac vein. The ureteric anastomosis is also variable according to the surgeon and may include an anti-reflux technique. The usual site for the anastomotic site is the dome of the bladder, although this may be altered if there is a large-capacity bladder in which the anastomosis may be lower.

TECHNIQUE OF EXAMINATION

Ultrasound (US) remains the mainstay for imaging the kidney in both the short- and long-term management of the renal transplant, its advantages being its portability,

cost and lack of ionising radiation and nephrotoxicity (see Fig. 13-1). The transplant kidney is ideally suited for US imaging; being superficially placed in the iliac fossa makes it possible for high-frequency probes to provide good-quality images. A full examination of the transplant relies upon a combination of grey scale, and Doppler US. The graft length should be measured and evaluated for evidence of hydronephrosis, calculi or focal abnormality. The peri-renal tissues should be evaluated for fluid collections, and the bladder examined for wall-thickening, calculi or tumour. The orientation of the kidney can vary depending on surgical technique and should be established in the axial plane so that true longitudinal images can be obtained. The presence of ureteric stents should be noted and reported. The bladder should be evaluated both before and after micturition, particularly if there is hydronephrosis or urinary tract infection.

Doppler US should routinely be used. Colour flow and spectral Doppler evaluation of the intra-renal blood flow and the extra-renal vessels should be undertaken if there is a history of hypertension. The spectral pattern of the normal renal transplant artery is similar to that in the native renal artery. Various measurements of the Doppler trace can be made, although there is limited clinical value in performing extensive measurements as they tend not to be specific enough to differentiate between rejection and acute tubular necrosis (ATN). The normal trace is a low-resistance circulation (ski slope pattern) with the diastolic flow measuring approximately a third of the systolic velocity. A reduction in the diastolic velocity is usually a sign of a pathological process. The resistive index (RI) is a useful simple measurement for qualitative analysis, and is useful for communicating with clinicians. RI is measured by

$$\frac{\text{peak systolic velocity} - \text{end diastolic velocity}}{\text{peak systolic velocity}}$$

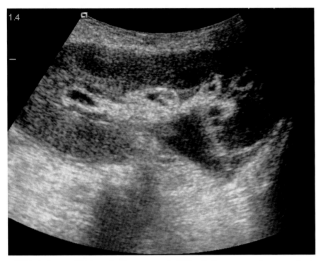

FIGURE 13-1 ■ **Normal ultrasound.** US of the normal transplant provides high-quality images of the kidney, allowing accurate measurement of renal length, and exclusion of a focal abnormality or hydronephrosis.

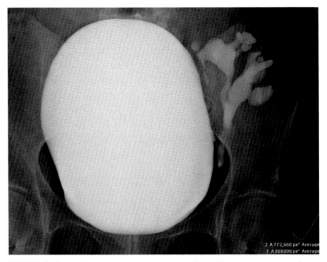

FIGURE 13-2 ■ **Transplant cystogram.** Voiding cystogram demonstrates the presence of reflux into the transplant kidney on voiding. The position and type of ureteric anastomosis may vary according to surgical technique used.

RIs exceeding 0.8 in the kidney transplant allograft have been defined as abnormal; however, multiple researchers have documented RI's lack of specificity considering the complex interaction between renal vascular resistance and compliance. Therefore, clinical assessment and associated sonographic findings remain integral in the assessment of graft dysfunction.[1,2]

In addition to intra-renal measurement of Doppler flow, a systematic assessment of colour flow in all regions of the kidney should be performed to assess differential blood flow. Although evaluation of colour flow is subjective, it is a useful tool and reassuring when normal. This is particularly important when multiple renal arteries are present at the time of transplant.

It is important to evaluate the native kidneys if the patient is being investigated for recurrent urinary tract infection, as these may be a source of sepsis or stones. Similarly, the investigation of haematuria post-transplant must include an assessment of the native kidneys for hydronephrosis or renal mass.

Computed tomography (CT) and magnetic resonance imaging (MRI) are both useful in the further evaluation of transplant complications where US cannot fully demonstrate an abnormality due to overlying bowel gas or when patients become systemically unwell and US is unable to demonstrate an abnormality. CT can be used to confirm vascular complications which have been detected by US, or where US has not been able to sufficiently exclude a vascular abnormality. A dedicated renal CT angiographic protocol with multiplanar reconstruction or a biphasic examination may be required to answer these questions.

Magnetic resonance (MR) angiography is an evolving technique that can be used to evaluate the transplant artery and vein. It is used predominantly when US evaluation is inconclusive. There are two main techniques of MR angiography—non-contrast and contrast-enhanced. Contrast-enhanced MR angiography relies upon the administration of gadolinium, which was widely used in the past in patients with renal dysfunction in preference to iodinated contrast agents. It is now contraindicated in patients with renal failure or severe dysfunction (i.e. with an estimated glomerular filtration rate of less than 30) due to the risk of nephrogenic systemic fibrosis. Contrast-enhanced MR angiography also relies upon a coronal three-dimensional (3D) fast multiplanar gradient-echo breath-hold sequence. This is performed after a timing bolus of contrast medium.

Many techniques are used to perform unenhanced MR angiography, the most frequently used being the time-of-flight (TOF) or phase-contrast method. TOF exploits the inflow effect of blood protons and uses flow-compensated 2D or 3D gradient-echo sequences. Phase contrast is independent of direction but is motion susceptible and time-consuming. Turbulent flow can cause loss of signal and may result in overestimation of narrowing.

Newer techniques which appear to offer significant improvement in image quality have been recently introduced. Steady-state free precession (SSFP) with or without arterial spin labelling can provide high-resolution images of blood vessels, including renal arteries, without the use of contrast agents. It relies upon a gradient-echo-based sequence that maintains steady-state longitudinal and transverse magnetisation by applying serial equidistant radiofrequency pulses. SSFP enables a short acquisition time and produces high signal-to-noise images which are independent of flow and direction. The images are susceptible to field heterogeneity.

Compared with CT angiography, MR angiography has a number of disadvantages, which include an increased time of imaging, a limited range and a range of complex artefacts. Conventional angiography is usually reserved as a prelude to intervention, or in cases where US and/or CT are unable to exclude or define an abnormality.

Cystography may be required in the evaluation of bladder abnormality immediately after surgery to evaluate bladder injury, or at a later date to investigate reflux following recurrent pain or infection (see Fig. 13-2).

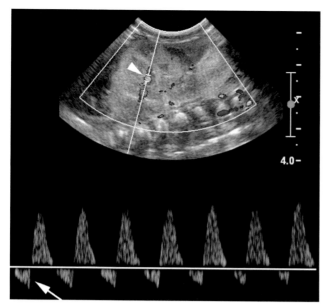

FIGURE 13-3 ■ **Renal vein thrombosis.** US of a kidney shortly after transplantation demonstrates poor colour flow in interlobar arteries (arrow head), and reversal of the diastolic blood flow in the vein (short arrow) consistent with renal vein thrombosis.

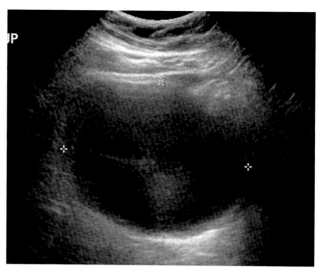

FIGURE 13-4 ■ **Post-transplant fluid collection.** US performed 2 weeks post-transplantation demonstrates a large collection adjacent to the transplant that was drained under US guidance for diagnostic and therapeutic purposes.

VASCULAR COMPLICATIONS: EARLY[3]

Infarction

Transplant thrombosis, either arterial or venous, is uncommon, occurring in 1–5% of transplants,[3] usually in the early postoperative period, and often complicating severe acute rejection, tubular necrosis and torsion or angulation of the surgical anastomosis. The assessment of renal venous flow can readily be obtained by Doppler US (see Fig. 13-3). In renal vein thrombosis, reverse diastolic flow within both main and intra-renal arteries is evident at spectral Doppler US. In renal artery thrombosis, flow in both main and intra-renal arteries is completely absent at colour Doppler. In intra-renal artery segmental infarction, a focal area of decreased echogenicity, typically wedge-shaped with associated diminished vascularity, is evident at colour Doppler. Confirmation, if necessary, can be achieved with gadolinium-enhanced MR, CT or selective angiography. Surgical thrombectomy with arterial or venous repair is typically performed once acute thrombosis has been confirmed; nephrectomy may be required if the kidney is non-viable. The role of endovascular management of graft thrombosis with mechanical and chemical thrombolytic techniques is currently evolving and may also be considered.[4,5]

Acute Rejection

Rejection, occurring as early as 1 week after transplantation, and peaking at 1–3 weeks, may be classified as either acute rejection or accelerated acute rejection. Whilst patients usually remain asymptomatic with deteriorating renal function, a myriad of US appearances may be demonstrated. The graft may be oedematous, with swelling of the medullary pyramids, reduced cortical echotexture and loss of normal corticomedullary differentiation; in severe cases, there may be complete absence of diastolic flow or flow reversal with associated elevation of the RI. Doppler findings are not specific for acute rejection and may be seen in ATN, renal vein thrombosis or drug toxicity. In patients with an appropriate clinical history and supporting sonographic findings, empirical immunosuppressive therapy may be commenced but percutaneous biopsy remains the gold standard for the diagnosis of rejection.

Acute Tubular Necrosis

ATN is the commonest cause of early failure of function following cadaveric transplantation. It relates to prolonged cold ischaemic times in cadaveric grafts when compared with living grafts. Clinical differentiation of ATN from acute rejection occurring in the first 10 days can be difficult. Similarly, the spectrum of sonographic appearances may vary from normal to those seen in acute rejection. As previously mentioned in relation to acute rejection, RIs are typically elevated; however, clinically significant ATN may also be demonstrated in conjunction with a normal RI. Serial radionuclide imaging studies have proven reliable in differentiating the entities by the time course of the findings. However, histological confirmation remains the standard and biopsy is frequently required.

NON-VASCULAR COMPLICATIONS

Postoperative pelvic collections following transplantation are common, and may be due to urinoma, lymphocele, haematoma or a seroma (see Figs. 13-4–13-7). Differentiation can often be made clinically according to

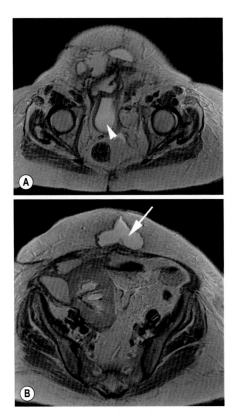

FIGURE 13-5 ■ MRI demonstration of postoperative peri-transplant fluid collection. Axial T2 MRI demonstrates (A) a complex pelvic collection (arrowhead) extending into (B) the abdominal wall (short arrow), which was confirmed as an abscess on percutaneous drainage.

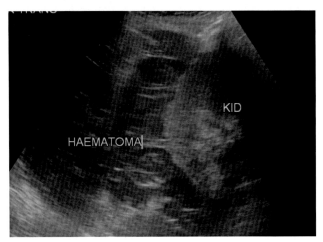

FIGURE 13-6 ■ Postoperative haematoma. US performed 2 days post-transplantation demonstrates a septated collection adjacent to the kidney secondary to postoperative haemorrhage.

symptoms and time since surgery. Urinoma formation usually occurs soon after surgery, whereas lymphocele formation usually develops at a slightly later stage.

Collections in the pelvis may be asymptomatic and picked up incidentally at the time of a routine US examination. CT or MRI may be used to plan drainage or further assess the distribution of a fluid collection. Collections can be associated with the development of pain if large and compression of adjacent structures.

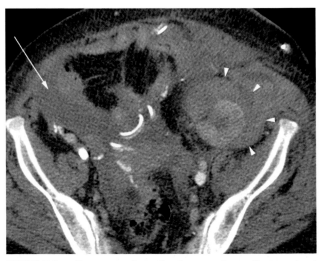

FIGURE 13-7 ■ Post-transplantation haemorrhage. Post-contrast CT demonstrates a peri-transplant haematoma (arrowheads) and significant intra-abdominal high-density fluid consistent with blood (long arrow).

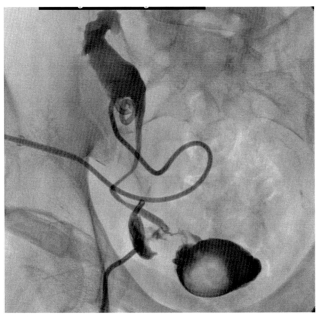

FIGURE 13-8 ■ Postoperative ureteric leak. A nephrostogram was performed following nephrostomy insertion for a postoperative urinoma. Contrast medium is leaking from the right side of the distal transplant ureter. A right-sided abdominal drain, inserted to drain the urinoma, is also evident.

Transplant hydronephrosis can also be caused by the compressive effects of a fluid collection. Although diagnosis can usually be made clinically and with the use of US, definitive diagnosis may rely upon the aspiration of fluid for analysis.

Urinoma

Urinoma usually develops soon after transplantation and is due to a disruption of the ureteric anastomosis or occasionally an infarcted segment in a patient with multiple renal arteries (see Fig. 13-8).

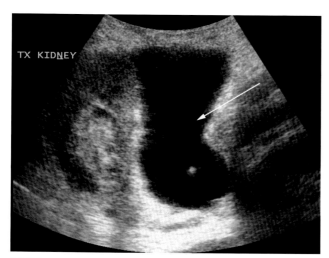

FIGURE 13-9 ■ **Lymphocele.** US performed 4 weeks post-transplantation demonstrates a large hypoechoic fluid collection (long arrow) medial to the kidney in keeping with a lymphocele.

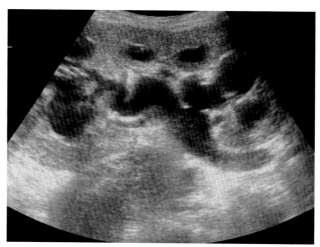

FIGURE 13-10 ■ **Transplant hydronephrosis.** US, performed because of a sudden rise in serum creatinine, demonstrated a markedly hydronephrotic transplant kidney. It is always important to exclude bladder dysfunction as a cause of hydronephrosis, and ultrasound should be performed both pre- and post-micturition.

It usually presents with a cystic collection in the pelvis adjacent to the transplant, although it can present with generalised ascites. Diagnosis can be made by US-guided aspiration of the fluid and measurement of the creatinine level, which will differentiate it from a lymphocele. Management is either conservative, involving the use of a stent and nephrostomy, or requires surgical intervention.

Lymphocele

Lymphocele is the commonest pelvic collection encountered after transplantation, occurring in between 0.6 and 18% of transplants. It is usually caused by leakage from lymphatics which are disturbed at the time of surgery and is more commonly seen in patients on tacrolimus (see Fig. 13-9).

US demonstrates a predominantly anechoic collection on the medial aspect of the transplant kidney. Internal septations can be present. Treatment is performed by either US-guided drainage with or without sclerosant or surgical (open or laparoscopic) marsupialisation. Simple aspiration is usually not efficacious.

Ureteric Strictures

Ureteric strictures occur in between 2 and 5% of renal transplants, and are usually due to ischaemia of the distal ureter. Diagnosis is usually made following a rise in the serum creatinine. US demonstrates dilatation of the renal collecting system with dilatation of the ureter. Comparison with previous imaging is important to confirm that the change is new. If the bladder is very full at the time of the examination, it is important to repeat the renal US following micturition to ensure the calyceal dilatation persists.

Hydronephrosis can also be caused by extrinsic ureteric compression from a perinephric or pelvic fluid collection or cystic mass, although this is usually evident at

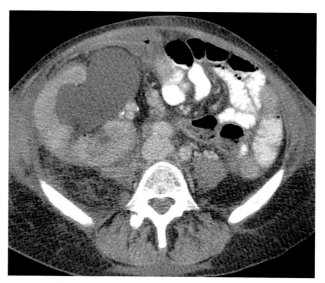

FIGURE 13-11 ■ **Transplant hydronephrosis.** CT demonstrates marked hydronephrosis of the transplant kidney, which was due to stricture at the ureteric anastomosis.

the time of US examination (see Figs. 13-10 and 13-11). In the early phase post-transplantation, hydronephrosis is more commonly seen as a consequence of a blood clot in the ureter or bladder, and tends to respond to bladder irrigation. Kinking of the ureter can also cause obstruction, as can intraluminal tumours, stones and fungal balls. Diagnosis can usually be revealed by US. Initial management is nephrostomy insertion followed by a nephrostogram, which will demonstrate the cause and level of obstruction (see Fig. 13-12). Although conservative management of ureteric strictures can be performed with stent insertion and balloon dilatation, definitive surgery which involves reimplantation of the ureter or anastomosis of the renal pelvis directly onto the bladder is frequently required.

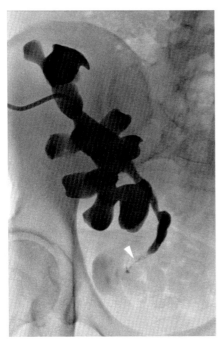

FIGURE 13-12 ■ **Post-transplantation ureteric stricture.** A ne-phrostogram performed in a patient presenting with hydrone-phrosis of the transplant kidney demonstrates a characteristic ischaemic stricture of the distal ureter (arrowhead) just above the bladder.

Renal Calculi

Renal stones can be seen in native or transplant kidneys following transplantation and may be asymptomatic or a cause of pain, recurrent urinary tract infection or even obstruction (see Fig. 13-13). Although ultrasound may be diagnostic, early use of non-enhanced CT should be considered.

VASCULAR COMPLICATIONS: INTERMEDIATE TO LATE

Renal Artery Stenosis

Renal artery stenosis is usually a late complication of transplantation. The stenosis normally occurs at the anastomosis between the donor and recipient artery. Clinical presentation is with severe hypertension or renal dysfunction. Screening for renal artery stenosis is best performed by a skilled technician. Knowledge of surgical anatomy is important for optimal ultrasonic evaluation of the graft.

Diagnosis is made by demonstration of a renal artery velocity greater than 2.5 m/s, a gradient of 2 : 1 between a stenotic and pre-stenotic segment and spectral broadening. Secondary findings can be useful, and include downstream turbulence and flow reversal distal to the stenotic segment (see Fig. 13-14 and 37-15). False-positive examinations may be due to kinking or tortuosity of vessels, which explains why best results are obtained with experienced technicians. If ultrasound and clinical features support a diagnosis of an arterial stenosis, formal

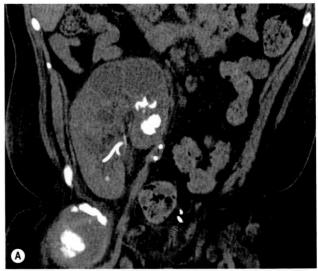

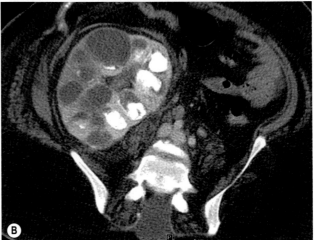

FIGURE 13-13 ■ **Renal transplant stones. (A)** Pre- and **(B)** post-contrast CT examinations demonstrate marked transplant hydronephrosis with multiple large renal calculi.

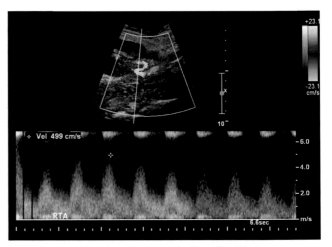

FIGURE 13-14 ■ **Renal artery stenosis.** Doppler US demonstrates abnormality of colour flow, elevated systolic velocities and spectral broadening in the renal transplant artery consistent with a significant artery stenosis.

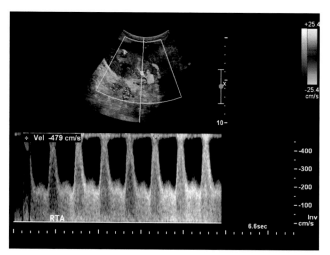

FIGURE 13-15 ■ **Renal artery stenosis.** Colour Doppler ultrasound performed of the transplant artery in a patient with hypertension and reduced renal function demonstrates markedly elevated peak systolic velocity in the artery consistent with stenosis of the transplant vessel.

angiography should be performed with a view to proceeding directly to angioplasty and stent insertion (see Fig. 13-16). If there is a discrepancy between the US and clinical appearance, non-invasive CT or MR angiography can be performed.[6–8]

Chronic Rejection

Chronic rejection is associated with intra-renal arterial segmental narrowing, which can be associated with segmental narrowing of the intra-renal vessels but normal waveforms in the main transplant artery. Chronic rejection is an insidious process involving deteriorating graft function, typically from 3 months to several years following transplantation. US examination at this stage demonstrates a small echobright kidney with parenchymal thinning and loss of corticomedullary differentiation. Global perfusion of the graft may be reduced with an elevated RI. Confirmation of the diagnosis is typically made at histological assessment (see Fig. 13-18).

Cancer and Transplant

The incidence of malignant tumours is significantly increased following transplantation as a consequence of immunosuppression (see Figs. 13-19-13-21).

Malignancy of the skin is the commonest encountered malignancy following transplantation. The most common solid organ malignancy is post-transplant lymphoproliferative disorder (PTLD). This malignancy is related to B-cell infection with Epstein–Barr virus and is most commonly seen in the first year following transplantation. The incidence is related to the degree of immunosuppression. Presentation is with nodal enlargement or systemic symptoms of fever and malaise. Treatment is initially based upon reduction of immunosuppression, which is usually sufficient to produce a response. Solid organ involvement, which can even involve the renal

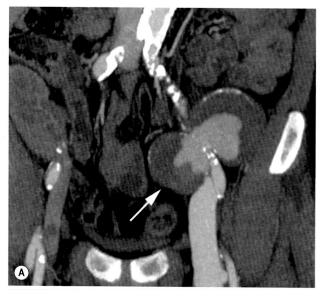

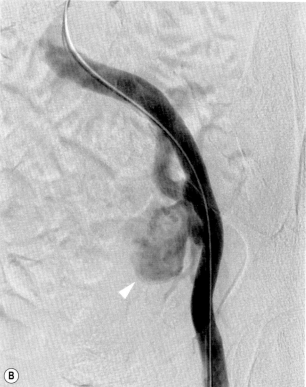

FIGURE 13-16 ■ **Post-transplant false aneurysm.** (A) CT (short arrow) and (B) angiogram (arrow head) demonstrate an incidentally discovered large false aneurysm arising from the left common iliac artery following a previous failed and resected renal graft.

graft, can be seen. The incidence of lymphoma is approximately 35 times higher than normal.

Other malignancies are also seen in increased incidence in patients with renal transplants, including cervical carcinoma and tumours of the hepatobiliary system. Renal cancer is also seen following transplantation and usually affects the native kidneys, particularly in the presence of renal cystic disease. Tumours can involve the transplant kidney as well as the urothelium.

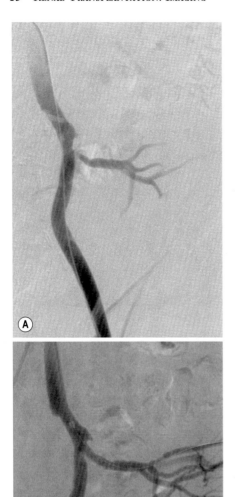

FIGURE 13-17 ■ **Renal artery stenosis.** Intra-arterial digital subtraction angiography (DSA) (A) pre- and (B) post-stent insertion demonstrates successful treatment of a stenosis at the arterial anastomosis.

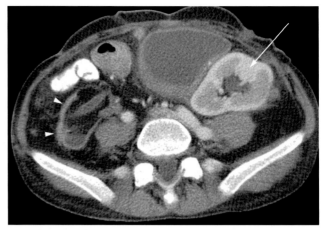

FIGURE 13-18 ■ **Appearance of a non-functioning transplant.** CT of the abdomen demonstrates an old and non-functioning transplant in the right iliac fossa (arrowheads). The normally functioning transplant is seen in the left iliac fossa (long arrow).

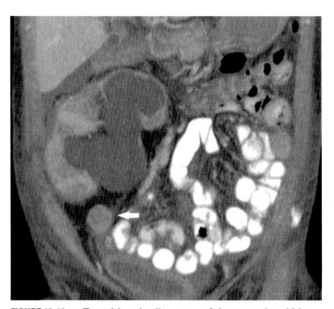

FIGURE 13-19 ■ **Transitional cell tumour of the transplant kidney.** Post-contrast CT of the transplant kidney in a patient with haematuria demonstrated marked hydronephrosis with a soft tissue mass in the ureter causing obstruction (see arrow). Ureteroscopy confirmed the presence of a high-grade tumour.

Infection and Renal Transplantation

Infections are more common in patients with transplant kidneys, secondary to immunosuppression. The presence of drains, catheters and lines at the time of transplantation also provide a source of sepsis. The most common infections following transplantation affect the urinary tract. They usually respond to antibiotics, although pyelonephritis of the graft is less responsive than a normal kidney. Pyelonephritis may also be associated with graft dysfunction. CT should be performed in severe infection to exclude abscess formation which may require percutaneous drainage (see Fig. 13-22). Other infections are seen following transplantation and include CMV, PCP and BK virus. Prophylaxis may be administered to prevent PCP. CMV infection is the commonest and may be due to reactivation of previous infection, or transmission of

the virus from the donor organ in a patient not previously exposed to the virus (see Fig. 13-23).

USE OF ISOTOPE STUDIES AND RENAL TRANSPLANT

Isotope studies can be used in the evaluation of early graft failure, although many centres now favour the use of US over isotope scintigraphy and tend to perform renal biopsy much more readily to establish the cause of post-transplant renal dysfunction in the absence of renal obstruction.

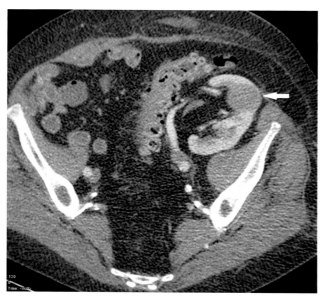

FIGURE 13-20 ■ **Tumour and the transplant kidney.** The poorly enhancing focal mass seen in the transplanted kidney is consistent with a papillary tumour (see arrow). The mass was biopsied, and subsequently treated with radiofrequency ablation.

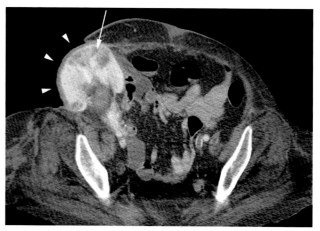

FIGURE 13-22 ■ **Transplant pyelonephritis.** Dynamic post-contrast CT demonstrates patchy enhancement in the kidney secondary to severe urinary sepsis (long arrow). The abdominal wall is deficient (arrowheads) secondary to a recent episode of necrotising fasciitis. The kidney function improved following antibiotic treatment.

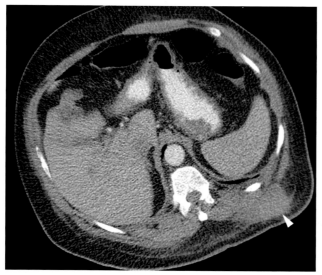

FIGURE 13-21 ■ **Post-transplant lymphoproliferative disorder (PTLD).** CT performed 6 months post-transplantation following the development of a mass in the left flank (arrowhead). Biopsy confirmed PTLD. Other sites of disease may include lymph nodes, solid organs or even the renal graft itself.

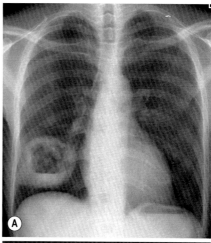

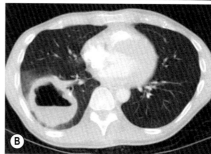

FIGURE 13-23 ■ **Infection and the renal transplant.** (A) Chest X-ray and (B) CT demonstrate an abscess in the right lower lobe of the lung in a patient with a cough and fever 6 months following renal transplantation.

Technetium-99m (Tc-99m) mercaptoacetyltriglycine (MAG3) may be used in the evaluation of renal transplant function. Baseline imaging is useful for assessment. ATN is characterised by delayed time to maximal activity (T_{max}), delayed time from maximum to one-half maximal activity ($T_{1/2}$) and a high 20-to-3 minute ratio.

The radionuclide imaging findings of acute rejection are characterised by diminished flow. These findings are similar to those of ATN, and the two entities can be differentiated by the time course of the findings. Acute rejection rarely develops in the first few days after transplantation and instead will manifest with a decrease in function on serial radionuclide imaging studies.

MAG3 renography may also be used in the assessment of transplant obstruction, although if there is hydronephrosis and reduced renal dysfunction, nephrostomy is usually performed as a diagnostic and therapeutic procedure.

In the work-up of potential live donors, Tc-99m dimercaptosuccinic acid (DMSA) can be used to assess split function if there is renal asymmetry on US or CT imaging. Technetium-99m mercaptoacetyltriglycine (Tc-99m MAG 3) can be used to exclude renal obstruction in patients with mild dilatation of the collecting system on pre-transplant imaging.

RENAL TRANSPLANT BIOPSY

Biopsy of transplants is commonly performed in the immediate postoperative phase in patients with poor or late-functioning transplants. As the transplant is superficially positioned, US-guided biopsy is relatively easy. A lower-pole approach is usually used, and complications can be reduced by obtaining the core from the cortex only.

Complications following biopsy are common and usually involve bleeding from the biopsy site into the calyceal system, perinephric tissues or retroperitoneum.[9] Anticoagulation is associated with a much higher risk of bleeding complications. If significant bleeding occurs following biopsy, a dynamic CT of the transplant is recommended to evaluate the presence of significant retroperitoneal haemorrhage, and to prove evidence of active bleeding on the angiographic phase of the CT (see Fig. 13-24). Formal angiography with a view to embolisation is advised if there are features of active arterial bleeding on CT.

Other vascular complications of biopsy include arteriovenous malformations (AVMs), which are frequently asymptomatic, and may often spontaneously resolve (see Fig. 13-25). Demonstration of an AVM can be seen on US as an arterialised venous trace, or a focal area of abnormal colour flow on colour Doppler imaging (CDI).

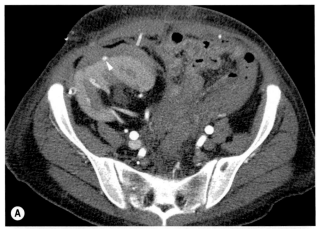

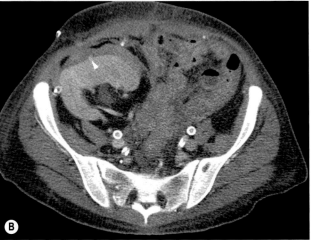

FIGURE 13-24 ■ **Post-transplant biopsy bleed.** (A) Arterial and (B) venous phase post-contrast CT performed following transplant biopsy demonstrates a small focal area of enhancement on the anterior aspect of the kidney, which is far less conspicuous on the later-phase examination (arrowheads). There is a small peri-renal haematoma. The acute bleeding point was subsequently embolised.

RADIOLOGICAL EVALUATION OF POTENTIAL DONOR KIDNEYS

With the increasing scarcity of cadaveric donors and the increased number of patients awaiting transplantation, there has been a significant increase in the use of live related and altruistic donors. This development has been aided by the improvement in immunosuppression, and the development of laparoscopy for nephrectomy, resulting in reduced morbidity for the donor.

Having evaluated the potential donor's medical and psychological suitability, assessment of the kidneys is performed to assess the donor's suitability.

A screening ultrasound can be performed to confirm the presence of two suitable kidneys with no obvious abnormality, although we now tend to perform CT evaluation only, as this can reduce the number of visits and investigations required.

An initial unenhanced CT data acquisition is performed through the kidneys to exclude renal calculi. Arterial phase imaging is then performed through the upper abdomen generally down to the aortic bifurcation to ensure that all accessory renal vessels are identified. Coronal reconstruction, and preferably curved in the plane of the arteries, is essential for demonstrating the vessels and identifying the site of bifurcation. Additional imaging phases at 60 s can also be performed to evaluate the renal veins, and cava, although we do not routinely perform these as the renal veins are usually adequately opacified on the early images. Immediately following CT, plain radiographs of the abdomen are obtained to demonstrate the renal collecting system and ureters and to exclude a duplex system or obstruction.

It is important to report relevant anatomical findings on the CT which should include accurate measurement of the kidneys to ensure that they are symmetrical in size. A discrepancy of more than 1 cm merits further evaluation with DMSA scintigraphy. It is obviously important to exclude an incidental and unexpected renal mass in the donor kidney, as well as any incidental and significant extra-renal abnormality. This is particularly important with the increased use of older donors, where the incidence of significant findings will be greater.

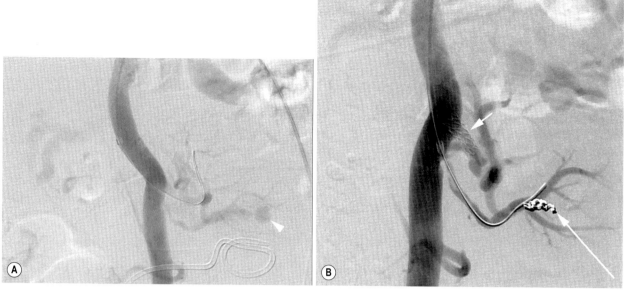

FIGURE 13-25 ■ **Post-biopsy arteriovenous malformation (AVM).** (A) Intra-arterial DSA performed in a patient with persistent haematuria post-biopsy demonstrates an AVM (arrowhead). (B) There is also a stent seen in the transplant renal artery (see short arrow). The AVM was successfully treated with embolisation (see long arrow).

The number and site of the renal arteries, as well as the presence of an early bifurcation close to the aorta, all of which may affect kidney selection, should be recorded. The renal venous anatomy, as well as the presence of enlarged lumbar or gonadal veins, should also be recorded.

Dynamic MRI of the abdomen can be used to assess potential donors, although MRI may not provide equivalent information on the presence of calculi and may not provide the same resolution of the renal vessels. Obviously, different transplant centres may have their own preferences which will depend on local resource availability and local expertise.

REFERENCES

1. Cosgrove D, Chan K. Renal transplant: what ultrasound can and cannot do. Ultrasound Q 2008;24:77–87.
2. Tublin ME, Bude RO, Platt JF. The resistive index in renal Doppler sonography: where do we stand? AJR Am J Roentgenol 2003;180:885–92.
3. Akbar SA, Jafri SZH, Amendola MA, et al. Complications of renal transplantation. Radiographics 2005;25:1335–56.
4. Melamed ML, Kim HS, Jaar BG, et al. Combined percutaneous mechanical and chemical thrombectomy for renal vein thrombosis in kidney transplant recipients. Am J Transplant 2005;5(3):621–6.
5. Kobayashi K, Censullo ML, Rossman LL, et al. Interventional radiologic management of renal transplant dysfunction: indications, limitations, and technical considerations. Radiographics 2007;27:1109–30.
6. Polak WG, Jezior D, Garcarek J, et al. Incidence and outcome of transplant renal artery stenosis: single center experience. Transplant Proc 2006;38(1):131–2.
7. Patel NH, Jindal RM, Wilkin T, et al. Renal arterial stenosis in renal allografts: retrospective study of predisposing factors and outcome after percutaneous transluminal angioplasty. Radiology 2001;219:663–7.
8. Beecroft JR, Rajan DK, Clark TW, et al. Transplant renal artery stenosis: outcome after percutaneous intervention. J Vasc Interv Radiol 2004;15:1407–13.
9. Boschiero LB, Saggin P, Galante O, et al. Renal needle biopsy of the transplant kidney: vascular and urologic complications. Urol Int 1992;48:130–3.

CHAPTER 14

UROTHELIAL CELL CANCER, UPPER TRACT AND LOWER TRACT

Nigel C. Cowan • Richard H. Cohan

UPPER TRACT UROTHELIAL CARCINOMA

DEFINITION

Upper tract urothelial carcinoma (UTUC) refers to malignant changes of the uroepithelial cells lining the urinary tract anywhere from the renal calyces to the ureteral orifice.

EPIDEMIOLOGY

Urothelial carcinomas are the fourth most common tumours, after prostate or breast cancer, lung cancer and colorectal cancer.[1-3] They may be located in the lower urinary tract; the bladder or urethra, or the upper urinary tract; renal calyces, renal pelvis and ureter. Bladder cancers (BCa) account for 90–95% of urothelial carcinomas and are the second most common malignancy of the urogenital tract after prostate cancer.[2] UTUCs are uncommon and account for only 5–10% of urothelial carcinomas. Urothelial carcinomas account for 90% of tumours of the renal pelvis; other epithelial cell types include squamous cell carcinoma, adenocarcinoma, carcinosarcoma, small cell carcinoma and papilloma.

The accuracy of incidence and mortality statistics for renal pelvic UTUC in the USA is limited by the fact that UTUC and renal cell carcinoma are grouped together for reporting purposes.[1] The estimated annual incidence of UTUCs in Western countries is approximately 1–2 new cases per 100,000 inhabitants. Pyelocalyceal tumours are about as twice as common as ureteral tumours. In

8–13% of cases a concurrent bladder cancer is present. Recurrence of disease in the bladder occurs in 30–51% of UTUC patients[4] and recurrences in the contralateral upper tract are observed in 6%.[5]

The natural history of UTUCs is different from that of bladder cancer; 60% of UTUCs are invasive at diagnosis compared with only 15% of bladder tumours.

Hereditary cases of UTUC are linked to hereditary non-polyposis colorectal carcinoma (HNPCC), which should be suspected if the patient is <60 years of age or has a history of an HNPCC-type cancer.[6-8]

RISK FACTORS

UTUC has a peak incidence in patients in their 70s and 80s. UTUC is three times more prevalent in men than in women predominantly because of the higher rates of smoking and occupational exposure to carcinogens among men.[9]

Chemical carcinogens predispose the entire urothelium to the development of multifocal urothelial carcinoma[10] by an effect sometimes referred to as field change of the urothelium. Smoking is the principal risk factor for UTUC.[11] Occupational exposure is most commonly caused by aromatic amines found in certain chemicals used in many industries, e.g. dyes, textiles, rubber, chemicals, petrochemical and coal and responsible for 'amino tumours'. Chemicals such as benzidine and β-naphthalene were banned in the 1960s in most industrialised countries. Usually a UTUC caused by occupational exposure to aromatic amines is also associated with a bladder tumour. The average duration of exposure needed for a UTUC to develop is 7 years.[10]

UTUCs resulting from the drug phenacetin have almost disappeared after the product was withdrawn in the 1970s.[10] UTUC is very common in patients and families afflicted with Balkan endemic nephropathy (BEN).[12] The incidence is highest in Croatia, Bosnia, Bulgaria, Romania and Serbia. Aristocholic acid (AA) contained in *Aristolochia fangchi* and *Aristolochia clematis*, plants endemic to the Balkans, is thought to play a role in the aetiology of UTUC. AA is the cause of Chinese herb nephropathy (aristocholic nephropathy or AAN), which is a rapidly progressing interstitial fibrosing renal disease with frequent urothelial malignancies.[13] A high incidence of UTUC has also been described in Taiwan, especially in the population of the southwest coast, representing 20–25% of urothelial carcinomas in the region.

Most urothelial carcinomas of the renal pelvis are of high histological grade and present in advanced stages, whereas most bladder cancers present as low grade and stage.[14,15]

In the region of 40% of renal pelvis urothelial carcinomas can show unusual atypical features and metaplastic phenomena.[15,16]

IDENTIFICATION OF PROGNOSTIC FACTORS

Prognostic factors are patient characteristics which predict the disease outcome including the chance of recovery or recurrence. Prognostic factors are significant and important in clinical practice as they can guide selection of treatment and the timing of surveillance. Identification of prognostic factors determining which patients can benefit from endoscopic versus radical nephroureterectomy, neoadjuvant or adjuvant chemotherapy and/or lymphadenectomy is urgently needed.

MANAGEMENT

Multiple treatment options are available for the management of patients with UTUC.

Open radical nephroureterectomy (ONU) with excision of an ipsilateral bladder cuff is the reference standard surgical treatment for UTUC in patients with a normal contralateral kidney regardless of the location of tumour in the upper tract. Nephroureterectomy can be performed by an open, laparoscopic (LNU) or hand-assisted technique (HARU). Resection of the distal ureter and its orifices is performed because it is a part of the urinary tract with especially high risk of recurrence and has been reported to be beneficial

Laparoscopic nephroureterectomy (LNU) is increasingly used in the management of UTUC.

Several studies have compared perioperative outcomes between ONU and LNU. LNU generally results in less blood loss, shorter hospital stay, decreased analgesic intake, a shorter interval to oral intake and decreased interval to convalescence, with no significant difference in the rate of perioperative complications.

Regarding oncological outcomes of ONU compared with LNU, emerging data support at least equivalent outcomes for LNU and ONU. In a prospective randomised trial, Simone et al. showed improved disease-specific and metastasis-free survival for ONU in patients with stage T3 tumours and high-grade disease. Long-term outcome data are awaited. ONU might improve cancer control in patients with high-grade/stage ureteral tumours. Port-site metastases following laparoscopic surgery for UTUC have been reported, which is another factor to be considered.

Traditionally, endoscopic management of UTUC was reserved for patients with solitary kidneys, bilateral synchronous tumours, baseline renal insufficiency, or comorbid diseases that preclude abdominal surgery. Recently, the use of endoscopic treatment via the retrograde ureteroscopic approach for patients with UTUC, normal renal function and low-grade, low-volume disease has been advocated, so long as patients are able to accept strict surveillance protocols. Opponents of ureteroscopic management argue that any delay in surgery might adversely affect prognosis but there is evidence suggesting that ureteroscopic biopsy/ablation before surgery does not adversely affect the outcomes compared with immediate surgery. Studies with longer follow-up are needed to assess the oncological efficacy of ureteroscopic treatments of UTUC.

Topical immunotherapy in addition to endoscopic management can be administered directly through a ureteral catheter or antegradely via a nephrostomy tube. Topical immunotherapy with BCG and chemotherapy with mitomycin C have a clear role in patients with bladder urothelial carcinoma; the data are not so clear for UTUC.

Consensus has not been reached regarding the therapeutic benefit of regional lymphadenectomy (LND) for UTUC. There is much clinical data supporting lymphadenectomy for bladder cancer but to date evidence with respect to lymphadenectomy for UTUC is mixed. Kondo et al. reported that preoperative imaging accurately identified lymph node positive patients in <50% of cases.[17] This means that some patients might be understaged and undergo suboptimal treatment without lymphadenectomy. Lughezzani et al. found no difference in cancer-specific mortality in patients with UTUC undergoing surgery with and without lymphadenectomy.[18] However, other studies have shown improvement in cancer-specific survival and disease-free survival in patients with stage T2 or greater disease who underwent lymph node dissection. Lymphadenectomy during radical NU remains controversial. Additional studies and the use of standardised dissection templates will help define the role of lymphadenectomy in the treatment of UTUC.[19]

Chemotherapeutic regimens for patients with advanced UTUC are based on those used for bladder urothelial carcinoma, of which cisplatin-based regimens are the most commonly used. In a large multicentre retrospective study on 140 patients, with locally advanced, node-positive disease and metastases, adjuvant chemotherapy with cisplatin-based regimens did not have any effect on overall or cancer-specific survival compared with the patients who did not undergo chemotherapy.

BIOPSY

For patients with suspected UTUC found by diagnostic imaging, ureteroscopic biopsy provides histopathological confirmation and information as to the histological grade of the UTUC, which is one of the best predictors of pathological stage, tumour recurrence and overall survival. The diagnostic accuracy of ureteroscopic biopsy for UTUC is high but recent work has shown that ureteroscopic biopsy of upper tract lesions tends to underestimate the tumour grade when compared with the grade determined by histopathological analysis of the nephrouretrectomy specimen. If ureteroscopic biopsy underestimates tumour grade, this may go some way in explaining the failure of some endoscopic management of UTUC. A high grade at biopsy could be used as supporting radical surgery.

IMAGING UPPER TRACT UROTHELIAL CARCINOMA

Diagnostic imaging plays a significant role in diagnosing and staging of UTUC. Previously, multiple imaging investigations were common with ultrasound, excretory urography and retrograde pyelography. Currently, CT urography is the most common imaging technique for imaging UTUC and MR urography is used only when CT urography is contraindicated. Clinical presentation of UTUC is usually with haematuria and so the imaging techniques used must not only be highly accurate for diagnosing UTUC but also be able detect other diseases responsible for haematuria.

Definition of CT Urography

CT urography is a developing diagnostic imaging technique made possible by recent advances in CT technology. It is defined as a CT examination of the kidneys, ureters and bladder with at least one series of images acquired during the excretory phase, after administration of intravenous contrast medium.[20]

Indications and Contraindications for CT Urography

Early reports of CT urography for detecting urinary tract abnormalities including stones,[21–24] renal masses[25–28] and UTUC have been very encouraging.[29–35] The first set of guidelines from the Upper Urinary Tract Imaging Group of the European Society of Urogenital Radiology was published in 2008.[20]

The indications for CT urography are controversial and consensus has still not been reached.[33] The principal indication is the investigation of haematuria suspected to be due to UTUC. Other indications will not be discussed further here. A working knowledge of the indications for a particular diagnostic test is essential before requesting the said test, but there are three other key pieces of information that should be understood in order to avoid requesting redundant diagnostic tests. First, the clinician should use existing clinical knowledge of the patient to estimate the probability that the patient has the disease in question (the pretest probability). Secondly, the clinician should be aware of the sensitivity and specificity of the diagnostic test, and thirdly, the physician must consider whether the results of the test will affect the patient's management.[36] Contraindications are few but centre around whether iodine-based contrast or radiation should be avoided.[37]

Optimisation of CT Urography Technique

There are three main protocols for the intravenous administration of contrast medium which depend on the number of boluses of contrast used, single, double or triple bolus.[38]

The single bolus protocol is optimised for patients with haematuria at high risk of UTUC, renal masses and stones. This protocol consists of three series of image acquisition: an unenhanced series optimised for detecting stones, a nephrographic series optimised for detecting renal masses and an excretory series optimised for detecting UTUC.

The double bolus protocol involves a slightly lower radiation dose than the single bolus protocol. It uses less contrast medium than the single bolus protocol for demonstration of the nephrographic and excretory phases and so may not produce such an intense nephrogram for demonstration of renal cell carcinoma or excretory series for diagnosing UTUC. If the unenhanced series is excluded, and the enhanced nephrographic and excretory phases are acquired in one series, a low-dose protocol is achieved which is commonly used for the follow-up of patients with known bladder cancer or UTUC.[32,39,40]

The triple bolus protocol is used for the assessment of living related kidney donors and patients undergoing percutaneous nephrolithotomy.[39] Although use of a triple bolus protocol for investigating haematuria has been described,[40] it is currently not recommended for routine use because the volume of contrast agent available for the excretory phase is reduced by bolus splitting, which is likely to compromise diagnostic accuracy.

Many studies have evaluated techniques aimed at promoting complete opacification of the urinary tract during CT urography, in order to optimise the contrast between urine and urothelial disease. Currently there is no consensus regarding the optimum technique. A number of manoeuvres have been suggested that are often interrelated in a complex fashion so that adjustment of one will impact on the others. Such manoeuvres include oral administration of water, intravenous furosemide or saline to encourage urine flow, abdominal compression, varying the timing of the image acquisition, acquiring a second series of images in the excretory phase, increasing the volume of contrast injected and encouraging patient movement (walking or log rolling on the CT table) to promote mixing of contrast agent and urine.

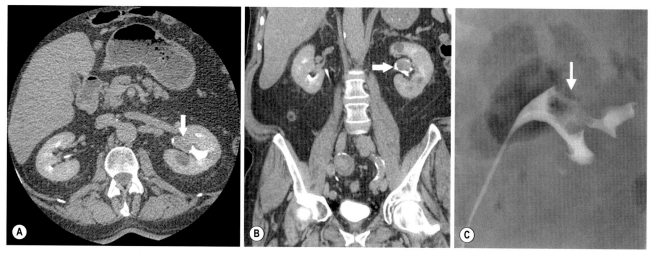

FIGURE 14-1 ■ **A 72-year-old man presenting with visible haematuria.** (A) Axial section of an excretory-phase CT urogram showing a filling defect in the left renal pelvis, white arrow, which was a urothelial carcinoma, G2 pT1. (B) A coronal reconstruction of the left renal pelvis urothelial carcinoma. (C) The extensive nature of the tumour at retrograde ureteropyelography.

Quality Control

Continuous audit of opacification is required to maintain the standard of CT urography from day to day. All users of CT urography should employ comparable scoring systems. In one such scoring system, the urinary tract is divided into four anatomical components (collecting system and renal pelvis; abdominal ureter; pelvic ureter; and bladder), and each is given a score of 0 (no opacification), 1 (partial opacification) or 2 (complete opacification). The bladder is scored slightly differently, with 0 representing no opacification, 1 is used for regions of interest within the bladder at less than 100 HU, and 2 corresponds to all regions of interest in the bladder over 100 HU. Only by using a similar scoring system across different centres will it be possible to accurately compare different CT urography techniques.[38]

Radiation Dose Optimisation Strategies

There has been much recent interest in radiation dose optimisation strategies.[41,42] There are many ways to reduce radiation exposure from CT while maintaining diagnostic accuracy. Such methods may be considered in three groups: reducing radiation exposure before the examination, during the examination and after the examination. The most effective way to reduce radiation exposure is to not perform the examination. Scrutiny of examination appropriateness is essential. Once the decision has been made to perform CT, there are many available strategies to reduce radiation exposure; these include the use of size-dependent protocols, automated tube current modulation, reduction of the number of passes, reduction in duplicate coverage, reduction of mAs and kVp where possible, optimisation of intravenous contrast medium administration and possible use of external shielding. Radiation exposure can also be reduced with better post-processing methods to decrease noise,

smoother kernels for reconstruction, reconstruction at larger slice thickness and iterative reconstruction.[43]

Diagnostic Accuracy of CT Urography for UTUC

Diagnosing UTUC ultimately depends on detection of small filling defects in the collecting system of the kidney and ureter (Figs. 14-1 and 14-2). Such tumours may be pedunculated or sessile, invasive or non-invasive, local or metastatic.[32]

The reasoning for using CT urography for the investigation of haematuria ultimately depends on the high diagnostic accuracy of the excretory phase series in identifying urothelial cancer. Other component image series, unenhanced and nephrographic, have high diagnostic accuracy for stones and renal masses, but by definition they do not provide CT urography. To justify its use in patients with haematuria, CT urography must be as good if not better, in terms of diagnostic accuracy and patient acceptability, than the alternative techniques for imaging UTUC. A number of studies have evaluated the accuracy of CT urography for UTUC.[30,44–49]

Although it is conceptually simple to design a study that compares two imaging techniques in the same patients, in practice it is very difficult to justify the increased radiation dose that such patients would receive. Studies using surrogate comparisons are now commonly reported, which require careful scrutiny to ensure that optimum CT urography is compared with optimal IVU to mimic genuine clinical practice. It is also important to ensure that there are a sufficient number of patients with UTUC in each clinical cohort for an assessment of diagnostic accuracy for UTUC to be meaningful.[50]

In 2010, Wang et al.[51] performed a retrospective study of adult patients with haematuria who underwent both CT urography and IVU over a 2.5-year period in a single institution; 19 of 60 patients had UTUC. The sensitivity,

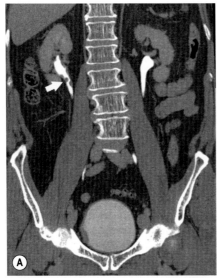

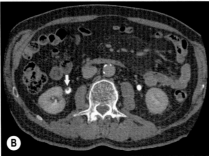

FIGURE 14-2 ■ **A 75-year-old man presenting with visible haematuria.** (A) A coronal reconstruction of a CT urogram demonstrating a multifocal filling defect in the upper right abdominal ureter. (B) An axial section through one of the filling defects. Following resection, the histopathological diagnosis was a multifocal grade 3 urothelial carcinoma.

specificity and accuracy of IVU were 0.750, 0.860 and 0.849, respectively, compared with 0.958, 1.000 and 0.996 using CT urography for UTUC. The authors concluded that CT urography should be the first-choice non-invasive imaging technique for diagnosing UTUC in patients with haematuria. A similar study was reported by Jinzaki et al. in 104 patients with haematuria, 46 of whom had UTUC.[49] Per-patient sensitivity, specificity and overall accuracy for the detection of UTUC with CT urography (93.5, 94.8 and 94.2%, respectively) were significantly greater than the corresponding values for excretory urography (80.4, 81.0 and 80.8%; $P = 0.041$, 0.027 and 0.001, respectively).[49] Although the designs of these studies are theoretically imperfect, the results suggest that the diagnostic accuracy of CT urography is greater than IVU for upper urinary tract disease, especially UTUC.

Several retrospective studies report on the diagnostic accuracy of CT urography for UTUC,[30,45–48] against the reference standard of histopathology, cytology and clinical follow-up. Despite the variation in CT urography technique, most report high sensitivities and specificities for UTUC. Many studies using a double bolus protocol give the majority of the contrast volume in the second

bolus, a move that is likely to reduce the opacification scoring of the upper tract in the excretory phase as much of the contrast agent will not have been excreted into the collecting systems and ureter at the time of image acquisition.

In 2007, Cowan et al. compared the diagnostic accuracy of CT urography and retrograde ureteropyelography for diagnosing UTUC.[44] The clinical cohort consisted of a selected group of 106 patients who presented with haematuria and initially underwent IVU and flexible cystoscopy. Patients with equivocal or positive IVU results and those with negative IVU and flexible cystoscopy results but with persistent haematuria were investigated with CT urography and retrograde ureteropyelography. The reference standard was histopathology from biopsy or resected specimens and 3–5-year clinical follow-up. The sensitivity, specificity, positive predictive value and negative predictive value of CT urography for diagnosing UTUC were 0.97, 0.93, 0.79 and 0.99, respectively. For retrograde ureteropyelography, the sensitivity, specificity, positive predictive value and negative predictive value were 0.96, 0.97, 0.87 and 0.97, respectively. Thus the diagnostic accuracy was similar for CT urography and retrograde ureteropyelography, which is an important result given that retrograde ureteropyelography is often regarded as the gold standard for imaging UTUC. The authors concluded that the quantitative evidence provided by the study validated the use of CT urography for diagnosing UTUC.[44]

Diagnostic Imaging Strategies for UTUC

Conventional diagnostic imaging pathways for haematuria—including ultrasound, IVU and CT urography—are complicated and lengthy. The principal aim of any new diagnostic strategy must be to simplify and shorten the time from presentation to diagnosis. The diagnostic accuracy of CT urography for urinary tract stones and solid renal masses surpasses that for ultrasound and IVU as described in the previous section. This means that CT urography has the potential to be a single replacement test for ultrasound and IVU. New evidence relating to the diagnostic accuracy of CT urography for diagnosis of UTUC suggests CT urography might also be the technique of choice for imaging the urothelium for suspected urothelial carcinoma.[44,47,49,51–53]

Whether all patients with haematuria should undergo CT urography, or whether there are subgoups of patients who are more likely to benefit from CT urography than others, remains under investigation. Some notable features of CT urography mean that it should be targeted towards a select patient population. These include the length of time required in the CT suite, the increased radiation dose compared to other CT studies, and the large bolus of intravenous contrast medium administered.

The ideal initial diagnostic imaging test should have high sensitivity and specificity for diseases at high prevalence in the test population. Deciding what constitutes a high prevalence is not just a clinical decision but also depends on economic and political factors. There is a 4.4–22 times greater prevalence for UTUC and a 1.8–5.1

greater prevalence for stones in a study using CT urography rather than US and/or IVU as the initial imaging investigation.[38,54-56] Although the populations cannot be exactly age matched in the three studies, the difference in prevalence is striking and is most likely to reflect that greater diagnostic accuracy of CT urography compared with ultrasound and IVU for investigating haematuria.

The prevalence of specific underlying diseases responsible for haematuria can be predicted with various risk factors. The two most readily identifiable risk factors that reflect the prevalence of urothelial carcinoma are the presence of visible or non-visible haematuria and increasing patient age. This knowledge can be used clinically for stratification into groups of patients at low risk and high risk for urothelial carcinoma.

The high-risk group consists of patients 50 years with visible haematuria and urinary tract infection excluded. UTUC is the most prevalent disease in this population, which justifies initial investigation with CT urography.

The low-risk group comprises patients >40 years with non-visible haematuria and those 50 years old with either non-visible or visible haematuria. The disease with the greatest prevalence in patients with non-visible haematuria under the age of 50 years is medical renal disease,[57] so renal tract ultrasound is recommended as the initial imaging test in these patients. Ultrasound can elucidate the presence, position and outline of the kidneys, cortical thickness, and the presence of large stones, large renal masses and hydronephrosis. Calculi represent the most common cause of haematuria in patients under the age of 50 years with visible haematuria and those older than 50 years of age with non-visible haematuria with urinary tract infection excluded. The prevalence of UTUC is very low in these patients. Given that unenhanced CT has the highest sensitivity for upper urinary tract stones, it is recommended as the initial imaging investigation in these patients. Unenhanced CT can detect small stones, hydronephrosis, hydroureter and some renal masses, upper tract urothelial cancers and bladder cancers.

For patients of any age in the low-risk group with persistent non-visible haematuria and normal imaging investigations, repeat imaging is only justified if there is a significant change in the risk score: for example, if urinary tract symptoms or visible haematuria are reported. The optimum diagnostic imaging strategy for patients at high risk for urothelial carcinoma consists of initial CT urography as a replacement for conventional upper tract imaging techniques[52] and as a triage test for bladder assessment. For patients at low risk of UTUC, ultrasound and unenhanced CT of the kidneys, ureters and bladder should be used instead.[20]

Problems and Solutions

The principal problems associated with CT urography for investigating haematuria are reader error, false-positive diagnoses and increased radiation dose. Other problems that are also important but are considered secondary issues include the length of time the patient is required to be in the CT room for the complete examination, availability of CT, cost compared with other imaging

TABLE 14-1 False-Positive Diagnoses for UTUC

1	Clot
2	Debris
3	Kink of the ureter (accentuated by respiration)
4	Fibroepithelial polyp
5	Injury to the ureter following passage of a stone, stent placement or ureteroscopy
6	Ureteritis cystica
7	Flow artefact following furosemide administration or layering effects
8	Unusual-looking papilla, a normal variant
9	Nephrogenic adenoma
10	Amyloid
11	Renal cell carcinoma
12	Lymphoma
13	Vascular impression
14	Inflammation, fibrosis

techniques, the need for special image-viewing hardware and software for optimum reporting, the diagnosis of unexpected extragenitourinary disease, the requirement for a quality assurance programme and the overutilisation of CT urography for inappropriate indications.

There are many ways to reduce reader error, but perhaps the best method of teaching radiologists to read CT urography is to introduce a formative teaching programme designed to simulate clinical reporting. Reader training, interpretation and certification has already been employed for CT colonography.[56,58] Various diagnostic accuracy studies have revealed that the positive predictive value of CT urography for UTUC is low, ranging from 0.50 to 0.82, which currently precludes the notion of referring patients for curative surgery as soon as they are diagnosed. A list of false-positive diagnoses is given in Table 14-1. Therefore, UTUC diagnosed with CT urography should be biopsied (by ureteroscopy or retrograde ureteropyelography), guided for histopathological confirmation of the diagnosis before proceeding to surgery.[59]

Overutilisation of high-technology imaging services such as multidetector CT, MR imaging and PET-CT is defined as performing imaging procedures that are unlikely to improve patient outcome.[60] Healthcare systems in which there is a fee-for-service payment process, self-referral practices and defensive medicine may be vulnerable to the overutilisation of imaging, which can be responsible for unnecessary healthcare costs and frequently exposes patients to unnecessary radiation. CT urography requires a higher dose of radiation than excretory urography, which can only be justified by its increased diagnostic accuracy in the correct clinical setting.[61] Individual patient radiation doses can be minimised by close attention to optimising image acquisition parameters and by using CT dose-reducing techniques.[62] The use of referral guidelines that incorporate appropriateness criteria based on objective clinical evidence and comparative effectiveness research makes an important contribution to reducing overutilisation. Further comparative effectiveness research of imaging technology is called for as a deterrent to overutilisation of medical imaging.

CONCLUSIONS AND SUMMARY

The principal indication for CT urography is the investigation of haematuria. Rapid developments in multi-detector CT technology make multiplanar review of isotropic data sets possible providing high-resolution CT urography studies. The high diagnostic accuracy of unenhanced CT for calculi, the nephrographic phase CT for renal masses and the excretory phase CT for urothelial cancer, compared with other techniques, makes CT urography the preferred initial imaging investigation for patients presenting with haematuria. To ensure maximum diagnostic accuracy, attention to detail of the CT urography technique is important. For patients at high risk for BCa and UTUC, CT urography should be used as a triage test before cystoscopy and as the initial imaging test for examination of the upper urinary tract. By careful attention to indications and technique, the radiation dose of CT urography can be optimised for those patients with haematuria who are at high risk of BCa and UTUC. Formative teaching programmes simulating clinical reporting are suggested as the preferred method of teaching radiologists to read CT urograms and to reduce reader error. As the positive predictive value of CT urography for UTUC is low, UTUC diagnosed with CT urography should be biopsied (by ureteroscopy or retrograde ureteropyelography) guided for histopathological confirmation of the diagnosis before proceeding to surgery.

In the future, MR imaging and dual-energy CT may have an important role in imaging UTUC. MR urography has some advantages over CT urography in that it does not use ionising radiation, but currently the spatial resolution of MR urography falls below CT urography, which is important when looking for small urothelial lesion in the upper urinary tract.[63–65] Dual-energy CT is currently being evaluated in clinical practice to determine its role in urinary tact imaging, and to address the issue of additional radiation exposure associated with dual-energy imaging.[66]

In conclusion, CT urography is recommended as the initial imaging test for patients presenting with haematuria who are at high risk of urothelial cancer, and specifically for imaging adult patients over 50 years of age presenting with visible haematuria, once infection is excluded.

BLADDER CANCER

INTRODUCTION

Bladder cancer is the fourth most common cancer in the developed world. The incidence of bladder cancer increases with increasing age. While genetic factors are also likely involved, bladder cancer is believed to develop in many individuals as a result of excretion of ingested carcinogens into the urine. Accordingly, there are a number of environmental risk factors for bladder cancer, the most substantial of which is smoking.[67] It has been estimated that cigarette smoking may be responsible for 50–60% of bladder cancers. Another 20% of bladder cancers are likely the result of occupational exposure (which result from working in the following areas: textiles or petrochemicals, bus/truck driving (due to diesel fumes), firefighting, hairdressing, plumbing and printing). There is also an increased risk of bladder cancer in patients who have been exposed to non-steroidal anti-inflammatory medication and to the chemotherapeutic agent cyclophosphamide. Primary bladder neoplasms are typically epithelial in origin, with urothelial cancer being the most common.

CLASSIFICATION OF UROTHELIAL CANCERS

By Growth Pattern

Urothelial cancers are generally divided into two major groups: those that are superficial (which do not invade the muscular layer of the bladder wall or the muscularis mucosa) and those that are invasive (which extend into the muscularis mucosa). Seventy to 80% of bladder tumours are superficial neoplasms, usually limited to the mucosa.[68] Superficial neoplasms are papillary neoplasms about 70% of the time. Papillary urothelial neoplasms are usually of low grade and have a good prognosis.[69] The remaining 30% of superficial urothelial tumours are flat neoplasms and are classified as carcinoma in situ. Flat tumours are typically of higher grade and are more likely to become invasive, if left untreated, with approximately 80% eventually progressing to invade the muscular layer of the bladder wall.[67] Some superficial tumours extend into the lamina propria. In general, superficial bladder tumours are treated topically by transuretheral resection (TURBT) and/or instillation of immunological (with bacille Calmette-Guérin (BCG)) or chemotherapeutic agents. Unfortunately, there is a 70% likelihood that any patient with a superficial bladder cancer will have a recurrence in the bladder within 3 years of presentation, with 10–20% of these recurrences being more aggressive.[68] About 20–30% of bladder neoplasms are muscle invasive at the time of presentation. Surgical resection (cystectomy) is required for cure of these patients.

By Histology

While most bladder cancers are composed entirely of transitional cells, a substantial minority (up to 40%) of urothelial cancers of the bladder, which were previously classified as transitional cell carcinomas, contain focal areas of atypical or divergent histology, with atypical features in addition to transitional cells, consisting of areas of poor differentiation, squamous cells, sarcomatoid cells, adenomatous cells and small cells.[70–72] Additional atypical histologies include clear cell, glandular cell, lymphoepithelial, micropapillary, plastmacytoid and neuroendocrine components.[70,73]

The presence of areas of atypical histology has been shown to affect patient prognosis poorly, as transitional cell tumours with divergent histology tend to behave more aggressively, both locally[71] and in terms of the likelihood of developing distant metastatic disease.[72] In a study by Shinagare et al., urothelial tumours containing areas of atypical histology were significantly more likely to spread to the peritoneum, with only 6 of 94 metastatic pure transitional cell cancers involving the peritoneum, in comparison to 18 of 56 neoplasms with divergent histology.[72]

Pure squamous cell carcinomas account for only 6–8% of all urothelial cancers.[74] These irritative cancers are more commonly encountered in areas where schistosomiasis is endemic or in patients with chronic urinary tract infections or bladder calculi. Bladder adenocarcinomas are even less common, being responsible for no more than 2% of all bladder cancers.[69,74] Squamous cell carcinomas and adenocarcinomas of the bladder will be discussed in more detail in later sections of this chapter.

By Grade

Grading of urothelial neoplasms is important, as it can affect treatment and predict patient outcome. According to the recent World Health Organisation classification,[75] papillary urothelial neoplasms are differentiated into four grades:

1. The lowest-grade superficial urothelial neoplasms are papillomas. These demonstrate normal nuclear size and shape, have no mitotic figures, and are generally considered to be benign.
2. Papillary urothelial neoplasms of low-malignant potential (PUNLMP) are of slightly higher grade. PUNLMP cells may have uniformly enlarged or elongated nuclei and rare mitotic figures. At the present time, some do not classify these neoplasms as benign or malignant.[76] PUNLMPs have an extremely low likelihood of recurrence and little to no risk of progression.[76]
3. Low-grade urothelial tumours contain cells that have some variation in nuclear shape and occasional mitoses.
4. High-grade urothelial tumours contain cells that demonstrate moderate variation in nuclear morphology and many mitoses.

CLINICAL DETECTION

The most common presentation of bladder cancer is painless haematuria, which may be macroscopic or microscopic.[77] This symptom is not specific, as it is frequently encountered in patients with cystitis and benign prostatic hyperplasia. In fact, most patients with haematuria do not have bladder cancer.[78] It is estimated that 12–20% of patients with macroscopic haematuria have bladder cancer,[78] while a much lower percentage of patients with microscopic haematuria have bladder cancer. Other less

common symptoms in patients with bladder cancer include dysuria, frequency and/or urgency.

While urine cytology may be positive in up to 90% of patients with carcinoma in situ, cytology is much less sensitive in patients with superficial papillary bladder cancers.[67] Thus, negative urine cytology cannot be utilised to rule out a diagnosis of bladder cancer definitively.

The gold standard for bladder cancer identification is cystoscopy, although, on occasion, some bladder neoplasms can be missed during this procedure. Initial cystoscopies can be performed as an outpatient office procedure using a flexible cystoscope. In the past, cystoscopy was performed using white light; however, some investigators have recently shown that fluorescent-light cystoscopy (performed after staining the bladder wall with fluorescent dyes) has higher sensitivity in detecting bladder cancer.[79]

IMAGING DETECTION

The ability of imaging studies to detect bladder cancer traditionally has been considered to be less important than their ability to detect upper tract urothelial cancers. This is because, as has already been mentioned, flexible cystoscopy is very sensitive and is an easily performed outpatient procedure. In comparison, upper tract evaluation by urologists requires ureteroscopy, a more involved procedure (usually performed under general anaesthesia). For this reason, the upper urinary tracts are frequently assessed with imaging studies.

Conventional excretory urography and cystography have long been known to have limited efficacy in detecting bladder cancers. In one study, only 60% of bladder cancers could be identified on excretory urograms.[78] With the recent emergence of CT urography and MR urography, however, imaging detection of bladder tumours has improved dramatically, with identification of even tiny urothelial bladder lesions now being possible.[53,81]

Technique of CT Urography and MR Urography

Both CT urography and MR urography are usually performed utilising thin-section reconstructed images obtained before and after the intravenous administration of iodinated (for CT) or gadolinium-based (for MRI) contrast media. At least one series of images is routinely obtained during the excretory phase of contrast material enhancement (which occurs 5–15 min after contrast material injection begins), at which time contrast material has usually been excreted into the renal collecting systems and ureters and has opacified the bladder. It has been generally accepted that sensitivity in detecting urothelial neoplasms on CT urography is maximised when excretory phase images are obtained.[81,82] This belief has recently been challenged in several studies,[83,84] where it has been observed that detection of upper and lower tract urothelial neoplasms is actually as good or greater when images are acquired 60 s after the initiation of the contrast media injection (during the corticomedullary phase of renal enhancement), at which time abnormally increased enhancement of even small urothelial neoplasms against a background of unopacified urine can be detected. The increased enhancement of urothelial cancers facilitates differentiation of these lesions from normally enhancing urothelium, urothelium that is thickened as a result of benign disease, or non-enhancing non-calcified filling defects within the urinary tract, such as blood clots, mucus, or fungus balls. In fact, it is most likely that the CT or MR urographic approach most sensitive for detecting bladder cancer is one where both early enhanced (corticomedullary phase) and delayed enhanced (excretory phase) series are obtained.

The above recommendations notwithstanding, a variety of contrast material injection techniques have been utilised for CT urography. Some investigators prefer a single bolus, with at least two series of contrast-enhanced images obtained (at least one during the corticomedullary and/or nephrographic phases, with the latter usually beginning 100 s after the initiation of the contrast material injection, and another during the excretory phase of contrast material enhancement). Some also obtain an additional enhanced series during the arterial phase. Another widely used technique is split-bolus injection, with each of two boluses administered separately, usually at least 5–10 min apart, before obtaining any contrast material-enhanced images.[85] Image acquisition of a single contrast-enhanced series is then performed at a time when the first bolus has been excreted into the renal collecting systems, ureters and bladder, while the second bolus is still opacifying the renal parenchyma and the bladder wall. Gadolinium-based contrast material injection during MR urography is generally performed as a single bolus, with multiple series of post-injection images obtained (often including the corticomedullary, nephrographic and excretory phase phases).

A variety of ancillary manoeuvres have been recommended to optimise urinary tract distension and opacification during CT and MR urography, including oral and/or intravenous hydration and administration of a diuretic.[82] Additionally, some experts have advocated that patients be physically moved between contrast material administration and excretory phase image acquisition, to ensure uniform mixing of any excreted contrast material in the bladder (by having them roll over on the CT table and/or even get off the CT table and walk around the room).[86] To date, no protocol has been universally accepted, nor has the ability of individual manoeuvres to detect a greater number of urinary tract cancers been demonstrated.

It is essential that CT or MR urographic images are reconstructed in at least two planes (most often in the axial and coronal planes). This reduces the likelihood that bladder tumours will be missed due to volume averaging with extravesical structures (particularly at the bladder dome and bladder base).[87] Additionally, CT or MR urographic images that are obtained after excretion of high attenuation contrast material into the urinary tract, including the bladder, must be reviewed using wide-windowing. If this is not done, small lesions can be obscured by high attenuation or high-signal-intensity

excreted contrast material in the adjacent bladder lumen.

Some investigators have performed virtual CT cystoscopy, with air or carbon dioxide instilled actively into the bladder via an inserted Foley catheter,[87–89] and have suggested that this may be the most sensitive imaging technique for bladder cancer detection. In one series, virtual CT cystoscopy detected 32 of 35 bladder cancers. The only missed lesions were two polypoid lesions that measured < 5 mm in size and one sessile lesion that measured < 1 cm in size.[87] Overall, this more invasive technique is felt to be unnecessary by most experts, however, as it is not believed to improve detection rates to a sufficient enough degree to warrant its routine performance.

CT and MR Urographic Appearance of Bladder Cancers

On CT and MR urography, bladder cancers have a variety of appearances. They can produce characteristic areas of focal asymmetric bladder wall thickening (Fig. 14-3), focal mass-like areas projecting into the bladder lumen (Fig. 14-4), or tiny round or frond-like filling defects (Figs. 14-5 and 14-6). Since bladder cancers are frequently multiple, it is important to assess an abnormal bladder and the upper tracts for additional focal lesions[90] (Fig. 14-7). While diffuse circumferential symmetric bladder wall thickening is most often seen in patients with cystitis, neurogenic bladders, or in cases of bladder

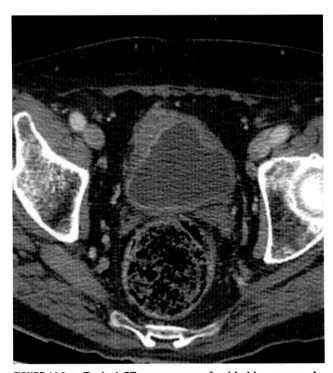

FIGURE 14-3 ■ **Typical CT appearance of a bladder cancer.** An early contrast-enhanced CT image through the pelvis, obtained before excretion of contrast material into the bladder, demonstrates a large irregularly lobulated mass along the anterior aspect of the bladder, with the thickening most pronounced on the right.

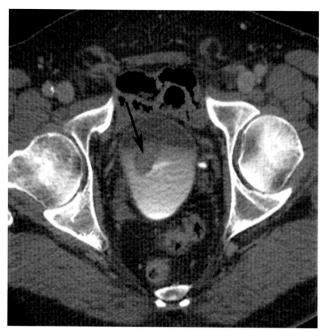

FIGURE 14-4 ▪ **Bladder cancer producing a focal mass projecting into the bladder lumen.** An excretory phase CT urographic image demonstrates an ovoid soft-tissue mass projecting into the bladder lumen from the bladder dome (arrow). As the patient remained supine throughout the study, the denser excreted contrast material has layered posteriorly in the bladder, with a fluid–fluid level present between it and the less dense unopacified urine.

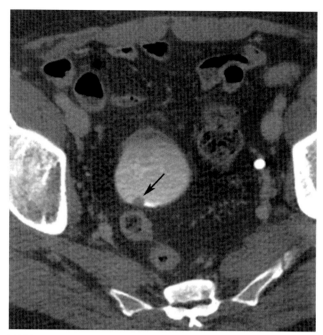

FIGURE 14-5 ▪ **CT of a papillary bladder cancer producing a tiny filling defect.** A small round soft-tissue mass is noted in the right posterolateral aspect of the bladder on this excretory phase contrast-enhanced CT urographic image (arrow).

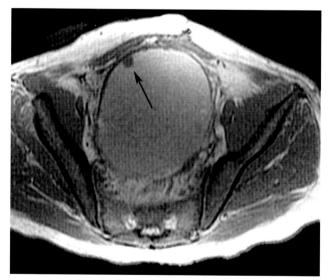

FIGURE 14-6 ▪ **MRI of a papillary bladder cancer producing a tiny filling defect.** A tiny round soft-tissue mass is noted along the right anterior bladder wall (arrow) on this T2-weighted axial MR image.

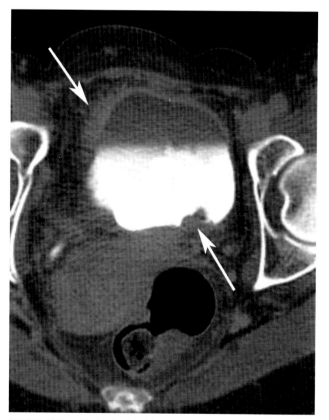

FIGURE 14-7 ▪ **Multiple bladder cancers.** An axial excretory phase CT urographic image demonstrates two bladder cancers in this patient (arrows), one producing irregular thickening along the right anterolateral bladder wall and the other appearing as a small mass projecting into the bladder lumen on the left, posteriorly.

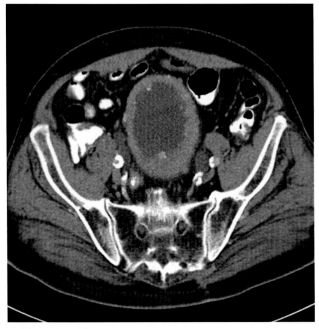

FIGURE 14-8 ■ **Infiltrative bladder cancer.** An excretory phase CT urographic image demonstrates pronounced circumferential bladder wall. Urothelial cancer was diagnosed at subsequent cystoscopic examination.

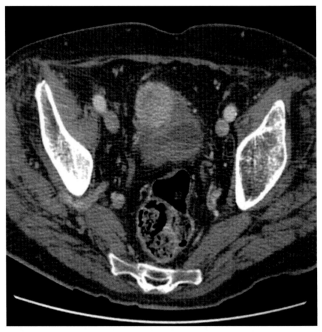

FIGURE 14-9 ■ **Enhancing urothelial cancer.** A contrast-enhanced CT image obtained through the pelvis at 70 s following the initiation of the contrast material injection demonstrates a large briskly enhancing ovoid urothelial neoplasm along the right anterolateral aspect of the bladder (arrow).

outlet obstruction, this appearance can occasionally be seen in patients with infiltrative bladder cancers[91] (Fig. 14-8).

On CT, bladder cancers have the same excretory phase attenuation as the bladder wall; however, as already mentioned, many bladder cancers demonstrate increased contrast enhancement on images obtained during the corticomedullary phase, with peak enhancement encountered at about 60 s.[83] This feature can assist in bladder cancer detection on multiphase or split-bolus CT[84,92] (Fig. 14-9). In one study, the bladder cancer detection rate on CT images obtained 60 s after initiation of contrast material injection was 97%.[81] Calcification can be identified in about 5% of bladder cancers[69] (Fig. 14-10).

On MRI, bladder cancers have soft-tissue signal intensity on T1- and T2-weighted images. On T1-weighted images this signal intensity is similar to that of the normal bladder wall; however, on T2-weighted images tumour signal intensity is intermediate between that of the very high-signal urine in the bladder lumen and the low-signal-intensity normal bladder wall.[79,93] Bladder cancers usually demonstrate brisk enhancement after gadolinium-based contrast material administration[65] (Fig. 14-11).

Diffusion-weighted MR imaging (DWI), which is based upon the detection of differences in the diffusion of water molecules in different tissues, has recently shown promise in the evaluation of patients with suspected or known bladder cancer. Studies have shown that DWI sequences can differentiate normal from abnormal urothelium, as well as benign from malignant urothelial abnormalities.[94-96] For example, in one study of 130

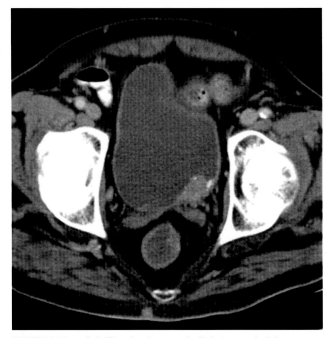

FIGURE 14-10 ■ **Calcification in a urothelial cancer.** Axial contrast-enhanced CT image through the pelvis demonstrates a urothelial cancer along the left posterior aspect of the bladder. There are tiny areas of calcification along the anterior and lateral surfaces of the cancer. Calcifications may be seen on ultrasound or CT in up to 5% of bladder cancers.

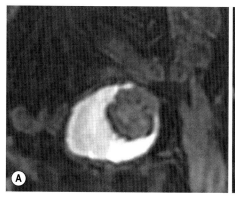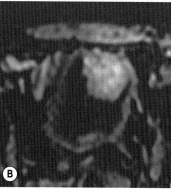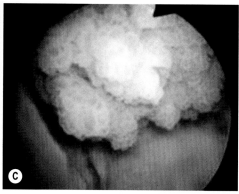

FIGURE 14-11 ■ **MRI of a papillary urothelial neoplasm.** (A) A large irregular mass along the left superior aspect of the bladder is outlined by high-signal-intensity urine on the unenhanced T2-weighted coronal MR image. (B) After administration of gadolinium-based contrast material, the mass demonstrates enhancement to a greater extent than the remainder of the bladder wall, as can be seen on this T1-weighted fat-suppressed axial image. (C) The large frond-like projections from the mass, indicating its papillary nature, are easily seen on a subsequently obtained cystoscopic image.

patients with gross haematuria,[94] DWI led to the detection of 104 of 106 (98% of) bladder cancers. In another investigation,[97] DWI images were obtained in 46 patients with malignant bladder lesions, 17 patients with benign bladder abnormalities and 20 patients with no bladder abnormalities. The apparent diffusion coefficient (ADC) values for normal bladder walls, benign bladder lesions and bladder malignancies were all different from one another. Most impressively, reviewers were able to detect all 46 bladder cancers by identifying restricted diffusion in these lesions (100% sensitivity and 100% negative predictive value). DWI may also be able to differentiate more aggressive from less aggressive tumours. Several studies have demonstrated that the ADC values in higher-stage and high-grade cancers are typically significantly lower than in those with lower-stage or low-grade cancers, although there is overlap.[96,97]

Sensitivity and Specificity of CT and MR Urography in Detecting Bladder Cancers

The reported sensitivity of CT urography in detecting bladder cancer has varied, depending upon the series,[46,73,98,99] but is clearly superior to that of excretory urography, with sensitivities in three studies ranging from 79%,[82] to 85%[100] to over 95%.[101] There is a paucity of data on the sensitivity of MR urography in detecting bladder cancers; however, MRI may be similarly sensitive. Studies indicate that occasional false-negative diagnoses with both CT and MR urography are to be expected (Fig. 14-12). Bladder cancers more likely to go undetected on both CT and MR urographic studies include flat lesions (carcinoma in situ),[101] small lesions (under 1 cm in maximal diameter),[79,87,101] and lesions at the bladder base (Fig. 14-13), where volume averaging with adjacent structures, including the prostate and perineum, can be a problem.

Since some bladder cancers can be missed by both CT and MR urography, a normal CT or MR urogram cannot exclude the diagnosis, and further assessment of patients

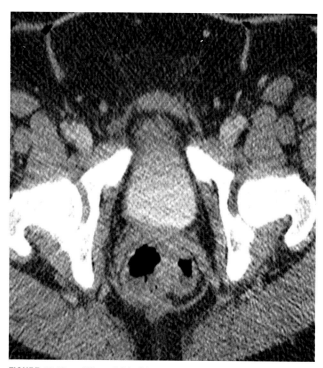

FIGURE 14-12 ■ **Missed bladder cancer on CT urography.** This axial excretory phase image from a CT urogram was interpreted as normal. At subsequent cystoscopy, a large urothelial cancer was identified along the right posterior bladder wall at this level.

at high risk for having bladder cancer (with risk factors being persistent haematuria, or a prior history of bladder cancer) with flexible cystoscopy is warranted.[101] However, when a possible bladder cancer is detected by CT or MR urography prior to flexible cystoscopy, a patient can be spared this procedure and can proceed directly to the more invasive rigid cystoscopy with biopsy and transurethral resection, as needed.[77] Unlike flexible cystoscopy, rigid cystoscopy is usually performed in an operative suite using general anaesthesia. This approach has been confirmed to be appropriate in a recent study that evaluated the use of CT urography in over 700 patients.[53]

Few studies have evaluated the positive predictive value of findings in the bladder. However, experience allows for several observations to be made concerning CT or MRI. Although most focal bladder abnormalities represent bladder cancers, benign bladder lesions can

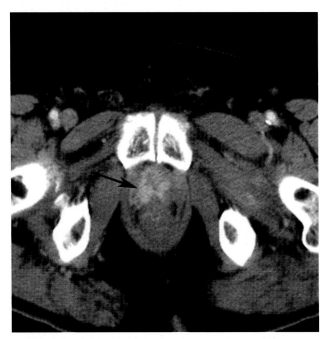

FIGURE 14-13 ■ Early enhanced axial CT image obtained at the bladder base demonstrates a small area of abnormal enhancement at the bladder base just posterior to the right symphysis pubis (arrow). This lesion could be easily missed at CT, particularly if only delayed-enhanced excretory phase images had been obtained, since its enhancement would no longer be evident. An invasive high-grade papillary bladder cancer was diagnosed subsequently at cystoscopy.

sometimes be focal and mimic bladder carcinomas. This includes benign neoplasms, such as papillomas and leiomyomas, as well as occasionally encountered focal bladder wall changes due to cystitis (Figs. 14-14 and 14-15). As previously mentioned, diffuse circumferential bladder wall thickening usually does not represent bladder cancer.

Risks of CT and MR Urography

One of the major risks of CT urography is the radiation dose, which generally exceeds that of excretory urography by a factor of at least 1.5.[77] Recently, dose reduction reconstruction algorithms (i.e. iterative reconstruction techniques) have been adopted, which may result in substantially decreased patient exposure in the near future. While MRI does not expose the patient to the potential risks of ionising radiation, properly performed CT and MR urographic studies each expose patients to contrast media. The iodinated contrast media used for CT can be nephrotoxic when administered to patients with pre-existing chronic renal disease (known as chronic kidney disease in the USA) or acute kidney injury. The gadolinium-based contrast material used for MRI must be administered with caution in patients with severe chronic renal failure (eGFR < 30 mL/min/1.73 m²) or acute kidney injury, due to the risks of nephrogenic systemic fibrosis (risks that are known to exist predominantly following administration of three specific MR contrast agents: gadodiamide, gadoversetamide and gadopentetate dimeglumine.

Use of Positron Emission Tomography for Detecting and Evaluating Bladder Cancers

Positron emission tomography (PET) with 18-fluorodeoxyglucose (FDG) may be used to detect bladder

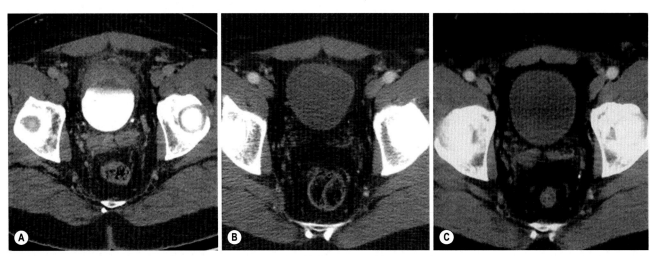

FIGURE 14-14 ■ **Focal bladder wall thickening due to cystitis.** This 47-year-old man developed urgency, frequency and microscopic haematuria. (A) An axial excretory phase image from a CT urogram shows pronounced asymmetric thickening along the anterior aspect of the bladder. Cystoscopy was performed and biopsies were obtained. Pathology revealed eosinophilic cystitis. The patient was placed on high-dose steroids. (B) An axial early enhanced CT image obtained 1 month later demonstrates only mild persistent bladder wall thickening. (C) An axial early enhanced CT image obtained 3 months after initial presentation demonstrates that the bladder wall thickening has resolved completely.

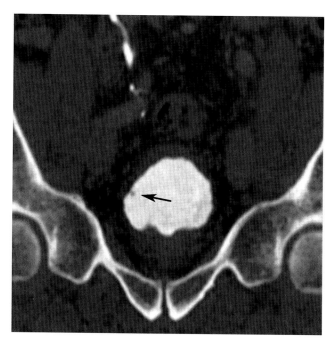

FIGURE 14-15 ▪ **Small filling defect due to cystitis.** A coronal excretory phase CT urographic image demonstrates moderate diffuse circumferential wall thickening. There is a tiny (3 mm) filling defect along the right superolateral aspect of the bladder lumen (arrow). This was felt to be suspicious for a small papillary urothelial neoplasm on this study, as well as during subsequent cystoscopy. A transurethral resection was performed with the final pathology revealing polypoid cystitis.

cancers, as well as to assess the degree of bladder cancer aggressiveness; however, the efficacy of PET is limited by the fact that FDG is normally excreted in the urine, a feature that can obscure measurements of bladder wall lesion standard uptake values (SUVs).[96] Some researchers have evaluated the roles of other more recently developed radiotracers that are not excreted into the bladder,[79] such as carbon-11-acetate, carbon-11-methionine, and carbon-11-choline;[93,102] however, preliminary studies have failed to demonstrate a consistent benefit of these new agents in comparison to FDG.[102] False-positive PET/CT cases have been encountered with all of the above radiotracers, with some due to the presence of granulomatous cystitis (as a result of prior BCG treatment).[79] Therefore, the utility of PET/CT in detecting bladder cancer has yet to be determined.[93]

STAGING

Bladder cancer is staged using the tumour–nodes–metastasis (TNM) system, with Ta tumours representing papillary neoplasms located only in the urothelium, Tis tumours representing flat tumours or carcinomas in situ that are non-invasive, T1 tumours invading the lamina propria, T2 tumours invading the muscularis mucosa (either superficially T2a or deeply T2b), T3 tumours spreading into the perivesical space (either microscopically T3a or grossly T3b), and T4 tumours invading the

TABLE 14-2 Staging of Bladder Cancer

Tx	Primary tumour cannot be assessed
T0	No evidence of residual primary tumour
Ta	Superficial (non-invasive) papillary carcinoma
Tis	Superficial flat tumour (carcinoma in situ)
T1	Invasion of subepithelial connective tissue (lamina propria)
T2a	Superficial invasion of muscularis mucosa (into inner half)
T2b	Deep invasion of muscularis mucosa (into outer half)
T3a	Microscopic pervesical spread
T3b	Macroscopic perivesical spread
T4a	Invasion of adjacent organs (prostate, seminal vesicles, uterus or vagina)
T4b	Invasion of pelvic sidewall or abdominal wall
Nx	Regional lymph nodes not assessed
N0	No lymph node involvement
N1	One affected lymph node in the true pelvis
N2	More than one affected true pelvic lymph node in the true pelvis
N3	Common iliac lymph node (or more central) involvement
Mx	Distant metastasis cannot be assessed
M0	No distant metastases
M1	Distant metastases

From <http://www.cancer.org/Cancer/BladderCancer/DetailedGuide/bladder-cancer-staging>.

adjacent organs or the pelvic sidewall. The TNM staging system is provided in detail in Table 14-2.

Imaging for Local Staging of Bladder Cancer

Cross-sectional imaging studies have limited accuracy for local staging of bladder cancer.[77] This is a particular problem when patients are imaged shortly after transurethral resection, since the perivesical tissue that may be present can be neoplastic or reactive/inflammatory (Fig. 14-14). Several studies have demonstrated that CT and MRI staging accuracy is highest when patients are imaged when the bladder is distended with fluid or air and also when groups of patients with similarly treated but differing stages of tumours are grouped together (such as might be done by combining patients with T2a, T2b and T3a tumours into one group, for example).[74]

Reported CT staging accuracy has generally been low, in some studies ranging from 40 to 60%,[69,73,74] with both overstaging and understaging being frequent problems.[93] In general, bladder cancers that produce pronounced bladder wall thickening on CT are likely to be at least stage T2 tumours (Fig. 14-16); however, it is not possible to determine depth of muscle invasion to allow distinction between stage T2a and T2b tumours.[93] It has also been suggested that most bladder tumours that produce an irregular outer bladder margin are more likely to have spread macroscopically into the perivesical fat (stage T3b); however, there is overlap.

MRI local staging accuracy has been higher than that of CT in a number of series, with accuracies of 73–96% reported.[77,93] Several researchers have found that MRI can often distinguish non-invasive from invasive bladder cancers, since the low signal intensity of the bladder wall

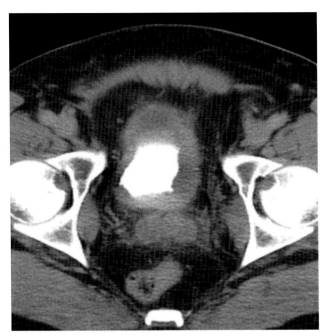

FIGURE 14-16 ■ **Perivesical stranding in a patient with bladder cancer.** This elderly patient has nearly circumferential bladder wall thickening, which is most pronounced on the left side, on this axial unenhanced CT image. Additionally, there is increased linear tissue in the perivesical space, which could represent oedema or tumour. This was subsequently determined to be high-grade muscle invasive papillary urothelial cancer containing signet ring, plasmacytoid and glandular components, which was fixed to the pelvic wall (T4 disease). In this case, the perivesical tissue represented infiltrative tumour.

is preserved adjacent to non-invasive bladder tumours, but disrupted adjacent to invasive bladder tumours on T2-weighted images[74] (Fig. 14-17). Use of this feature is not completely reliable, however. In one recent study evaluating the accuracy of MRI in staging bladder cancers, 12 of 55 patients with superficial bladder cancer were overstaged as having T2 disease.[103] This is an important error, as such overstaging would have changed treatment from local management with organ preservation to cystectomy. A few studies have shown that use of DWI improves staging accuracy,[104,105] but there are still problems.[69] Specifically, DWI has limited ability to determine the depth of muscularis mucosal invasion (if such invasion is present), and DWI cannot assess whether there is perivesical spread of tumour, when such spread is not extensive.[74,76]

On some occasions, other ancillary findings can be identified on CT or MRI that assist appropriate bladder cancer staging and/or predict patient prognosis. Identification of preoperative pelvocaliectasis and ureterectasis is associated with more aggressive disease, predicating higher-stage (T3) tumours, lymphovascular invasion, higher-grade tumours and poor prognosis.[106,107] In addition, when perivesical spread of tumour is extensive, stage T3b or T4 disease often can be appropriately identified (Fig. 14-18).

Imaging for Detection of Regional and Distant Metastatic Disease

Bladder cancer most frequently metastasises distantly first to pelvic and retroperitoneal lymph nodes. In one

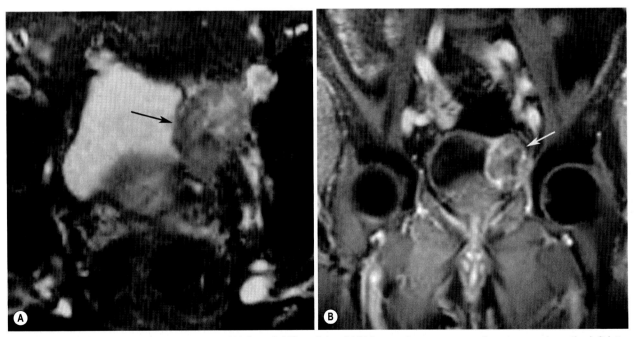

FIGURE 14-17 ■ **Muscle invasive bladder cancer.** (A) An axial T2-weighted MR image demonstrates a large mass along the left lateral aspect of the bladder (arrow). The low signal intensity of the bladder wall is disrupted along the periphery of the mass, while it can be seen surrounding the high-signal-intensity urine in the remainder of the bladder. This disruption is strongly suggestive of muscularis mucosa invasion. (B) The coronal gadolinium-based contrast material-enhanced T1-weighted image obtained with fat suppression demonstrates the mass, which is located along the left superolateral aspect of the bladder to be heterogeneously enhancing (arrow). The midline mass at the bladder base represents prostatic enlargement due to benign prostatic hyperplasia.

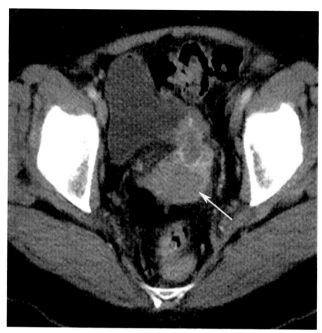

FIGURE 14-18 ■ **Stage T4 urothelial cancer.** Axial early enhanced CT image through the pelvis demonstrate a heterogeneous mass along the left posterolateral aspect of the bladder. The mass can be seen to extend directly into an enlarged fibroid uterus (arrow), indicating gross local organ invasion and T4 disease.

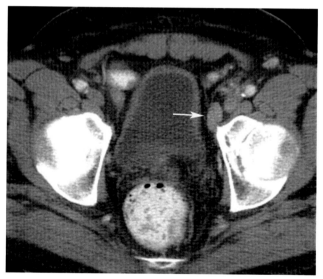

FIGURE 14-19 ■ **Lymph node metastases from bladder cancer.** An early enhanced axial CT image through the pelvis shows a mildly enlarged metastatic lymph node in the left external iliac region (arrow).

recent study 69% of detected distant metastases were to lymph nodes[72] (Fig. 14-19). On cross-sectional imaging studies, lymph node metastases from bladder cancer are generally detected only when they produce lymph node enlargement, with lymph nodes considered enlarged once they exceed 8–10 mm in maximal short-axis diameter.[108] Unfortunately, in many cases, bladder cancers spread to lymph nodes without producing any detectable

enlargement. Thus, lymph node metastases in normal-sized lymph nodes will frequently be missed by both CT and MRI. There has been a large variation in the reported accuracy of relying upon size criteria to identify lymph node metastases, with a reported range in sensitivity of 24 to 78%.[108] As can be seen, sensitivity in detecting bladder cancer lymph node metastases is limited, even in those studies that show the highest sensitivities.

It has been suggested that FDG-PET/CT or C-11 acetate, choline, or methionine PET/CT might have greater accuracy in detecting lymph node metastases from bladder cancer, since PET/CT might be able to identify abnormal activity in normal-sized lymph nodes. While some studies have demonstrated the ability of FDG-PET to detect metastatic disease in occasional patients in whom other preoperative evaluations have been negative (Fig. 14-20),[109] other series evaluating the utility of FDG-PET/CT for this purpose have had disappointing results. In one study, 13 of 51 patients with bladder cancer had metastatic lymph nodes identified at surgery; however, lymph node metastases had been identified on preoperative PET/CT in only 6 of these 13 patients (46%).[110] There was also one false-positive result. In this study, the accuracy of FDG-PET/CT, which was likely still limited by the very small size of many of the metastatic lymph nodes, was not significantly different from that of CT alone, leading the authors to conclude that there is no advantage of FDG-PET/CT for detecting lymph node metastases, at least with currently available techniques. To date, preliminary studies with carbon-11-acetate, carbon-11 choline and carbon-11-methionine PET/CT have also been disappointing.[79,93,102]

Other distant metastatic disease from bladder cancer (aside from metastases to lymph nodes) usually develops late in the course of the disease. Additional sites of distant metastatic disease are often detected with CT, MRI and/or nuclear scintigraphy, with distant metastases to sites other than lymph nodes encountered most commonly in the lungs, bones (with bone metastases being either lytic or sclerotic) (Fig. 14-21), brain, liver (Fig. 14-22) and peritoneum. Compared with its limited utility in detecting lymph node metastases, PET/CT may be more effective in this setting[111] (Fig. 14-23). Still, both false-positive and false-negative PET/CT results have been encountered.[112,113]

UPPER TRACT EVALUATION

A small percentage of patients with bladder cancer will also have synchronous upper tract urothelial neoplasms. For this reason, many urologists routinely evaluate the upper tracts prior to rigid cystoscopy, so that they can determine whether or not ureteroscopy is also needed. Upper tract imaging evaluation is now most commonly performed with CT urography, although MR urography can be obtained as an alternative, particularly in patients who have had prior reactions to iodinated contrast material or in whom radiation exposure is a concern. If an upper tract abnormality is identified on CT or MR urography, the patient can then undergo ureteroscopy at the time of rigid cystoscopy.

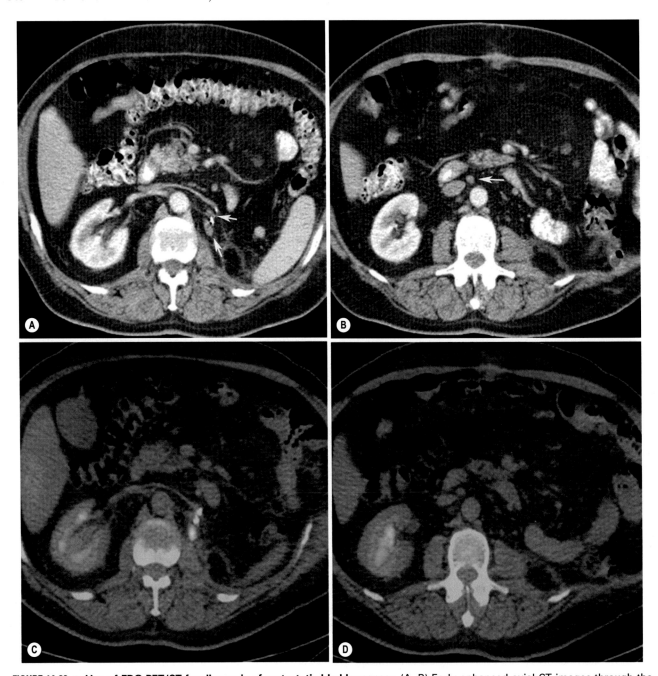

FIGURE 14-20 ■ **Use of FDG-PET/CT for diagnosis of metastatic bladder cancer.** (A, B) Early enhanced axial CT images through the mid abdomen were obtained in this patient with bladder cancer who had a prior nephrectomy for an upper tract neoplasm. (A) Two small normal-sized lymph nodes are noted in the left para-aortic region (arrows). (B) There is also a normal-sized aortocaval lymph node on the second image (arrow). Subsequently, an 18-fluorodeoxyglucose positron emission tomography–computed tomographic image was obtained. Fusion images reveal that (C) lymph nodes in the left para-aortic region have brisk radiotracer uptake, consistent with metastases. In comparison, the aortocaval lymph node (D) does not demonstrate increased uptake. This was a reactive lymph node.

On imaging studies, upper tract neoplasms have a similar appearance to bladder cancers. They produce focal mural thickening, circumferential mural thickening, or large or small filling defects. Several recent studies have analysed the positive predictive value of different upper tract findings on CT urography. In one report, 29 of 35 masses 5 mm or larger in diameter, were urothelial cancers, while none of 17 masses smaller than 5 mm were neoplasms.[114] In comparison, urothelial thickening was due to malignancy in just under half of cases (11 of 24 studies). In another study, which included 21 patients with 38 upper tract urothelial tumours, upper tract findings were divided into those seen in the proximal collecting systems and those seen in the ureters.[115] Urothelial thickening nearly always represented neoplasms in the proximal renal collecting systems, but this was the case only one-third of the time in the ureters. Conversely, filling defects in the ureters usually represented urothelial

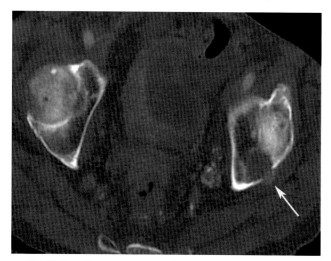

FIGURE 14-21 ■ **Bone metastasis from bladder cancer.** An axial early enhanced image through the pelvis, viewed utilising wide windows, demonstrates a large area of asymmetric bladder wall thickening on the right, corresponding to a large muscle invasive bladder cancer. There is also an ovoid lytic lesion in the posterior aspect of the left ischium (arrow), which was subsequently confirmed to represent a metastasis.

neoplasms, but were neoplastic in only 50% of the proximal renal collecting systems in which they were found. Additional discussion of upper tract urothelial imaging has been provided earlier in this chapter.

TREATMENT AND FOLLOW-UP

Urothelial neoplasms of all grades are usually treated, even papillomas and PUNLMPs. This is because even benign and low-grade lesions can produce symptoms (most commonly haematuria) and definitive diagnosis must be made pathologically. Superficial low- and high-grade bladder cancers are generally treated by transurethral resection, often followed by topical treatment with BCG or other agents. Although initial local treatment response to superficial bladder tumours is generally excellent, with 70 to 80% of patients responding, about 70% of patients with non-muscle invasive bladder cancer develop new bladder neoplasms within a few years of treatment, a minority of which will be muscle invasive at the time of detection.[68] This is why patients with non-muscle invasive bladder cancer must be followed closely after initial therapy.

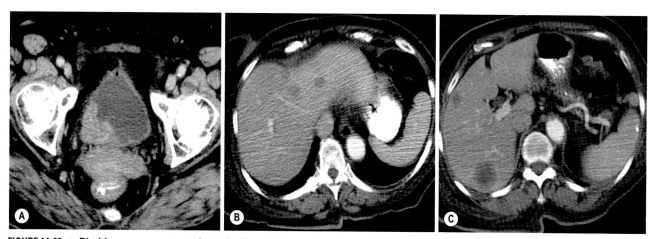

FIGURE 14-22 ■ **Bladder cancer metastatis to the liver.** (A) An early enhanced axial image through the pelvis demonstrates a lobulated mass along the right posterior aspect of the bladder, corresponding to a large muscle invasive bladder cancer. (B, C) Images through the liver demonstrate multiple solid low-attenuation masses, which were subsequently confirmed (by biopsy) to represent metastases.

FIGURE 14-23 ■ **Use of FDG-PET to evaluate patients for metastatic disease.** (A) An early enhanced axial image through the upper abdomen of a patient with newly diagnosed bladder cancer shows a large heterogeneous centrally located liver mass. (B) A fusion image obtained during a subsequent FDG-PET/CT examination fails to demonstrate any increased uptake. This lesion was a haemangioma.

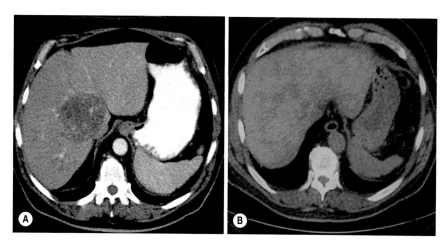

Treatment of muscle invasive bladder cancers is typically radical cystectomy, with bladder removal, pelvic lymph node dissection and creation of a urinary neobladder. Neobladders typically consist of a segment of detubularised ileum, which serves as a reservoir for urine and which is connected to an isolated tubularised ileal afferent limb. The afferent limb is anastomosed proximally to the ureters. The distal portion of the reservoir is anastomosed to the urethra. This surgery is preferred, because most patients who have it remain continent and do not need to have a stoma created on the anterior abdominal wall. In patients in whom less extensive surgery is preferable (such as the elderly or other patients with significant comorbidities who may not be able to tolerate a complex surgical procedure), an ileal loop urinary diversion is performed, with the ureters anastomosed to an isolated loop of ileum, which then exits the anterior abdominal wall, usually in the right lower quadrant, at an ostomy site. This is not a continent diversion, and a drainage bag must be attached to the ostomy site at all times. Less commonly, some urologists perform cutaneous continent diversions, whereby the ureters are anastomosed to a reservoir created from right colon and/or ileum (Kock or Indiana pouches), which is then connected to the anterior abdominal wall at a continent catheterisable stoma site.

Unfortunately, some patients present for treatment after their tumours have spread outside of the bladder, a point at which cystectomy will not be curative. About 25% of bladder cancer patients have positive lymph nodes at the time of cystectomy. Once bladder cancers have spread to lymph nodes (>N0 disease), patient prognosis is much worse. Five-year survival is between 40 and 80% for patients with N0 disease, but decreases to only 20 to 25% once any lymph nodes are involved (N1, N2 or N3 disease). In these patients, chemotherapy and/or radiotherapy will be needed, either before, following, or instead of cystectomy (depending upon the time when the extravesical spread has been detected, as well as the extent of the metastatic disease).

Clinical and Imaging Follow-up of Patients after Topical Treatment of Bladder Cancer

It is crucial that patients be monitored closely after topical treatment of non-invasive bladder cancers. Such follow-up is generally performed with regular urinalysis, urine cytology and cystoscopy. Periodic upper tract imaging is also recommended (every 1–2 years for the remainder of a patient's life), as a small minority of patients will eventually develop upper tract tumours.[116] As a result, urothelial cancer has been determined to be the most expensive cancer to treat and follow from the time of diagnosis, because many patients live for years after initial presentation, during which time regular monitoring and periodic treatment of any recurrences that develop must be performed.[117]

Imaging evaluation of topically treated bladders can be problematic, since scarring and/or wall thickening may develop in areas where there has been a prior transurethral resection. Additionally, some patients develop

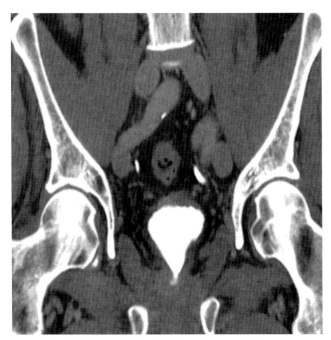

FIGURE 14-24 ■ Diffuse bladder wall thickening following topical treatment of bladder cancer. A coronally reconstructed excretory phase CT urographic image was obtained in this patient who has been treated for a bladder cancer, with transurethral resection and bacille Calmette-Guérin. There is moderate diffuse bladder wall thickening. It is difficult to determine whether any component of this thickening could be due to recurrent tumour. Although no recurrent neoplasm was detected during subsequent cystoscopic examination, cystoscopic distinction of inflammation/scarring from tumour can also be difficult.

reactions to BCG, which can produce irregular bladder wall thickening.[118] In one study, complications of BCG therapy were identified in 3% of topically treated patients, with some of these being visible on imaging studies, the most common of which was bladder wall thickening with areas of focal nodularity (in 11 of 16 affected patients).[118] In such a setting it can be difficult to determine whether subsequently detected bladder abnormalities are due to post-treatment change, recurrent tumour, or a combination of both (Fig. 14-24).

Imaging of Patients Following Neoadjuvant Chemoradiation and before Surgery

In recent years, neoadjuvant chemotherapy and/or radiation therapy has been performed in some patients before cystectomy in order to reduce the operative tumour burden and to potentially make initially locally unresectable neoplasms resectable. Imaging can be performed to follow patients undergoing such preoperative protocols in order to determine whether there has been a successful tumour response. While it is not yet clear how effective such follow-up imaging can be, preliminary studies have demonstrated that some techniques may be able to predict tumour responses to treatment. In one study, diffusion-weighted MR imaging was able to predict a complete response to chemoradiation in 13 of 20 patients with stages T2–T4a bladder cancer.[105]

Imaging Follow-up of Patients after Cystectomy

Approximately 6% of patients develop locally recurrent disease after cystectomy for bladder cancer, with the mean time to recurrence being about 7–8 months.[119,120] Patient survival after a recurrence develops is generally poor, underscoring the importance of optimal initial treatment.[119] In addition, 1–9% of patients develop upper tract tumours after cystectomy.[120] In one study, the incidence of metachronous upper tract urothelial tumours was 4% at 3 years and 7% at 5 years.[121]

A variety of imaging tests are obtained to evaluate patients for recurrent and metastatic disease after cystectomy, including chest X-rays, chest CTs, abdominal and pelvic CTs (standard abdominal pelvic CT or CT urography) and MRI examinations. At the present time, evidence that careful patient surveillance for metastatic disease after cystectomy improves patient survival is limited. In one study, for example, 2-year survival was 10% in asymptomatic patients undergoing routine imaging follow-up, as opposed to 8% in patients who were evaluated only when they became symptomatic.[122]

Thus, to date, there is no consensus of opinion among urological oncologists as to which patients should be imaged after cystectomy, as well as when patients should be imaged.[120] While CT urography is much more sensitive than excretory urography in its ability to detect upper tract urothelial neoplasms, it is not yet clear that the performance of CT urography provides any significant benefit in terms of patient prognosis and survival. Specifically, it has not yet been determined whether CT urography can detect upper tract lesions at a time when patient survival would be improved as a result of that detection (in comparison to patients whose tumours would only be detected when they present with symptoms).[120]

Imaging can also be performed after cystectomy to assess patients for post-surgical complications. The most common post-surgical complication is anastomotic stricture (usually developing at the ureteroileal anastomoses). Benign anastomotic strictures and strictures resulting from recurrent tumour and metachronous tumours developing at the distal anastomoses can be difficult to distinguish from one another (although the former are more likely). Less frequently observed complications include bowel obstructions (Fig. 14-25), usually due to strictures at the bowel re-anastomoses site, and fistulae (Fig. 14-26).

Use of Imaging to Identify Tumour Response to Chemotherapy

Patients have also been evaluated to assess tumour response to chemotherapy performed following cystectomy or instead of cystectomy (in patients who have presented with distant metastatic disease). Of course, decreased size of the primary cancer and of identified metastases on CT or MRI indicates that there has been

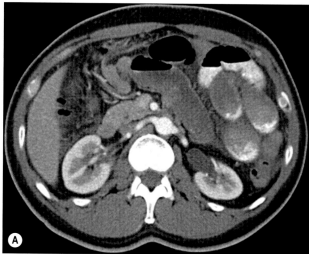

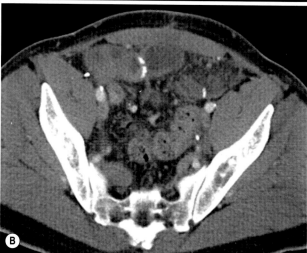

FIGURE 14-25 ■ **Obstruction at bowel anastomosis following cystectomy and creation of an ileal neobladder.** (A) Early enhanced axial CT images demonstrate multiple moderately dilated small bowel loops in this patient with worsening abdominal pain. (B) A transition is present in the right lower quadrant, at the ileal re-anastomosis, which is demarcated by a line of high-attenuation surgical staples.

a response to treatment. According to the Response Evaluation Criteria in Solid Tumours (RECIST), version 1.1, an overall net decrease in the sum of lesion diameters of at least 30% is required to indicate partial tumour response.[123] An increase in net size of at least 20% is required to indicate tumour progression (Fig. 14-27). In those instances in which positron emission tomography is performed, and in which the tumour and metastases are FDG-avid, decreased metabolic activity can also be used to indicate tumour response.

Although work in this area is preliminary, some investigators have demonstrated that changes in diffusion detected on diffusion-weighted MRI images[105] or of tumour perfusion, as determined on dynamic enhanced CT or MRI,[124] can also be used to indicate whether a chemotherapy regimen is effective, with these techniques perhaps being helpful at an earlier stage, before a decrease in tumour size has occurred.[124] If this is true, then patients in whom a chemotherapeutic regimen turns out to be ineffective, could be spared unnecessary chemotoxicity. Alternative, potentially more effective, regimens could be instituted more quickly.

UNCOMMON BLADDER NEOPLASMS

Squamous Cell Carcinomas

In comparison to urothelial malignancies containing focal areas of mixed or divergent histology, bladder

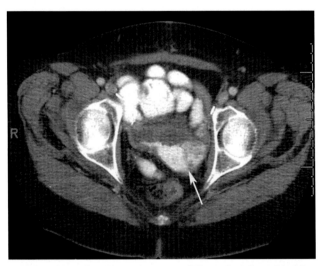

FIGURE 14-26 ■ **Fistula between small bowel and neobladder.** Early enhanced axial CT image through the pelvis demonstrates orally administered contrast material in the reservoir of a neobladder (arrow). This is diagnostic of a fistula, which can be seen in 1–5% of patients. The intravenously administered contrast material has not yet been excreted into the renal collecting systems.

cancers are now considered to be squamous cell carcinomas only if they are composed entirely of squamous cells. Squamous cell carcinomas are irritative neoplasms, generally arising in patients with ongoing urinary tract infections. Thus, they are the most common bladder malignancies in areas where schistosomiasis is endemic. Most squamous cell carcinomas are high grade and present at higher stages than the previously discussed urothelial malignancies. As a result, there is poor 5-year survival. On cross-sectional imaging studies, squamous cell carcinomas cannot be distinguished from other urothelial neoplasms (Fig. 14-28); however, many are large and heterogeneous at the time of presentation (Fig. 14-29).

Adenocarcinomas

Bladder cancers are now classified as adenocarcinomas only when they consist entirely of adenomatous cells. While adenocarcinomas can be encountered in occasional patients with no suggestive history, these rare neoplasms are most commonly diagnosed in patients with urachal carcinomas, bladder exstrophy, and in patients with cystitis glandularis.

Urachal cancers arise in a urachal remnant, which is a muscular and/or fibrous band of tissue that extends from the anterior and superior aspect of the dome of the bladder to the umbilicus. In many patients, there is a residual lining of transitional cells within the urachal remnant, which may become metaplastic and differentiate into mucin-producing adenomatous cells. These cells can then dedifferentiate further into adenomatous cancer cells. While most urachal cancers are adenocarcinomas, urachal transitional cell and squamous cell cancers, and urachal sarcomas have also been encountered.

Patients with urachal carcinoma often present with haematuria.[125] Mucus may be found in the urine, a finding

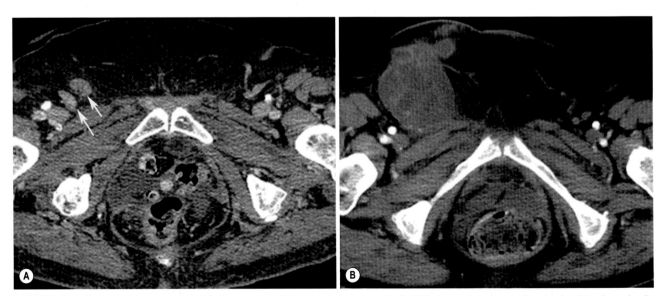

FIGURE 14-27 ■ **Progressive metastatic bladder cancer.** (A) An early enhanced axial CT shows two borderline in size lymph nodes in the right inguinal region in this patient who previously had a cystectomy for bladder cancer (arrows). (B) An early enhanced axial CT image obtained 5 months later shows that there has been pronounced progression of disease, with a single bulky enlarged necrotic lymph node mass now noted in the right inguinal region.

that can suggest the diagnosis. Some patients may also or alternatively have abdominal pain and/or pain on urination.[125]

On imaging studies, urachal cancers have a characteristic location at the bladder dome anteriorly and in the midline. While they often contain hypervascular enhancing components, many also have cystic areas.

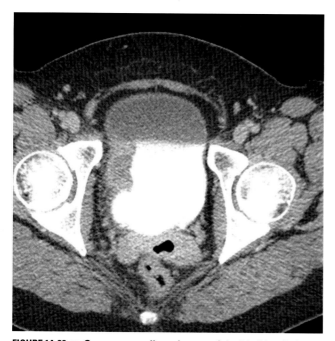

FIGURE 14-28 ■ **Squamous cell carcinoma of the bladder.** Delayed enhanced axial image from a CT urogram shows a lobulated mass along the right lateral aspect of the bladder. Subsequent biopsy demonstrated this to be a squamous cell carcinoma. The appearance of the mass is identical to that of the more common transitional cell predominant urothelial cancers.

They frequently contain stippled or granular calcifications, which can be seen easily on CT[125] (Fig. 14-30). As with squamous cell carcinomas, prognosis in patients with urachal cancers tends to be poor. Many patients develop lung and bone metastatic lesions either before or shortly after presentation.

Cancers in Bladder Diverticula

Most bladder diverticula are pseudodiverticula, representing projections of urothelium through defects in the bladder wall musculature (muscularis mucosa). Patients with bladder diverticula are at increased risk for developing a number of complications, including urinary tract infections, stones and bladder cancer. This may be due to the urinary stasis that develops in these structures (since these usually false diverticula have no muscular lining and cannot contract during voiding). On imaging studies, cancers in bladder diverticula usually appear as soft-tissue masses (Fig. 14-31). Cancers in bladder diverticula have a worse prognosis than cancers in the normal bladder wall, a feature that may be due, in part, to delayed diagnosis, but also to the fact that since most bladder diverticula are not surrounded by all of the layers of the bladder wall, it is much easier for these cancers to spread quickly beyond the bladder, both locally and distantly.[69,126]

Other Bladder Malignancies

A variety of other malignant neoplasms can affect the bladder, including lymphoma, carcinosarcomas, sarcomas and metastases. In most patients, lymphoma involves the bladder secondarily.[127] Urinary bladder involvement can be seen in up to 10–20% of patients with end-stage non-Hodgkin's lymphoma. In these patients, the diagnosis

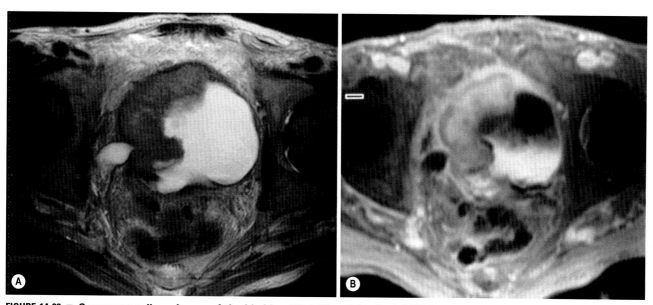

FIGURE 14-29 ■ **Squamous cell carcinoma of the bladder.** (A) A T2-weighted axial MR image through the pelvis of an elderly man with haematuria demonstrates a large lobulated mass along the right lateral and anterior bladder wall, which was eventually diagnosed as a squamous cell carcinoma. (B) A T1-weighted gadolinium-enhanced axial image obtained at the same level shows pronounced mass enhancement.

has usually already been made. In comparison, primary bladder lymphoma is exceedingly rare, accounting for 0.2% of extranodal lymphoma.[127] The most frequently encountered symptom in patients with bladder lymphoma is haematuria. On imaging studies, bladder lymphoma can produce a focal mural mass (which may be indistinguishable from primary urothelial neoplasms) or diffuse bladder wall thickening (which may be indistinguishable from cystitis).

Mesenchymal malignancies occur rarely in the bladder wall. The two most common cell types are leiomysarcomas and rhabdomyosarcomas. Sarcomas are often large at presentation. On CT and MRI, they typically produce large heterogeneous ulcerated and necrotic masses (Fig. 14-32). While leiomyosarcomas and rhabdomyosarcomas are often encountered in older patients, rhabdomyosarcomas can also be seen in the paediatric population. On imaging studies, paediatric rhabdomyosarcomas often have a lobulated appearance, resembling a cluster of grapes.

Metastases to the bladder are quite rare, but have been reported with a variety of primary malignancies. Most commonly, the bladder tends to be secondarily involved, with tumour resulting from direct spread of a malignancy from an adjacent organ (rather than by hematogenous seeding).

Benign Bladder Lesions

A number of benign lesions can be encountered in the bladder. These include benign epithelial tumours, such as the previously described papillomas, as well as non-epithelial tumours, such as leiomyomas (which represent the most common benign bladder neoplasm), paragangiomas, fibromas, haemangiomas and neurofibromas,[69] and inflammatory lesions (such as nephrogenic adenomas and inflammatory myofibroblastic tumours). Several of these entities are described in more detail in the paragraphs that follow.

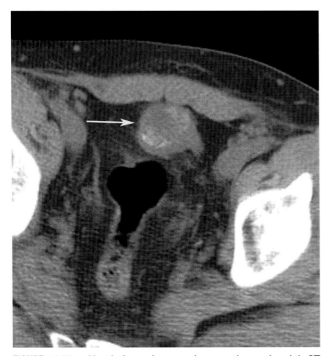

FIGURE 14-30 ■ **Urachal carcinoma.** An unenhanced axial CT image through the pelvis reveals a small ovoid midline urachal cancer (arrow), with peripheral calcification, which was seen to be located just cephalad to the bladder dome.

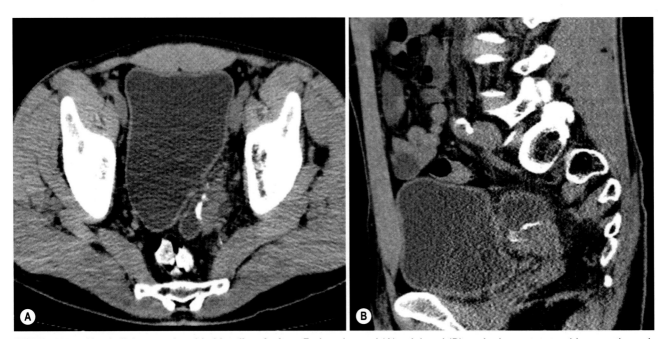

FIGURE 14-31 ■ **Urothelial cancer in a bladder diverticulum.** Early enhanced (A) axial and (B) sagittal reconstructed images through the lower abdomen and pelvis in this elderly man with gross haematuria show a solid mass in the inferolateral aspect of a left-sided bladder diverticulum. Calcification has developed along the periphery of the neoplasm, at its interface with the urine in the lumen of the diverticulum.

Leiomyomas are most commonly encountered in women. Most patients are asymptomatic; however, affected patients may complain of urinary frequency and can develop haematuria. On imaging studies, these tumours appear as soft-tissue masses with smooth margins, with the appearance often being characteristic and suggestive (Fig. 14-33). Their appearance is not specific and they can be confused with malignant urothelial neoplasms on CT; however, on MRI they may have low signal intensity on T2-weighted images, a finding which should raise suspicion for this diagnosis.[69,128] Since these tumours are subepithelial in origin, cystoscopy usually demonstrates intact overlying epithelium.

Paragangliomas arise from chromaffin cells located in the sympathetic nerves near or even within the bladder wall. Although many paragangliomas are asymptomatic, paragangliomas can release catecholamines during micturition, resulting in headache, anxiety or syncope during voiding. As with paragangliomas located elsewhere, most patients with bladder wall paragangliomas have hypertension (which may or may not already have been diagnosed), although the hypertension need not be episodic. While the majority of paragangliomas are benign, occasional paragangliomas are malignant. Although these masses are often smoothly marginated, the US, CT and MR imaging appearance is non-diagnostic, since malignant urothelial neoplasms can have an identical appearance (Fig. 14-34). Paragangliomas often (although not always) demonstrate increased uptake on iodine-131 metaiodobenzylguanidine (MIBG) scintigraphy.

Nephrogenic adenomas are benign growths of the urinary tract, usually occurring in the urinary bladder. These usually develop as a result of chronic inflammation. On histology, their appearance is similar to that of proximal renal tubules in the nephron, thus explaining their name. On imaging studies, nephrogenic adenomas may have a variety of appearances. They can produce areas of irregular bladder wall thickening or lobulated masses. Their appearance is indistinguishable from that of bladder cancers and biopsy is required for diagnosis.

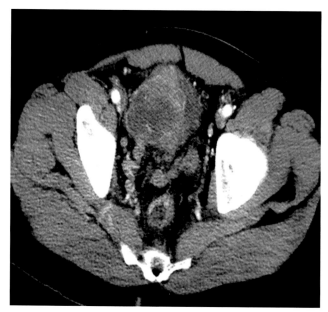

FIGURE 14-32 ■ **Bladder sarcoma.** An early enhanced axial CT image obtained through the pelvis in a 32-year-old man with neurofibromatosis shows a large heterogeneous bladder mass, which was subsequently diagnosed as a fibromyxosarcoma. While most patients with bladder sarcomas present with similarly large lesions, a high-grade aggressive urothelial cancer could also have this appearance.

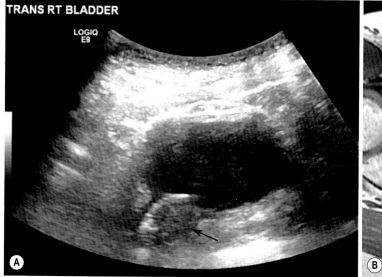 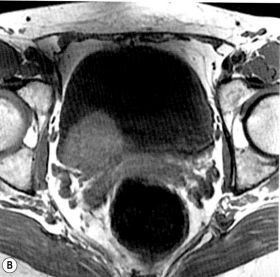

FIGURE 14-33 ■ **Bladder leiomyoma.** (A) A transverse ultrasound image through the bladder demonstrates a mass along the right posterolateral aspect of the bladder (arrow). (B) A T1-weighted axial MR image again shows the soft-tissue mass outlined centrally by the low-signal-intensity urine in the bladder lumen.

Continued on following page

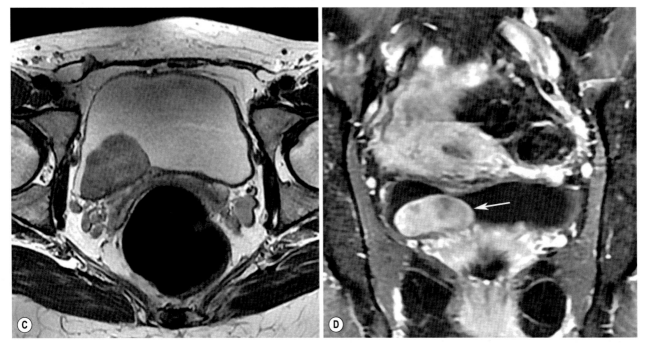

FIGURE 14-33, Continued ■ (C) A T2-weighted axial image again shows the mass, this time outlined by the high-signal-intensity urine. (D) A gadolinium-based contrast material-enhanced T1-weighted coronal image shows that the mass is briskly enhancing (arrow). On all of the images, the mass is well-defined, an appearance typical of leiomyoma, although urothelial cancer can also have this appearance.

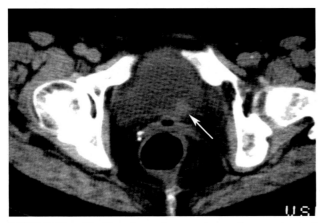

FIGURE 14-34 ■ Bladder phaeochromocytoma. An unenhanced CT image in a woman with a history of hypertension shows small rounded mass along the left posterolateral aspect of the bladder (arrow).

Inflammatory myofibroblastic tumours are rare spindle cell tumours that can occur in many different organs, including the bladder (Fig. 14-35). These lesions, which have also been called inflammatory pseudotumours, usually appear in middle-aged adults. Due to their spindle cell components, they can be confused with sarcomas. The most common presenting symptom is haematuria. Approximately 20% of affected patients have a history of prior instrumentation. Patients with these lesions usually have an unremarkable course following local resection; however, 10–25% of patients develop recurrences. There have been a few reports of patients developing simultaneous sarcomatoid urothelial cancers.[129]

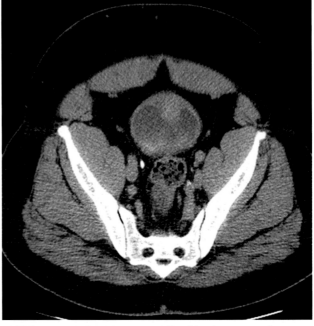

FIGURE 14-35 ■ Inflammatory myofibroblastic tumour. An excretory phase CT urographic image through the pelvis, with only a small amount of contrast material layering dependently in the bladder shows a small ovoid mass projecting into the bladder lumen from an otherwise thickened anterior bladder wall. Cystoscopic biopsy led to the appropriate diagnosis of this benign lesion (also referred to as an inflammatory pseudotumour).

REFERENCES

1. Jemal A, Siegel R, Xu J, Ward E. Cancer statistics, 2010. CA Cancer J Clin 2010;60:277–300.
2. Ferlay J, Autier P, Boniol M, et al. Estimates of the cancer incidence and mortality in Europe in 2006. Ann Oncol 2007;18: 581–92.
3. Ploeg M, Aben K, Kiemeney L. The present and future burden of urinary bladder cancer in the world. World J Urol 2009;27: 289–93.
4. Azémar MD, Comperat E, Richard F, et al. Bladder recurrence after surgery for upper urinary tract urothelial cell carcinoma: Frequency, risk factors, and surveillance. Urol Oncol 2011;29: 130–6.
5. Novara G, De Marco V, Dalpiaz O, et al. Independent predictors of contralateral metachronous upper urinary tract transitional cell carcinoma after nephroureterectomy: Multi-institutional dataset from three European centers. Int J Urol 2009;16:187–91.
6. Acher P, Kiela G, Thomas K, O'Brien T. Towards a rational strategy for the surveillance of patients with Lynch syndrome (hereditary non-polyposis colon cancer) for upper tract transitional cell carcinoma. BJU Int 2010;106:300–2.
7. Roupret M, Catto J, Coulet F, et al. Microsatellite instability as indicator of MSH2 gene mutation in patients with upper urinary tract transitional cell carcinoma. J Med Genet 2004; 41(7):e91.
8. Rouprêt M, Yates DR, Comperat E, Cussenot O. Upper urinary tract urothelial cell carcinomas and other urological malignancies involved in the hereditary nonpolyposis colorectal cancer (Lynch syndrome) tumor spectrum. Eur Urol 2008;54:1226–36.
9. Wong-You-Cheong JJ, Wagner BJ, Davis CJ Jr. Transitional cell carcinoma of the urinary tract: radiologic-pathologic correlation. Radiographics 1998;18:123–4.
10. Colin P, Koenig P, Ouzzane A, et al. Environmental factors involved in carcinogenesis of urothelial cell carcinomas of the upper urinary tract. BJU Int 2009;104:1436–40.
11. McLaughlin JK, Silverman DT, Hsing AW, et al. Cigarette smoking and cancers of the renal pelvis and ureter. Cancer Res 1992;52:254–7.
12. Stefanovic V, Polenakovic M, Toncheva D. Urothelial carcinoma associated with Balkan endemic nephropathy. A worldwide disease. Pathol Biol (Paris) 2011;59:286–91.
13. Nortier JL, Martinez MC, Schmeiser HH, et al. Urothelial carcinoma associated with the use of a Chinese herb (*Aristolochia fangchi*). N Engl J Med 2000;342:1686–92.
14. Perez-Montiel D, Wakely PEJ, Hes O, et al. High-grade urothelial carcinoma of the renal pelvis: clinicopathologic study of 108 cases with emphasis on unusual morphologic variants. Mod Pathol 2006;19:494–503.
15. Olgac S, Mazumdar M, Dalbagni G, Reuter VE. Urothelial carcinoma of the renal pelvis: a clinicopathologic study of 130 cases. Am J Surg Pathol 2004;28:1545–52.
16. Chromecki TF, Bensalah K, Remzi M, et al. Prognostic factors for upper urinary tract urothelial carcinoma. Nat Rev Urol 2011;8: 440–7.
17. Kondo T, Nakazawa H, Ito F, et al. Primary site and incidence of lymph node metastases in urothelial carcinoma of upper urinary tract. Urology 2007;69:265–9.
18. Lughezzani G, Jeldres C, Isbarn H, et al. A critical appraisal of the value of lymph node dissection at nephroureterectomy for upper tract urothelial carcinoma. Urology 2010;75(1):118–24.
19. Ristau BT, Tomaszewski JJ, Ost MC. Upper tract urothelial carcinoma: current treatment and outcomes. Urology 2012;79(4): 749–56.
20. Van Der Molen A, Cowan N, Mueller-Lisse U, et al. CT urography: definition, indications and techniques. A guideline for clinical practice. Eur Radiol 2008;18:4–17.
21. Smith RC, Rosenfield AT, Choe KA, et al. Acute flank pain: comparison of noncontrast enhanced CT and intravenous urography. Radiology 1995;194:789–94.
22. Sourtzis S, Thibeau JF, Damry N, et al. Radiologic investigation of renal colic: unenhanced helical CT compared with excretory urography. Am J Roentgenol 1999;172:1491–4.
23. Fielding JR, Silverman SG, Samuel S, et al. Unenhanced helical CT of ureteral stones: a replacement for excretory urography in planning treatment. Am J Roentgenol 1998;171:1051–3.
24. Smith RC, Verga M, McCarthy S, Rosenfield AT. Diagnosis of acute flank pain: value of unenhanced helical CT. Am J Roentgenol 1996;166:97–101.
25. Bosniak MA. The small (less than or equal to 3.0 cm) renal parenchymal tumor: detection, diagnosis, and controversies. Radiology 1991;179:307–17.
26. Silverman SG, Lee BY, Seltzer SE, et al. Small (< or = 3 cm) renal masses: correlation of spiral CT features and pathologic findings. Am J Roentgenol 1994;163:597–605.
27. Zagoria RJ. Imaging of small renal masses. Am J Roentgenol 2000;175:945–55.
28. Warshauer DM, McCarthy SM, Street L, et al. Detection of renal masses: sensitivities and specificities of excretory urography/linear tomography, US, and CT. Radiology 1988;169:363–5.
29. Caoili EM, Cohan RH, Korobkin M, et al. Urinary tract abnormalities: initial experience with multi-detector row CT urography. Radiology 2002;222:353–60.
30. Chow LC, Kwan SW, Olcott EW, Sommer G. Split-bolus MDCT urography with synchronous nephrographic and excretory phase enhancement. Am J Roentgenol 2007;189:314–22.
31. Kawashima A, Vrtiska TJ, LeRoy AJ, et al. CT urography. Radiographics 2004;24:235–54.
32. Anderson EM, Murphy RM, Rennie ATM, Cowan NC. Multidetector computed tomography urography (MDCTU) for diagnosing urothelial malignancy. Clin Radiol 2006;62:324–32.
33. Nolte-Ernsting C, Cowan N. Understanding multi-slice CT urography techniques: Many roads lead to Rome. Eur Radiol 2006;16:2670–86.
34. Dillman JR, Caoili EM, Cohan RH. Multi-detector CT urography: a one-stop renal and urinary tract imaging modality. Abdom Imaging 2007;32:519–29.
35. Silverman SG, Lyendecker JR, Amis ES. What is the current role of CT urography and MR urography in the evaluation of the urinary tract? Radiology 2009;250:309–23.
36. Weinstein S, Obuchowski NA, Lieber ML. Clinical evaluation of diagnostic tests. Am J Roentgenol 2005;184:14–19.
37. Stacul F, Van Der Molen A, Reimer P, et al. Contrast induced nephropathy: updated ESUR Contrast Media Safety Committee guidelines. Eur Radiol 2011;21:2527–41.
38. Cowan NC. CT urography for haematuria. Nat Rev Urol 2012;9: 218–26.
39. Knox MK, Rivers-Bowerman MD, Bardgett HP, Cowan NC. Multidetector computed tomography with triple-bolus contrast medium administration protocol for preoperative anatomical and functional assessment of potential living renal donors. Eur Radiol 2010;20:2590–9.
40. Kekelidze M, Dwarkasing RS, Dijkshoorn ML, et al. Kidney and urinary tract imaging: triple-bolus multidetector CT urography as a one-stop shop–protocol design, opacification, and image quality analysis. Radiology 2010;255:508–16.
41. Brenner DJ, Hall EJ. Computed tomography—an increasing source of radiation exposure. N Engl J Med 2007;357:2277–84.
42. Brenner DJ, Shuryak I, Einstein AJ. Impact of reduced patient life expectancy on potential cancer risks from radiologic imaging. Radiology 2011;261:193–8.
43. Sodickson A. Strategies for reducing radiation exposure in multi-detector row CT. Radiol Clin N Am 2012;50:1–14.
44. Cowan NC, Turney BW, Taylor NJ, et al. Multidetector computed tomography urography (MDCTU) for diagnosing upper urinary tract tumour. BJU Int 2007;99:1363–70.
45. Fritz GA, Schoellnast H, Deutschmann HA, et al. Multiphasic multidetector-row CT (MDCT) in detection and staging of transitional cell carcinomas of the upper urinary tract. Eur Radiol 2006;16:1244–52.
46. Sudakoff GS, Dunn DP, Guralnick ML, et al. Multidetector computerized tomography urography as the primary imaging modality for detecting urinary tract neoplasms in patients with asymptomatic haematuria. J Urol 2008;179:862–7.
47. Wang LJ, Wong YC, Chuang CK, et al. Diagnostic accuracy of transitional cell carcinoma on multidetector computerized tomography urography in patients with gross hematuria. J Urol 2009;181:524–31.
48. Maheshwari E, O'Malley ME, Ghai S, et al. Split-bolus MDCT urography: upper tract opacification and performance for upper tract tumors in patients with haematuria. Am J Roentgenol 2010;194:453–8.

49. Jinzaki M, Matsumoto K, Kikuchi E, et al. Comparison of CT urography and excretory urography in the detection and localization of urothelial carcinoma of the upper urinary tract. Am J Roentgenol 2011;196:1102–9.

50. O'Malley ME, Hahn PF, Yoder IC, et al. Comparision of excretory phase, helical computed tomography with intravenous urography in patients with painless haematuria. Clin Radiol 2003;58: 294–300.

51. Wang LJ, Wong YC, Huang CC, et al. Multidetector computerized tomography urography is more accurate than excretory urography for diagnosing transitional cell carcinoma of the upper urinary tract in adults with haematuria. J Urol 2010;183:48–55.

52. Cowan NC, Mallett S, Crew JP. Justification for using CT urography as the first-line diagnostic imaging test for investigating haematuria in patients at high risk of upper urinary tract cancer. The Thirty-Sixth Scientific Assembly of the Society of Uroradiology, Carlsbad, California, USA, 2011;50.

53. Blick CG, Nazir SA, Mallett S, et al. Evaluation of diagnostic strategies for bladder cancer using computed tomography (CT) urography, flexible cystoscopy and voided urine cytology: results for 778 patients from a hospital haematuria clinic. BJU Int 2012; 110(1):84–94.

54. Khadra MH, Pickard RS, Charlton M, et al. A prospective analysis of 1,939 patients with haematuria to evaluate current diagnostic practice. J Urol 1999;163:524–7.

55. Edwards TJ, Dickinson AJ, Natale S, et al. A prospective analysis of the diagnostic yield resulting from the attendance of 4020 patients at a protocol-driven haematuria clinic. BJU Int 2006;97: 301–5.

56. Dachman AH, Kelly KB, Zintsmaster MP, et al. Formative evaluation of standardized training for CT colonographic image interpretation by novice readers. Radiology 2008;249:167–77.

57. Tomson C, Porter T. Asymptomatic microscopic or dipstick haematuria in adults: which investigations for which patients? A review of the evidence. BJU Int 2002;90:185–98.

58. Soto JA, Barish MA, Yee J. Reader training in CT colonography: how much is enough? Radiology 2005;237:26–7.

59. Roupret M, Babjuk M, Comperat E, et al. European guidelines on upper tract urothelial carcinomas: 2013 update. Eur Urol 2013;63:1059–71.

60. Hendee WR, Becker GJ, Borgstede JP, et al. Addressing overutilization in medical imaging. Radiology 2010;257:240–5.

61. Vrtiska TJ, Hartman RP, Kofler JM, et al. Spatial resolution and radiation dose of a 64-MDCT scanner compared with published CT urography protocols. Am J Roentgenol 2009;192:941–8.

62. Toth T, Hsieh J. Strategies to reduce radiation dose in CT. In: Mahesh M, editors. MDCT Physics The Basics—Technology, Image Quality and Radiation Dose. 1st ed. Philadelphia: Lippincott Williams & Wilkins; 2009. pp. 115–43.

63. Nolte-Ernsting CC, Staatz G, Tacke J, Gunther RW. MR urography today. Abdom Imaging 2003;28:191–209.

64. Leyendecker JR, Barnes CE, Zagoria RJ. MR urography: techniques and clinical applications. Radiographics 2008;28: 23–46.

65. Takahashi N, Kawashima A, Glockner JF, et al. Small (<2-cm) upper-tract urothelial carcinoma: evaluation with gadolinium-enhanced three-dimensional spoiled gradient-recalled echo MR urography. Radiology 2008;247:451–7.

66. Coursey C, Nelson RC, Boll DT, et al. Dual-energy multidetector CT: how does it work, what can it tell us, and when can we use it in abdominopelvic imaging? Radiographics 2010;30:1037–55.

67. Stone R, Sabichi AL, Gill J, et al. Identification of genes correlated with early-stage bladder cancer progression. Cancer Prev Res 2010;3:776–86.

68. Ng CS. Radiologic diagnosis and staging of renal and bladder cancer. Semin Roentgenol 2006;41:121–37.

69. Dighe MK, Bhargava P, Wright J. Urinary bladder masses: techniques, imaging spectrum, and staging. J Comput Assist Tomogr 2011;35:411–24.

70. Lopez-Beltran A, Requena MJ, Cheng L, Montironi R. Pathological variants of invasive bladder cancer according to their suggested clinical significance. BJU Int 2007;101:275–81.

71. Wasco MJ, Daignault S, Zhang Y, et al. Urothelial carcinoma with divergent histologic differentiation (mixed histologic features) predicts the presence of locally advanced bladder cancer when detected at transurethral resection. Urology 2007;70:69–74.

72. Shinagare AB, Ramaiya NH, Jagannathan JP, et al. Metastatic pattern of bladder cancer: correlation with the characteristics of the primary tumor. Am J Roentgenol 2011;196:117–22.

73. Cohan RH, Caoili EM, Cowan NC, et al. MDCT urography: exploring a new paradigm for imaging of bladder cancer. Am J Roentgenol 2009;192:1501–8.

74. Zhang J, Gerst S, Lefkowitz RA, Bach A. Imaging of bladder cancer. Radiol Clin N Am 2006;45:184–205.

75. Miyamoto H, Miller JS, Fajardo DA, et al. Non-invasive papillary urothelial neoplasms: the 2004 WHO/ISUP classification system. Pathol International 2010;60:1–8.

76. Pan CC, Chang YH, Chen KK, et al. Prognostic significance of the 2004 WHO/ISUP classification for prediction of recurrence, progression, and cancer-specific mortality of non-muscle, invasive urothelial tumors of the urinary bladder: a clinicopathologic study of 1,515 cases. Am J Clin Pathol 2010;133:788–95.

77. Cowan NC, Crew JP. Imaging of bladder cancer. Curr Opin Urol 2010;20:409–13.

78. Beyersdorff D, Zhang J, Schoder H, et al. Bladder cancer: can imaging change patient management? Cur Opin Urol 2008;18: 98–104.

79. Moses KA, Zhang J, Hricak H, Bochner BH. Bladder cancer imaging: an update. Curr Opin Urol 2011;21:393–7.

80. Hillman BJ, Silvert M, Cook G. Recognition of bladder tumors by excretory urography. Radiology 1981;138:319–23.

81. Turney BW, Willatt JMC, Nixon D, et al. Computed tomography urography for diagnosing bladder cancer. BJU Int 2006;98:345–8.

82. Sadow CA, Silverman SG, O'Leary MP, Signorovitch JE. Bladder cancer detection with CT urography in an academic medical center. Radiology 2008;249:195–202.

83. Kim JK, Park SY, Ahn HJ, et al. Bladder cancer: analysis of multi-detector row helical CT enhancement pattern and accuracy in tumor detection and perivesical staging. Radiology 2004;231: 725–31.

84. Mester U, Goldstein MA, Chawla TP, et al. Detection of urothelial tumors: comparison of urothelial phase with excretory phase CT urography—a prospective study. Radiology 2012;264: 110–18.

85. Noroozian M, Cohan RH, Caoili EM, et al. Multislice CT urography: state of the art. Br J Radiol 2004;77:S74–86.

86. Knox MK, Cowan NC, Rivers-Bowerman MD. Evaluation of multi-detector computed tomography urography and ultrasonography in diagnosing bladder cancer. Clin Radiol 2008;63: 1317–25.

87. Koplay M, Kantarci M, Guven F, et al. Diagnostic efficiency of multidetector computed tomography with multiplanar reformatted imaging and virtual cystoscopy in the assessment of bladder tumors after transurethral resection. J Comput Assist Tomogr 2010;34:121–6.

88. Song JH, Francis IR, Platt JF, et al. Bladder tumor detection at virtual cystoscopy. Radiology 2001;218:95–100.

89. Panebianco B, Sciarra A, Di Martino M, et al. Bladder carcinoma: MDCT cystograohy and virtual cystoscopy. Abdom Imaging 2010;35:257–64.

90. Vikram R, Sandler CM, Ng CSD. Imaging and staging of transitional cell carcinoma: part 1. Lower urinary tract. Am J Roentgenol 2009;192:1481–7.

91. Cohan RH. CT urography of the bladder. In: Silverman SG, Cohan RH, editors. CT Urography: An Atlas. Philadelphia: Lippincott, Williams & Wilkins; 2007. pp. 209–50.

92. Jinzaki M, Tanimoto A, Shinmoto H, et al. Detection of bladder tumors with dynamic contrast-enhanced MDCT. Am J Roentgenol 2007;188:913–18.

93. Totaro A, Brescia A, Cappa E, et al. Imaging in bladder cancer: present role and future perspectives. Urol Int 2010;85:373–80.

94. Abou-El-Ghar ME, El-Assmy A, Refaie HF, El-Diasty T. Bladder cancer: diagnosis with diffusion-weighted MR imaging in patients with gross hematuria. Radiology 2009;251:415–21.

95. Watanabe H, Kanematsu M, Kondo H, et al. Preoperative T staging of urinary bladder cancer: does diffusion-weighted MRI have supplementary value? Am J Roentgenol 2009;192:1361–6.

96. Kobayashi S, Koga F, Yoshida S, et al. Diagnostic performance of diffusion-weighted magnetic resonance imaging in bladder cancer: potential utility of apparent diffusion coefficient values as a biomarker to predict clinical aggressiveness. Eur Radiol 2011;21: 2178–86.

97. Avcu S, Koseoglu MN, Ceylan K, et al. The value of diffusion-weighted MRI in the diagnosis of malignant and benign urinary bladder lesions. Br J Radiol 2011;84:875–82.

98. O'Malley ME, Hahn PH, Yoder IC, et al. Comparison of execretory phase helical computed tomography with intravenous urography in patients with painless hematuria. Clin Radiol 2003;58:294–300.

99. Mueller-Lisse UG, Mueller-Lisse UL, Hinterberger J, et al. Multidetector-row computed tomography (MDCT) in patients with a history of previous urothelial cancer or painless macroscopic hematuria. Eur Radiol 2007;17:1046–54.

100. Martingano P, Stacul F, Carllaro M, et al. 64-slice CT urography: 30 months of clinical experience Radiol Med 2010;115:920–35.

101. Wang LJ, Wong YC, Ng KF, et al. Tumor characteristics of urothelial carcinoma on multidetector computerized tomography urography. J Urol 2010;183:2154–60.

102. Golan S, Sopov V, Baniel J, Groshar D. Comparison of ^{11}C-choline with ^{18}F-FDG in positron emission tomography/computerized tomography for staging urothelial carcinoma: a prospective study. J Urol 2011;186(2):436–41.

103. Rajesh A, Sokhi HK, Fung R, et al. Bladder cancer: evaluation of staging accuracy using dynamic MRI. Clin Radiol 2011;66:1135–40.

104. Takeuchi M, Sasaki S, Ito M, et al. Urinary bladder cancer: diffusion-weighted MR imaging—accuracy for diagnosing T stage and estimating histologic grade. Radiology 2009;251:112–21.

105. Yoshida S, Saito K, Masua H, et al. Initial experience with diffusion-weighted magnetic resonance imaging to assess therapeutic response to induction chemoradiotherapy against muscle-invasive bladder cancer. Urology 2010;75:387–91.

106. Chapman DM, Pohar KS, Gong MC, Bahnson RR. Preoperative hydronephrosis as an indicator of survival after radical cystectomy. Urol Oncol 2009;27:491–5.

107. Ito Y, Kikuchi E, Tanaka N, et al. Preoperative hydronephrosis grade independently predicts worse pathological outcomes in patients undergoing nephroureterectomy for upper tract urothelial carcinoma. J Urol 2011;185:1621–6.

108. Feldman AS, Siddiqui MM. Advances in the evaluation and management of lymph node involvement in urothelial carcinoma of the bladder. Exp Rev Anticancer Ther 2010;10:1855–60.

109. Kibel AS, Dehdashti F, Katz MD, et al. Prospective study of [18F] fluorodeoxyglucose positron emission tomography/computed tomography for staging of muscle-invasive bladder carcinoma. J Clin Oncol 2009;27:4314–20.

110. Swinnen G, Maes A, Pottel H, et al. FDG-PET/CT for the preoperative lymph node staging of invasive bladder cancer. Eur Urol 2010;57:641–7.

111. Drieskens O, Oyen R, van Poppel H, et al. FDG-PET for preoperative staging of bladder cancer before radical cystectomy. Eur J Nucl Med Mol Imaging 2005;32:1412–17.

112. Jadvar H, Quan V, Henderson RW. [F-18]-fluorodeoxyglucose PET and PET-CT in diagnostic imaging evaluation of locally recurrent and metastatic bladder transitional cell carcinoma. Int J Clin Oncol 2008;13:42–7.

113. Bouchelouche K, Oehr P. Positron emission tomography and positron emission tomography/computerized tomography of urological malignancies: an update review. J Urol 2008;179:34–45.

114. Sadow CA, Wheeler SC, Kim J, et al. Positive predictive value of CT urography in the evaluation of upper tract urothelial cancer. Am J Roentgenol 2010;195:W337–43.

115. Xu AD, Ng CS, Kamat A, et al. Significance of upper urinary tract urothelial thickening and filling defect seen on MDCT urography in patients with a history of urothelial neoplasms. Am J Roentgenol 2010;195:959–65.

116. Bradford TJ, Montie JE, Hafez KS. The role of imaging in the surveillance of urologic malignancies. Urol Clin North Am 2006;33:377–96.

117. Steiner H, Bergmesiter M, Verdorfer I, et al. Early results of bladder cancer screening in a high-risk population of heavy smokers. BJU Int 2008;102:291–6.

118. Ma W, Kang SK, Hricak H, et al. Imaging appearance of granulomatous disease after intravesical Bacille Calmette-Guerin (BCG) treatment of bladder carcinoma. Am J Roentgenol 2009;192:1494–500.

119. Dhar NB, Jones JS, Reuther AM, et al. Presentation, location and overall survival of pelvic recurrence after radical cystectomy for transitional cell carcinoma of the bladder. BJU Int 2007;101:969–72.

120. Dalbagni G, Bochner BH, Cronin A, et al. A plea for a uniform surveillance schedule after radical cystectomy. J Urol 2011;185:2091–6.

121. Tran W, Serio AM, Raj GV, et al. Longitudinal risk of upper tract recurrence following radical cystectomy for urothelial cancer and the potential implications for long-term surveillance. J Urol 2008;179:96–100.

122. Volkmer BG, Kuefer R, Bartsch GC Jr, et al. Oncological followup after radical cystectomy for bladder cancer—is there any benefit? J Urol 2009;181:1587–93.

123. Eisenhauer EA, Therasse P, Bogaerts J, et al. New response evaluation criteria in solid tumours: revised RECIST guideline (version 1.1). Eur J Cancer 2009;45:228–47.

124. Naish JH, McGrath DM, Bains LJ, et al. Comparison of dynamic contrast-enhanced MRI and dynamic contrast-enhanced CT biomarkers in bladder cancer. Magn Reson Med 2011;66:219–26.

125. Yu JS, Kim KW, Lee HJ, et al. Urachal remnant diseases: Spectrum of CT and US findings. Radiographics 2001;21:451–61.

126. Lowe FC, Goldman SM, Oesterling JE. Computerized tomography in evaluation of transitional cell carcinoma in bladder diverticula. Urology 1989;6:390–5.

127. Maninderpal K, Amir FH, Azad HAR, Mun KS. Imaging findings of a primary bladder maltoma. Br J Radiol 2011;84:e186–90.

128. Chen M, Lipson SA, Hricak H. MR imaging evaluation of benign mesenchymal tumors of the urinary bladder. Am J Roentgenol 1997;168:399–403.

129. Montgomery EA, Shuster DD, Burkhart AL, et al. Inflammatory myoblastic tumors of the urinary tract: a clinicopathologic study of 46 cases, including a malignant example inflammatory fibrosarcoma and a subset associated with high-grade urothelial carcinoma. Am J Surg Pathol 2006;30:1502–12.

CHAPTER 15

PROSTATE

Joyce G.R. Bomers • Leonardo Kayat Bittencourt • Geert Villeirs • Jelle O. Barentsz

---

CHAPTER OUTLINE

MULTI-PARAMETRIC PROSTATE MRI

Introduction

With almost 240,000 new cases and approximately 30,000 deaths in the USA predicted for 2013, prostate cancer (PCa) is the most common non-cutaneous male cancer, and the second cause of cancer-related death.[1] Presently, one in six men will be diagnosed with PCa at a certain moment in their life.

The past three decades have seen a steep rise in PCa incidence. To a certain extent this can be explained by the introduction of prostate specific antigen (PSA) level measurement, by the development of improved diagnostic imaging and by the improvement in demographic information systems. The improvement in overall life expectancy and the trend to apply lower cut-off levels for the PSA blood level test will further increase the number of men diagnosed with PCa.[2]

Nowadays, an abnormal digital rectal examination (DRE), an elevated PSA level or anomalous changes in PSA level and dynamics (i.e. doubling time or PSA velocity) are biological signs indicating an increased risk of PCa. However, these techniques are being considered of restricted accuracy in PCa detection. DRE is affected by considerable inter-observer variability, and is limited to the evaluation of lesions in the posterior and lateral peripheral zone. The specificity of PSA testing is of limited value, as 70–80% of patients with slight PSA elevation (>4.0 ng/mL) have benign prostatic hyperplasia (BPH) or prostatitis rather than PCa.

In general, when there is an increased risk of PCa, systematic random transrectal ultrasound (TRUS) biopsies are performed. However, undersampling is a large limitation. Even with the most aggressive biopsy schemes, detection rates of only 23–42% after the first biopsy session, until 18% after the fourth biopsy session, are reported.[3] Furthermore, significant underscoring of tumour aggression is a notable limitation of systematic biopsies.[4] These results are caused by sampling errors, tumour multifocality and heterogeneity of the lesion or a combination of these factors. As histopathology results obtained from TRUS-guided biopsy are commonly used in nomograms for risk assessment and prognosis in PCa, an inaccurate assessment of the true tumour aggression will lead to wrong treatment options.

The limitations of DRE, PSA, TRUS and systematic biopsy schemes have raised interest in the development of prostate magnetic resonance imaging (MRI). In the assessment of PCa, MRI can be used for multiple purposes: screening, detection of primary or recurrent cancer, localisation and staging of local and distant disease.

Since the first prostate MR examinations in the 1980s, prostate MRI has evolved to a mature imaging technique. The development of additional functional and metabolic techniques, such as dynamic contrast-enhanced MRI (DCE-MRI),[5] diffusion-weighted imaging (DWI)[6] and proton MR spectroscopy imaging (MRSI),[7] has made MRI an even more powerful modality in the detection and localisation of PCa. Next to high-resolution T2-weighted imaging, which is mainly used to depict the prostate anatomy, DCE-MRI improves the sensitivity in PCa detection[8–10] and DWI[11–14] and MRSI[15,16] add specificity in characterisation of PCa.[95]

For these reasons, a group of prostate MRI experts of the European Society of Urogenital Radiology (ESUR) recommends a multi-parametric approach, combining high-resolution T2-weighted images with at least two functional MR techniques for improving detection and characterisation of PCa.[17]

At this moment, multi-parametric magnetic resonance imaging (MP-MRI) is the most sensitive and specific imaging technique for localising prostate cancer.[18]

Anatomy

The prostate gland surrounds the proximal part of the urethra and is located directly caudal from the bladder and ventral of the rectum (Fig. 15-1). The seminal vesicles lie posterosuperiorly between the bladder and the rectum. The ejaculatory ducts pass through the gland and end in the prostatic urethra at the verumontanum. The

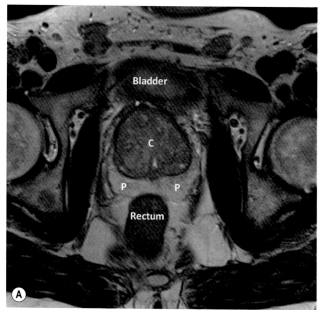

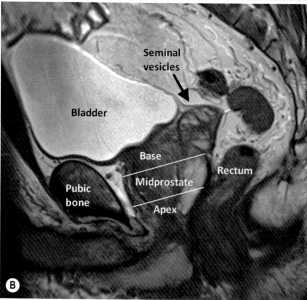

FIGURE 15-1 ■ (A) Axial T2-weighted MR image showing the prostate and its zonal anatomy. The peripheral zone (P) is shown as a crescent-shaped hyperintense structure; the central gland (C) is depicted as a structure with heterogeneous signal intensity. (B) Sagittal T2-weighted image showing the craniocaudal segmentation of the prostate and its relation to the adjacent structures.

neurovascular bundles, responsible for erectile function, pass from superior to inferior along both posterolateral sides of the prostate.

In craniocaudal direction, the prostate can be divided into three parts (Fig. 15-1B). The cranial part of the prostate is referred to as the *base*, the middle part is the *midprostate* and the caudal part is called the *apex*. Anatomically, the prostate consists of three different zones: the peripheral zone, the transition zone and the central zone. Ventral to the prostate lies the anterior fibromuscular stroma, mainly composed of smooth

muscle cells and connective tissue; it does not contain glandular tissue.

The peripheral zone is located posteriorly and inferiorly and around 70–80% of the tumour foci are located in this zone.[19,20] The transition zone is located interiorly and surrounds the prostatic urethra. The central zone is located posterior and superior of the transition zone. Approximately 20% of PCa foci arise from the transition zone and 10% arises from the central zone.[21]

In young men, the transition and central zone are usually indistinguishable from each other, being usually referred together as the 'central or internal gland'.[22] With increasing age, the prostate zonal anatomy changes. In young men, the central gland is composed mainly of the central zone. In older men the central gland is composed mainly of the transition zone, due to the development of benign prostatic hyperplasia. BPH leads to the formation of adenomatous nodules in the transition zone. Mostly, the central zone becomes compressed and will be displaced towards the prostatic base, making it a difficult task to accurately define the zonal anatomy of the central gland by MR imaging.[23] As for the peripheral zone, it is generally not affected by BPH and retains its histological features.

Areas of prostatitis are almost exclusively derived from the peripheral zone, and in the specific clinical context of MR imaging, chronic prostatitis is a much more relevant condition than acute prostatitis, because it is usually of asymptomatic course or shares manifestations similar to that of BPH, being often associated with increased PSA levels, and constituting an important differential diagnosis for PCa.

Histology

The prostate is a histologically heterogeneous structure, with a diversity of cellular types. Ninety per cent of malignant prostate tumours consist of adenocarcinoma. Other prevalent tumour types are ductal, cystic adenoid, signet-ring cell, small-cell and neuroendocrine tumours.[24] Unlike most other solid tumours, PCa usually does not manifest itself as a discrete nodule. The neoplastic tumour cells are usually intermingled with normal cells.[25] For this reason, it can be understood why DRE is incapable of detecting a significant number of lesions, and also why PSA testing, being a marker of prostate activity, is not specific enough to rule out other more frequent benign conditions.[26] The final diagnosis of PCa is exclusively histopathological.

The gold standard for the determination of the biological aggressiveness of PCa is the Gleason grading system.[27] This system is based on a description of cancer cell architecture at low-power optic microscopy. Five different microscopic patterns can be described, increasing from less (Gleason grade 1; well-differentiated uniform glands) to most aggressive (Gleason grade 5; poorly differentiated, anaplastic or even no presence of prostate gland cells).

After radical prostatectomy the Gleason score (GS) is calculated by the sum of the two most prevalent patterns, ranging from 2 to 10: for example, Gleason 3 + 4 = 7. After a prostate biopsy session, the sum of the most prevalent pattern and the most aggressive pattern are given. The GS is considered a strong clinical predictor for the prognosis of the patient and is used for decisions in further patient treatment.[28] Gleason grades 4 and 5 and GS >7 have the worst prognosis.[27,29]

MR IMAGING

T2-Weighted MR Imaging

In general, high-resolution T2-weighted images are used to depict the anatomy of the prostate and its surrounding structures as the seminal vesicles, bladder and rectal wall.

The normal peripheral zone has a homogeneous intermediate to high signal intensity, clearly distinguishable from the transition and central zones (Fig. 15-2). It is usually surrounded by a thin hypointense rim, which represents the anatomical capsule and is an important landmark in tumour staging.[22]

In T2-weighted images PCa can appear as an area of low signal intensity (Fig. 15-3). High-grade tumours, with a Gleason grade 4 or 5, usually present with a lower signal intensity.[30] Low-grade tumours, with a Gleason grade 2 or 3, can present as T2-isointense areas, or even as non-focal mildly hypointense abnormalities.

Non-malignant conditions, such as (post-biopsy) haematomas, (granulomatous) prostatitis (Fig. 15-4), scar tissue, atrophy, post-radiation changes and hormonal therapy effects, also manifest as T2-hypointense lesions in the peripheral zone.[31,32] However, wedge-shaped lesions with low signal intensity or diffuse extensions without mass effect are highly likely to be benign.[33]

The central gland is characterised by low signal intensity on T2-weighted images, frequently intermingled by round, well-circumscribed heterogeneous BPH nodules with a mixed heterogeneous high and low signal intensity, in a pattern described as 'organised chaos' (Fig. 15-2). Encircling the central gland lies the pseudo-capsule, a thin T2-hypointense rim that separates the central gland from the peripheral zone.[22]

Given the heterogeneity of the region and the wide spectrum of changes attributable to BPH, the diagnosis of PCa in the central gland (Fig. 15-5) imposes an even greater challenge than in the peripheral zone. In the literature a number of findings that can be helpful in the detection of PCa in the central gland have been described. If there is an ill-defined homogeneous T2-hypointense focal lesion ('erased charcoal drawing sign'), a lesion with spiculated or undefined margins, an anteriorly located lesion with a lenticular or fusiform shape, loss of the T2-hypointense contour of BPH nodules, loss of

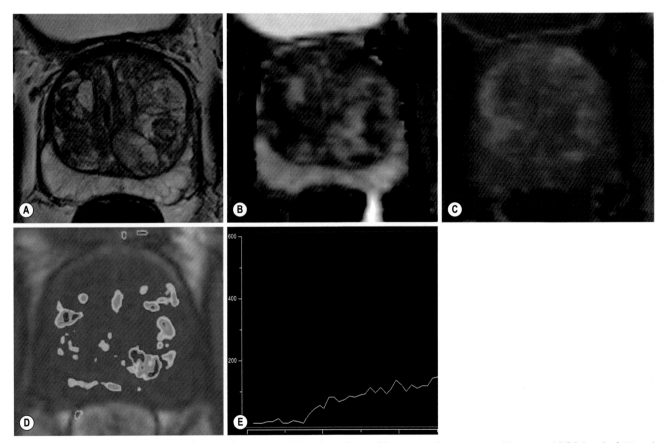

FIGURE 15-2 ■ **Multi-parametric MR images of a 68-year-old male patient with a normal prostate and increased PSA level of 17 ng/mL and 4 negative TRUS biopsy sessions.** The peripheral zone is depicted with high signal intensity on the T2-weighted images and ADC map. In the central gland typical signs of BPH are shown. (A) Axial T2-weighted image. (B) Axial ADC map. (C) Axial DWI with b = 1400. (D) Axial DCE image. (E) Curve of the DCE image.

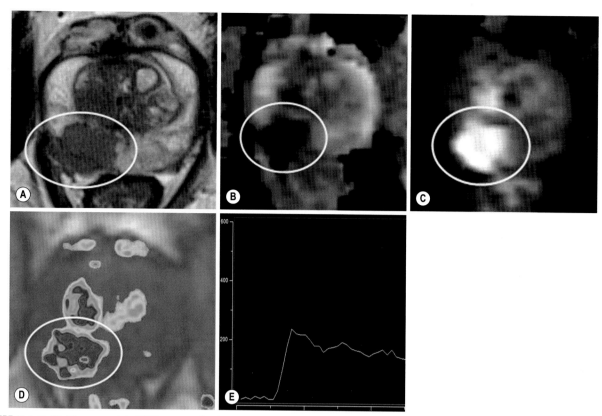

FIGURE 15-3 ■ **Multi-parametric MR images of a 64 year old man with a PSA level of 13 ng/mL and 1 negative TRUS biopsy session, showing a typical case of a peripheral zone tumor.** With MR-guided biopsy a GS 4 + 4 = 8 was found. (A) Axial T2-weighted image. (B) Axial ADC map. (C) Axial DWI with b = 1400. (D) Axial DCE image. (E) Curve of the DCE image.

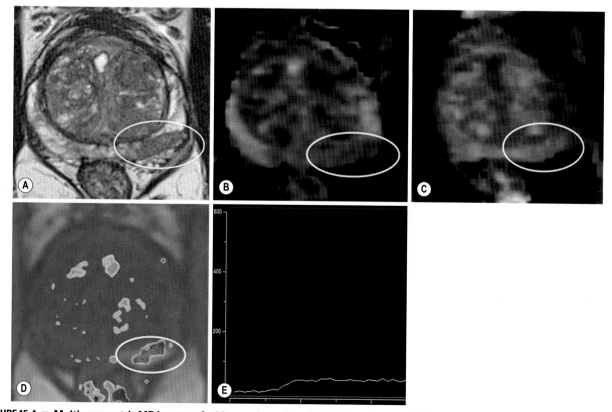

FIGURE 15-4 ■ **Multi-parametric MR images of a 68 year old male patient with an increased PSA level of 22 ng/mL and 4 negative TRUS biopsy sessions.** In the left peripheral zone a typical prostatitis (white circle) is shown. (A) Axial T2-weighted image. (B) Axial ADC map. (C) Axial DWI with b = 1400. (D) Axial DCE image. (E) Curve of the DCE image.

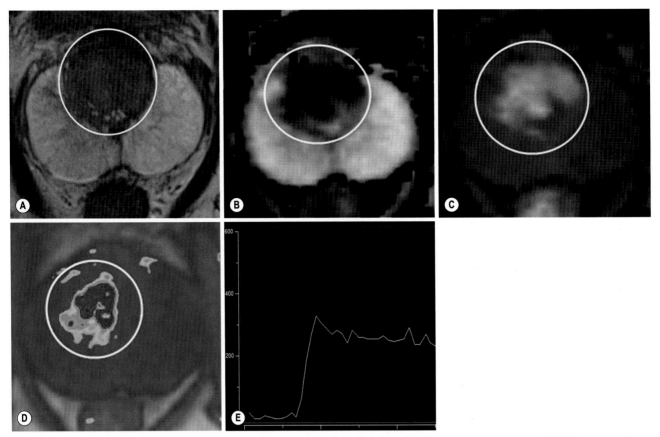

FIGURE 15-5 ■ **Multi-parametric MR images of a 65-year-old man with a PSA level of 37 ng/mL and 4 negative TRUS biopsy sessions, showing a typical case of a transition zone tumour (white circle).** With MR-guided biopsy a GS 4 + 4 = 8 was found. (A) Axial T2-weighted image. (B) Axial ADC map. (C) Axial DWI with b = 1400. (D) Axial DCE image. (E) Curve of the DCE image.

definition of the pseudo-capsule, or signs of urethral invasion, PCa might be present. On the other hand, focal T2-hypointense areas may still be normally observed in the central gland either as predominantly stromal BPH or as protrusion of the anterior fibromuscular stroma.[34]

The reported diagnostic performance of T2-weighted imaging in the detection and localisation of PCa has a wide range, with sensitivities and specificities between 48–88% and 44–67% for detection[8,35,36] and between 58–67% and 60–81% for localisation.[37–39]

T1-Weighted MR Imaging

T1-weighted images show little to no utility for the detection of suspicious lesions in the prostate, since the normal parenchyma is homogeneously isointense in this sequence, and therefore does not allow for the detailed evaluation of its architecture. This sequence is predominantly used for the assessment of haemorrhagic foci, which present as T1-hyperintense areas (Fig. 15-6). Even so, considering that haemorrhage is a potentially confounding factor for PCa, due to its low signal intensity on T2-weighted images, an interval of 8 weeks between the biopsy session and MRI examination is usually advised,[40] in order to reduce the incidence of false-positive findings.

DCE MR Imaging

Dynamic contrast-enhanced MRI is a functional MR imaging technique that shows the dynamic uptake and rapid washout of a gadolinium-based contrast agent to exploit the typical pharmacokinetic properties of normal and tumour tissue.

Technically, DCE MR imaging is based on fast axial T1-weighted sequences which are repeatedly acquired before, during and after IV bolus injection (2–4 mL/s) of a gadolinium-based contrast medium, encompassing the whole prostate gland and seminal vesicles, with a temporal resolution preferably lower than 15 s per acquisition.[17]

Originally, DCE evaluation based on T1-weighted images is a technique derived from the initial studies in dynamic breast MR imaging,[41] consequently also bringing its post-processing techniques and concepts such as contrast medium 'wash-in' and 'washout' from the classic curve types I, II and III, in a qualitative, quantitative or even semi-quantitative approach.

In most of the neoplastic conditions, PCa included, angiogenesis is induced by secretion of vascular growth factors in reaction to local hypoxia or lack of nutrients.[42] An increase in tumour vascularity leads to an enhancement pattern with peaks earlier and higher than those of

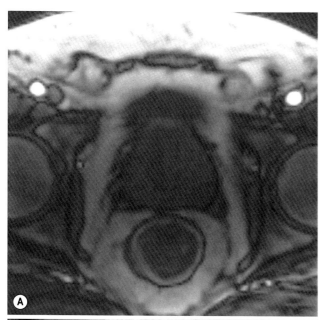

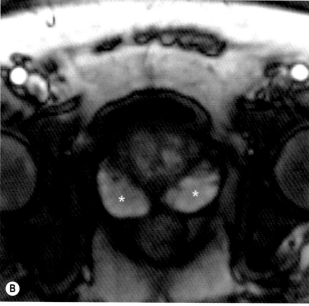

FIGURE 15-6 ▪ (A) T1-weighted image of the prostate. Detailed evaluation of the architecture is not possible due to homogeneously isointense signal. (B) T1-weighted image of the prostate with hyperintense signal (*) in the peripheral zone caused by haemorrhage.

the normal surrounding tissue, combined also with early and pronounced contrast media washout (Figs. 15-3 and 15-5).[42,43]

Other benign conditions such as prostatitis (Fig. 15-4) in the peripheral zone and BPH in the central gland (Fig. 15-2) also lead to regional changes in the enhancement pattern. Therefore, PCa is hard to detect with DCE-MRI alone. Granulomatous prostatitis of the peripheral zone is only shown by moderate enhancement, which can be lower than usually observed in PCa.[44]

Regardless of the choice between a semi-quantitative and a quantitative model, DCE evaluation shows strong evidence of good performance in the management of PCa. It has been shown that DCE is significantly better

than conventional T2-weighted imaging alone in the localisation of tumour foci,[45-47] and that it increases the accuracy of less experienced radiologists in the detection of extracapsular extension and seminal vesicle involvement.[48] Because of this, the use of DCE is definitely well indicated, and is a fundamental part of multi-parametric prostate MR imaging.

DWI MR Imaging

In diffusion-weighted imaging (DWI) the random movement of water molecules in tissue is shown. In an environment of totally unrestricted diffusion, the movement of water molecules is completely random, constituting a phenomenon known as Brownian movement, or 'free diffusion'. Restricted diffusion is seen in tissues with a high cellular density and intact cell membranes. Tissue types associated with restricted diffusion comprise cancer, abscess, cytotoxic oedema and fibrosis.[49]

In the clinical setting, thanks to those properties, DWI has become one of the most important non-invasive biomarkers in oncology, with many already proven applications such as tumour detection, staging and evaluation of therapy response.[50]

On diffusion-weighted images areas with restricted diffusion have a hyperintense signal. The sensitivity of DWI to water movement is variable, depending on the MR field strength and on the time/amplitude relation of the movement-encoding gradient, also known as b-value. For local prostate imaging, DWI should be performed with at least 2 b-values, including a low b-value of 0 s/mm^2 and a higher b-value of 500–1000 s/mm^2.

Based on the diffusion-weighted images, a so-called apparent diffusion coefficient (ADC) map can be calculated. ADC is measured in millimetre per second squared (mm/s^2), and provides quantitative information that is inversely proportional to the degree of diffusion restriction. Low ADC values, which are hypointense on the ADC map, represent tissue with restricted diffusion. More detailed technical information about DWI is given in the article of Qayyum et al.[49]

Healthy prostate tissue in the peripheral zone is rich in tubular fluid-filled structures, allowing for unrestricted diffusion of water molecules, manifesting through low signal intensity on the diffusion-weighted images and high ADC values (Fig. 15-2). In the majority of cases, the peripheral zone can be easily discerned from the central gland, owing to its homogeneously higher ADC values.[51] Upon microscopic observation, the central gland exhibits a greater proportion of compact smooth muscle and concurrently a smaller proportion of glandular elements than the peripheral zone, with this probably responding for a higher percentage of intracellular than extracellular fluid.[23] Additionally, with the ageing of the patient, there is an increase in the ADC values of both the peripheral zone and central gland,[51] which is probably due to atrophic changes, causing a decrease in cell volume, and simultaneous enlargement of the gland ducts.

BPH is histologically characterised by hyperplasia of central gland cells, with variable degrees of involvement of the glandular, muscular and fibrous components.[52] This heterogeneity is also manifested in water diffusion properties in BPH, being classically expressed in MRI as foci of low ADC values interspersed with areas of high values (Fig. 15-2).[53]

Histologically, prostatitis is characterised by extracellular oedema surrounding the prostate cells, associated with lymphocyte aggregates, plasma cells, macrophages and neutrophils in the stroma.[32] In a recent study it has been shown that although there is a significant overlap, ADC values of prostatitis are lower than normal prostate tissue, and significantly higher than low- and high-grade PCa.[14] However, due to a very high cell density, granulomatous prostatitis can present itself by ADC values lower than the ADC values of PCa.[54]

PCa is histologically characterised by a higher cell density and a higher nucleus/cytoplasm ratio than the surrounding normal prostate tissue, with substitution of the glandular parenchyma by tumour cells. This causes a marked reduction in the ADC values relative to the normal prostate (Figs. 15-3 and 15-5).[6,55]

Moreover, while well-differentiated tumours may in some way preserve their tubular architecture, poorly differentiated or aggressive tumours exhibit prominent cellular components, with derangement of tubular architecture and, consequently, generating potential differences in diffusion properties and ADC measurements between those two categories.[11–13,56,57]

MRSI

Proton MR spectroscopic imaging (MRSI) is based on the quantification of differences in proton precessing frequency of different compounds. The latter consist of protons surrounded by a molecular cloud that insulates the protons from the external electromagnetic field (B_0). This compound-specific insulation from B_0 causes a specific precessing frequency shift, also called 'chemical shift', and is measured in hertz (Hz) or parts per million (ppm).

The amount of chemical shift is unique to a given compound or its composing elements, and enables the assessment of the molecular signature of a given sample in biochemical analyses. The same principle applies to clinical MR spectroscopy, allowing in vivo assessment of the presence or absence of relevant compounds such as citrate and choline in the detection and characterisation of prostate cancer. It involves the acquisition of a 3D data set of spectroscopic voxels, using a 3D chemical shift imaging acquisition protocol.[16,58] Signal contributions from water and fat are selectively suppressed, and several outer-voxel saturation bands are applied close to the prostate margins to reduce contamination from surrounding structures, especially periprostatic fat.

Among the metabolites usually studied in prostate spectroscopy, citrate is found in high concentrations (>60 mM) in normal prostate epithelium and prostatic fluid, being also observed in low concentrations in other locations of the gland.[59] Lipids cover a broad spectral range on the right side of the citrate peak (mean resonance frequency around 1.3 ppm). To avoid lipid contamination of the citrate peak, it is of fundamental importance to correctly position fat saturation bands close to the prostatic margin. The normal prostate spectrum has a prominent citrate peak at a frequency of 2.6 ppm (Fig. 15-7). Reduced levels of citrate are characteristically seen in PCa, but also in areas of prostatitis.

Choline presents as a peak precessing at 3.2 ppm. It actually consists of a mix of different choline compounds, including free choline, phosphocholine and glycerocholine, which are involved in the cellular membrane synthesis and degradation. Choline concentrations are generally elevated in PCa due to a higher cell-membrane turnover[60,61] (Fig. 15-7), although it may also be observed in conditions such as prostatitis.[32]

Creatine is related to by-products of metabolism, and its peak is found at a frequency of 3.0 ppm. The creatine concentration in the prostate tends to be low and is not substantially different in normal prostate tissue than in prostate cancer.[58,62] However, at 1.5 tesla (T) MRSI, the creatine peak cannot be entirely resolved from the choline peak, so both peaks are usually evaluated together. Moreover, the polyamine peak, resonating at 3.1 ppm, can fill the potential gap between both peaks. Polyamines play a role in the regulation of cell proliferation and differentiation and are present in normal prostatic tissue and benign hyperplastic nodules, but reduced or absent in prostate cancer.[63]

A choline plus creatine-to-citrate (CC/C) ratio has generally been used to predict the presence or absence of prostate cancer, with higher CC/C ratios being suggestive of prostate cancer.[58,64,65] Metabolite peaks and ratios can be evaluated quantitatively or qualitatively. In the quantitative analysis, the CC/C ratio is calculated on the basis of the area under the curve below each individual peak, and a 5-point scale according to the number of standard deviations above the normal ratio has been proposed for the assessment of the likeliness of PCa.[66–68] In the qualitative analysis, the peak heights of citrate and choline are visually compared using a 5-point pattern recognition diagnostic scale.[15,17,69]

For the diagnosis and localisation of prostate cancer of any Gleason grade, diagnostic accuracies between 70 and 90% have been reported for MRSI, combined with T2-weighted MRI.[7,25,45,70–73]

LOCAL STAGING

Local staging involves the assessment of the anatomical extent of PCa at the time of diagnosis. In the locoregional staging of PCa, the single most relevant aspect for treatment choice is the differentiation between organ-confined disease (stages T1–T2) and extracapsular extension (stage T3a), invasion of the seminal vesicle(s) (stage T3b) or invasion of the bladder, rectum or periprostatic muscles (stage T4). Clinical staging based on PSA level, digital rectal examination and transrectal ultrasound imaging results in frequent understaging (59%) and sometimes overstaging (5%).[74] Adding MR images to this clinical data resulted in significantly increased accuracy of predicting tumour stage, and the presence of extracapsular extension or seminal vesicle invasion (SVI).[75,76]

The identification of minimal extracapsular extension requires high-resolution anatomical T2-weighted images in at least two directions. Most of the time these images

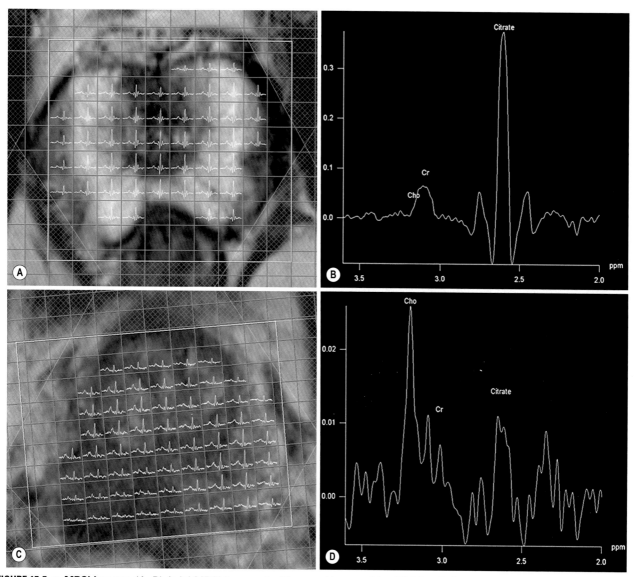

FIGURE 15-7 ■ **MRSI images.** (A, B) Axial MRSI image of a 60-year-old man with a PSA level of 11 ng/mL and no tumour, showing a normal spectrum, with the typical citrate peak at 2.6 ppm. (C, D) Axial MRSI image of a 77-year-old man, with a PSA level of 18 ng/mL and a GS 4 + 3 = 7 in his right peripheral zone (white arrow). The spectrum (D) shows an elevated choline peak and a decreased citrate peak.

are acquired with the help of an endorectal coil. The criteria for extracapsular extension include asymmetry of the neurovascular bundle, obliteration of the recto-prostatic angle, irregularity and/or bulging of the prostatic contour, broad contact (>1 cm) of the tumour focus with the prostatic capsule and signs of capsular rupture with direct tumour extension to the periprostatic fat (Fig. 15-8).

The characteristic findings of SVI include focal low signal intensity in the seminal vesicle (Fig. 15-8), T2 hypointense and enlarged seminal vesicle, T2 hypointense and enlarged ejaculatory duct, obliteration of the vesico-prostatic angle and direct tumour extension from the prostatic base to the seminal vesicle, this last one being the finding with the highest positive predictive value.[77] However, many conditions mimic SVI, and

therefore, a diagnosis of SVI should be made on MP-MRI and not on T2-weighted images alone.

In a meta-analysis published in 2002,[78] a maximum combined sensitivity and specificity of 71% in differenti-ating clinical stages T2 and T3 was reported for conven-tional anatomical T2-weighted imaging at 1.5 T with an endorectal coil (ERC). More recent studies, describing a multi-parametric approach, combining T2-weighted imaging with DCE or MRSI using a 3-T MR system with an ERC, report maximum sensitivities and specificities of 75–88% and 92–100%, respectively.[45,79] For the detection of SVI, sensitivities and specificities of, respectively, 57–65% and 89–91% were reported for T2-weighted images alone. When combining T2-weighted imaging with DCE and DWI the sensitivities and specificities increased to 61–78% and 96–98%, respectively.[80] These

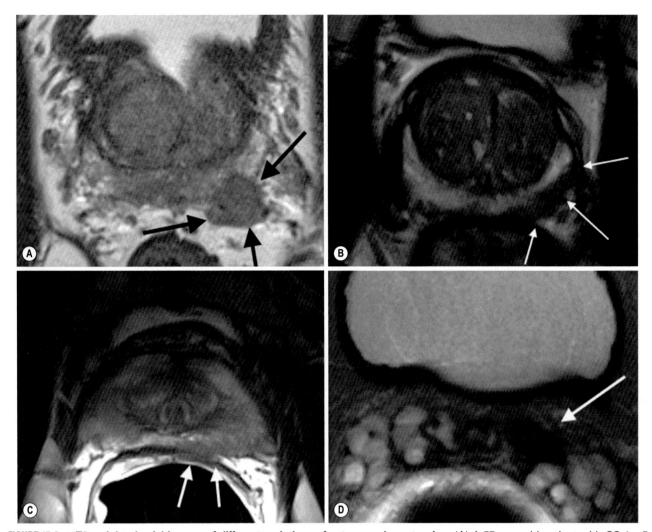

FIGURE 15-8 ■ **T2-weighted axial images of different variations of extracapsular extension.** (A) A 57-year-old patient with GS 4 + 5 = 9, with a bulging tumour in the left peripheral zone (black arrows). (B) A 63-year-old patient with GS 3 + 3 = 6, with a tumour in the left peripheral zone with an irregular border and broad contact with the capsule (white arrows). (C) A 55-year-old patient with GS 3 + 4 = 7, with obliteration of the recto-prostatic angle (white arrows). (D) A 68-year-old patient with GS 4 + 3 = 7, with seminal vesicle infiltration, shown by the low signal intensity in the left seminal vesicle (white arrow).

results underscore the need for a multi-parametric approach in prostate MRI, combining the anatomical findings with those of the functional techniques.

AGGRESSIVENESS

As mentioned earlier, prostate cancer aggressiveness is pathologically graded by the Gleason score,[27] and is, in combination with PSA level and clinical stage, one of the most important prognostic factors in PCa.

On T2-weighted images, areas with low signal intensities have been correlated with higher Gleason grades.[30] Furthermore, several studies on DWI have reported a negative correlation between ADC values and tissue type.[81–83] Healthy prostate tissue has significant higher ADC values than PCa tissue and high-grade (Gleason grade 4 or 5) tumours have significant lower ADC values than low-grade (Gleason grade 3) tumours. In DCE

(semi-)quantitative parameters may have the potential to discriminate low-grade from intermediate-grade plus high-grade PCa in the peripheral zone.[97] In MRSI, a correlation between choline plus creatine-to-citrate ratios and Gleason grade has been reported.[25,84,96]

In conclusion, MP-MRI may help facilitate non-invasive assessment of prostate cancer aggressiveness; however, it will never replace biopsy, because histopathological verification is always required.

1.5 VERSUS 3.0

Multi-parametric prostate MR imaging can be performed at either 1.5 or 3 T. Image acquisition at 3 T results in images with a higher signal-to-noise ratio (SNR), and facilitates high-quality imaging within a short time, without the use of an ERC. Drawbacks of this higher field strength are longer T1 and shorter T2 relaxation times, increased susceptibility artefacts and dielectric effects, higher specific absorption rates and the homogeneity of the magnetic field. However, most of the problems are solved by improvement of the hardware, coils and imaging techniques.

RECURRENCE

Local recurrence of PCa after radical prostatectomy (RP) or radiotherapy (RT) is very frequent, affecting, respectively, 20–50% and 10–60% of the patients after previous treatment.[85,86] Currently, a rise in PSA level is the only major indicator for PCa recurrence, because both DRE and TRUS are of diminished value because of the difficulty in differentiation between recurrent disease or fibrotic changes. MP-MRI can be helpful in the detection of recurrent disease.

After RP, the bladder is usually funnel-shaped, occupying the space created by the absent prostate (Fig. 15-9). In some patients the seminal vesicles might still be present. In the prostatic bed some postoperative fibrosis and granulation tissue can be seen. Postoperative fibrosis presents itself with hypointense signal on the T2- and T1-weighted images, low ADC values and no enhancement on the DCE. Granulation tissue can mimic tumour tissue, because it has hyperintense signal on the T2-weighted images. Furthermore, surgical clips can be shown as hypointensity structures on T2- and T1-weighted images and can produce susceptibility artifacts on DWI and MRSI.

A typical local recurrence (Fig. 15-10) may appear with hyperintense signal on T2-weighted images, low ADC values and high signal intensity on the high b-value images, and enhances early on the DCE images. MRSI of the prostatectomy bed usually suffers from susceptibility artefacts caused by surgical clips, and from the absence of citrate in a properly removed prostate, with difficulty to calculate a CC/C ratio.

Typical locations of local recurrence after RP are around the anastomosis (where the urinary bladder is attached to the membranous urethra), retrovesical (between the urinary bladder and rectum), within the bladder wall, within the seminal vesicles or at the anterior or lateral surgical margins of the prostatectomy bed.[87] A potential pitfall is when there is residual prostate left due to partial or incomplete surgery. This tissue should not be mistaken for local recurrence; however, tumour tissue still might be present.

Radiation therapy can be applied in different forms: external beam radiation therapy (EBRT) or by brachytherapy. During EBRT an external beam of ionising radiation is focused on the prostate. Sometimes a few gold markers are inserted into the prostate to optimise treatment planning (Fig. 15-9). During brachytherapy radioactive seeds are permanently implanted in the prostate (Fig. 15-9). Radiation therapy causes atrophy and fibrosis. For this reason, the entire prostate and seminal vesicles are reduced in size and demonstrate diffusely low signal intensity on T2-weighted images, with an indistinct zonal anatomy.[88]

Local recurrence after RT appears often at the same location as the initial tumour.[89] The detection of local recurrence can be difficult on the T2-weighted images alone. It may present itself as a lesion with a signal intensity lower than that of the surrounding normal prostate tissue; however, it can be unapparent as well, because of decreased contrast between benign irradiated tissue and tumour recurrence, and eventually by decreased image quality as a result of the implanted gold markers or radioactive brachyseeds. However, the latter will influence the quality of DWI in particular. On diffusion-weighted images restricted diffusion might be seen, represented as areas with low ADC values and/or high signal intensity on the high b-value images. On the DCE images recurrent tumour can show early enhancement and early washout (Fig. 15-10). MRSI of the irradiated prostate usually shows high CC/C ratios even in non-malignant cells, because of reparative phenomena that alter the

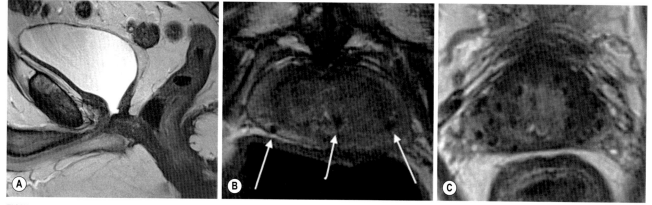

FIGURE 15-9 ■ MRI after previous therapy. (A) T2-weighted sagittal image of the prostatic bed of a 67-year-old patient after radical prostatectomy. (B) T2-weighted axial image of a 76-year-old patient after radiotherapy and 3 inserted gold markers (white arrows). Typical is the diffuse low signal intensity and the indistinct zonal anatomy. (C) T2-weighted axial image of a 72-year-old patient with inserted brachyseeds, shown as little black signal voids. Again, there is diffuse low signal intensity and zonal anatomy is lost.

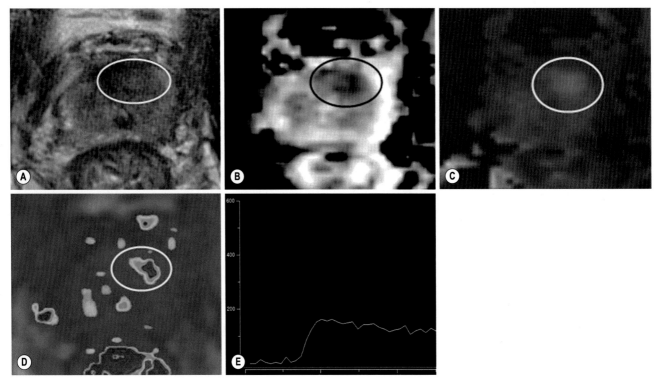

FIGURE 15-10 ■ **(A–E) Multi-parametric MRI of a 72-year-old man with a suspicion of PCa recurrence (white circle) in the left ventral part of the prostate after previous radiotherapy.** The tumour is not visible on the T2-weighted images. On the ADC map and the B1400 image an area of restricted diffusion is seen and on the DCE a small enhancing area is shown. (A) Axial T2-weighted image. (B) Axial ADC map. (C) Axial DWI with b = 1400. (D) Axial DCE image. (E) Curve of the DCE image.

cellular energy requirements (with oxidation of citrate). On the other hand, absence of significant metabolite peaks (also known as 'metabolic atrophy') has been reported to indicate absence of local recurrence, which can be valuable for reassuring patients with rising or repeatedly elevated ('bouncing') post-treatment PSA.[90,91]

Evaluation of extracapsular extension might be hindered by RT-induced irregularity of the capsule.[87]

BIOPSY

As mentioned earlier, random systematic TRUS-guided biopsies have relatively low detection rates and are affected by undersampling and underscoring of PCa.[3,4] As MP-MRI is the most sensitive and specific imaging technique for localising prostate cancer,[18] it can be used to target biopsies towards regions previously determined to be suspicious for cancer.

MR image-guided biopsy can be performed in three different ways and each method has its own benefits and limitations. For each of these methods the MP-MRI for tumour detection and localisation and the biopsy procedure need to be performed in two different sessions, because image post-processing and accurate localisation require time. At the moment there is no consensus as to which is the best method; however, MRI-targeted biopsies result in fewer biopsies in fewer men, with a decreased amount of clinically insignificant cancers compared to standard TRUS biopsy.[92]

The first method is visual targeting, where the urologist performs a TRUS-guided biopsy and aims for specific cancer-suspicious regions (CSR) previously detected on MR images. An advantage of this method is that it needs no additional equipment; however, especially anterior and apical CSRs could be hard to identify on ultrasound images, and can therefore be missed.

The second method is by using rigid or elastic registration or fusion software, where MR images are fused with real-time TRUS images. The crucial factor in this method is accurate fusion of the images, which can be affected by, for example, prostate deformation or patient movement.

The third method is completely MR-guided, so the complete biopsy is performed in the MR scanner itself (Fig. 15-11). A needle guide is inserted in the rectum and the radiologist has to manually adjust the needle guide to aim to the CSR. This procedure needs a trained radiologist and takes more time than a systematic TRUS biopsy. For these reasons MR-compatible robots for needle placement have been developed.[93,94] The first results are promising and in the future these robots might also play a role in MR-guided therapies as focal laser ablation and cryoablation.

PROTOCOLS

In 2012 a group of prostate MRI experts from the ESUR published a set of guidelines for MRI in prostate cancer.[17] Two different MRI protocols are recommended in these guidelines: one for detection and localisation of primary or recurrent PCa, and one for local staging of PCa.

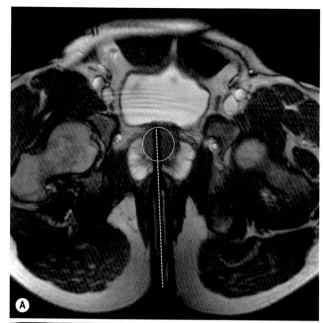

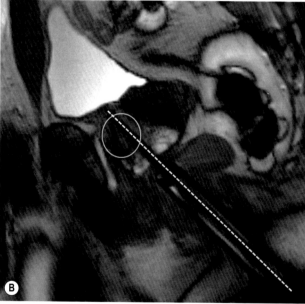

FIGURE 15-11 ■ Same patient as described and depicted in Fig. 15-5. MRI-guided biopsy of the cancer suspicious region (white circle) revealed a GS 4 + 4 = 8. (A) Axial oblique image with the needle (white dashed line) in the prostate. (B) Sagittal image of the same needle (white dashed line).

Detection and Localisation of Primary or Recurrent PCa

The detection protocol is a fast (<30 min) protocol without involvement of an ERC. Imaging can adequately be performed at 1.5 T, always using a good 8- to 16-channel pelvic phased array (PPA). Anti-peristaltic drugs (Buscopan, glucagon) should be administered to provide optimal imaging with fewer motion artefacts, both in 1.5 and 3 T. Optionally, MRSI can be added to the detection protocol. This requires an additional

10–15 min of examination time and the use of an ERC is mandatory at 1.5 T and optional at 3 T.

The minimum requirements should include images covering the entire prostate:

- T2-weighted axial and sagittal images with a slice thickness of 4 mm at 1.5 T and 3 mm at 3 T: the in-plane resolution should be at least 0.5 × 0.5 to 0.7 × 0.7 mm at both 1.5 and 3 T. The phase-encoding direction should be from left to right to minimise motion artefacts.
- DWI axial images with a slice thickness of 5 mm at 1.5 T and 4 mm at 3 T: the in-plane resolution should be at least 1.5 × 1.5 to 2.0 × 2.0 mm at 1.5 T and 1.0 × 1.0 to 1.5 × 1.5 mm at 3 T. At least 3 b-values (0, 100 and 800–1000 s/mm^2) should be acquired in three orthogonal directions and adapted to quality of SNR. An ADC map should be calculated and the highest b-value used for that should be 1000 s/mm^2.
- DCE-MRI axial images with a slice thickness of 4 mm at both 1.5 and 3 T: the in-plane resolution should be at least 1.0 × 1.0 mm at 1.5 T and 0.7 × 0.7 mm at 3 T. Quantitative or semi-quantitative DCE-MRI analysis is not mandatory. The maximum temporal resolution should be 15 s following a single dose of contrast agent, with an injection rate of 3 mL/s. Imaging acquisition should be prolonged for 5 min to detect washout. Unenhanced T1-weighted images can be used to detect post-biopsy haematomas.
- MRSI: The volume of interest (VOI) should cover the whole prostate and should be aligned to the axial T2-weighted images. The field of view (FOV) should be at least 1.5 voxels larger than the VOI in all directions to avoid back folding or wrap-around. A matrix of at least 8 × 8 × 8 phase-encoding steps with nominal voxel size <0.5 cc should be used. Spectral selective suppression of water and lipid signals. At least six fat-saturation bands should be positioned close to the prostatic margin (inside the VOI is allowed) to conform to the prostatic shape as closely as possible; Automatic or manual shimming should be performed up to a line width at half-height of the water resonance peak between 15 and 20 Hz at 1.5 T and between 20 and 25 Hz at 3 T.

Staging of PCa

The staging protocol takes 45 min and is generally used for evaluating minimal extracapsular extension. The use of an ERC is highly preferred in this examination. Images should include the entire prostate and anti-peristaltic drugs should be given.

- T2-weighted axial, sagittal and coronal images with a slice thickness of 3 mm at 1.5 and 3 T. The in-plane resolution should be at least 0.3 × 0.3 to 0.7 × 0.7 mm at 1.5 T and 0.3 × 0.3 to 0.5 × 0.5 mm at 3 T.
- DWI and DCE-MRI: same requirements as in the detection protocol.
- MRSI optional.

370 **15** PROSTATE

REFERENCES

1. Siegel R, Naishadham D, Jemal A. Cancer statistics, 2013. CA Cancer J Clin 2013;63(1):11–30.
2. Max W, Rice DP, Sung HY, et al. The economic burden of prostate cancer, California, 1998. Cancer 2002;94(11):2906–13.
3. Chun FK, Epstein JI, Ficarra V, et al. Optimizing performance and interpretation of prostate biopsy: a critical analysis of the literature. Eur Urol 2010;58(6):851–64.
4. Hambrock T, Hoeks C, Hulsbergen-van de KC, et al. Prospective assessment of prostate cancer aggressiveness using 3-T diffusion-weighted magnetic resonance imaging-guided biopsies versus a systematic 10-core transrectal ultrasound prostate biopsy cohort. Eur Urol 2012;61(1):177–84.
5. Franiel T, Hamm B, Hricak H. Dynamic contrast-enhanced magnetic resonance imaging and pharmacokinetic models in prostate cancer. Eur Radiol 2010;21(3):616–26.
6. Tan CH, Wang J, Kundra V. Diffusion weighted imaging in prostate cancer. Eur Radiol 2010;593–603.
7. Weinreb JC, Blume JD, Coakley FV, et al. Prostate cancer: sextant localization at MR imaging and MR spectroscopic imaging before prostatectomy—results of ACRIN prospective multi-institutional clinicopathologic study. Radiology 2009;251(1):122–33.
8. Tanimoto A, Nakashima J, Kohno H, et al. Prostate cancer screening: the clinical value of diffusion-weighted imaging and dynamic MR imaging in combination with T2-weighted imaging. J Magn Reson Imaging 2007;25(1):146–52.
9. Girouin N, Mege-Lechevallier F, Tonina Senes A, et al. Prostate dynamic contrast-enhanced MRI with simple visual diagnostic criteria: is it reasonable? Eur Radiol 2007;17(6):1498–509.
10. Ben CA, Girouin N, Ryon-Taponnier P, et al. [MR detection of local prostate cancer recurrence after transrectal high-intensity focused US treatment: preliminary results]. J Radiol 2008;89(5. Pt 1):571–7.
11. Tamada T, Sone T, Jo Y, et al. Apparent diffusion coefficient values in peripheral and transition zones of the prostate: comparison between normal and malignant prostatic tissues and correlation with histologic grade. J Magn Reson Imaging 2008;28(3):720–6.
12. Turkbey B, Shah VP, Pang Y, et al. Is apparent diffusion coefficient associated with clinical risk scores for prostate cancers that are visible on 3-T MR images? Radiology 2011;258(2):488–95.
13. Hambrock T, Somford DM, Huisman HJ, et al. Relationship between apparent diffusion coefficients at 3.0-T MR imaging and Gleason grade in peripheral zone prostate cancer. Radiology 2011;259(2):453–61.
14. Nagel KN, Schouten MG, Hambrock T, et al. Differentiation of prostatitis and prostate cancer by using diffusion-weighted MR imaging and MR-guided biopsy at 3 T. Radiology 2013;267(1):164–72.
15. Villeirs GM, Oosterlinck W, Vanherreweghe E, De Meerleer GO. A qualitative approach to combined magnetic resonance imaging and spectroscopy in the diagnosis of prostate cancer. Eur J Radiol 2010;73(2):352–6.
16. Scheenen TW, Klomp DW, Roll SA, et al. Fast acquisition-weighted three-dimensional proton MR spectroscopic imaging of the human prostate. Magn Reson Med 2004;52(1):80–8.
17. Barentsz JO, Richenberg J, Clements R, et al. ESUR prostate MR guidelines 2012. Eur Radiol 2012;22(4):746–57.
18. Sciarra A, Barentsz J, Bjartell A, et al. Advances in magnetic resonance imaging: how they are changing the management of prostate cancer. Eur Urol 2011;59(6):962–77.
19. Chen ME, Johnston DA, Tang K, et al. Detailed mapping of prostate carcinoma foci: biopsy strategy implications. Cancer 2000;89(8):1800–9.
20. McNeal JE, Redwine EA, Freiha FS, Stamey TA. Zonal distribution of prostatic adenocarcinoma. Correlation with histologic pattern and direction of spread. Am J Surg Pathol 1988;12(12):897–906.
21. McNeal JE. Normal anatomy of the prostate and changes in benign prostatic hypertrophy and carcinoma. Semin Ultrasound CT MR 1988;9(5):329–34.
22. Coakley FV, Hricak H. Radiologic anatomy of the prostate gland: a clinical approach. Radiol Clin North Am 2000;38(1):15–30.
23. Hricak H, Dooms GC, Mcneal JE, et al. MR imaging of the prostate gland: normal anatomy. Am J Roentgenol 1987;148(1):51–8.
24. Ross JS, Jennings TA, Nazeer T, et al. Prognostic factors in prostate cancer. Am J Clin Pathol 2003;120:85–100.
25. Zakian KL, Sircar K, Hricak H, et al. Correlation of proton MR spectroscopic imaging with Gleason score based on step-section pathologic analysis after radical prostatectomy. Radiology 2005;234(3):804–14.
26. Wolf A, Wender RC, Etzioni RB, et al. American Cancer Society guideline for the early detection of prostate cancer: update 2010. CA Cancer J Clin 2010;60(2):70–98.
27. Gleason DF, Mellinger GT. Prediction of prognosis for prostatic adenocarcinoma by combined histological grading and clinical staging. J Urol 1974;111(1):58–64.
28. Falzarano SM, Magi-Galluzzi C. Staging prostate cancer and its relationship to prognosis. Diagnostic Histopathology 2010;16(9):432–8.
29. Epstein J, Allsbrook W Jr, Amin M, Egevad L. The 2005 International Society of Urological Pathology (ISUP) consensus conference on Gleason grading of prostatic carcinoma. Am J Surg Pathol 2005;29(9):1228–42.
30. Wang L, Mazaheri Y, Zhang J, et al. Assessment of biologic aggressiveness of prostate cancer: correlation of MR signal intensity with Gleason grade after radical prostatectomy. Radiology 2008;246(1):168–76.
31. Quint LE, Van Erp JS, Bland PH, et al. Prostate cancer: correlation of MR images with tissue optical density at pathologic examination. Radiology 1991;179(3):837–42.
32. Shukla-Dave A, Hricak H, Eberhardt SC, et al. Chronic prostatitis: MR imaging and ^{1}H MR spectroscopic imaging findings—initial observations. Radiology 2004;231(3):717–24.
33. Cruz M, Tsuda K, Narumi Y, et al. Characterization of low-intensity lesions in the peripheral zone of prostate on pre-biopsy endorectal coil MR imaging. Eur Radiol 2002;12(2):357–65.
34. Akin O, Sala E, Moskowitz CS, et al. Transition zone prostate cancers: features, detection, localization, and staging at endorectal MR imaging. Radiology 2006;239(3):784–92.
35. Cheikh AB, Girouin N, Colombel M, et al. Evaluation of T2-weighted and dynamic contrast-enhanced MRI in localizing prostate cancer before repeat biopsy. Eur Radiol 2009;19(3):770–8.
36. Chen M, Dang HD, Wang JY, et al. Prostate cancer detection: comparison of T2-weighted imaging, diffusion-weighted imaging, proton magnetic resonance spectroscopic imaging, and the three techniques combined. Acta Radiol 2008;49(5):602–10.
37. Jager GJ, Ruijter ET, van de Kaa CA, et al. Local staging of prostate cancer with endorectal MR imaging: correlation with histopathology. Am J Roentgenol 1996;166(4):845–52.
38. Kim JK, Hong SS, Choi YJ, et al. Wash-in rate on the basis of dynamic contrast-enhanced MRI: usefulness for prostate cancer detection and localization. J Magn Reson Imaging 2005;22(5):639–46.
39. Bianco FJ Jr, Scardino PT, Stephenson AJ, et al. Long-term oncologic results of salvage radical prostatectomy for locally recurrent prostate cancer after radiotherapy. Int J Radiat Oncol Biol Phys 2005;62(2):448–53.
40. Qayyum A, Coakley FV, Lu Y, et al. Organ-confined prostate cancer: effect of prior transrectal biopsy on endorectal MRI and MR spectroscopic imaging. Am J Roentgenol 2004;183(4):1079–83.
41. Kuhl CK, Mielcareck P, Klaschik S, et al. Dynamic breast MR imaging: are signal intensity time course data useful for differential diagnosis of enhancing lesions? Radiology 1999;211(1):101–10.
42. Franiel T, Ludemann L, Rudolph B, et al. Evaluation of normal prostate tissue, chronic prostatitis, and prostate cancer by quantitative perfusion analysis using a dynamic contrast-enhanced inversion-prepared dual-contrast gradient echo sequence. Invest Radiol 2008;43(7):481–7.
43. Barentsz JO, Engelbrecht M, Jager GJ, et al. Fast dynamic gadolinium-enhanced MR imaging of urinary bladder and prostate cancer. J Magn Reson Imaging 1999;10(3):295–304.
44. Bott SR, Ahmed HU, Hindley RG, et al. The index lesion and focal therapy: an analysis of the pathological characteristics of prostate cancer. BJU Int 2010;106(11):1607–11.
45. Fütterer JJ, Heijmink SW, Scheenen TWJ, et al. Prostate cancer localization with dynamic contrast-enhanced MR imaging and proton MR spectroscopic imaging. Radiology 2006;241(2):449–58.

46. Ocak I, Bernardo M, Metzger G, et al. Dynamic contrast-enhanced MRI of prostate cancer at 3 T: a study of pharmacokinetic parameters. Am J Roentgenol 2007;189(4):W192.

47. Tanaka N, Samma S, Joko M, et al. Diagnostic usefulness of endorectal magnetic resonance imaging with dynamic contrast enhancement in patients with localized prostate cancer: mapping studies with biopsy specimens. Int J Urol 1999;6(12):593–9.

48. Fütterer JJ, Engelbrecht MR, Huisman HJ, et al. Staging prostate cancer with dynamic contrast-enhanced endorectal MR imaging prior to radical prostatectomy: experienced versus less experienced readers. Radiology 2005;237(2):541–9.

49. Qayyum A. Diffusion-weighted imaging in the abdomen and pelvis: concepts and applications. Radiographics 2009;29(6): 1797–810.

50. Padhani AR, Liu G, Mu-Koh D, et al. Diffusion-weighted magnetic resonance imaging as a cancer biomarker: consensus and recommendations. Neoplasia 2009;11(2):102–25.

51. Tamada T, Sone T, Toshimitsu S, et al. Age related and zonal anatomical changes of apparent diffusion coefficient values in normal human prostatic tissues. J Magn Reson Imaging 2008;27(3): 552–6.

52. Somford DM, Futterer JJ, Hambrock T, Barentsz JO. Diffusion and perfusion MR imaging of the prostate. Magn Reson Imaging Clin North Am 2008;16(4):685–95, ix.

53. Ren J, Huan Y, Wang H, et al. Diffusion-weighted imaging in normal prostate and differential diagnosis of prostate diseases. Abdom Imaging 2008;33(6):724–8.

54. Bour L, Schull A, Delongchamps NB, et al. Multiparametric MRI features of granulomatous prostatitis and tubercular prostate abscess. Diagn Interv Imaging 2013;94(1):84–90.

55. Anderson A, Xie J, Pizzonia J, et al. Effects of cell volume fraction changes on apparent diffusion in human cells. Magn Reson Imaging 2000;18(6):689–95.

56. Verma S, Rajesh A, Morales H, et al. Assessment of aggressiveness of prostate cancer: correlation of apparent diffusion coefficient with histologic grade after radical prostatectomy. Am J Roentgenol 2011;196(2):374–81.

57. Woodfield CA, Tung GA, Grand DJ, et al. Diffusion-weighted MRI of peripheral zone prostate cancer: comparison of tumor apparent diffusion coefficient with Gleason score and percentage of tumor on core biopsy. Am J Roentgenol 2010;194(4):W316.

58. Kurhanewicz J, Vigneron DB, Hricak H, et al. Three-dimensional H-1 MR spectroscopic imaging of the in situ human prostate with high (0.24–0.7-cm³) spatial resolution. Radiology 1996;198(3): 795–805.

59. Costello LC, Franklin RB. The intermediary metabolism of the prostate: a key to understanding the pathogenesis and progression of prostate malignancy. Oncology 2000;59(4):269–82.

60. Podo F. Tumour phospholipid metabolism. NMR Biomed 1999;12(7):413–39.

61. Glunde K, Ackerstaff E, Mori N, et al. Choline phospholipid metabolism in cancer: consequences for molecular pharmaceutical interventions. Mol Pharm 2006;3(5):496–506.

62. Fuchsjager M, Shukla-Dave A, Akin O, et al. Prostate cancer imaging. Acta Radiol 2008;49(1):107–20.

63. Shukla-Dave A, Hricak H, Moskowitz C, et al. Detection of prostate cancer with MR spectroscopic imaging: an expanded paradigm incorporating polyamines. Radiology 2007;245(2):499–506.

64. Jung JA, Coakley FV, Vigneron DB, et al. Prostate depiction at endorectal MR spectroscopic imaging: investigation of a standardized evaluation system. Radiology 2004;233(3):701–8.

65. Scheenen TW, Futterer J, Weiland E, et al. Discriminating cancer from noncancer tissue in the prostate by 3-dimensional proton magnetic resonance spectroscopic imaging: a prospective multicenter validation study. Invest Radiol 2011;46(1):25–33.

66. Futterer JJ, Scheenen TW, Heijmink SW, et al. Standardized threshold approach using three-dimensional proton magnetic resonance spectroscopic imaging in prostate cancer localization of the entire prostate. Invest Radiol 2007;42(2):116–22.

67. Testa C, Schiavina R, Lodi R, et al. Prostate cancer: sextant localization with MR imaging, MR spectroscopy, and ¹¹C-choline PET/CT. Radiology 2007;244(3):797–806.

68. Sciarra A, Panebianco V, Ciccariello M, et al. Value of magnetic resonance spectroscopy imaging and dynamic contrast-enhanced imaging for detecting prostate cancer foci in men with prior negative biopsy. Clin Cancer Res 2010;16(6):1875–83.

69. Yuen JS, Thng CH, Tan PH, et al. Endorectal magnetic resonance imaging and spectroscopy for the detection of tumor foci in men with prior negative transrectal ultrasound prostate biopsy. J Urol 2004;171(4):1482–6.

70. Wefer AE, Hricak H, Vigneron DB, et al. Sextant localization of prostate cancer: comparison of sextant biopsy, magnetic resonance imaging and magnetic resonance spectroscopic imaging with step section histology. J Urol 2000;164(2):400–4.

71. Umbehr M, Bachmann LM, Held U, et al. Combined magnetic resonance imaging and magnetic resonance spectroscopy imaging in the diagnosis of prostate cancer: a systematic review and meta-analysis. Eur Urol 2009;55(3):575–90.

72. Seitz M, Shukla-Dave A, Bjartell A, et al. Functional magnetic resonance imaging in prostate cancer. Eur Urol 2009;55(4): 801–14.

73. Scheidler J, Hricak H, Vigneron DB, et al. Prostate cancer: localization with three-dimensional proton MR spectroscopic imaging—clinicopathologic study. Radiology 1999;213(2):473–80.

74. Bostwick DG. Staging prostate cancer—1997: current methods and limitations. Eur Urol 1997;32(Suppl. 3):2–14.

75. Wang L, Hricak H, Kattan MW, et al. Prediction of seminal vesicle invasion in prostate cancer: incremental value of adding endorectal MR imaging to the Kattan nomogram. Radiology 2007;242(1): 182–8.

76. Wang L, Hricak H, Kattan MW, et al. Prediction of organ-confined prostate cancer: incremental value of MR imaging and MR spectroscopic imaging to staging nomograms. Radiology 2006;238(2): 597–603.

77. Sala E, Akin O, Moskowitz CS, et al. Endorectal MR imaging in the evaluation of seminal vesicle invasion: diagnostic accuracy and multivariate feature analysis. Radiology 2006;238(3):929–37.

78. Engelbrecht MR, Jager GJ, Laheij RJ, et al. Local staging of prostate cancer using magnetic resonance imaging: a meta-analysis. Eur Radiol 2002;12(9):2294–302.

79. Bloch BN, Genega EM, Costa DN, et al. Prediction of prostate cancer extracapsular extension with high spatial resolution dynamic contrast-enhanced 3-T MRI. Eur Radiol 2012;22(10): 2201–10.

80. Soylu FN, Peng Y, Jiang Y, et al. Seminal vesicle invasion in prostate cancer: evaluation by using multiparametric endorectal MR imaging. Radiology 2013;267(3):797–806.

81. Vargas HA, Akin O, Franiel T, et al. Diffusion-weighted endorectal MR imaging at 3 T for prostate cancer: tumor detection and assessment of aggressiveness. Radiology 2011;259(3):775–84.

82. Hambrock T, Somford DM, Huisman HJ, et al. Relationship between apparent diffusion coefficients at 3.0-T MR imaging and Gleason grade in peripheral zone prostate cancer. Radiology 2011;259(2):453–61.

83. Oto A, Yang C, Kayhan A, et al. Diffusion-weighted and dynamic contrast-enhanced MRI of prostate cancer: correlation of quantitative MR parameters with Gleason score and tumor angiogenesis. Am J Roentgenol 2011;197(6):1382–90.

84. Villeirs GM, De Meerleer GO, De Visschere PJ, et al. Combined magnetic resonance imaging and spectroscopy in the assessment of high grade prostate carcinoma in patients with elevated PSA: a single-institution experience of 356 patients. Eur J Radiol 2011; 77(2):340–5.

85. Allen GW, Howard AR, Jarrard DF, Ritter MA. Management of prostate cancer recurrences after radiation therapy-brachytherapy as a salvage option. Cancer 2007;110(7):1405–16.

86. Panebianco V, Barchetti F, Sciarra A, et al. Prostate cancer recurrence after radical prostatectomy: the role of 3-T diffusion imaging in multi-parametric magnetic resonance imaging. Eur Radiol 2013;23(6):1745–52.

87. Vargas HA, Wassberg C, Akin O, Hricak H. MR imaging of treated prostate cancer. Radiology 2012;262(1):26–42.

88. Chan TW, Kressel HY. Prostate and seminal vesicles after irradiation: MR appearance. J Magn Reson Imaging 1991;1(5): 503–11.

89. Pucar D, Hricak H, Shukla-Dave A, et al. Clinically significant prostate cancer local recurrence after radiation therapy occurs at the site of primary tumor: magnetic resonance imaging and step-section pathology evidence. Int J Radiat Oncol Biol Phys 2007; 69(1):62–9.

90. Coakley FV, Teh HS, Qayyum A, et al. Endorectal MR imaging and MR spectroscopic imaging for locally recurrent prostate cancer

after external beam radiation therapy: preliminary experience. Radiology 2004;233(2):441–8.

91. Pickett B, Kurhanewicz J, Coakley F, et al. Use of MRI and spectroscopy in evaluation of external beam radiotherapy for prostate cancer. Int J Radiat Oncol Biol Phys 2004;60(4): 1047–55.

92. Moore CM, Robertson NL, Arsanious N, et al. Image-guided prostate biopsy using magnetic resonance imaging-derived targets: a systematic review. Eur Urol 2013;63(1):125–40.

93. Yakar D, Schouten MG, Bosboom DGH, et al. Feasibility of a pneumatically actuated MR-compatible robot for transrectal prostate biopsy guidance. Radiology 2011;260(1): 241–7.

94. Tokuda J, Fischer GS, DiMaio SP, et al. Integrated navigation and control software system for MRI-guided robotic prostate interventions. Comput Med Imaging Graph 2010;34(1):3–8.

95. Hoeks CM, Barentsz JO, Hambrock T, et al. Prostate cancer: multi-parametric MR imaging for detection, localization, and staging. Radiology 2011;261(1):46–66.

96. Kobus T, Vos PC, Hambrock T, et al. Prostate cancer aggressiveness: in vivo assessment of MR spectroscopy and diffusion-weighted imaging at 3T. Radiology 2012;265(2):457–67.

97. Vos EK, Litjens GJS, Kobus T, et al. Assessment of prostate cancer aggressiveness using dynamic contrast-enhanced magnetic resonance imaging at 3T. Eur Urol 2013;64(3):448–55.

CHAPTER 16

MALE GENITOURINARY TRACT

Nadeem Shaida • Lol Berman

METHODS OF EXAMINATION

Although ultrasound (US) is the method of choice for imaging the scrotal contents, an increasing number of publications now describe magnetic resonance imaging (MRI) in the evaluation of testicular masses. MRI has been assessed in patients following an inconclusive US study with a claimed role as a problem-solving tool with particular benefit in differentiating paratesticular from testicular masses and in helping to further characterise masses as solid, cystic or containing fat.[1]

Computed tomography (CT) and MRI are the investigations of choice in the staging of testicular malignancy and are used in the evaluation of undescended testes that have not been demonstrated sonographically. Radionuclide imaging is still employed in some centres in the evaluation of acute testicular torsion but in practice has now been superseded by colour Doppler US studies. Contrast venography is undertaken to define the anatomy of varicoceles and is often supplemented by embolic techniques, thereby reducing the need for operative intervention in this situation. Intravascular studies with iodinated contrast agents, both venous and arterial, continue to play a part in the assessment of male impotence but Doppler ultrasound may well be able to replace many of these invasive investigations.

ANATOMY

The testicular parenchyma consists almost entirely of seminiferous tubules enclosed by the fibrous tunica albuginea which extends as septations between lobules of testicular tissue, dividing the testis into several hundred lobules. These septations cannot be imaged except where they converge at the mediastinum testis to produce a linear structure which is reflective on US. The seminiferous tubules merge centrally to form the rete testis, from which efferent tubules perforate the tunica albuginea and convey seminal fluid to the epididymis. The adult testis is 3–5 cm in length and 2–3 cm in transverse diameter and depth. The normal adult testicular volume is 15–20 mL, calculated from the formula: length × width × depth × 0.52 = volume. At the superior pole is a remnant of the Müllerian duct, the appendix of the testis or hydatid of Morgagni, a 3- to 5-mm appendage of similar reflectivity to the testis. A further appendage, the appendix of the epididymis, is situated adjacent to the testicular appendix at the upper pole of the testis (Figs. 16-1–16-3). The epididymis is usually described and illustrated as a tubular structure posterior to the testis. This is far from universal as it may be demonstrated on US laterally or even anterior to the testis. The epididymis comprises a head, tail and body. The head lies adjacent to the superior pole of the testis; the body is formed from the confluence of the ductules of the rete testis to form a single ductus epididymis; this continues as the tail of the epididymis at the inferior aspect of the testis. At the tail of the epididymis, the duct courses cephalad to form the vas deferens. In its developmental descent through the inguinal canal, the testis is invested by a layer of visceral and parietal peritoneum, the processus vaginalis. In normal development the processus obliterates with no residual connection with the peritoneal cavity. The layers of peritoneum surrounding the testis and appendages persist as the tunica vaginalis.

The scrotal contents have a triple arterial supply. The deferential artery is a branch of the inferior vesical artery and accompanies the vas deferens, branching into a capillary network at the tail of the epididymis and is the main blood supply to that organ. The testis is predominantly supplied by the testicular artery, which originates directly from the abdominal aorta, inferior to the renal arteries, passing through the inguinal canal with the spermatic cord. The distal testicular artery branches into capsular arteries surrounded by tunica albuginea. Centripetal

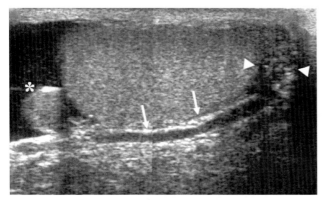

FIGURE 16-1 ■ Normal testis, montaged longitudinal US view showing tail (arrowheads), body (arrows) and appendix (asterisk) of the epididymis.

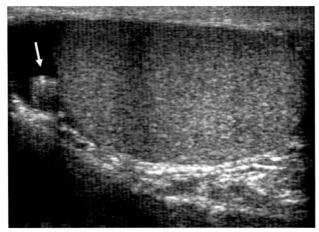

FIGURE 16-2 ■ Normal testis, slightly more medial view of same subject as in Fig. 16-1, demonstrating the appendix of the testis (arrow).

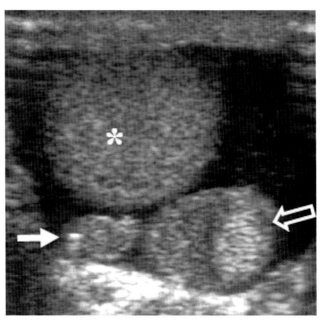

FIGURE 16-3 ■ Transverse US view demonstrating both appendages adjacent to the upper pole of the testis. Epididymis (open arrow), appendix testis (closed arrow) and testis (asterisk) are shown.

arteries arise from the capsular arteries, flow towards the mediastinum testis and thence into the testicular parenchyma as arterioles and capillaries. The cremasteric arteries are branches of the inferior epigastric artery, and after accompanying the spermatic cord, anastomose with the testicular and deferential arteries.

The venous drainage of the testis is via the pampiniform plexus, draining to the gonadal vein. The scrotal wall and epididymis drain via the cremasteric plexus.[2,3]

SCROTAL MASSES

Scrotal masses can be considered as abnormalities arising from the testis and masses arising from adjacent structures. The distinction is frequently obvious to the referring clinician and can usually be made with ease on the ultrasound study with a claimed sensitivity of 100%.[4] The specificity for distinguishing malignant from benign intratesticular lesions is less reliable. A false-positive rate of 22% for malignancy was reported in the sonographic evaluation of 23 scrotal masses. The abnormalities contributing to this overdiagnosis of malignancy included testicular infarction, epididymal tumour, organised haematoma and epididymo-orchitis.[5] Occasionally, the testicular parenchyma may be compressed and distorted by a large extratesticular lesion to the extent that the distinction between testicular and extratesticular origin is difficult without surgical exploration. Numerous early descriptions of the role of US have advised that intratesticular lesions are to be regarded as malignant until surgically proven to be otherwise.[6] This impression has not altered in the intervening years with the proviso that percutaneous biopsy under US guidance may emerge as

an alternative to open surgery for defining indeterminate lesions.[7] More recent advances in US technology such as the development of sonoelastography to assess the 'stiffness' of focal intratesticular lesions have also demonstrated promising early results.[8]

TESTICULAR MASSES

Malignant Testicular Pathology

Testicular malignancies include primary testicular germ cell tumours, non germ cell tumours, metastases, lymphoma and adrenal rest tumours.

Primary testicular malignancy comprises approximately 1% of malignancies in men, with an incidence of 3 : 100,000 per annum. This peaks between the age of 15 and 45 years where it accounts from approximately 9% of deaths from malignant disease. The most publicised risk factor is cryptorchidism which appears to be a factor in 10% of primary testicular malignancy. This increased risk persists after orchidopexy and, mysteriously, includes an increased risk of malignancy in the normal contralateral testis in men with unilateral cryptorchidism. Other reported associations include mumps orchitis, testicular microlithiasis, infective orchitis and infertility. The risk of developing a further malignancy in the contralateral testis several years after initial treatment of testicular malignancy is 500–700 times the incidence in the normal population. At present there is no common policy regarding screening any of the at-risk populations although there is an emerging consensus regarding microlithiasis. There is an unexplained rising incidence and geographical variation to testicular malignancy. An incidence of 8 : 100,000 is reported in Denmark compared with 2 : 100,000 in Israel.[9]

Testicular tumours usually present with a painless unilateral scrotal mass noticed by the patient on self-examination. Approximately 10% present with acute pain thought to be due to haemorrhage. A small group present with metastases from an undeclared primary, which may be demonstrated by US when still clinically impalpable. In this setting the reported negative predictive value of 100% for excluding testicular malignancy is reassuring but should be considered in the light of a recent report of US negative intratubular germ cell neoplasms discovered at orchiectomy in patients with the rare presentation of paraneoplastic meningitis.[10]

Approximately 95% of primary testicular tumours are of germ cell origin, the remainder arising from Leydig, Sertoli or theca cells that comprise the gonadal stroma. Most germ cell tumours are of single histological type and are seminomas. In order of frequency, other histological types comprise embryonal tumours, yolk sac tumours and teratomas. Approximately 40% of tumours are of mixed cellularity. The peak incidence of seminoma is in the fourth and fifth decades, while the incidence of other germ cell tumours peak approximately a decade earlier. All testicular tumours are rare in childhood, where yolk sac tumours, followed by teratomas, are the most common. Seminomas are generally extremely radiosensitive; they are associated with high levels of alphafeto-protein (AFP) but less often with human chorionic gonadotrophin (hCG). Teratomas respond well to a number of chemotherapeutic agents and are associated with elevated AFP and hCG. They are characteristically less responsive to radiotherapy.

The differentiation of seminoma from the other histological types is important clinically but, despite some variation in the 'textbook' appearances, there are generally insufficient features to make the distinction using direct imaging or Doppler features. Seminomas are characteristically hyporeflective compared with the surrounding parenchyma and are well-defined and homogeneous (Fig. 16-4). They may also be apparently multifocal on presentation. The typical embryonal cell tumour is less homogeneous and well-defined, while teratomas are of mixed reflectivity and more likely than seminoma to contain cystic spaces and calcifications (Figs. 16-5 and 16-6).

Increased tumour flow on Doppler ultrasound is common but not invariable and in practice this cannot be used to differentiate neoplastic from non-neoplastic, benign from malignant or one cell type from another.[11]

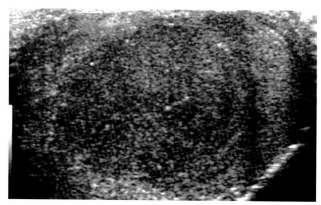

FIGURE 16-4 ■ **Seminoma: longitudinal US view.** The slightly hyporeflective lesion is almost replacing the entire testis. Microcalcifications are seen in the normal and abnormal parenchyma.

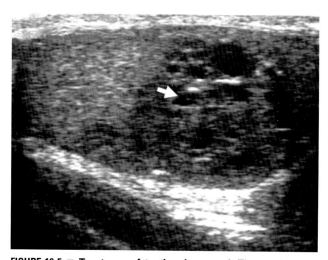

FIGURE 16-5 ■ **Teratoma of testis, ultrasound.** The cystic areas (arrows) within the lesion are characteristic.

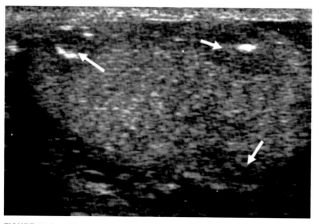

FIGURE 16-6 ■ **Teratoma, ultrasound.** The malignancy is multifocal with macrocalcifications (arrows).

Staging Testicular Malignancy

Testicular tumours extend into the surrounding testicular parenchyma and from the mediastinum testis to the epididymis. The lymphatics accompany the venous drainage to retroperitoneal nodes at the level of the renal hila.

The local inguinal nodes are not typically involved unless there has been invasion of the scrotal wall. Although up to 96% accuracy has been claimed for ultrasound in the diagnosis of retroperitoneal metastases,[12] the widespread availability of more accurate cross-sectional techniques has increased since this report, and in practice ultrasound would no longer be primarily used, although it may still have a role in evaluating visceral metastases. Current best practice suggests the use of CT to assess the retroperitoneal and mediastinal lymph nodes.[13] MRI of the retroperitoneum is feasible but as yet has not been widely adopted, due to cost, and instead serves a role in selected patients where repeat CT examinations may be undesirable.[14] 18-FDG-PET or 18-FDG-PET/CT examinations do not form part of the diagnostic algorithm for initial staging but may be helpful in the evaluation of residual disease after chemotherapy.[15]

Computed Tomography

Although a chest radiograph will demonstrate the larger pulmonary and mediastinal metastases, CT reliably demonstrates pulmonary lesions of 3–4 mm in diameter. These are frequently peripheral (subpleural and basal—in line with maximal ventilation and perfusion) but no lung segment is exempt. In the relatively younger age group susceptible to testicular malignancy, pulmonary lesions that may mimic lung metastases such as old granulomata are not common. Nevertheless, care should be taken before assuming that a lung lesion is a metastasis, especially in the absence of mediastinal lymphadenopathy. Mediastinal deposits are less common than pulmonary metastases but care should be taken in the subcarinal region. It is debatable whether iodinated intravenous contrast enhancement should be used routinely. However, close attention should be paid to the mediastinum at soft-tissue settings. Unexpected lesions in the hila or mediastinum with absent tumour markers, favourable histology and a normal retroperitoneum should raise the possibility of coincidental disease such as sarcoidosis.

There are few pitfalls in the evaluation of the para-aortic chain apart from the generic problems common to all CT studies of the retroperitoneum such as underfilled bowel loops, anomalous venous anatomy, etc. The spread of testicular malignancy is predictable. Left-sided lesions spread to the upper left para-aortic chain closer to the left renal vein than the aortic bifurcation. Metastases from right-sided lesions tend to be situated slightly more caudad and are usually seen in the anterior interaortico-caval recess. Right-sided lesions may, however, be situated at a more superior level and, when located just posterior to the third part of the duodenum, can prove problematic to the surgeon should resection of a residual mass at this site be required.

Only when nodal disease is well established in the ipsilateral side does crossover to the contralateral side and inferior spread to the inguinal nodes occur. Isolated contralateral lymphadenopathy should be viewed with extreme suspicion. Isolated pelvic disease is slightly more common but still rare in uncomplicated testicular tumours. Naturally it can occur where there has been previous testicular maldescent or scrotal involvement.

The whole pelvis should be examined at initial staging but it is controversial whether this needs to be undertaken at follow-up in straightforward cases; radiation dose is a consideration in these usually young patients. The accurate staging of testicular malignancy is important and can influence treatment (surveillance, radiotherapy, chemotherapy, etc.). The radiological findings should be considered with other diagnostic features such as cell type and tumour markers. If staging uncertainty persists, a limited repeated CT study at, say, 6 weeks can often resolve the matter. The lung nodule or para-aortic mass may have enlarged and involvement can be assumed.

Non-Primary Testicular Malignancies, Lymphoma and Leukaemia

A testicular mass in a patient older than 50 years should raise the suspicion of a metastasis. These are more common in this age group than primary malignancies. Primary sites include the prostate, kidney, bronchus, pancreas bladder and thyroid.[6] Although overt clinical involvement is rare in leukaemia, over 50% of men with acute leukaemia and 25% with chronic leukaemia have testicular involvement. The testis is a common site for the occurrence of leukaemia relapse following treatment explained by the theory that there is limited penetration by chemotherapeutic agents at this site. The US features are not specific but are typically of a diffuse multifocal infiltrating lesion which may be of increased reflectivity compared with surrounding testicular parenchyma. Non-Hodgkin's lymphoma involves the testes in up to 20% of men and may be the 'primary site' as well as occurring bilaterally in a proportion of cases. In Hodgkin's lymphoma, testicular involvement is rare. US patterns of multifocal discrete hypo- as well as hyper-reflective lesions have been described.

Non-Malignant Focal Testicular Lesions

Cystic lesions, both unicameral and multiseptate, are occasionally encountered, usually as chance findings, and have been reported in up to 10% of testicular ultrasound studies (Fig. 16-7). They are more common in older

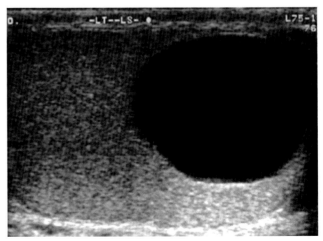

FIGURE 16-7 ■ Ultrasound of an intratesticular cyst of unknown aetiology in a male patient referred with clinical diagnosis of epididymal cyst.

men.[16] Previous trauma, inflammation and embryonal remnants have been described in their aetiology. They should be carefully differentiated from tumours with a cystic component. Epidermoid cysts of the testis have been described varyingly cystic, mixed and solid lesions with a characteristic whorled appearance on US[17] (Fig. 16-8). In addition they exhibit no vascular enhancement and appear 'stiff' on real-time elastography.[18] This has recently been correlated with alternating high- and low-signal layers on T2-weighted MRI images. This is a rare instance where a combination of laboratory tests and imaging findings may suggest that testicle sparing surgery is a possibility.[19]

Testicular abscess may result from many infective agents and usually demonstrates a low or mixed reflectivity pattern. Although the clinical presentation, often associated with epididymitis, is acute, indolent infections such as tuberculous disease of the testis may have a more insidious onset and be indistinguishable from malignancy (Fig. 16-9). In chronic cases, the presence of calcification within the lesion has been a clue to diagnosis. Percutaneous fine needle aspirate has given the diagnosis without resorting to exploration or orchidectomy where there was clinical suspicion that a lesion was due to tuberculosis.[20]

Non-Focal Testicular Abnormalities

Tubular Ectasia

This condition is seen in older men and is thought to be due to cystic dilatation of the rete testis. Coexisting epididymal abnormalities, usually consisting of epididymal cysts, have been noted in 85% of cases, leading to the theory that the condition is secondary to obstruction of the epidymis[21] (Fig. 16-10). The importance of this finding lies in the recognition of its benign nature. Unnecessary orchiectomy has been undertaken for this entity. In equivocal cases, MRI may be helpful. Characteristic findings have been described as hypointense signal relative to the normal testis on T1 and proton density-weighted sequences, the lesions being undetectable (unlike tumours) and non-enhancing on T2-weighted images.[22]

Testicular Microlithiasis

The discovery, usually by chance, of multiple sub 1-mm highly reflective foci in one or both testes indicates testicular microlithiasis (Fig. 16-11). The condition is thought to result from degenerating cells in the seminiferous tubules and is currently the subject of much speculation as to its association with testicular malignancy. Microlithiasis has also been reported in association with cryptorchidism, infertility, Klinefelter's syndrome,

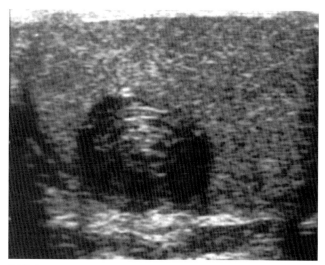

FIGURE 16-8 ■ **Ultrasound of epidermoid cyst of testis in young adult**.

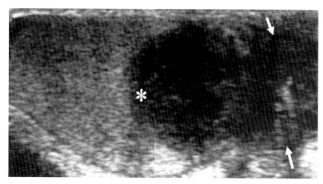

FIGURE 16-9 ■ **Tuberculous epididymo-orchitis**. The tail of the epididymis (arrowed) is hyporeflective and swollen. The testicular lesion (asterisk) is indistinguishable from tumour.

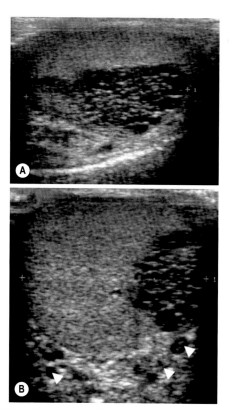

FIGURE 16-10 ■ **Tubular ectasia of the rete testis**. Longitudinal (A) and transverse (B) ultrasound views. There is a superficial resemblance to testicular teratoma. Typical cystic lesions of the epididymis are demonstrated (arrowheads).

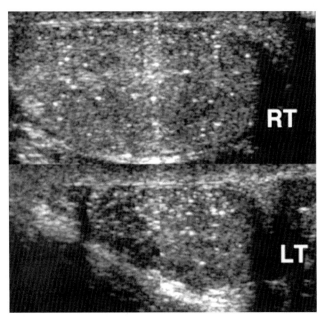

FIGURE 16-11 ■ **Microlithiasis of the testes.** Longitudinal US views demonstrate unilateral atrophy. The cause was unknown. Microlithiasis involves both the normal and atrophic testis.

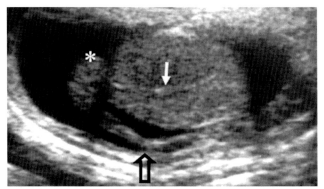

FIGURE 16-12 ■ **Congenital hydrocele in a neonate.** Ultrasound: the epididymal appendix (asterisk), body of epididymis (open arrow) and mediastinum testis (arrow) are clearly demonstrated.

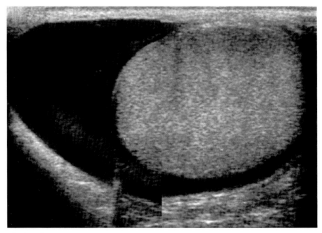

FIGURE 16-13 ■ **Longitudinal US view of normal testis and moderately sized hydrocele.**

testicular infarction, alveolar microlithiasis and numerous other conditions.[23]

Numerous cases of microlithiasis in association with germ cell tumours have been reported but the exact premalignant potential of this condition is unknown. Case reports of malignancy arising in testes under surveillance for this condition are rare.[24] The debate over the premalignant potential of this condition continues. A study of asymptomatic Turkish army recruits reported a prevalence of 2.4% in normal adult men, with a mean age of 23 years, and concluded that there is no association with malignancy.[25] Conversely, others have concluded that subjects with this condition should be followed up regularly.[26] A recent literature review has suggested that clarification to the exact definition of what constitutes microlithiasis would be helpful. The authors also conclude that whilst microlithiasis alone does not require follow-up, in the presence of another risk factor it may be advisable to perform testicular biopsy.[27]

EXTRATESTICULAR SCROTAL LESIONS

These lesions arise from many structures within the scrotum and can be considered as cystic or solid lesions.

Hypoechoic Lesions

These are far more common than solid lesions. A small amount of fluid surrounding the testicle is a normal finding in most asymptomatic men. A hydrocele may be congenital or acquired and is the commonest cause of scrotal enlargement. Hydroceles also occur in infancy as a result of a patent processus vaginalis and usually resolve spontaneously (Fig. 16-12). On US, hydroceles characteristically appear as fluid collections surrounding one or both testes and are either non-reflective or may contain swirling low-reflectivity echoes due to cholesterol crystals (Fig. 16-13). The fluid surrounds the anterior and lateral aspects of the testis. Hydroceles are usually obvious clinically. Imaging is requested when their size prevents adequate examination of the testis and there is a query about underlying malignancy, a rare association. Multiloculated hydroceles are recognised and may be indistinguishable from an organising haematoma (Fig. 16-14).

Spermatoceles and epididymal cysts are related lesions in that they are caused by dilated epididymal tubules (Fig. 16-15). Spermatoceles are retention cysts of the head of the epididymis and contain sperm, unlike their counterparts, which may be demonstrated in other locations within the epididymis. Epididymal cysts may be single or multiple and are discrete well-defined structures usually containing non-reflective fluid. They are easily distinguished from hydroceles but confusion may arise in the case of extremely large cysts, which may bear a superficial resemblance to a hydrocele.

Varicoceles are dilated tortuous veins of the pampiniform plexus, which can be demonstrated superior and

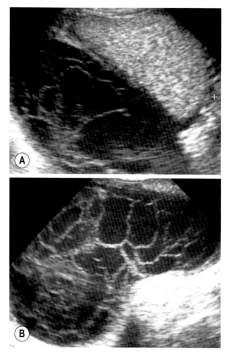

FIGURE 16-14 ■ **Longitudinal (A) and transverse (B) US views of organising scrotal haematoma following trauma.** The adjacent testis is compressed but otherwise normal. A septated hydrocele may present a similar appearance.

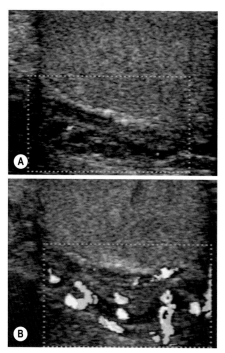

FIGURE 16-16 ■ **US of asymptomatiic left varicocele.** At rest (A), there is little detectable flow on colour Doppler. During Valsalva manoeuvre the flow is enhanced (B).

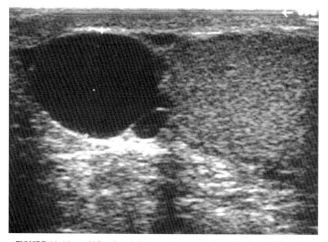

FIGURE 16-15 ■ **US of epididymal cyst in head of epididymis.**

posterior to the testis. They may be idiopathic or secondary to incompetent valves in the spermatic vein and are associated with male infertility. Early claims that varicoceles are the commonest treatable cause of male infertility[28] have been challenged by more recent critical reviews,[29] although there is evidence of demonstrable improvement in testicular function following treatment.[30] Idiopathic varicoceles are almost invariably left-sided, thought to be due to the more indirect drainage of the left testis into the left renal vein. Isolated right-sided varicoceles, particularly in an older age group, raise the possibility of an intra-abdominal mass. The US diagnosis

involves the identification of multiple serpiginous tubules of more than 2 mm in diameter posterior to the testis which may extend to the inferior pole of the testis. Although spontaneous flow may not be demonstrated even on low-flow colour or power Doppler settings, requesting the patient to cough, inhale rapidly or perform a Valsalva manoeuvre are all effective in producing detectable flow (Fig. 16-16). Standing the patient up increases the prominence of the vessels. Although normal patients are said not to have demonstrable veins in the spermatic cord or epididymis,[9] in the authors' experience, the prevalence of varicoceles as a chance finding appears to increase with each generation of improved ultrasound equipment. While 2 mm is a widely used cut-off between normal and abnormal veins, other studies have suggested diameters of 2.7 for subclinical and 3.6 mm for clinical varicoceles.[31]

Internal spermatic venography is not commonly used for the diagnosis of varicoceles but is undertaken for venous mapping in the treatment of varicoceles by embolotherapy (Fig. 16-17). Treatment is indicated mainly for subfertility but also for large symptomatic varicoceles. The gonadal vein is selectively catheterised from either a femoral, jugular or transbrachial approach and injection of iodinated contrast medium performed. Anatomical variations consisting of anastomoses with other retroperitoneal veins may affect the success of embolotherapy. The procedure has been undertaken using a variety of coils, plugs, Gelfoam and sclerosants. Success rates for coil embolisation have been reported in 73% of aberrantly fed and 97% of normally supplied varicoceles.[32] Distal coil migration is a recognised but uncommon complication of the procedure.

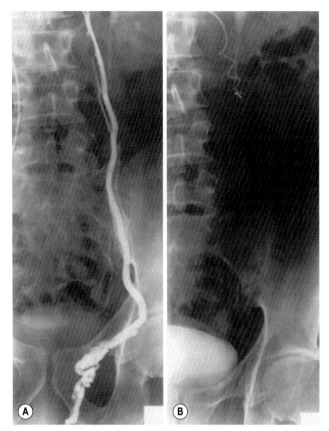

FIGURE 16-17 ■ Varicogram (A) of left varicocele, catheter in left testicular vein. (B) Following therapeutic embolisation with a Gianturco coil.

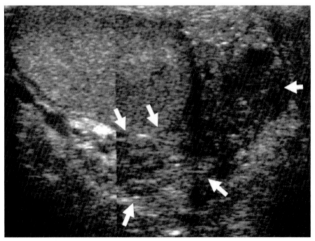

FIGURE 16-18 ■ **Acute bacterial epididymitis.** Ultrasound: the body and tail of the epididymis (arrows) are heterogeneous and enlarged. The testis is normal.

Solid Extratesticular Lesions

Extratesticular tumours may arise from the spermatic cord and epididymis and are extremely rare. An enlarged epididymis, from any cause, produces an extratesticular swelling. This is usually the result of acute or chronic infection (Fig. 16-18), but may also be seen as a normal

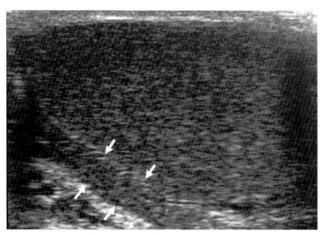

FIGURE 16-19 ■ **US showing normal post-vasectomy enlargement of the epididymis (arrows).**

late post-vasectomy appearance in approximately 45% of men undergoing this procedure (Fig. 16-19).

Acute Epididymitis

Numerous organisms cause acute epididymitis, including *Escherichia coli*, *Pseudomonas*, *Aerobacter*, gonococcus and *Chlamydia*. On US the entire epididymis may be enlarged but occasionally only the head. The epididymal reflectivity may be heterogeneous but is usually of lower reflectivity than normal.[33] Colour Doppler US studies have been shown to be useful in differentiating epididymitis and orchitis from other causes of acute scrotal pain and, in particular, from testicular torsion. All cases of acute epididymitis demonstrate an increase in colour flow. None of the cases of scrotal pain other than epididymitis demonstrate this finding.[34] Tuberculous epididymitis is considered to be secondary to prostatic tuberculosis. The testis may be involved by direct extension and the resulting lesion may be difficult to distinguish from tumour (Fig. 16-9).

Sperm granulomas occur within the epididymis with a recognised increased incidence following vasectomy (Fig. 16-20).

The distinction between the generally benign nature of solid extratesticular masses in adults, and the far more sinister nature of this finding in children, has been emphasised. Fifty per cent of paediatric extratesticular masses are malignant, usually rhabdomyosarcomas.[35]

Testicular Atrophy

The incidental chance finding of unequally sized testes is a frequent occurrence on ultrasound studies. Usually there is no clue in the history as to the aetiology. Many causes of atrophy have been described and include epididymo-orchitis, testicular torsion, cryptorchidism, varicoceles, mumps, trauma and oestrogen therapy. Testicular atrophy is also a normal ageing process.

Atrophic testes may be iso- or hyporeflective compared with the normal side. The parenchyma may be homogeneous or of mixed reflectivity and this pattern may be related to the cause of atrophy (Fig. 16-21).

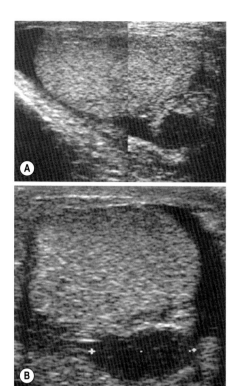

FIGURE 16-20 ■ **Post-vasectomy sperm granuloma.** Longitudinal (A) and transverse (B) views.

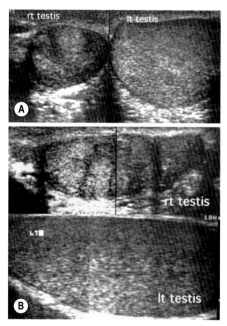

FIGURE 16-21 ■ **Unilateral testicular atrophy three months after blunt scrotal trauma.** Transverse (A) and longitudinal (B) US views.

Testicular Trauma

The characterisation of scrotal trauma is an important step in defining correct management of the patient and, in particular, in deciding whether emergency surgery is indicated. In one series the orchiectomy rate was 9% in

patients undergoing exploration in the first 72 h compared with 45% where this was delayed.[36] The distinction between ruptured and non-ruptured testis can be made extremely accurately with US. Surgical exploration may be avoided if the testis has a normal appearance.[37] US will demonstrate whether scrotal enlargement is due to a testicular fracture, testicular rupture, an adjacent haematoma (Fig. 16-14), or a combination of these findings. Testicular atrophy as a late complication of trauma, even in the presence of an undisrupted testis, has been documented (Fig. 16-21).

Cryptorchidism

Undescended testes are common as an isolated abnormality as well as occurring in association with other abnormalities such as prune-belly syndrome, Beckwith–Wiedemann syndrome, congenital rubella and renal agenesis. The incidence closely parallels gestational age, with 100% of premature males less than 900 g birthweight affected. In males weighing more than 2500 g the incidence is 3–4% and this decreases to less than 1% by the age of one year as most of these testes will descend spontaneously. The condition is bilateral in 10–25% of affected patients. In normal development the testis is drawn caudad towards the inguinal canal by the gubernaculum attached to its lower pole. This migration is said to be due to differential growth of the gubernaculum and the abdominal wall. Testicular descent commences at 28 weeks, reaching the scrotum at 32 weeks. In those cases where the testis does not eventually descend into its normal intrascrotal position, the testis may be found anywhere along its normal course of descent from retroperitoneum to the inguinal canal. In practice, 80% lie in the inguinal region where they are usually palpable. The rationale that underpins the quest for the undescended testes is an association with subfertility (even when unilateral) and even more importantly a greatly increased risk of malignancy. Seminoma is the most common associated tumour. This increased risk is not decreased by subsequent orchidopexy and even persists in the contralateral normal testis of male patients who have undergone orchidopexy. There are many descriptions of the success of US in demonstrating undescended testes in the inguinal region. A sensitivity of 97% for palpable testes and 75% of impalpable testes has been demonstrated.[38] The examination requires a high-resolution linear array transducer and should begin with an initial study of the scrotum to ensure that both testes are not present within. The testes are best demonstrated by US on axial imaging, the search requiring patience and care as the testis may be atrophic (Figs. 16-22 and 16-23).

CT or MRI studies which have the advantage of imaging the retroperitoneum have been used to demonstrate undescended testes not apparently located in the inguinal region.

Five CT patterns of findings in undescended testes have been described, and these depend on a combination of observations of the spermatic cord and testis.[39] Detection of testes in the pelvis and abdomen may be hampered by adjacent bowel loops and the paucity of fat in infants. MRI studies have disadvantages in terms of the need for

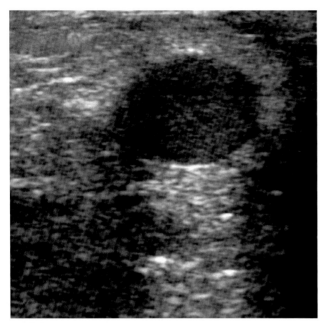

FIGURE 16-22 ■ **US of an undescended testis in an infant.** The testis lies in the inguinal canal surrounded by suprapubic fat.

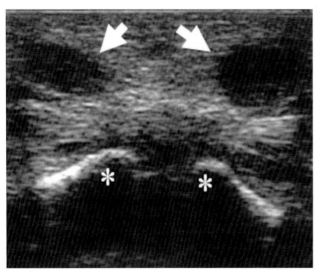

FIGURE 16-23 ■ **Bilateral undescended testes, transverse view.** The testes (arrowed) are demonstrated at the level of the superior pubic rami (asterisks).

sedation, high cost and problems with identifying intra-abdominal testes. The testes are characteristically of low signal on T1-weighted images and high signal on T2-weighted images. Sensitivities similar to ultrasound have been reported,[40] the detection rate being improved by the addition of diffusion-weighted imaging series.[41] An interesting recent meta-analysis of studies describing magnetic resonance angiography (MRA) in the management of patients with a non-palpable testis explored the cost in relation to the risk of cancer. The authors concluded that the protocol of MRA and subsequent observation (rather than removal) of the testicular nubbin results in a third of boys avoiding surgery without any significant risk of developing cancer.[42]

The role of imaging in the work-up of cryptorchidism is the subject of debate and practice varies according to clinical preference and prejudice as much as to published data. A study attempting to assess these ergonomic aspects of the available imaging techniques in 18 boys concluded 'in no case did radiographic assessment influence the decision to operate, the surgical approach, or the viability/salvageability of the involved testes. Preoperative radiography for undescended testes is neither necessary nor helpful'.[43] Despite advances in US apparatus, this view was reiterated in a study published a decade later.[44]

Testicular Torsion

A clinical diagnosis of testicular (spermatic cord) torsion is often difficult. Clinical examination is effective in differentiating this entity from other causes of acute scrotal pain in only 50% of cases.[45] The incidence peaks in peripubertal boys but there is a smaller peak in infancy. In the former group, torsion occurs within the tunica vaginalis due to a 'bell clapper' deformity. Normally the tunica vaginalis converges posteriorly, fixing the testis to the scrotal wall. This attachment may be deficient or patulous, allowing the testis to rotate. Painless torsion is a recognised entity but the classic presentation is of an afebrile boy with acute scrotal pain and vomiting. Acute torsion has been defined as lasting from 24 h to 10 days. Thereafter the condition is considered to be subacute and then progresses to chronic torsion. Other classifications define torsion of greater than 24 h duration as missed torsion. Testicular salvage rates are closely related to time to diagnosis. Salvage rates of 80% in the first 6 h drop to 20% if surgery is delayed for 24 h.[46]

The need for early surgery has resulted in many surgeons accepting a number of unnecessary explorations as the price for a higher salvage rate, and at the authors' institute imaging studies of any description are the exception rather than the rule. Grey-scale US appearances have been described which include an enlarged heterogeneous testis and epididymis in the acute phase,[45] along with other features such as a visibly torted cord, scrotal oedema and reactive hydroceles.[47] Nevertheless these features have been considered non-specific and unhelpful. As a working rule it is suggested that a swollen hypoechoic testis is usually not salvageable whereas a normal testis on grey-scale image often is.[48] Colour Doppler studies have resulted in an improvement in the US evaluation of testicular torsion with a claimed sensitivity and specificity of 100%.[49,50] Testicular torsion was diagnosed when blood flow in the symptomatic testis was absent or markedly reduced compared with the normal side. In five of seven patients subsequently shown to have torsion, flow was absent. In two cases, a single small vessel was demonstrated. The authors concluded that depending on local availability, colour Doppler US could supersede scintigraphy as the primary imaging study for excluding testicular torsion. This prophesy has proved correct, and, as the use of radionuclide studies for the diagnosis of torsion has essentially ceased, a detailed description of dose, imaging sequence and interpretation is no longer appropriate.

There are parallels between the imaging of testicular torsion and acute appendicitis. Early intervention is of such importance that clinical concern should override imaging findings.

The demonstration of normal blood flow in a testis does not exclude torsion, as evidenced by a study where of seven patients with surgically proven torsion, one patient with acute 360° torsion had relatively normal intratesticular flow on colour Doppler study compared with the contralateral side.[51]

Torsion of the testicular appendages, the most common cause of acute scrotal pain in children, may also produce misleading US findings. Of 29 boys with surgically proven torsion of the testicular appendages, 14 of the US studies suggested inflammatory change without a characteristic scrotal nodule.[52]

IMAGING OF MALE SEXUAL DYSFUNCTION

This subject can be considered in two main sections. First is the role of imaging in subfertility. This implies that normal sexual activity is achievable and, in those cases where imaging is indicated, it will usually provide information regarding physical structure. The second area involves imaging where normal sexual intercourse is impaired, usually by erectile failure. In this latter group, both structural and functional imaging are important. A further application of imaging, still in its infancy, has emerged comprising cerebral functional studies, mapping areas of cerebral cortex during sexual arousal using positron emission tomography[53] or functional MRI.[54] Whether this line of research proves useful remains to be defined. Similar studies on subjects with erectile dysfunction have failed to demonstrate a deviation from normal responses.[55] This esoteric application of functional neuroimaging will not be considered further here.

SUBFERTILITY WITH NORMAL SEXUAL FUNCTION

The investigation of subfertility goes well beyond imaging and includes endocrine and, if necessary, chromosomal studies. Sperm quality will also be evaluated. The US diagnosis and interventional radiological therapy of varicoceles has been discussed above. In the context of subfertility, several further points are worth emphasising. In a study of 150 men with infertility and varicoceles it has been shown that the size of the varicocele does not correlate with the degree of impaired spermatogenesis.[56] There is a therapeutic dilemma revolving around the fact that subclinical varicoceles have been estimated to occur in the general population in 20–80% of normal fertile men, yet profoundly impaired spermatogenesis may be caused by a small subclinical varicocele only detected by imaging studies.[57] Data-assessing the value of treating subclinical varicoceles are controversial as various criteria have been used by authors to describe this abnormality. There is evidence that when a subclinical right-sided varicocele is demonstrated where there is a clinically obvious left-sided varicocele, fertility is improved by correcting both abnormalities.[58]

Testicular atrophy from whatever cause is an obvious structural parameter that can be assessed in the setting of subfertility. An increase (as measured by US) in the volume of the ipsilateral testis following varicocele treatment has been shown to parallel an improvement in sperm count.[59]

The epididymis is of concern in subfertility and should be examined for features of chronic epididymitis. The normal epididymis has a mean diameter of 7 mm. Epididymal cysts, when large, have been reported as the cause of epididymal obstruction and the finding of an enlarged epididymis proximal to the cyst is indirect evidence of this.

The seminal vesicles, ejaculatory ducts, ampullae of the vas deferens and the prostate can be imaged by transrectal ultrasound. The normal ejaculatory duct is not demonstrated and, if dilated, appears as a hyporeflective tube traversing the prostate to enter the urethra at the verumontanum.[57] Contrast vasography is still considered the gold standard for the demonstration of distal ductal abnormalities. This is an invasive technique requiring incision of the scrotal skin, catheterisation of the distal afferent vas and distal injection of iodinated contrast medium sometimes mixed with a dye such as indigo carmine. An unobstructed distal vas and ejaculatory duct system demonstrates a low injection pressure and normal dimensions to the ejaculatory ducts, seminal vesicles and contrast in the bladder. Bladder catheterisation returns coloured urine.[57]

Ejaculatory duct obstruction may be responsible for subfertility. The findings at transrectal US of ejaculatory duct cysts, calcification or dilatation are consistent with obstruction. Transrectal US is an excellent technique for demonstrating seminal vesicle anatomy and may be coupled with contrast medium instillation in seminal vesiculography. MRI with an endorectal coil can also be used to delineate the anatomy of the distal seminal tract but as yet is largely reserved for use after transrectal US.[60] Seminal vesicle abnormalities have been reported in 100% of patients with agenesis of the vas deferens, with renal anomalies such as agenesis, crossed ectopia or pelvic kidney present in 16–43%.[61]

Congenital absence of the vas deferens is also associated with the genetic carrier state for cystic fibrosis. Transrectal US has been reported to be of value in the investigation of chronic haematospermia. Of 26 patients with this condition, significant US abnormalities were demonstrated in 24, including dilated seminal vesicles, ejaculatory duct and seminal vesicle cysts, duct or vesicle calculi and agenesis of the vas. No abnormalities were found in an age-matched control group.[62] Transrectal ultrasound of the prostate in the evaluation of prostatic malignancy and infection is described in Chapter 15.

ERECTILE FAILURE

The numerous risk factors for erectile dysfunction include endocrine abnormalities, renal failure, chronic liver disease, neurological disorders such as Parkinson's disease and multiple sclerosis, smoking, depression and HIV/AIDS. There are few data concerning the epidemiology of erectile abnormalities. The Massachusetts Male Aging Study found that complete erectile dysfunction was reported in 5% of males aged 40 years and 15% of men aged 70 years.[63]

Apart from documenting soft-tissue abnormalities of the penis such as the plaques of Peyronie's disease, advances in the role of imaging in erectile dysfunction have concerned the demonstration of vasogenic causes of impotence. The arterial supply to the corpora cavernosa is derived from the internal pudendal artery, a branch of the internal iliac artery. The internal pudendal artery gives off the perineal artery and then continues as the common penile artery, which pierces the pelvic floor adjacent to the bulbar urethra, giving off bulbar, urethral, dorsal and cavernosal branches. The paired cavernosal arteries run distally within the corpora, giving off numerous helicine arteries which open directly into lacunar spaces within the corpora.

Venous drainage of the erectile corpora cavernosa of the penis occurs via emmisary veins communicating with circumflex veins, which eventually join the deep dorsal vein of the penis. The proximal cavernosa drain via cavernosal veins into the internal pudendal veins.

In terms of vascular physiology, normal erection is paradoxically a process of relaxation. Penile flaccidity is maintained by smooth muscle tone within the thick-walled helicine arteries. In response to humoral and neurogenic stimuli there is reduced vasoconstriction activity resulting in increased flow to the cavernosal arteries. Relaxation of the smooth muscle in the walls of the helicine arteries and lacunar spaces allows increased inflow which compresses the subtunical venules against the tunica albuginea, resulting in a rise in intracavernosal pressure to approximate to systolic pressure.

The radiology of impotence involves a fairly simplistic model of the demonstration of adequate inflow and also the confirmation of a normal reduction in venous outflow, assessing relatively major arteries and veins. Dynamic infusion cavernosometry is frequently combined with cavernosography. There are various techniques for cavernosometry. Following insertion of a needle into the corpus cavernosum, the amount of saline flow required to maintain an erection can be measured. Without using smooth muscle relaxants, a figure of 120 mL min^{-1} has been quoted.[64] An alternative method, consisting of four phases, utilises an intracavernosal injection of papaverine, followed by monitoring of the intracavernosal pressure. With a normal response, the intracavernosal pressure should approach mean arterial blood pressure within 5–10 min. Failure to achieve this may be due to impaired inflow or inability to reduce outflow.

With arteriogenic impotence but normal veno-oclussive function, there is a slow rise in pressure, which never reaches systemic blood pressure. Patients with normal inflow and impaired veno-occlusion show an initial rapid rise in pressure which equilibrates early in the study well below systemic pressure.[65] The final phase of this approach involves an iodinated contrast cavernosogram. In a normal study no venous drainage should occur. Abnormal patterns of drainage involve demonstration of leakage from the dorsal, crural or cavernosal veins.

Duplex and triplex Doppler US has been extensively studied in the assessment of erectile dysfunction. In a comparison of US with internal pudendal arteriography in 20 men, cavernosal arteries with peak systolic velocities (PSV) less than 25 cm s^{-1} were associated with angiographic arterial disease. Thirteen of 17 cavernosal arteries with PSV of 25–34 cm s^{-1} had arterial disease and only 1 of 12 with a PSV greater than 35 cm s^{-1} had arterial disease. The authors recommended a cut-off PSV of 35 cm s^{-1} for distinguishing normal from abnormal.[66]

There is a debate concerning which Doppler parameters to measure. There have also been questions over the simplistic view that an analysis of large vessel inflow and outflow is the key to understanding vasogenic impotence.[67,68] The former commentary speculated that venous leakage and arterial insufficiency may be incidental and the underlying structural or functional abnormality may be at arteriolar level. The latter study concluded that Doppler ultrasound of the cavernosal arteries may not be reliable if PSV alone is assessed and that acceleration in the cavernosal arteries (defined as (PSV—end diastolic velocity)/ pulse rise time) was a more sensitive indicator of arterial disease.

There is some consensus that Doppler US has not been demonstrated to be a successful method of assessing abnormal venous leakage (as opposed to arterial inflow). In 13 men with cavernosometric and cavernosographic evidence of venous leakage who were examined with Doppler studies of the dorsal and cavernosal veins after intracorporeal papaverine injection, only five of the 12 with proven dorsal leaks had sonographically detectable flow in the dorsal vein. In all 11 cases with cavernous vein leaks, it proved impossible to insonate these veins successfully.[69]

EVALUATION OF THE SOFT TISSUES OF THE PENIS

Peyronie's disease is characterised by fibrotic plaques in the tunica albuginea of the corpora cavernosa. Sexual intercourse may be impossible due to penile deformity as a direct effect of fibrosis. Vasogenic erectile failure also occurs due to the plaques obstructing distal flow in the corpora cavernosa. Venous leakages are also a feature of Peyronie's disease. The diagnosis is usually made on the basis of symptoms of pain, penile curvature and palpable plaques. The initiating problem is thought to be a vasculitis of the subtunica connective tissue. The plaques are characteristically hyper- or hyporeflective peripheral lesions in the corpora cavernosa. Plaque calcification with acoustic shadowing may be present. Contrast cavernosograms demonstrate the plaques as filling defects or deformity of the normal contour of the corpus (Fig. 16-24). US is claimed to be more sensitive than palpation for the detection of plaques. Occult Peyronie's disease was found in 45 out of 280 men undergoing Doppler sonography for erectile dysfunction.[70] Conversely other workers found no correlation between the degree of

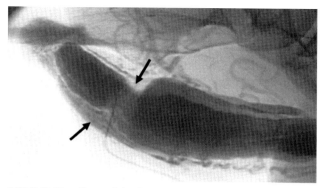

FIGURE 16-24 ■ **Peyronie's disease.** Cavernosogram in a patient with erectile failure confined to the distal penis. There is a circumferential stricture (arrowed) of the mid-shaft of both corpora cavernosa.

symptoms of the disease and the plaque burden as demonstrated by US or with soft-tissue radiography, and favoured clinical examination rather than imaging for the diagnosis and management of Peyronie's disease.[71] Inevitably, the role of MRI in Peyronie's disease has been investigated. A study comparing MRI, US and palpation in 57 men concluded that US is the method of choice for the evaluation of Peyronie's disease but noted that plaques at the base of the penis were better demonstrated by MRI. In addition, post-gadolinium enhancement patterns suggestive of inflammatory change were demonstrated by MRI where there were no US abnormalities.[72]

Penile trauma has been assessed with US and MRI in several studies. Trauma may be penetrating or blunt, the latter usually occurring during sexual activity. Disruption to the corpora cavernosa and tunica albuginea may occur, sometimes associated with urethral damage. In a study of seven men with penile fractures who underwent surgery, the exact site of the tunica tear was demonstrated with grey-scale US in six patients. In a patient with a tunical tear but no fracture, this lesion was not defined by US preoperatively.[73] MRI was evaluated in five patients with suspected penile fractures. In all cases a unilateral fracture of a corpus cavernosum, confirmed surgically, was demonstrated.[74] Nevertheless the diagnosis remains largely clinical in most situations, with US usually preferred as the initial investigation of choice in doubtful cases.[75]

Until recently, imaging of **penile carcinoma** has generally involved staging the disease rather than direct imaging of the tumour. Stage I tumours are confined to the glans or foreskin. Stage II tumours have invaded the shaft. Stage III and IV tumours demonstrate regional lymph nodes and distant metastases, respectively. Penile malignancy may also be staged using the TNM classification. US studies to assess the extent of the primary lesion have been attempted. It has been claimed that the margins of the tumour are easily demonstrated.[76] However, a study comparing US with histological examination found that in the region of the glans, US was not able to differentiate between invasion of the subepithelial tissue and invasion into the spongiosum. Invasion into the tunica albuginea was easily demonstrated. Accurate measurements of the tumour dimensions were only possible

in seven of 16 patients.[77] MRI may be helpful with imaging of the primary penile lesion and this has recently been comprehensively reviewed. In this study, primary penile carcinomas were usually solitary, ill-defined and infiltrating lesions, hypointense on both T1- and T2-weighted sequences, relative to the corpora cavernosa. The tumour margin and extension into the penile shaft was better evaluated on T2-weighted images or gadolinium-enhanced T1 sequences.[78] Overall it has been suggested that a combination of clinical staging and MRI may be the best approach for local staging.[79]

REFERENCES

1. Kim W, Rosen MA, Langer JE, et al. US MR imaging correlation in pathologic conditions of the scrotum. Radiographics 2007;27: 1239–53.
2. Middleton WD, Bell MW. Analysis of intratesticular arterial anatomy with emphasis on transmediastinal arteries. Radiology 1993;189(1):157–60.
3. Horstman WG. Scrotal imaging. Urol Clin N Am 1997;24(3): 653–71.
4. Rifkin MD, Kurtz AB, Pasto ME, et al. Diagnostic capabilities of high-resolution scrotal ultrasonography: prospective evaluation. J Ultrasound Med 1985;4(1):13–19.
5. Van Dijk R, Doesburg WH, Verbeek ALM, et al. Ultrasonography versus clinical examination in evaluation of testicular tumours. J Clin Ultrasound 1994;22(3):179–82.
6. Krone KD, Carroll BA. Scrotal ultrasound. Radiol Clin N Am 1985;23(1):121–39.
7. Soh E, Berman LH, Grant JW, et al. Ultrasound guided core needle biopsy of the testis for focal indeterminate intra-testicular lesions. Eur Radiol 2008;18(12):2990–6.
8. Aigner F, De Zordo T, Pallwein-Prettner L, et al. Real time sono-elastography for the evaluation of testicular lesions. Radiology 2012;263(2):584–9.
9. Gescovich EO. Scrotum and testes. In: McGahan JP, Goldberg BB, editors. Diagnostic Ultrasound: A Logical Approach. 1st ed. Philadelphia: Lippincott-Raven; 1998.
10. Mathew RM, Vandenberghe R, Garcia-Merino A, et al. Orchiectomy for suspected microscopic tumor in patients with anti-Ma2-associated encephalitis. Neurology 2007;68(12):900–5.
11. Horstman WG, Melson GI, Middleton WD, et al. Testicular tumours: findings with color Doppler ultrasound. Radiology 1992;185(3):733–7.
12. Schwerk WB, Schwerk WN, Rodeck G. Testicular tumours: prospective analysis of real-time US patterns and abdominal staging. Radiology 1987;164(2):369–74.
13. Albers P, Albrecht W, Algaba F, et al. EAU guidelines on testicular cancer: 2011 update. European Urology 2011;60:304–19.
14. Souchon R, Hartmann M, Krege S, et al. Interdisciplinary evidence based recommendations for the follow up of early stage seminomatous testicular germ cell cancer patients. Strahlenther Onkol 2011;187(3):158–66.
15. Bachner M, Loriot Y, Gross-Goupil M, et al. 2-18fluoro-deoxy-D-glucose positron emission tomography (FDG-PET) for post-chemotherapy seminoma lesions: a retrospective validation of the SEMPET trial. Ann Oncol 2012;23(1):59–64.
16. Gooding GA, Leonhardt W, Stein R. Testicular cysts: US findings. Radiology 1987;163(2):537–8.
17. Cittadini G, Gauglio C, Pretolesi F, et al. Bilateral epidermoid cysts of the testis: Sonographic and MRI findings. J Clin Ultrasound 2004;32(7):370–2.
18. Patel K, Sellars ME, Clarke JL, et al. Features of testicular epidermoid cysts on contrast enhanced sonography and real-time tissue elastography. J Ultrasound Med 2012;31(1):115–22.
19. Nichols J, Kandzari S, Elyadfrani MK, et al. Epidermoid cyst of the testis: a report of three cases. J Urol 1985;133(2):286–7.
20. Wolf JS Jr, McAninch JW. Tuberculous epididymo-orchitis: diagnosis by fine needle aspiration. J Urol 1991;145(4):836–8.
21. Brown DR, Benson CB, Doherty FJ, et al. Cystic testicular mass caused by dilated rete testis: sonographic findings in 31 cases. Am J Roentgenol 1992;158(6):1257–9.

22. Tartar VM, Trambert MA, Balsara ZN, Mattrey RF. Tubular ectasia of the testicle: sonographic and MR imaging appearance. Am J Roentgenol 1993;160(3):539–42.

23. Janzen DL, Mathieson JR, Marsh H, et al. Testicular microlithiasis: sonographic and clinical features. Am J Roentgenol 1992;158(5): 1057–60.

24. McEnnif N, Doherty F, Katz J, et al. Yolk sac tumour of the testis discovered on a routine annual sonogram in a boy with testicular microlithiasis. Am J Roentgenol 1995;1164:971–2.

25. Serter S, Gumus B, Unlu M, et al. Prevalence of testicular microlithiasis in an asymptomatic population. Scand J Urol Nephrol 2006;40(3):212–14.

26. Zastrow S, Hakenberg O, Wirth MP. Significance of testicular microlothiasis. Urol Int 2005;75:3–7.

27. Van Casteren NJ, Looijenga JH, Dohle GR. Testicular microlithiasis and carcinoma in situ overview and proposed clinical guideline. Int J Androl 2009;32(4):279–87.

28. Cockett ATK, Urry RL, Dougherty KA. The varicocele and semen characteristics. J Urol 1979;121(4):435–6.

29. Schlesinger MH, Wilets IF, Nagler HM. Treatment outcome after varicocelectomy: a critical analysis. Urol Clin N Am 1994;21(3): 517–29.

30. Li F, Yue H, Yamaguchi K, et al. Effect of surgical repair on testosterone production in infertile men with varicocoele: a meta-analysis. Int J Urol 2012;19(2):149–54.

31. Eskew AL, Bechtold R, Watson NE, et al. Ultrasonographic diagnosis of varicoceles. Fertil Steril 1993;60(4):693–7.

32. Marsman JW. The aberrantly fed varicocele: frequency, venographic appearance, and results of transcatheter embolization. Am J Roentgenol 1995;164(3):649–57.

33. Benson CB, Doubilet PM, Richie JP. Sonography of the male genital tract. Am J Roentgenol 1989;153(4):705–13.

34. Ralls PW, Jensen MC, Lee KP, et al. Color Doppler sonography in acute epididymitis and orchitis. J Clin Ultrasound 1990;18(5): 383–6.

35. Sung T, Reidlinger WF, Diamond DA, Chow JS. Solid extratesticular masses in children: radiographic and pathologic correlation. Am J Roentgenol 2006;186:483–90.

36. Del Villar RG, Ireland GW, Cass AS. Early exploration following trauma to the testicle. J Trauma 1973;13(7):600–1.

37. Jeffrey RB, Laing FC, Hricak H, et al. Sonography of testicular trauma. Am J Roentgenol 1983;141(5):993–5.

38. Graif M, Czerniak A, Avigdad I, et al. High-resolution sonography of the undescended testis in childhood: an analysis of 45 cases. Isr J Med Sci 1990;26(7):382–5.

39. Lee JKT, Glazer HS. Computed tomography in the localisation of the nonpalpable testis. Urol Clin N Am 1982;9(3):397–404.

40. Kier R, McCarthy S, Rosenfield AT, et al. Nonpalpable testes in young boys: evaluation with magnetic resonance imaging. Radiology 1988;169(2):429–33.

41. Kantarci M, Doganay S, Yalcin A, et al. Diagnostic performance of diffusion weighted MRI in the detection of nonpalpable undescended testes: comparison with conventional MRI and surgical findings. Am J Roentgenol 2010;195(4):268–73.

42. Eggener SE, Lotan Y, Cheng EY. Magnetic resonance angiography for the nonpalpable testis: A cost and cancer risk analysis. J Urol 2005;173(5):1745–9.

43. Hrebinko RL, Bellinger MF. The limited role of imaging techniques in managing children with undescended testes. J Urol 1993;150(2 P+1):458–60.

44. Elder JS. Ultrasonography is unnecessary in evaluating boys with a nonpalpable testis. Pediatrics 2002;110(4):748–51.

45. Mueller DL, Amundson GM, Rubin SZ, et al. Acute scrotal abnormalities in children: diagnosis by combined sonography and scintigraphy. Am J Roentgenol 1988;150(3):643–6.

46. Donohue RE, Utley WL. Torsion of spermatic cord. Urology 1978;11(1):33–6.

47. Sung EK, Setty B, Castro-Aragon I. Sonography of the pediatric scrotum: emphasis on the Ts—Torsion, trauma, and tumors. Am J Roentgenol 2012;198(5):996–1003.

48. Chmelnik M, Schenk JP, Hinz U, et al. Testicular torsion: sono-morphological appearances as a predictor for testicular viability and outcomes in neonates and children. Paediatr Surg Int 2010;26: 281–6.

49. Lerner RM, Mevorach RA, Hulbert WC, et al. Color Doppler US in the evaluation of acute scrotal disease. Radiology 1990;176(2): 355–8.

50. Middleton WM, Siegel BA, Melson GL, et al. Acute scrotal disorders: prospective comparison of color Doppler US and testicular scintigraphy. Radiology 1990;177(1):177–81.

51. Burks DD, Markey BJ, Burkhard TK, et al. Suspected testicular torsion and ischemia: evaluation with color Doppler sonography. Radiology 1990;175(3):815–21.

52. Karmazyn B, Steinberg R, Livne P, et al. Duplex sonographic findings in children with torsion of the testicular appendages: overlap with epididymitis and epididimoorchitis. Pediatr Surg 2006;41(3): 500–4.

53. Bocher M, Chisin R, Parag Y, et al. Cerebral activation associated with sexual arousal in response to a pornographic clip: A ^{15}O-H$_2$O PET study in heterosexual men. Neuroimage 2001; 14:105–17.

54. Ferretti A, Cauler M, Del Gratta C, et al. Dynamics of male sexual arousal: distinct components of brain activation. Revealed by fMRI. Neuroimage 2005;26(4):1086–96.

55. Hagemann JH, Berding G, Bergh S, et al. Effect of visual sexual stimuli and apomorphine SL on cerebral activity in men with erectile dysfunction. Eur Urol 2003;43(4):412–42.

56. Dubin L, Amelar R. Varicocele size and the results of varicocelectomy in selected subfertile men with varicocele. Fertil Steril 1970;21(8):606–9.

57. Honig SC. New diagnostic techniques in the evaluation of anatomic abnormalities of the infertile male. Urol Clin N Am 1994;21(3):417–32.

58. Gat Y, Bachar GN, Everaert K, et al. Induction of spermatogenesis in azoospermic men after internal spermatic vein embolization for the treatment of varicocoele. Hum Reprod 2005;20(4): 1013–17.

59. Zucchi A, Mearini E, Fioretti F, et al. Varicocele and fertility: relationship between testicular volume and seminal parameters before and after treatment. J Androl 2006;27:548–51.

60. Donkol RH. Imaging in male factor obstructive infertility. World J Radiol 2010;28(5):172–9.

61. Kuligowska E, Pomeroy OH. Prostate. In: McGahan JP, Goldberg BB, editors. Diagnostic Ultrasound: A Logical Approach. 1st ed. Philadelphia: Lippincott-Raven; 1998.

62. Worischeck JH, Parra RO. Chronic hematospermia: assessment by transrectal ultrasound. Urology 1993;43:515–20.

63. Kirby RS. An Atlas of Erectile Dysfunction. 1st ed. New York: Parthenon; 1999.

64. Jeffcoate WJ. The investigation of impotence. Br J Urol 1991;68: 449–53.

65. Rosen MP, Schwartz AN, Levine FJ, et al. Radiologic assessment of impotence: angiography, sonography, cavernosography, and scintigraphy. Am J Roentgenol 1991;157:923–31.

66. Benson CB, Aruny JE, Vickers MA Jnr. Correlation of duplex sonography with arteriography in patients with erectile dysfunction. Am J Roentgenol 1993;160:71–3.

67. Bookstein JJ, Valji K. The arteriolar component in impotence: a possible paradigm shift. Am J Roentgenol 1991;157:932–4.

68. Valji K, Bookstein JJ. The diagnosis of arteriogenic impotence: efficacy of duplex sonography as a screening tool. Am J Roentgenol 1993;160:65–9.

69. Vickers MA Jnr, Benson CB, Richie JP. High resolution ultrasonography and pulsed wave Doppler for detection of corporovenous incompetence in erectile dysfunction. J Urol 1990;143: 1125–7.

70. Amin Z, Patel U, Friedman EP, et al. Colour Doppler and duplex ultrasound assessment of Peyronie's disease in impotent men. Br J Radiol 1993;66:398–402.

71. Pohar SS, Jackson FI, Glazebrook GA. Ultrasonography and radiography in the diagnosis of Peyronie's disease. Can Assoc Radiol J 1990;41:369–71.

72. Hauk EW, Hackstein N, Vosshenrich R, et al. Diagnostic value of magnetic resonance in Peyronie's disease—a comparison with palpation and ultrasound in the evaluation of plaque formation. Eur Urol 2003;43:293–9.

73. Koga S, Saito Y, Arakaki N, et al. Sonography in fracture of the penis. Br J Urol 1993;72:228–9.

74. De Lucchi R, Rizzo, Rubino A, Tola E. Magnetic resonance diagnosis of traumatic penile fracture. Radiol Med (Torino) 2004;107: 234–40.

75. Koifman L, Barros R, Junior RA, et al. Penile fracture: Diagnosis, treatment and outcomes of 150 patients. Urology 2010;76(6): 1488–92.

76. King BF. The penis. In: Rumack CM, Wilson SR, Charboneau JW, editors. Diagnostic Ultrasound. 2d ed. St Louis: Mosby; 1997.

77. Horenblas S, Kroger R, Gallee MPW, et al. Ultrasound in squamous cell carcinoma of the penis: A useful addition to clinical staging? A comparison of ultrasound and histology. Urology 1994;43:702–7.

78. Singh AK, Saokar A, Hahn P, Haringhani MG. Imaging of penile neoplasms. Radiographics 2005;25:1629–38.

79. Heyns CF, Mendoza-Valdes A, Pompeo AC. Diagnosis and staging of penile cancer. Urology 2010;76(2):S15–23.

CHAPTER 17

GYNAECOLOGICAL CANCER

Evis Sala • Susan Freeman • Susan M. Ascher • Hedvig Hricak

The results of diagnostic imaging tests frequently change treatment strategies and affect our understanding of disease processes. This chapter gives a brief review of common gynaecological malignancies and presents indications for each imaging technique used (Table 17-1) while focusing on advances in ultrasound (US), computed tomography (CT), magnetic resonance imaging (MRI) and positron emission tomography/computed tomography (PET/CT). As with any changing technological arena, imaging strategies are not static and require ongoing updates and re-evaluation.

IMAGING TECHNIQUES

Ultrasound

Ultrasound (transabdominal or transvaginal) is accepted as the primary imaging technique for examining the female pelvis. Currently, the main role of US in gynaecological oncology includes evaluation of a suspected pelvic mass, evaluation of causes of uterine enlargement, identification of endometrial abnormalities in a patient with postmenopausal bleeding and characterisation of ovarian masses. In addition, US has become invaluable in guiding a wide selection of invasive procedures such as transabdominal and transvaginal guidance of fluid or tissue sampling,[1] transvaginal-guided drain placement and guidance for placement of brachytherapy devices for cervical and endometrial malignancies.

A full bladder is mandatory for transabdominal US, as it provides a sonic window to image the pelvic organs. It is usual to employ 3.5–5.0 MHz transducers. Transvaginal US, which is optimally performed with an empty bladder, provides greater detail of the anatomy and pathology due to the closer apposition to the pelvic organs, as well as the higher frequencies of insonation (5.0–7.5 MHz). Colour, power and spectral Doppler provide additional information regarding associated vascularity.

Ultrasound has many advantages: it is relatively inexpensive, provides multiplanar views, is widely available and lacks ionising radiation. Its portability allows use in virtually any setting, including the ultrasound suite, operating room, patient bedside or radiotherapy suite. However, US also has a number of limitations: it is operator dependent and image quality varies with patient body habitus. Although transvaginal, sonohysterography and endorectal US provide improved spatial resolution, they are not as useful as either CT or MRI in the staging of pelvic malignancies, including the evaluation of regional extent or metastatic spread.

Computed Tomography

CT is the most commonly used primary imaging study for evaluating the extent of gynaecological malignancies and for detecting persistent and recurrent disease although there is increasing use of MRI. CT-guided biopsy of omental cake or pelvic mass can be used to obtain histological confirmation of ovarian cancer and to confirm pelvic recurrence.[1] Advantages of CT include wide availability, fast data acquisition and high spatial resolution. Disadvantages of CT include the use of ionising radiation, degradation of image quality by body habitus or metallic hip prosthesis and the risk of morbidity and mortality associated with iodinated contrast agents. Although CT is useful in the advanced stages of pelvic malignancy, it often has limited utility in characterising early-stage disease.

CT images of the abdomen and pelvis are acquired in the portal venous phase, 70 s following an injection of intravenous low osmolar contrast medium; this enhances blood vessels and viscera, allowing easier identification of enlarged lymph nodes and parenchymal lesions. Oral contrast medium is utilised to opacify the small and large bowel, which allows detection of bowel serosal deposits and the differentiation of bowel loops from pelvic and nodal disease.

TABLE 17-1 The Choice of Imaging Investigation in Endometrial, Cervical and Ovarian Cancer

Pathology	Imaging Techniques			
	US (TA/TV/SHG)	CT	MRI	PET/CT
Endometrial cancer	• Evaluation of endometrium in patients presenting with postmenopausal bleeding • Double-layer endometrial thickness > 5 mm on TV US determines the need for endometrial sampling	• Detection of enlarged lymph nodes • Detection of distant metastases (lung, liver, etc.) • Identification of peritoneal nodules in serous papillary and clear cell carcinoma • Detection of recurrent pelvic and distant metastatic disease	• Delineating the origin of the primary tumour (endometrial vs cervical) when the biopsy results are inconclusive • Assess depth of myometrial invasion and cervical stromal invasion (improves pre-treatment risk stratification) • Evaluation of disease extent in the pelvis • Detection of enlarged lymph nodes • Evaluation of surgical resectability, if pelvis is the sole site of recurrence	• Detection of extrauterine disease • Monitoring treatment response in selected cases • Detection of distant metastases in patients with suspected recurrence within the pelvis; detecting unsuspected distant metastases significantly alters treatment choices
Cervical cancer	• No role in diagnosis of cervical cancer • Evaluation of complications including hydronephrosis and guiding interventional procedures (e.g. nephrostomy)	• Evaluation of extent of disease in advanced cases (especially if no access to MRI) • Detection of enlarged lymph nodes • Detection of distant metastases (lung, liver, etc.)	• Accurate evaluation of tumour size (FIGO staging, risk stratification and when considering trachelectomy) • Evaluation of parametrial invasion • Evaluation of pelvic side-wall invasion and bladder/rectal mucosa invasion • Detection of enlarged lymph nodes • Brachytherapy treatment planning • Monitoring response to chemoradiotherapy • Evaluation of surgical resectability, if pelvis is the sole site of recurrence • May distinguish radiation fibrosis from recurrent disease	• Evaluation of patients with advanced cervical cancer, especially the detection of lymph node metastases • Radiotherapy field planning • Evaluation of response to treatment • May distinguish radiation fibrosis from recurrent disease • Detection of distant metastases in patients with suspected recurrence within the pelvis; significantly alters treatment choices
Ovarian cancer	• Detection and characterisation of adnexal masses • Screening of women at high risk for ovarian carcinoma • Guide omental/peritoneal biopsy and drainage of ascites	• Characterisation of ovarian lesions that are detected incidentally on CT • Accurate evaluation of the extent and anatomical location of peritoneal spread (dictates the feasibility of optimal cytoreductive surgery vs need for adjuvant chemotherapy) • Detect enlarged lymph nodes • Detect complications such as small bowel obstruction • Evaluation of residual disease following surgery • Evaluate treatment response and assess suspected relapse with rising CA-125 levels or clinically suspicious symptoms • Guide omental/peritoneal biopsy	• Characterisation of indeterminate adnexal lesions on US • Evaluation of disease extent, particularly where CT is contraindicated (allergy to contrast media, renal insufficiency and pregnancy) • Evaluate resectability of a pelvic recurrence, if surgery is planned	• May play a role in evaluation of the extent of disease • Evaluation of recurrent ovarian cancer especially in patients with elevated CA-125 but negative CT findings

TA, transabdominal; TV, transvaginal; SHG, sonohysterography.

Magnetic Resonance Imaging

The role of MRI in the evaluation of gynaecological malignancies has evolved during the past two decades. MRI has been shown to be superior to CT in the work-up of endometrial and cervical cancer and may be a useful problem-solving tool in the evaluation of ovarian cancer. In addition, there is evidence that MRI may aid the differentiation of radiation fibrosis from recurrent tumour. The accuracy of MRI assessment of lymph node invasion is similar to that of CT; both rely primarily on size criteria to detect lymph node metastases.

Although MRI is still relatively expensive, it has been shown to minimise costs in some clinical settings by limiting or eliminating the need for further expensive and/ or more invasive diagnostic or surgical procedures. Advantages of MRI include superb spatial and tissue contrast resolution, no use of ionising radiation, multiplanar capability and fast (i.e. breath-hold and breathing-independent) techniques. MRI is the technique of choice for patients with previous reactions to iodinated IV contrast media or impaired renal function. However, MRI is contraindicated in patients with implants such as pacemakers, neural stimulators or cochlear implants, certain vascular clips and metallic objects. Some patients may experience claustrophobia, causing difficulty in completing the examination or requiring sedative premedication in subsequent MR examinations.

The basic imaging protocol for gynaecological MRI includes T1-weighted images (T1WI) of the pelvis in the axial plane and T2-weighted images (T2WI) in the axial and sagittal planes. When high signal intensity is seen within the adnexa on T1WI, which may represent fat or haemorrhage, fat-saturation T1-weighted images (T1W FS) are mandatory to differentiate between the two. Staging of gynaecological malignancies requires large field-of-view axial T1WI and/or T2WI of the pelvis and abdomen to identify enlarged lymph nodes, hydronephrosis and bone marrow changes.[2,3] High-resolution, small field-of-view, axial oblique (short-axis) T2W fast spin-echo (T2W FSE) images taken parallel to the short axis of the uterine corpus are essential in evaluating accurate depth of myometrial invasion in endometrial carcinoma. In the assessment of patients with cervical cancer, high-resolution, small field-of-view, axial oblique (short-axis) T2W FSE images parallel to the short axis of the cervix are crucial for identification of parametrial invasion.

Dynamic multiphase contrast-enhanced MRI using a three-dimensional (3D) gradient echo T1WI after intravenous gadolinium is often utilised in staging patients with endometrial cancer; it is also useful in the characterisation of complex adnexal lesions and can aid in the detection of small peritoneal and serosal implants, when ovarian cancer is suspected. Routine use of dynamic multiphase contrast-enhanced 3D T1-weighted sequences is not recommended for staging of patients with cervical carcinoma. However, they may be very useful for accurate delineation of small cervical tumours in patients being considered for fertility sparing surgery (i.e. trachelectomy) and differentiation of tumour recurrence from radiation fibrosis in patients with cervical cancer.

Increasingly, diffusion-weighted MRI (DW-MRI) is routinely incorporated in MRI staging protocols for uterine malignancies. DW-MRI can be useful for accurately determining the depth of myometrial invasion in patients with endometrial cancer, which can be particularly helpful in cases of tumours that are either iso- or hyperintense relative to the myometrium on T2WI or when the use of intravenous contrast medium is contraindicated, and may replace dynamic imaging in the future.[4] DW-MRI may also improve detection of drop metastases in the cervix or metastatic foci outside the uterus, such as adnexa or peritoneum.[4]

Positron Emission Tomography/ Computed Tomography

The main applications of 2-[^{18}F]-fluoro-2-deoxy-D-glucose (FDG) PET/CT in gynaecological oncology are the staging of cervical cancer and detection of recurrent ovarian, cervical and endometrial cancer. PET/CT takes advantage of the biochemical changes associated with malignancy that are more specific than, and often precede, the structural changes visualised by conventional means. Specifically, FDG-PET/CT exploits the accelerated rate of glycolysis that is common to neoplastic cells to image tumours. FDG-PET/CT does not have the same spatial resolution or soft-tissue contrast as US or MRI, but image fusion techniques that overlay FDG-PET images onto MR images are available. There are several disadvantages of FDG-PET/CT. False negatives can occur with lesions smaller than 0.5 cm and with certain tumour types that demonstrate low metabolic activity. False-positive results can be seen with inflammatory or infective aetiology, postoperative changes or reactive lymphadenopathy, including chronic inflammatory disorders such as granulomatous disease.

ENDOMETRIAL CARCINOMA

Endometrial cancer is the most commonly diagnosed gynaecological malignancy in affluent societies. Presenting as postmenopausal bleeding, the disease has a peak incidence between the ages of 55 and 65 years. Risk factors include unopposed oestrogen intake, nulliparity, obesity and diabetes. The prognosis of endometrial carcinoma depends on a number of factors, including stage, depth of myometrial invasion, nodal status and tumour grade. Preoperative evaluation of prognostic factors helps in subspecialist treatment planning.

Detection, Diagnosis and Staging

Endometrial carcinoma is typically diagnosed at endometrial biopsy or dilatation and curettage, with imaging being reserved to evaluate the extent of disease.[5] Imaging criteria for staging of endometrial cancer are based on the International Federation of Gynecology and Obstetrics (FIGO) surgical-pathological staging system, revised in 2009 (Table 17-2).[6] Full FIGO staging comprises a total abdominal hysterectomy (TAH), bilateral salpingo-oophorectomy (BSO), peritoneal washings and

TABLE 17-2   FIGO Staging of Endometrial Carcinoma with Corresponding MR Findings

FIGO Stage	Description of Stage	MRI Findings
Stage I	Tumour confined to the corpus uteri	
Ia	Tumour extending to <50% of myometrial depth	Abnormal signal intensity extends into <50% of the myometrium
Ib	Tumour extending to ≥50% of myometrial depth	Abnormal signal intensity extends into ≥50% of the myometrium
Stage II	Tumour invades cervical stroma, but does not extend beyond the uterus	Disruption of low signal intensity cervical stroma by tumour. A widened internal os with tumour protruding into the endocervical canal does not represent stromal invasion
Stage III	Local and/or regional spread of the tumour	
IIIa*	Tumour invades the serosa of the corpus uteri and/or adnexa	Disruption of continuity of outer myometrium. Irregular uterine configuration
IIIb	Vaginal and/or parametrial involvement	Segmental loss of hypointense vaginal wall
IIIc	Metastases to pelvic and/or para-aortic lymph nodes	Regional or para-aortic nodes >1 cm in short-axis diameter. Additional suspicious features include multiple small rounded lymph nodes, irregular lymph node contour, abnormal signal intensity similar to that of the primary tumour, presence of necrosis
IIIc1	Positive pelvic nodes	
IIIc2	Positive para-aortic lymph nodes ± positive pelvic lymph nodes	
Stage IV	Tumour invades bladder and/or bowel mucosa, and/or distant metastases	
IVa	Tumour invades bladder and/or bowel mucosa (biopsy proven)	Abnormal signal intensity disrupts normal low signal intensity bladder/rectal mucosa. Note that bullous oedema does not indicate stage IVa
IVb	Distant metastases, including intra-abdominal metastases and/or inguinal lymph nodes	Tumour in distant sites or organs

*Positive cytology obtained at peritoneal washings should be recorded but does not alter any stage.

retroperitoneal lymph node dissection. Imaging is not part of the FIGO staging system for endometrial cancer; however, both MRI and CT are increasingly playing a crucial role in risk stratification and surgical treatment planning.[5]

Ultrasound

Transvaginal (TVUS) is superior to transabdominal US for imaging endometrial abnormalities.[7] The most common appearance of endometrial cancer is non-specific thickening of the endometrium. Endometrial thickening in endometrial carcinoma is indistinguishable from that found with hyperplasia or a polyp. However, the diagnosis of endometrial cancer should be considered when the endometrial/myometrial junction is disrupted or the endometrial surface is irregular (Fig. 17-1). In postmenopausal women, the threshold value for a thickened endometrium is 5 mm.[8] In sonohysterography, endometrial cancer may appear as an intracavitary polyp or as asymmetric thickening of the endometrial lining. Doppler, colour and 3D US have been advocated to improve endometrial carcinoma detection.

The use of US is limited to the evaluation of stage I disease with emphasis on the evaluation of the depth of myometrial invasion. For the evaluation of myometrial invasion, the presence and continuity of the hypoechoic halo that surrounds the outer layer of the endometrium are assessed (i.e. intact, focally disrupted or totally disrupted). The extent of myometrial invasion is then estimated by measuring the distance from the central lumen of the uterus to the distal junction between tumour and normal myometrium. Transvaginal ultrasound has been reported to have a sensitivity of 77 to 100%, a specificity of 65 to 93% and an overall accuracy of 60 to 76% in assessing the degree of myometrial invasion.[3]

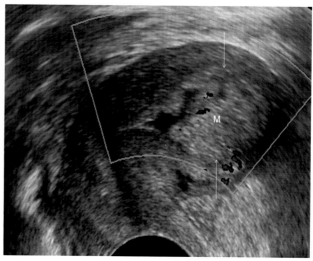

FIGURE 17-1 ■ Endometrial carcinoma, transvaginal US. The endometrium is thickened and irregular in this postmenopausal patient. A polypoid mass (M) which demonstrates internal vascularity on power Doppler is seen distending the endometrial cavity. The anterior and posterior endometrial–myometrial junction is indistinct, indicating myometrial invasion (white arrows).

Computed Tomography

On contrast-enhanced CT, endometrial cancer is seen as a hypodense mass relative to normal myometrium but delineation of the tumour is difficult as there is relatively little contrast difference between tumour and the myometrium.[9]

CT is most commonly used in the assessment of advanced disease and performs as well as MRI in identifying extrauterine spread and enlarged lymph nodes.[3] Its greatest clinical impact is in confirming parametrial and side-wall extension in stage III tumours and in detecting pelvic lymphadenopathy. Limitations of CT include a tendency to understage endometrial carcinoma because of limited soft-tissue resolution which leads to inaccurate estimation of depth of myometrial invasion. In addition, CT has a limited accuracy in evaluation of cervical stroma invasion and bladder or rectal mucosa invasion.

Magnetic Resonance Imaging

MRI is considered the most accurate imaging technique for preoperative assessment of endometrial carcinoma due to its excellent soft-tissue contrast resolution. The National Cancer Institute in France[10] has recently incorporated MRI into the standard preoperative assessment of patients with endometrial carcinoma. The European Society of Urogenital Imaging (ESUR) and the Royal College of Radiologists cancer imaging guidelines also recommend MRI for staging of high-grade endometrioid adenocarcinomas (type I histology) as well as serous papillary and clear cell adenocarcinomas (type II histology).[11]

Although endometrial cancer may demonstrate high signal intensity on T2-weighted sequences, it is more typically heterogeneous and may even be of low signal intensity. Following IV contrast medium administration, there is early avid enhancement of normal myometrium. Endometrial cancer enhances more slowly than the adjacent myometrium, allowing identification of small tumours, even those contained by the endometrium.[12] In the later phases of enhancement, tumour appears hypointense relative to the myometrium (Fig. 17-2).

MRI is significantly superior to US and CT in the evaluation of both depth of myometrial invasion and tumour invasion into the cervical stroma. The overall staging accuracy of MRI has been reported to be between 85 and 93%.

Stage I. Stage I endometrial cancers include tumours confined to the corpus. Stage Ia tumours invade less than 50% into the myometrium with associated disruption or irregularity of the junctional zone (JZ). If the JZ is indistinct, stage Ia tumour is suggested by an irregular

tumour–myometrium interface. The presence of low signal intensity tumour within the outer myometrium or beyond indicates deep myometrial invasion—stage Ib disease (Fig. 17-3).

Stage II. Stage II is indicated by the presence of cervical stroma invasion. Disruption of the low signal intensity fibrocervical stroma by high signal intensity tumour on T2-weighted images, together with disruption of normal enhancement of the cervical mucosa by low signal intensity tumour on late dynamic contrast-enhanced MRI, indicates cervical stroma invasion. Widening of the internal os and endocervical canal with preservation of the

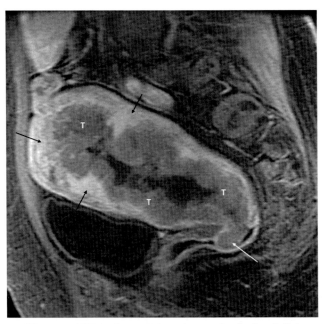

FIGURE 17-2 ■ **MRI, endometrial carcinoma.** Sagittal gadolinium-enhanced T1-weighted fat-suppressed MR image shows the endometrial tumour (T) relatively hypointense to the avidly enhancing myometrium (black arrows), revealing deep myometrial invasion. The disease extends to the upper third of the vagina (white arrow).

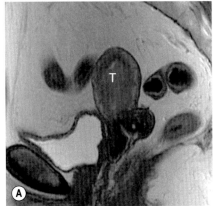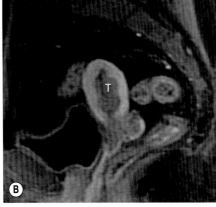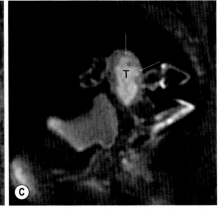

FIGURE 17-3 ■ **Endometrial carcinoma, MRI.** Sagittal T2-weighted (A) MR image shows an intermediate signal intensity endometrial cancer (T) relatively isointense to the adjacent myometrium. The depth of myometrial invasion is difficult to determine. However, sagittal gadolinium-enhanced T1-weighted fat-suppressed (B) and diffusion-weighted MR images (C) clearly reveal the endometrial cancer (T) with deep (≥50%) myometrial invasion (arrows). The cervical stroma is intact, excluding stage II disease.

normal low signal intensity fibrocervical stroma does not change the staging.

Stage III. In stage III disease, tumour extends outside the uterus but not beyond the true pelvis. Serosal involvement—stage IIIa—appears as disruption of the uterine serosa, irregular uterine contour, tumour deposits along the serosa of sigmoid colon (Fig. 17-4A), in the surface of one or both ovaries (Fig. 17-4B) or tumour extension into the fallopian tubes. In stage IIIb disease,

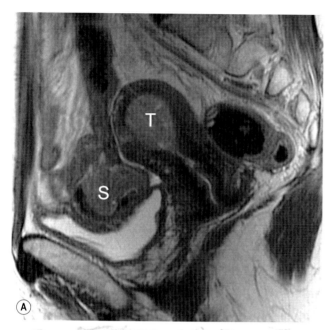

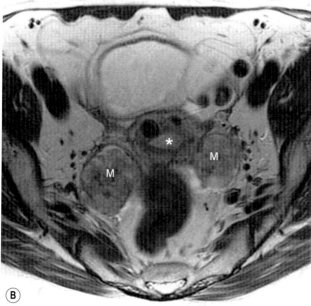

FIGURE 17-4 ■ **Stage IIIa endometrial carcinoma, MRI—two different cases.** (A) Sagittal T2-weighted MR image demonstrates a heterogeneous intermediate signal intensity endometrial tumour (T) distending the endometrial cavity. A serosal deposit (S) is seen on the sigmoid colon, superior to the bladder. In a different patient (B), the axial T2-weighted MR image shows mild endometrial thickening (asterisk) secondary to an endometrial tumour and heterogeneous bilateral adnexal masses (M).

tumour extends into the upper vagina and there is segmental loss of the low signal intensity vaginal wall. In stage IIIc disease, lymphadenopathy is present in the pelvis (stage IIIc1) or para-aortic region (stage IIIc2).

Stage IV. Stage IV disease is tumour that extends beyond the true pelvis or invades the bladder or rectal mucosa. On MRI, loss of low signal intensity of the bladder or rectal wall and tumour invading the mucosa indicates stage IVa disease. Bullous oedema of the bladder is a frequent sign of tumour in the subserosal or muscular layer of the bladder, but does not qualify for stage IVa disease. In stage IVb disease, distant metastases (including nodal enlargement above renal veins or inguinal region), malignant ascites or peritoneal deposits are present. The latter are more common with high-grade, clear cell or serous papillary tumours, as clinically they behave like ovarian cancer with a propensity to spread along the serosal and peritoneal surfaces. Distant spread to lung, liver and bone is rare at presentation.

Positron Emission Tomography/ Computed Tomography

FDG-PET/CT has a limited role in the initial staging of patients with endometrial carcinoma. However, FDG-PET/CT is helpful in assessing patients with suspected disease recurrence within the pelvis, by detecting unsuspected distant metastases, which significantly alters treatment choices.

Recommended Imaging Approach

US, especially transvaginal US, is often considered to be the primary imaging approach for evaluation of women presenting with postmenopausal bleeding. CT is very useful in screening for lymph nodes or peritoneal metastases in patients with a serous papillary and clear cell endometrial carcinoma and for confirmation of stage IVb disease. MRI is the imaging technique of choice for the accurate assessment of the depth of myometrial and cervical stromal invasion. These, in combination with tumour histology and grade, can help to determine a patient's preoperative risk stratification and ultimately guide treatment planning. PET/CT imaging is promising in the post-treatment surveillance of endometrial cancer patients.

CARCINOMA OF THE CERVIX

Cervical cancer is the second most common cancer in women worldwide, predominantly in developing countries in regions such as Central and South America, parts of Africa and South Central Asia. The peak incidence is between 30 and 40 years. Established risk factors for cervical cancer include early sexual activity (especially with multiple partners), cigarette smoking, immunosuppression and infection with human papilloma viruses 16 and 18. Abnormal uterine bleeding (especially after intercourse) and vaginal discharge may be symptoms leading to the diagnosis. In colposcopy, a lesion may be detected and vaginal cytology is usually positive.

Detection, Diagnosis and Staging

Cervical cancer is typically detected clinically (Papanicolaou smear and/or physical examination), with imaging being reserved for evaluating of extent of disease, monitoring treatment response and detecting tumour recurrence. Recommendations for the diagnostic evaluation of tumour staging derive from the FIGO clinical staging system (Table 17-3). Accurate tumour staging is important not only for prognosis but also in determining appropriate therapy. Among the various prognostic indicators, the most critical include tumour grade, tumour size, depth of stromal invasion, parametrial extension and lymph node involvement. Due to a relatively high likelihood of parametrial invasion and/or lymph node metastases, cross-sectional imaging is recommended in evaluating patients with cervical carcinoma with clinical stage Ib disease or greater, when the primary lesion is larger than 2 cm.[13,14]

Ultrasound

Transabdominal US can show the presence of hydronephrosis but has a limited role in the evaluation of the local extent of cervical cancer. Transrectal and transvaginal US have been used in the assessment of local disease but are limited in the detection of parametrial disease and pelvic side-wall involvement due to poor soft-tissue contrast, small field-of-view and operator dependence. More advanced cervical cancer can be visualised with TVUS. The cervix appears as an enlarged, irregular, hypoechoic mass that may mimic a cervical leiomyoma. If tumour obstructs the endocervical canal, hydro- and/or haematometra result.

Computed Tomography

Typically, CT findings in cervical cancer include enlargement of the cervix. After the administration of IV contrast medium, low attenuation areas may be seen within the tumour. These regions of decreased attenuation are a function of tumour necrosis/ulceration and/or inherent differences in the attenuation between tumour and normal cervical tissue. Distinguishing tumour from normal cervix and parametrium may be problematic. Obstruction of the endocervical canal can result in uterine enlargement with a fluid-filled endometrial cavity. CT

TABLE 17-3   FIGO Staging of Cervical Carcinoma with Corresponding MR Findings

FIGO Stage	Description of Stage	MRI Findings
Stage I	The carcinoma is strictly confined to the cervix	
Ia	Invasive carcinoma which can be diagnosed only by microscopy, with deepest invasion <5 mm and largest extension >7 mm	MRI is not indicated in stage Ia as tumour is not seen (except in cases considered for fertility sparing surgery such as trachelectomy)
Ia1	Measured stromal invasion of <3 mm in depth and extension <7 mm	
Ia2	Measured stromal invasion of >3 mm and not >5 mm with an extension of not >7 mm	
Ib	Clinically visible lesions limited to the cervix uteri or preclinical cancers greater than stage Ia	Intermediate signal intensity mass on T2WI. MRI can accurately delineate the tumour and its location and provide accurate size measurement (including distance from the internal os and cervical length in cases considered for trachelectomy)
Ib1	Clinically visible lesions <4 cm in greatest dimension	
Ib2	Clinically visible lesions >4 cm in greatest dimension	
Stage II	Cervical carcinoma invades beyond the uterus, but not to the pelvic wall or to the lower third of the vagina	Accurate evaluation of tumour location and tumour size. Invasion of the upper two-thirds of vagina is indicated by disruption of the low signal intensity vaginal wall by high signal intensity tumour on T2WI
IIa	Without parametrial invasion	
IIa1	Clinically visible lesion <4 cm in greatest dimension	
IIa2	Clinically visible lesion >4 cm in greatest dimension	
IIb	With obvious parametrial invasion	Parametrial invasion is indicated by disruption of the low signal intensity stromal ring, presence of a spiculated tumour/parametrium interface, gross nodular tumour extension into the parametrium or encasement of the uterine vessels by tumour
Stage III	The tumour extends to the pelvic wall and/or involves the lower third of the vagina and/or causes hydronephrosis or non-functioning kidney	
IIIa	Tumour involves lower third vagina, no extension to pelvic wall	Invasion of the lower third of vagina is indicated by disruption of the low signal intensity vaginal wall by high signal intensity tumour on T2WI
IIIb	Extension to the pelvic wall and/or hydronephrosis/non-functioning kidney	Pelvic side-wall invasion is indicated by tumour extension within 3 mm of pelvic side wall. Hydronephrosis is an indication of ureteral and/or bladder invasion
Stage IV	The carcinoma has extended beyond the true pelvis or has involved (biopsy proven) the mucosa of the bladder or rectum	Bladder or rectal invasion is indicated by loss of perivesical/perirectal fat planes and disruption of the normal low signal intensity bladder/rectal mucosa. Note that bullous oedema does not indicate stage IVa
IVa	Spread to adjacent organs	
IVb	Distant metastases (including intra-abdominal metastases) and/or inguinal lymph nodes	Tumour in distant sites or organs

T2WI, T2-weighted image.

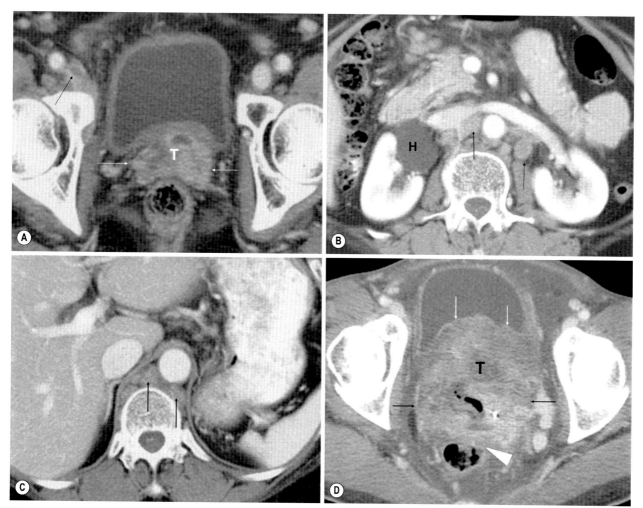

FIGURE 17-5 ■ **Cervical cancer, CT.** Axial CT images (A–C) show a cervical cancer (T, A) which is contiguous with the adjacent parametrial fat, indicating parametrial invasion (white arrows, A). Note the presence of a filling defect within the right external femoral vein suggesting deep venous thrombosis (black arrow, A). There is bilateral para-aortic (black arrows, B) and retrocrural lymphadenopathy (black arrows, C). Also, note the presence of right hydronephrosis (H, B). Axial CT image (D) of extensive cervical cancer (T, D) in a different patient. The tumour extends to both parametria (black arrows, D) and invades the posterior aspect of the bladder (white arrows, D) and anterior rectal wall (white arrowhead, D).

has limited value (a positive predictive value of 58%) in the evaluation of early parametrial invasion;[15,16] however, CT has an accuracy of 92% in the depiction of advanced disease (Fig. 17-5).

Magnetic Resonance Imaging

MRI can accurately determine tumour location (exophytic or endocervical), tumour size, depth of stromal invasion, presence of parametrial invasion and extension into the lower uterine segment.[13] The most important issue in staging cervical cancer is to distinguish early disease that can be treated with surgery from advanced disease that must be treated with chemoradiotherapy. MRI is the best single imaging investigation for this purpose, since it is better than either CT or physical examination in demonstrating parametrial invasion and as good as CT in detecting nodal metastases.[17] The

staging accuracy of MRI ranges from 75 to 96%. The reported sensitivity of MRI in the evaluation of parametrial invasion is 69% and the specificity is 93%.[13,17]

On T1-weighted images, tumours are usually isointense with the normal cervix and may not be visible. On T2-weighted images, cervical cancer appears as a relatively hyperintense mass and is easily distinguishable from low signal intensity cervical stroma.

Stage I. Stage I tumours are confined to the uterus. Stage Ia is defined as a microinvasive tumour that cannot be demonstrated at MRI. Stage Ib carcinoma appears as a high signal intensity mass relative to the low signal intensity fibrocervical stroma on T2-weighted images. Stage Ib is defined as clinically visible tumour limited to the cervix and is subdivided by size into Ib1 (<4 cm in greatest dimension) (Fig. 17-6) and Ib2 (>4 cm in greatest dimension).

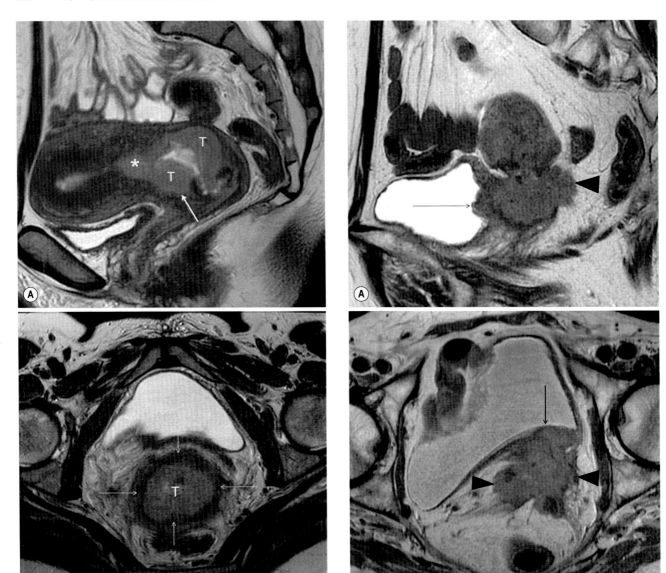

FIGURE 17-6 ■ **Cervical cancer, MRI.** Sagittal (A) and axial oblique (B) T2-weighted images show a large cervical cancer (T) involving the anterior fornix of the vagina (arrow, A). The fibrocervical stroma (arrows, B) is intact, which excludes parametrial invasion. The tumour extends into the lower endometrial canal (asterisk, A).

FIGURE 17-7 ■ **Cervical cancer, MRI.** Sagittal (A) and axial (B) T2-weighted images show a large cervical cancer (T) invading the posterior aspect of the bladder (arrows, A and B). Bilateral parametrial invasion and posterior tumour extension is seen (arrowheads, A and B).

Stage II. Stage II is defined as tumour growth beyond the cervix but without extension to the pelvic side wall or the lower third of the vagina. In stage IIa tumours, segmental disruption of the upper two-thirds of the vaginal wall without parametrial invasion is demonstrated on T2-weighted images. Stage IIa is again subdivided by size into IIa1 (<4 cm in greatest dimension) and IIa2 (>4 cm in greatest dimension); this subdivision has an effect on prognosis similar to that observed in stage Ib1 versus Ib2, which is reflected in the differing treatment strategies.[18] On MRI, stage IIb disease is seen as disruption of the low signal intensity stromal ring on T2WI, with the additional signs of a spiculated tumour to parametrium

interface, overt soft-tissue extension into the parametria (Fig. 17-7) or encasement of the peri-uterine vessels.[19]

Stages III and IV. Stage III is defined as tumour extension into the lower third of the vagina and/or pelvic side wall. In stage IIIa, vaginal involvement reaches the lower third of the vaginal canal without extending to the pelvic side wall. When the tumour extends to the pelvic side wall (pelvic musculature or iliac vessels) or causes hydronephrosis, it is defined as stage IIIb. Once tumour invades the adjacent organs such as the bladder and rectal mucosa, or distant metastasis occurs, it is defined as stage IV. Although pelvic node metastases do not change the

FIGO stage, para-aortic lymphadenopathy above the renal hila or inguinal node metastases are classified as stage IVb.

Positron Emission Tomography/ Computed Tomography

FDG-PET/CT is useful in staging of patients with advanced cervical cancer, especially the detection of lymph node metastases. Although lymphadenopathy is not part of the FIGO staging system, it can be considered indicative of stage IVb disease and its presence is therefore when developing a treatment plan. Conventional cross-sectional imaging techniques rely on size criteria for the diagnosis of lymphadenopathy and, as such, microscopic disease is often not detected. FDG-PET is better than the conventional imaging techniques for the detection of lymph node metastases in patients with cervical cancer, with sensitivities of 75–100% and specificities of 87–100%.[20] FDG-PET/CT also improves initial staging in cases of advanced disease by demonstrating unexpected sites of disease beyond the pelvis or retroperitoneum, such as supraclavicular nodal metastases. In patients with advanced disease at presentation (FIGO IIb to IVb), PET or PET/CT has been found to alter management in a significant number of patients.[21] By contrast, the value of FDG-PET in early-stage disease (FIGO I to IIa) is questionable.

FDG-PET has a prognostic value in patients with cervical cancer.[22] Kidd et al. found that the maximum standardised uptake value (SUVmax) of the primary cervical tumour at diagnosis was a sensitive biomarker of treatment response and prognosis for patients with cervical cancer.[23] Recently, the same group reported that the SUV of pelvic lymph nodes is a prognostic biomarker, predicting treatment response, pelvic recurrence risk and disease-specific survival in patients with cervical cancer.[24]

Recommended Imaging Approach

Transvaginal US has poor soft-tissue contrast and thus limited value in cervical cancer detection and in the determination of stromal invasion or parametrial extension. Contrast-enhanced CT may be helpful in local staging; however, it is mainly used in advanced disease and in the assessment of lymph nodes. CT is also performed to detect distant metastases, for radiotherapy planning and for guiding interventional procedures. For locoregional staging, MRI is the method of choice because it can accurately determine tumour size, location (exophytic or endocervical), depth of stromal invasion and the local extent of the tumour. PET/CT is useful for primary staging (mainly in assessing nodal disease) as well as evaluating distant metastatic disease in patients with recurrent cervical cancer before they undergo pelvic exenteresis (Fig. 17-8).

OVARIAN CARCINOMA

Ovarian neoplasms account for more cancer-related deaths than all other primary cancers of the female reproductive system. In general, ovarian cancer is a disease of postmenopausal women and, occasionally, prepubescent girls. The cause of ovarian cancer is unknown, although a number of risk factors have been identified. Chronic anovulation, multiparity and a history of breast-feeding seem to be protective, whereas genetic factors appear to play an important role in the development of progression of ovarian cancer. Ten per cent of ovarian cancers are due to hereditary syndromes such as BRCA-1 and BRCA-2 mutations (risk of breast cancer) and Lynch syndrome II (risk of colon cancer). Approximately 90% of ovarian cancers are of epithelial origin. Epithelial tumours are subtyped as serous (50%), mucinous (20%),

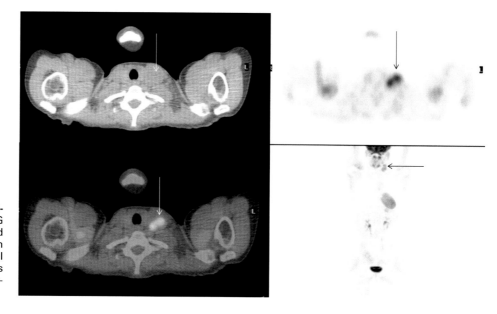

FIGURE 17-8 ■ Recurrent cervical carcinoma, PET/CT. FDG uptake is seen within left-sided supraclavicular lymph nodes on axial CT, PET and fused axial and coronal PET/CT images (arrows) of a patient with recurrent cervical cancer.

endometrioid (20%), clear cell (10%) or undifferentiated (1%). Non-epithelial cancers include malignant granulosa cell tumour, dysgerminoma, immature teratoma, endodermal sinus tumour and metastases to the ovary.

Detection, Diagnosis and Staging

The detection of early ovarian cancer is difficult for a variety of reasons and currently involves a combination of physical examination, serum CA125 levels and transvaginal US. Imaging by means of US, CT, MRI and FDG-PET/CT plays a crucial role in detection, characterisation, staging and follow-up of patients with ovarian cancer.

Early ovarian cancer is treated with comprehensive staging laparotomy, which includes transabdominal hysterectomy and bilateral salpingo-oophorectomy (TAH/BSO), omentectomy, retroperitoneal lymph node sampling, peritoneal and diaphragmatic biopsies and cytology of peritoneal washings. Advanced but operable disease is treated with primary cytoreductive surgery (debulking) followed by adjuvant chemotherapy. Patients with non-resectable disease may benefit from neoadjuvant (preoperative) chemotherapy before debulking. Imaging is of paramount importance in helping triage patients for appropriate management. Accurately evaluating the extent and anatomical location of peritoneal spread dictates the feasibility of cytoreductive surgery and predicts the likelihood of optimal primary cytoreduction.

Accurate imaging will help guide the surgeon to areas of disease that may be difficult to identify surgically and describe the volume and extent of disease for optimal cytoreductive surgery. Relative criteria for 'non-optimally resectable disease' have been developed.[25] They include:
- In the pelvis: invasion of pelvic side wall or urinary bladder, or urinary obstruction.
- In the upper abdomen: tumour deposits greater than 1 cm in size in the gastrosplenic ligament, lesser sac, falciform ligament, porta hepatis, subphrenic space, small bowel mesentery or retroperitoneal nodes above the renal hila.
- Distant metastases (i.e. liver, spleen, lung).

Imaging by US and CT is also used to guide ovarian mass/omental biopsy, which is needed before neoadjuvant chemotherapy.

Ultrasound

Combined transabdominal and transvaginal US has been advocated for the detection of ovarian carcinoma. These studies provide superb morphological detail of the adnexa, allowing detection of masses before they are clinically apparent. Ultrasound features that suggest benignancy and malignancy have been well described. Although several scoring systems have been devised to predict the nature of an adnexal mass, most researchers agree that wall irregularity, thick septations (>3 mm), papillary projections, solid components and size (>9 cm) are suspicious for malignancy[26] (Fig. 17-9).

Malignant tumours often have neovascularity that consists of blood vessels with walls that have little or no smooth muscle support. As a result, these vessels

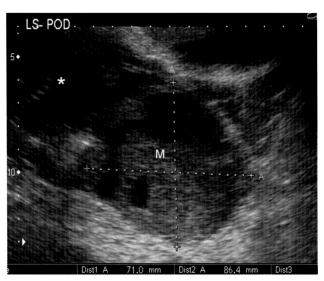

FIGURE 17-9 ■ **Clear cell ovarian carcinoma, US.** Transabdominal US reveals a predominantly solid mass (M) with some cystic areas, within the pouch of Douglas. Small amount of ascites also shown (asterisk).

frequently have a characteristic waveform with a low resistive index (RI <0.4) (peak systolic – end diastolic Doppler shift/peak systolic Doppler shift). A meta-analysis of the literature demonstrated that the best adnexal lesion characterisation is achieved by the combined use of grey scale and colour Doppler US.[27]

Computed Tomography

CT is the most commonly performed study for preoperative staging of a suspected ovarian carcinoma. The FIGO staging system and its corresponding CT findings are outlined in Table 17-4. CT is particularly useful in determining the extent of cytoreductive surgery required to optimise subsequent chemotherapeutic response.[25] On CT, ovarian cancer demonstrates varied morphological patterns, including a multilocular cyst with thick internal septations and solid mural or septal components, a partially cystic and solid mass (Fig. 17-10) and a lobulated papillary heterogeneous solid mass. The outer border of the mass may be irregular and poorly defined, and amorphous coarse calcifications and contrast enhancement may be seen in the cyst wall or soft-tissue components.[28] It is possible to suggest the histological subtype of the epithelial cancer based on the imaging findings. Calcification suggests a serous tumour, whereas high density within the locules of a multilocular tumour is suggestive of proteinaceous fluid in a mucinous tumour. Endometrioid carcinomas are associated with endometrial hyperplasia or carcinoma in 20–30% of cases.

Intraperitoneal dissemination is the most common route of spread of ovarian cancer. Peritoneal implants appear as nodular or plaque-like enhancing soft-tissue masses of varying size (Fig. 17-10). Ascitic fluid may outline small implants, facilitating detection. Although peritoneal implants may occur anywhere in the peritoneal cavity, the most common sites include the pouch of Douglas, paracolic gutters, surface of the small and large

TABLE 17-4 **FIGO Staging of Ovarian Carcinoma with Corresponding CT Findings**

FIGO Stage	Description of Stage	CT Findings
Stage I	Tumour limited to ovaries (one/both)	
Ia	Tumour limited to one ovary, capsule intact, no tumour on ovarian surface, no malignant cells in ascites or peritoneal washings[a]	Enlarged or normal ovary and ascites may be present
Ib	Tumour limited to both ovaries, capsule intact, no tumour on ovarian surface, no malignant cells in ascites or peritoneal washings[a]	Enlarged or normal ovaries and ascites may be present
Ic	Tumour limited to one or both ovaries with any of the following: capsular rupture, tumour on ovarian surface, malignant cells in ascites or peritoneal washings[a]	Unilateral or bilateral mixed cystic/solid or solid adnexal mass with irregular contour, heterogeneous enhancement of solid components and thick septa. Ascites
Stage II	Tumour involves one or both ovaries with pelvic extensions or implants	
IIa	Tumour extension and/or implants on uterus/fallopian tube(s), no malignant cells in ascites or peritoneal washings[a]	Irregularity or obliteration of the fat plane between the uterus and the adnexal mass. Dilated fallopian tubes which may contain enhancing soft-tissue nodules. Ascites
IIb	Tumour extension and/or implants on other pelvic tissue, no malignant cells in ascites or peritoneal washings	Loss of the normal fat plane around the rectum or bladder, less than 3 mm between the tumour and the pelvic side wall, and/or displacement or encasement of the iliac vessels. Ascites
Stage III	Tumour involves one or both ovaries with microscopically confirmed peritoneal metastasis outside the pelvis	
IIIa	Microscopically confirmed peritoneal metastasis[b] outside the pelvis (no macroscopic tumour)	Microscopic extra-pelvic peritoneal implants are not detectable with CT
IIIb	Macroscopically peritoneal metastasis outside the pelvis is 2 cm or less in dimension	Peritoneal/serosal deposits <2 cm outside the pelvis
IIIc	Macroscopically peritoneal metastasis outside the pelvis is >2 cm and/or involved regional lymph nodes	Peritoneal implants of >2 cm. Omental cake. Note that subcapsular liver implants and those along the diaphragm, lesser sac, porta hepatis, intersegmental fissure, gall bladder fossa; gastrosplenic, gastrohepatic ligament and small bowel mesentery are 'difficult to resect'. Enlarged inguinal and retroperitoneal lymph nodes
Stage IV	Distant metastasis beyond the peritoneal cavity. Enlarged lymph nodes above the level of the renal hilum	Liver parenchymal metastases, pleural effusion.[c] Enlarged lymph nodes above the level of the renal hilum

[a]The presence of ascites does not affect staging unless malignant cells are present.
[b]Liver capsule metastasis is stage III; liver parenchymal metastasis is stage IV.
[c]Stage IV: pleural effusion must have positive cytology.

bowel, greater omentum, surface of the liver (perihepatic implants) and subphrenic space. CT is useful in differentiating between subcapsular and parenchymal liver metastasis, which alters staging and therapy.[28] Ascites is a non-specific finding but, in a patient with ovarian cancer, usually indicates peritoneal metastases.

In addition to peritoneal implantation, ovarian cancer also spreads by local continuity to the ovary, uterus and other pelvic organs. Surgically important features of local spread that may be detected by imaging are invasion of the pelvic side wall, rectum, sigmoid colon or urinary bladder. Pelvic side-wall invasion should be suspected when the primary tumour lies within 3 mm of the pelvic side wall or when the iliac vessels are surrounded or distorted by tumour. The ovarian lymphatic vessels are another important route of metastatic spread. While enlarged nodes are likely to be involved, CT is unable to exclude disease in normal-sized nodes.

The CT appearance of ovarian metastasis is indistinguishable from that of a primary ovarian neoplasm, and the stomach and colon should be carefully examined as potential primary tumour sites. Occasionally, it is not

possible to determine whether the origin of a pelvic mass is ovarian or uterine on CT.

Magnetic Resonance Imaging

The role of MRI in patients with suspected or known ovarian carcinoma is still evolving. To optimise MR detection and characterisation of an adnexal mass, contrast-enhanced protocols and attention to eliminating, or at least limiting, bowel motion are needed. Both transvaginal US and contrast-enhanced MRI have high sensitivity (97 and 100%, respectively) in the identification of solid components within an adnexal mass. MRI, however, shows higher accuracy (93%).[29]

Primary and ancillary criteria for characterising an adnexal mass as malignant have been established. Primary criteria for malignancy include (A) size larger than 4 cm, (B) a cystic lesion with a solid component, (C) irregular wall thickness greater than 3 mm, (D) septa greater than 3 mm and/or the presence of vegetations or nodularity and (E) a solid mass with the presence of necrosis. Ancillary criteria for malignancy include (A) involvement of

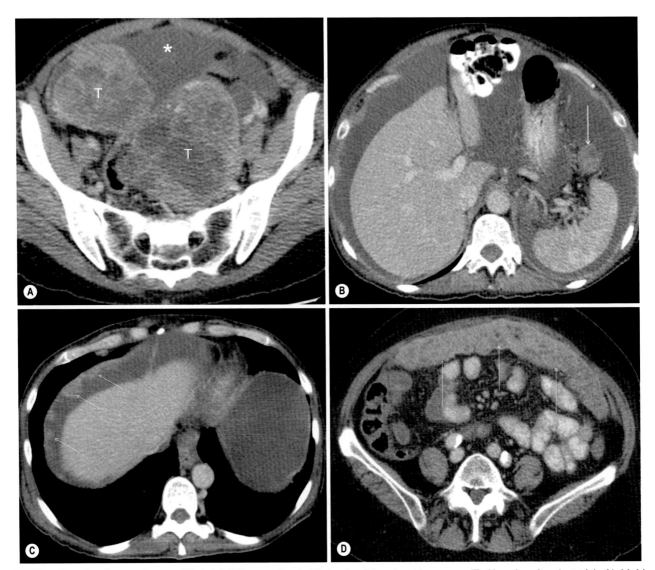

FIGURE 17-10 ■ **Ovarian carcinoma, CT.** Axial CT image shows bilateral solid and cystic masses (T, A) and ascites (asterisk, A), highly suggestive of ovarian carcinoma. Axial CT images of the upper abdomen demonstrate the presence of peritoneal deposits on the gastrosplenic ligament (arrow, B) and around the right hemidiaphragm (arrows, C). The presence of an omental cake is noted (arrows, D).

pelvic organs or side wall, (B) peritoneal, mesenteric or omental disease, (C) ascites or (D) adenopathy. Utilising unenhanced T1-, T2- and contrast-enhanced T1-weighted sequences, the presence of at least one of the primary criteria coupled with a single criterion from the ancillary group correctly characterises 95% of malignant lesions (Fig. 17-11).[30]

Peritoneal/serosal implants and omental cake are best seen on delayed (5-min) images. However, longer delays beyond 5 min should be avoided as ascites may also enhance, impairing visualisation of subtle peritoneal implants. Recently, there has been a growing awareness of the potential of DW-MRI in improving the mapping of the extent of ovarian cancer and quantifying its early treatment response.[31–33] The omental cake and peritoneal deposits retain high signal intensity with increasing b values against a background of suppressed signal from surrounding ascites, bowel contents and fat, increasing conspicuity.[31]

Positron Emission Tomography/Computed Tomography

Currently, there is no established role for PET/CT in preoperative staging of patients with advanced ovarian cancer. However, PET/CT plays an important role in evaluating patients for recurrent ovarian cancer, particularly those with negative CT or MRI findings and rising tumour marker levels.[34] PET/CT is also useful in the detection of implants that are difficult to assess by conventional imaging studies, such as serosal bowel implants or tumour deposits within the small bowel mesentery (Fig. 17-12).

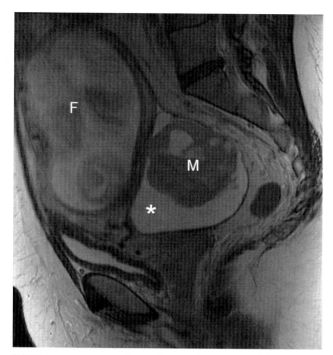

FIGURE 17-11 ■ **Clear cell ovarian carcinoma, MRI.** T2-weighted sagittal MR image in a pregnant patient. Gravid uterus is identified (F). Posterior to the uterus, in the pouch of Douglas, is a heterogeneous solid and cystic rounded mass (M). The mass is surrounded by ascites (*).

Recommended Imaging Approach

US is the primary technique for the detection and characterisation of adnexal masses. MRI is a problem-solving investigation in cases of indeterminate adnexal masses and the best technique for assessing pelvic side-wall invasion. CT is the imaging technique of choice for pre-operative staging and for follow-up. CT is the primary technique for prediction of tumour resectability, tumour extent into the upper abdomen and related complications such as hydronephrosis and bowel obstruction. PET/CT is very valuable in the setting of recurrent disease and particularly useful for detecting tumour deposits in mesentery and bowel serosa.

CONCLUSION

Increased use of CT, MRI and PET/CT for staging gynaecological malignancies has led to a significant decline in the use of conventional radiological studies such as intravenous urography and barium enema that have now become obsolete in most institutions. US is the primary imaging technique for characterising ovarian masses and evaluating endometrial thickness. CT is the technique of choice for the staging of ovarian cancer, detection of distant metastases and lymphadenopathy in

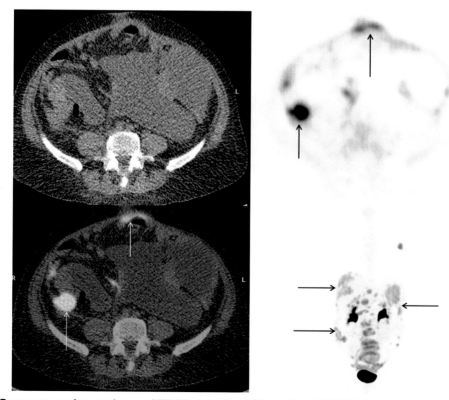

FIGURE 17-12 ■ **Recurrent ovarian carcinoma, PET/CT.** Axial CT, PET and fused PET/CT in axial and coronal planes show multiple areas of increased FDG uptake in the anterior peritoneum and paracolic gutters.

endometrial and cervical cancer, and evaluation of recurrent pelvic malignancies. Both US and CT are used to guide percutaneous drainage and biopsy.

MRI plays an important role in the patient journey from the initial evaluation of the extent of the disease to appropriate treatment selection and follow-up. In patients with endometrial cancer, MRI enables accurate surgical planning and selection of patients for pelvic or para-aortic lymph node dissection in high-risk disease, whilst obviating the need for extended surgery in patients with low-risk disease. In patients with cervical cancer, MRI improves FIGO clinical staging accuracy, leading to better treatment selection and planning. In patients with recurrent ovarian cancer, MRI plays an important role by assessing resectability in cases of solitary pelvic recurrences. FDG-PET/CT is increasingly being used to evaluate gynaecological malignancies. It is useful in the primary staging of cervical cancer as well as the detection of recurrent ovarian, cervical and endometrial cancer.

ACKNOWLEDGEMENTS

We acknowledge the contribution of Sandra Allison to the chapter in the previous edition of this book.

REFERENCES

1. Griffin N, Grant LA, Freeman SJ, et al. Image-guided biopsy in patients with suspected ovarian carcinoma: a safe and effective technique? Eur Radiol 2009;19(1):230–5.
2. Balleyguier C, Sala E, Da CT, et al. Staging of uterine cervical cancer with MRI: guidelines of the European Society of Urogenital Radiology. Eur Radiol 2011;21(5):1102–10.
3. Kinkel K, Kaji Y, Yu KK, et al. Radiologic staging in patients with endometrial cancer: a meta-analysis. Radiology 1999;212(3):711–18.
4. Beddy P, Moyle P, Kataoka M, et al. Evaluation of depth of myometrial invasion and overall staging in endometrial cancer: comparison of diffusion-weighted and dynamic contrast-enhanced MR imaging. Radiology 2012;262(2):530–7.
5. Sala E, Wakely S, Senior E, Lomas D. MRI of malignant neoplasms of the uterine corpus and cervix. AJR Am J Roentgenol 2007;188(6):1577–87.
6. Pecorelli S. Revised FIGO staging for carcinoma of the vulva, cervix, and endometrium. Int J Gynaecol Obstet 2009;105(2):103–4.
7. Arko D, Takac I. High frequency transvaginal ultrasonography in preoperative assessment of myometrial invasion in endometrial cancer. J Ultrasound Med 2000;19(9):639–43.
8. Smith-Bindman R, Kerlikowske K, Feldstein VA, et al. Endovaginal ultrasound to exclude endometrial cancer and other endometrial abnormalities. JAMA 1998;280(17):1510–17.
9. Ascher SM, Reinhold C. Imaging of cancer of the endometrium. Radiol Clin North Am 2002;40(3):563–76.
10. Querleu D, Planchamp F, Narducci F, et al. Clinical practice guidelines for the management of patients with endometrial cancer in France: recommendations of the Institut National du Cancer and the Societe Francaise d'Oncologie Gynecologique. Int J Gynecol Cancer 2011;21(5):945–50.
11. Kinkel K, Forstner R, Danza FM, et al. Staging of endometrial cancer with MRI: guidelines of the European Society of Urogenital Imaging. Eur Radiol 2009;19(7):1565–74.
12. Manfredi R, Mirk P, Maresca G, et al. Local-regional staging of endometrial carcinoma: role of MR imaging in surgical planning. Radiology 2004;231(2):372–8.
13. Okamoto Y, Tanaka YO, Nishida M, et al. MR imaging of the uterine cervix: imaging–pathologic correlation. Radiographics 2003;23(2):425–45.
14. Scheidler J, Heuck AF. Imaging of cancer of the cervix. Radiol Clin North Am 2002;40(3):577–90, vii.
15. Hricak H, Gatsonis C, Coakley FV, et al. Early invasive cervical cancer: CT and MR imaging in preoperative evaluation—ACRIN/GOG comparative study of diagnostic performance and interobserver variability. Radiology 2007;245(2):491–8.
16. Mitchell DG, Snyder B, Coakley F, et al. Early invasive cervical cancer: tumor delineation by magnetic resonance imaging, computed tomography, and clinical examination, verified by pathologic results, in the ACRIN 6651/GOG 183 Intergroup Study. J Clin Oncol 2006;24(36):5687–94.
17. Hricak H, Yu KK. Radiology in invasive cervical cancer. AJR Am J Roentgenol 1996;167(5):1101–8.
18. Pecorelli S, Zigliani L, Odicino F. Revised FIGO staging for carcinoma of the cervix. Int J Gynaecol Obstet 2009;105(2):107–8.
19. Nicolet V, Carignan L, Bourdon F, Prosmanne O. MR imaging of cervical carcinoma: a practical staging approach. Radiographics 2000;20(6):1539–49.
20. Reinhardt MJ, Ehritt-Braun C, Vogelgesang D, et al. Metastatic lymph nodes in patients with cervical cancer: detection with MR imaging and FDG PET. Radiology 2001;218(3):776–82.
21. Chao A, Ho KC, Wang CC, et al. Positron emission tomography in evaluating the feasibility of curative intent in cervical cancer patients with limited distant lymph node metastases. Gynecol Oncol 2008;110(2):172–8.
22. Kidd EA, Siegel BA, Dehdashti F, et al. Lymph node staging by positron emission tomography in cervical cancer: relationship to prognosis. J Clin Oncol 2010;28(12):2108–13.
23. Kidd EA, Siegel BA, Dehdashti F, Grigsby PW. The standardized uptake value for F-18 fluorodeoxyglucose is a sensitive predictive biomarker for cervical cancer treatment response and survival. Cancer 2007;110(8):1738–44.
24. Kidd EA, Siegel BA, Dehdashti F, Grigsby PW. Pelvic lymph node F-18 fluorodeoxyglucose uptake as a prognostic biomarker in newly diagnosed patients with locally advanced cervical cancer. Cancer 2010;116(6):1469–75.
25. Qayyum A, Coakley FV, Westphalen AC, et al. Role of CT and MR imaging in predicting optimal cytoreduction of newly diagnosed primary epithelial ovarian cancer. Gynecol Oncol 2005;96(2):301–6.
26. Brown DL, Doubilet PM, Miller FH, et al. Benign and malignant ovarian masses: selection of the most discriminating gray-scale and Doppler sonographic features. Radiology 1998;208(1):103–10.
27. Kinkel K, Hricak H, Lu Y, et al. US characterization of ovarian masses: a meta-analysis. Radiology 2000;217(3):803–11.
28. Coakley FV. Staging ovarian cancer: role of imaging. Radiol Clin North Am 2002;40(3):609–36.
29. Hricak H, Chen M, Coakley FV, et al. Complex adnexal masses: detection and characterization with MR imaging—multivariate analysis. Radiology 2000;214(1):39–46.
30. Stevens SK, Hricak H, Stern JL. Ovarian lesions: detection and characterization with gadolinium-enhanced MR imaging at 1.5 T. Radiology 1991;181(2):481–8.
31. Fujii S, Kakite S, Nishihara K, et al. Diagnostic accuracy of diffusion-weighted imaging in differentiating benign from malignant ovarian lesions. J Magn Reson Imaging 2008;28(5):1149–56.
32. Sala E, Priest AN, Kataoka M, et al. Apparent diffusion coefficient and vascular signal fraction measurements with magnetic resonance imaging: feasibility in metastatic ovarian cancer at 3 Tesla: technical development. Eur Radiol 2010;20(2):491–6.
33. Kyriazi S, Nye E, Stamp G, et al. Value of diffusion-weighted imaging for assessing site-specific response of advanced ovarian cancer to neoadjuvant chemotherapy: correlation of apparent diffusion coefficients with epithelial and stromal densities on histology. Cancer Biomark 2010;7(4):201–10.
34. Sala E, Kataoka M, Pandit-Taskar N, et al. Recurrent ovarian cancer: use of contrast-enhanced CT and PET/CT to accurately localize tumor recurrence and to predict patients' survival. Radiology 2010;257(1):125–34.

CHAPTER 18

BENIGN GYNAECOLOGICAL DISEASE

Sue J. Barter • Fleur Kilburn-Toppin

This chapter gives a brief review of common benign gynaecological disorders and presents indications for the role of ultrasound (US), computed tomography (CT) and magnetic resonance imaging (MRI) in investigation, problem solving and management.

IMAGING TECHNIQUES

Ultrasound

Ultrasound (transabdominal and transvaginal) is accepted as the primary imaging technique for examining the female pelvis. Indications include evaluation of a suspected pelvic mass, acute pelvic pain, causes of uterine enlargement, investigation of postmenopausal bleeding and characterisation of ovarian masses, as well as guiding invasive procedures such as biopsy and drainage.

Ultrasound has many advantages in routine pelvic imaging: it is relatively inexpensive, provides multiplanar views, is widely available and lacks ionising radiation or contrast media (Fig. 18-1).

Computed Tomography

The role of CT in benign gynaecological conditions has largely been replaced by MRI, although it may be used to investigate acute pelvic pain where US has been unhelpful (Fig. 18-2).

Magnetic Resonance Imaging

The role of MRI in gynaecology has evolved rapidly, and it is now commonly used for the investigation of Müllerian duct anomalies and benign conditions such as endometriosis and evaluation of fibroids especially before possible embolisation. It is invaluable in investigation of the indeterminate adnexal mass (Fig. 18-3).

Hysterosalpingography and Fallopian Tube Catheterisation

Hysterosalpingography (HSG) is used mainly to investigate infertility. It is best performed in the first 10 days of the cycle, but not during active bleeding. Contraindications are pregnancy and active pelvic infection. Complications include pain, pelvic infection, haemorrhage and vasovagal attacks (Fig. 18-4).

Fallopian tube catheterisation is a technique using small catheters and guidewires to cannulate the fallopian tubes and establish patency if there is cornual occlusion in an otherwise normal pelvis. Pregnancy rates of around 60% have been reported following the procedure[1] (Fig. 18-5).

Sonohysterography

This technique involves placement of a 5F balloon catheter through the cervix and instilling sterile saline or a microbubble solution under direct ultrasound visualisation (Fig. 18-6). The procedure is well tolerated, with contraindications and complications similar to HSG.

It is indicated for evaluation of masses detected in the uterine cavity at US, and fallopian tube patency. Some fertility centres prefer HSG because of the additional information obtained despite the radiation dose.

CONGENITAL ANOMALIES OF THE FEMALE GENITAL TRACT

Congenital uterine anomalies comprise a wide spectrum of disorders, occurring in 1–15% of women. Embryologically, they result from abnormal development and fusion of the paired Müllerian ducts from which the uterus, the upper two-thirds of the vagina and the

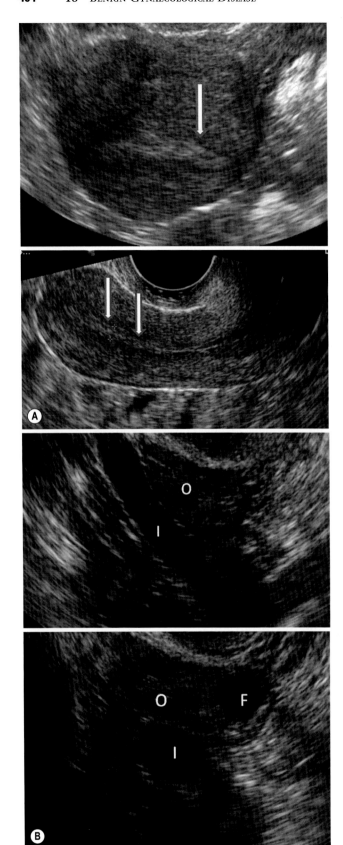

FIGURE 18-1 ■ **Normal US anatomy.** (A) Sagittal and axial transvaginal US shows normal endometrium (arrows). (B) Sagittal and axial transvaginal US shows a normal ovary (O) with a follicle (F). Note the location of the ovary anterior and medial to the internal iliac vessels (I) within the ovarian fossa.

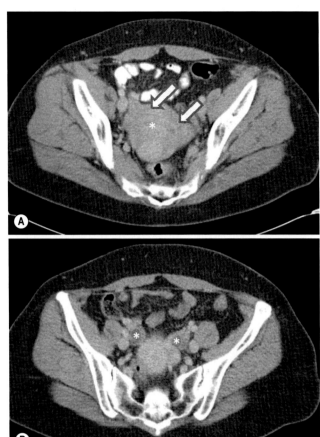

FIGURE 18-2 ■ **Helical CT of the normal uterus and adnexa.** (A) Low-attenuation endometrial cavity (*) surrounded by enhancing myometrium (arrows). (B) Normal ovaries. CT shows bilateral follicles (*). The ovaries are in their expected location, anterior to the internal iliac vessels and posterior to the external iliac vessels.

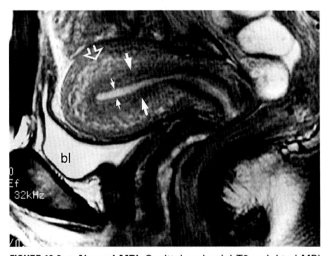

FIGURE 18-3 ■ **Normal MRI.** Sagittal and axial T2-weighted MRI demonstrating zonal anatomy of the uterus. The central, high-signal intensity stripe represents the endometrium (small arrows); the band of low signal intensity subjacent to the endometrial stripe represents the inner myometrium or junctional zone (arrows). The outer layer of the myometrium is of intermediate signal intensity (open arrow). bl = bladder.

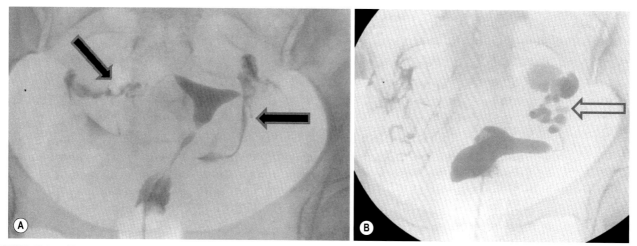

FIGURE 18-4 ■ **Hysterosalpingogram.** (A) Normal hysterosalpingogram demonstrating a normal uterine cavity and fallopian tubes with bilateral spill of contrast into the peritoneal cavity (arrows). (B) Hysterosalpingogram showing bilateral hydrosalpinges.

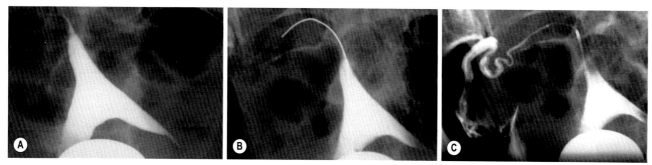

FIGURE 18-5 ■ **Fallopian tube catheterisation.** (A) Initial HSG confirms bilateral corneal occlusion. (B) A catheter has been introduced into the right cornu, and a guidewire passed to the obstruction. (C) The guidewire is manipulated across the occlusion and tubal patency restored.

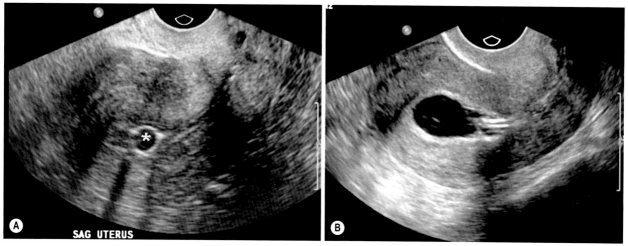

FIGURE 18-6 ■ **Sonohysterography.** (A) Sagittal transvaginal US demonstrates the inflated balloon of the sonohysterographic catheter (*) within the endometrial canal. (B) Following the instillation of 40 mL of sterile saline, fluid distends the endometrial canal.

fallopian tubes are derived. They are associated with menstrual disorders, infertility and obstetric complications, and a high incidence of renal anomalies, particularly agenesis and ectopia. Often, more minor Müllerian duct abnormalities are detected incidentally during investigations for other conditions.

MRI, which provides exquisite detail of pelvic anatomy, is the most accurate imaging technique for investigating and classifying congenital anomalies; classification is important as fertility outcomes and surgical management vary considerably. In addition to standard MR imaging planes, coronal oblique planes (parallel to the long axis of the uterus) and axial oblique planes (perpendicular to the long axis of the uterus) should be obtained for optimal imaging to allow for variation in uterine flexion.[2] T2-weighted images are best for uterine zonal anatomy, whereas coronal oblique T1-weighted images best depict the fundal contour. A standard coronal T1-weighted image through the kidneys is important due to the high association of renal abnormalities.

Müllerian Duct Anomalies

These disorders are classified according to Buttram and Gibbons and the American Fertility Society.[3]

Class I: Uterine Agenesis or Hypoplasia

Uterine agenesis or hypoplasia results from failure of normal development of both Müllerian ducts. The ovaries are normal most patients, helping to distinguish the condition from other syndromes such as androgen insensitivity and gonadal dysgenesis.[4]

The commonest subtype of uterine agenesis is the Mayer–Rokitansky–Küster–Hauser (MRKH) syndrome. There is uterine and vaginal agenesis or hypoplasia with intact ovaries and fallopian tubes with variable anomalies of the urinary tract and skeletal system.

Detection of uterine remnants may be difficult on US and sagittal and axial MR images can more reliably detect the absence or anomalies of the uterus and vagina, respectively[5] (Fig. 18-7).

Class II: Unicornuate Uterus

This results from failure of normal development of one Müllerian duct, and is associated with increased spontaneous abortion and obstetric complications, and renal abnormalities.

On T2-weighted MR images, the unicornuate uterus demonstrates a curved, elongated uterus with tapering of the fundal segment off midline (the 'banana-like' configuration) best seen on the axial oblique (long axis) images (Fig. 18-8).

Normal uterine zonal anatomy is maintained. If a rudimentary horn is present, it usually demonstrates lower signal intensity.

Class III: Uterus Didelphys

Non-fusion of the Müllerian ducts results in uterus didelphys with two separate normal-sized uterine horns and

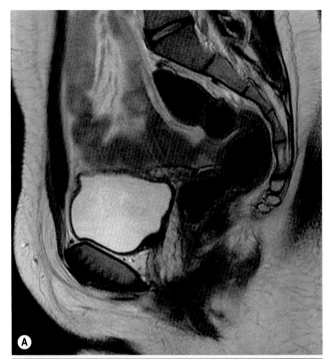

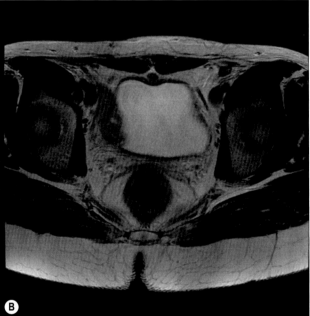

FIGURE 18-7 ■ **Uterine and vaginal agenesis.** (A) Sagittal and (B) axial T2-weighted MRI of the pelvis showing absent uterus and vagina.

cervices. A longitudinal vaginal septum is present in 75% of cases. On coronal oblique T2-weighted images the two uterine horns can be appreciated, which are usually widely separated with preservation of the endometrial and myometrial widths (Fig. 18-9).

Class IV: Bicornuate Uterus

Incomplete fusion of the cephalad extent of the uterovaginal horns with resorption of the uterovaginal septum gives rise to a bicornuate uterus. Obstetric complications

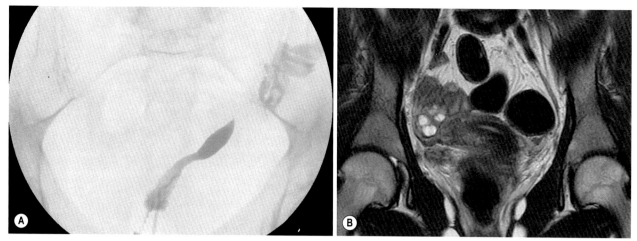

FIGURE 18-8 ■ **Unicornuate uterus.** (A) Hysterosalpingogram and (B) T2-weighted axial oblique MRI showing the 'banana-like' configuration.

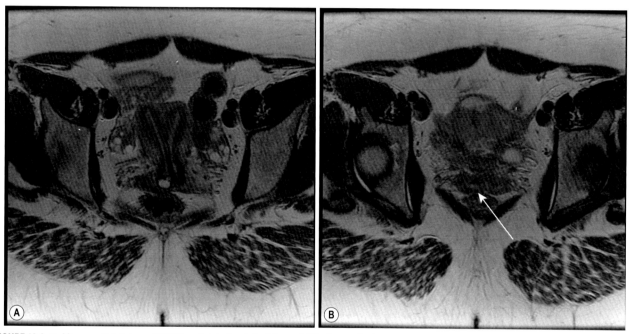

FIGURE 18-9 ■ **Uterus didelphys.** (A) T2-weighted axial oblique MRI elegantly demonstrates two separate normal-sized uterine horns and cervices. (B) T2-weighted axial image at the level of the vagina demonstrates a longitudinal vaginal septum (arrow).

relate to the degree of non-fusion of the horns. T2-weighted coronal images show the communicating uterine horns with a concave fundus. They are separated by an intervening cleft longer than 1 cm in the external fundal myometrium, which demonstrates signal intensity the same as that of myometrium on all sequences. Normal zonal anatomy is seen in each horn (Fig. 18-10).

Class V: Septate Uterus

This is the commonest Müllerian duct abnormality, with incomplete resorption of the fibrous septum between the two uterine horns. The septum may be partial or complete, extending to the external cervical os. The

differentiation between the septate and the bicornuate uterus is clinically important because the septate uterus has the worst obstetric outcome of all Müllerian duct abnormalities. The fibrous septum is best demonstrated on coronal oblique T2-weighted MR images, with the key differentiating factor being the external uterine contour, which is convex, flat or concave (<1 cm) in contrast to the bicornuate uterus[6] (Fig. 18-11).

Class VI: Arcuate Uterus

This is considered a normal variant, and is thought to have no significant effects on fertility or pregnancy. On imaging there is a smooth, broad indentation of the

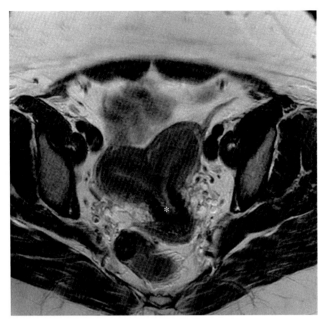

FIGURE 18-10 ■ **Bicornuate uterus.** Coronal T2-weighted MRI demonstrating two endometrial cavities and single cervical canal (*). Note the communicating uterine horns with a concave fundus.

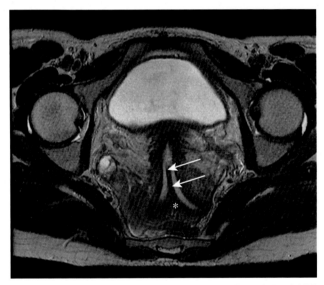

FIGURE 18-11 ■ **Septate uterus.** Axial oblique T2-weighted MRI shows a partially septate retroverted uterus. The fibrous septum (arrows) and muscular septum (*) are clearly demonstrated.

fundus of the uterine cavity, with a normal external uterine contour (Fig. 18-12).

Class VII: Diethylstilbestrol Related

Diethylstilbestrol is a synthetic oestrogen which can produce uterine abnormalities secondary to in utero exposure. A T-shaped uterine cavity is the commonest finding, with uterine hypoplasia, irregular constrictions and intraluminal filling defects also seen.

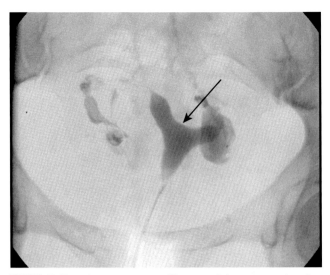

FIGURE 18-12 ■ **Arcuate uterus.** Hysterosalpingogram showing the typical smooth, broad indentation of the fundus of the uterine cavity.

Vaginal Anomalies

Defects in vertical and lateral fusion of the Müllerian ducts can result in vaginal septae formation. Along with vaginal agenesis, as seen in MRKH syndrome, these may cause obstruction, preventing loss of menstrual blood and leading to haematocolpos or haematometrocolpos.

On MRI, the septum is identified as low signal intensity fibrous tissue on T2-weighted sagittal images, with loss of vaginal zonal anatomy (Fig. 18-9B). Dilatation of the vagina with intraluminal fluid of intermediate or high signal intensity and the occasional presence of fluid/debris levels can also be shown. T1-weighted images with fat suppression confirm blood products in haematometrocolpos.

Imaging of Ambiguous Genitalia

This is a broad spectrum of disorders, including male (46 XY) and female (46 XX) pseudo and true hermaphroditism and gonadal dysgenesis, including Turner's syndrome. Imaging is important for depicting internal genitalia and identifying gonads. US is the initial imaging investigation of choice, but MR is often used as a problem-solving tool. Streak ovaries, as seen in Turner's syndrome, are particularly difficult to detect and appear as low signal stripes on T2-weighted MR. Additional high signal intensity foci should raise the suspicion of malignant change.[7]

BENIGN UTERINE CONDITIONS

Fibroids

Fibroids, or leiomyomas, are benign smooth muscle tumours found in up to 40% of women. They are usually multiple and are classified according to their location:

- Submucosal (projecting into and distorting the uterine cavity);

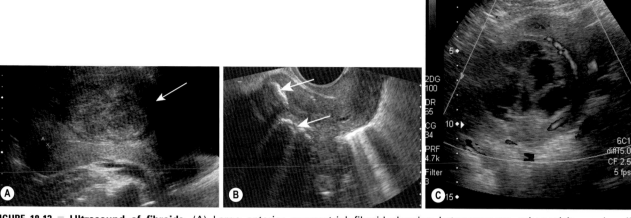

FIGURE 18-13 ■ **Ultrasound of fibroids.** (A) Large anterior myometrial fibroid showing heterogeneous echogenicity, and well-circumscribed margins (arrow). (B) Calcified fibroid with pronounced acoustic shadowing (arrows). (C) Degenerate fibroid. Note echo-poor areas and lack of vascularity.

- Intramural (within the myometrium); and
- Subserosal (protruding out of the serosal surface of the uterus).

Symptoms may be caused by mass effect and location of the fibroids, and include menorrhagia, pain, urinary symptoms, infertility and obstetric complications.

Alternative procedures to hysterectomy such as myomectomy, uterine arterial embolisation (UAE) and MR-guided high intensity focused ultrasound (HIFU) ablation may be appropriate for some patients wishing to preserve fertility.[8,9]

Ultrasound is often the initial radiological investigation in these patients, with MRI reserved for patients with inconclusive US results or for patient selection and pre-treatment planning before myomectomy and UAE.[10]

Ultrasound

US can accurately detect fibroids, but up to 20% of small fibroids may be occult. The fibroid uterus is typically enlarged with an irregular or lobulated outline. Fibroids commonly appear as well-marginated, hypoechoic, rounded or oval masses within the uterine body. Depending on the proportion of smooth muscle, fibrosis and degeneration, the appearance ranges from hypoechoic to echogenic, homogeneous to heterogeneous, with or without acoustic shadowing. Calcification secondary to necrosis or degeneration appears as shadowing echogenic foci (Fig. 18-13).

Magnetic Resonance Imaging

MRI allows precise determination of the size, location and number of fibroids, and is useful in evaluation and monitoring response in patients undergoing myomectomy and UAE. It is the most accurate non-invasive imaging method for differentiation of a fibroid from adenomyosis.[11]

The commonest appearances are of well-circumscribed, rounded masses with lower signal intensity than

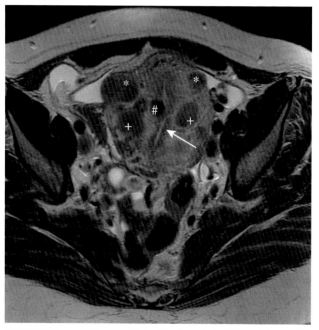

FIGURE 18-14 ■ **MRI of multiple fibroids.** Axial T2-weighted MRI of the uterus demonstrates multiple fibroids of lower signal intensity than the myometrium. Subserosal (*), intramural (+) and submucosal (#) fibroids are shown. Their precise location in relation to the endometrial cavity (arrow) is clearly demonstrated.

myometrium on T2-weighted images and intermediate signal intensity on T1-weighted images (Fig. 18-14). Most enhance less than adjacent myometrium following contrast; however, a variety of degenerative processes can alter the characteristic appearances, making differential diagnosis more difficult.[12] Cystic degeneration results in well-demarcated areas with fluid signal intensity, which do not enhance post-IV contrast medium (Fig. 18-15). Myxoid degeneration may show very high signal on T2-weighted images with minimal enhancement. Red

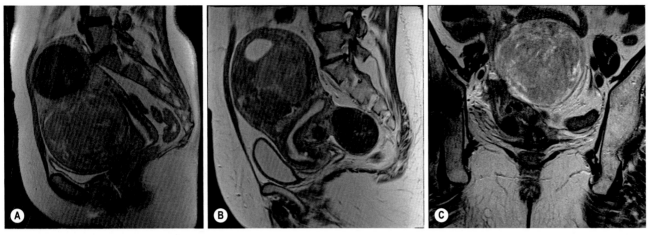

FIGURE 18-15 ■ **Variable appearance of fibroids on MRI.** (A) Sagittal T2-weighted MRI showing an intermediate signal anterior myometrial fibroid. Patchy high signal areas indicate degeneration. A second fibroid at the fundus is of characteristic low signal. (B) There is cystic degeneration in the anterior fibroid, and a low signal intensity posterior fibroid that has displaced the rectum. Note retroverted uterus. (C) A large pedunculated fibroid is of mixed signal, indicating degeneration. Note multiple small low signal fibroids in the myometrium.

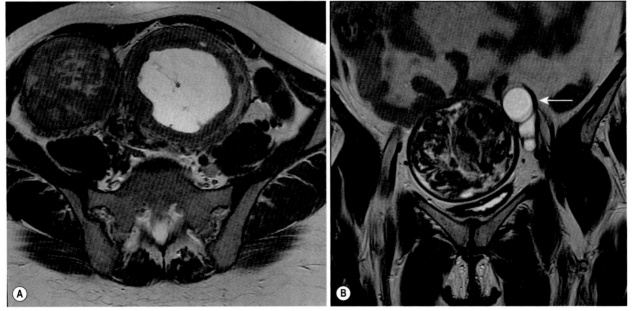

FIGURE 18-16 ■ **Myxoid and red degeneration of fibroids on MRI.** (A) Axial T2-weighted image. There is myxoid degeneration of a large fibroid with central very high signal. (*) A second fibroid on the right is of mixed signal. (B) Red degeneration with massive haemorrhagic infarction and necrosis of the entire leiomyoma, with a peripheral rim of low signal on this coronal T2-weighted image. Note also left hydrosalpinx (arrow).

degeneration involves massive haemorrhagic infarction and necrosis of the entire fibroid, with a peripheral rim of low signal on T2- and high signal on T1-weighted images, with no enhancement (Fig. 18-16). Fat saturation T1-weighted images may be helpful in cases of haemorrhage. Calcification usually results in areas of signal void on both T1- and T2-weighted images.

Computed Tomography

CT is not used for routine evaluation of fibroids. They are often an incidental finding on CT performed for

other reasons, and usually have a soft-tissue density similar to that of normal myometrium, although necrosis or degeneration may result in low attenuation. Contour deformity is the most common sign on CT; calcification is the most specific finding.

Hysterosalpingography

HSG is no longer recommended for the evaluation of submucosal fibroids, although distortion of the cavity may been seen at HSG performed for investigation of infertility. Appearances range from a smooth and rounded

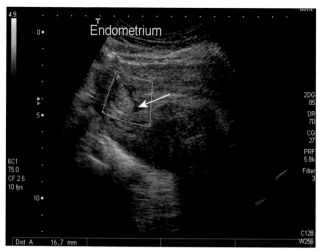

FIGURE 18-17 ▪ **Endometrial polyp.** Sagittal US showing an endometrial polyp with a thin rim of surrounding fluid (arrow).

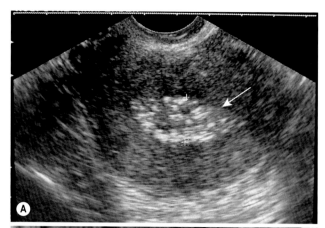

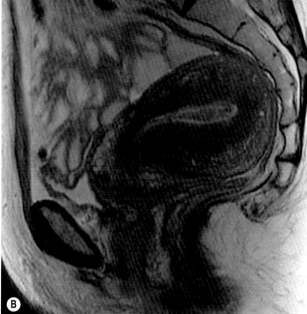

FIGURE 18-18 ▪ **Endometrial hyperplasia.** US in a patient with postmenopausal bleeding who is taking tamoxifen following breast cancer surgery. The endometrium (A) is thickened and hyperechoic, measuring more than 10 mm. (B) Sagittal T2-weighted MRI shows non-specific heterogeneous endometrial thickening. Endometrial biopsy is indicated to exclude endometrial cancer. In this case the histological diagnosis was endometrial hyperplasia.

filling defect of the uterine contour, to gross distortion of the cavity.

Endometrial Polyps

Benign endometrial polyps commonly occur at all ages, with their greatest prevalence after age 50. They are a common cause of postmenopausal bleeding and are often seen in patients taking tamoxifen. They must be differentiated from submucosal fibroids and malignancy. Polyps are well seen on sonohysterography. They are typically homogeneous, isoechoic to and continuous with the endometrium and preserve the endomyometrial interface. They may be centrally cystic, corresponding to dilated, fluid-filled glands. Colour Doppler may reveal a characteristic feeding vessel (Fig. 18-17).

On MR imaging, polyps are generally intermediate signal on T1-weighted images, with heterogeneous high signal on T2-weighted imagines. Hysteroscopy and biopsy are required to exclude malignancy and foci of atypical hyperplasia within polyps.[13]

Endometrial Hyperplasia

Endometrial hyperplasia is characterised histologically by the proliferation of endometrial glands, usually secondary to chronic unopposed oestrogen stimulation or in patients taking tamoxifen. It often presents with postmenopausal or irregular uterine bleeding.

Transvaginal US is the initial method of investigation, which reveals thickening of the echogenic endometrial stripe (Fig. 18-18A). In postmenopausal women, the threshold value for further intervention such as hysteroscopy and endometrial biopsy on transvaginal US is 5 mm. If the endometrial thickness is less than 5 mm in postmenopausal women, endometrial biopsy may be avoided.[14]

On MR, two distinct imaging patterns are seen; homogeneous high signal on T2-weighted images, and heterogeneous T2-weighted signal with lattice-like enhancement traversing the endometrial canal on post-contrast images, particularly in women taking tamoxifen[15] (Fig. 18-18B).

A definitive diagnosis requires biopsy, as imaging cannot reliably differentiate between hyperplasia and carcinoma.[16]

Adenomyosis

Adenomyosis is characterised pathologically as the presence of endometrial tissue within the myometrium and secondary smooth muscle hyperplasia. It most commonly occurs as a diffuse abnormality, with less common focal disease referred to as an adenomyoma. The most frequent symptoms are dysmenorrhoea and dysfunctional uterine bleeding. It is found in 15–27% of hysterectomy specimens. Transvaginal US is the initial imaging investigation, with MRI reserved for indeterminate cases or those undergoing uterus-sparing surgery.[11,17]

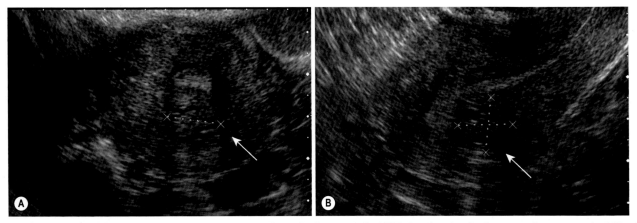

FIGURE 18-19 ■ **US of focal adenomyosis.** (A) Axial and (B) sagittal transvaginal US showing focal adenomyosis as a poorly defined echogenic nodule (arrows).

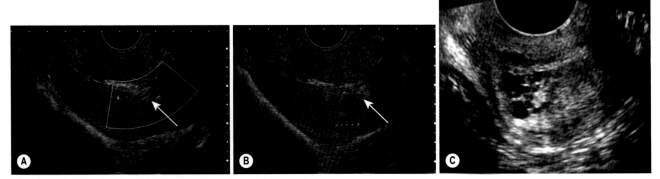

FIGURE 18-20 ■ **Ultrasound of adenomyosis.** (A) Sagittal and (B) axial transvaginal US of a retroverted uterus with subendometrial echogenic linear striations and nodules. (C) There is poor definition of the endomyometrial interface.

Ultrasound

Transvaginal US has an accuracy of 68–86% in the diagnosis of diffuse adenomyosis. Typically, the uterus has an enlarged but globular configuration, often with asymmetry of the anterior and posterior uterine walls. The implants present as diffuse echogenic nodules (Fig. 18-19), subendometrial echogenic linear striations and nodules and 2- to 6-mm subendometrial cysts (present in 50% of cases) representing haemorrhagic areas (Fig. 18-20). Other features include endometrial pseudo-widening, poor definition of the endomyometrial interface and multiple fine areas of attenuation throughout the lesion—the 'rain shower' appearance. Colour Doppler examination demonstrates a speckled pattern of increased vascularity within the heterogeneous areas.[18] While the diagnosis of diffuse adenomyosis can be suggested on transvaginal US, the findings of focal adenomyosis are hard to distinguish from fibroids.

Magnetic Resonance Imaging

MRI is useful in distinguishing adenomyosis from other uterine diseases, in particular fibroids, which is clinically important in management. On T2-weighted MRI, adenomyosis appears as areas of low myometrial signal intensity, due to smooth muscle hyperplasia, which presents as focal or diffuse thickening of the junctional zone (JZ).

When diffuse, a widened low intensity JZ > 12 mm predicts adenomyosis with high accuracy, while a JZ < 8 mm **excludes** it with high accuracy (Fig. 18-21). For indeterminate cases (JZ 8–12 mm), ancillary criteria are used. These include high signal intensity foci within low signal myometrium on T2-weighted images, representing islands of ectopic endometrial tissue and cystic dilatation of glands (Figs. 18-22 and 18-23). High signal linear striations (finger-like projections) extending out from endometrium into myometrium may also be seen, representing direct myometrial invasion. Less commonly, high signal intensity foci on T1-weighted images can be seen, which represent small punctate haemorrhage within ectopic endometrial tissue.[11,17]

MR is highly accurate in the diagnosis of adenomyosis, but various diagnostic pitfalls do occur, including myometrial contractions, endometrial carcinoma and fibroids.

PELVIC PAIN

Common causes of pelvic pain are endometriosis, adenomyosis, fibroids, pelvic varices and pelvic inflammatory disease (PID).

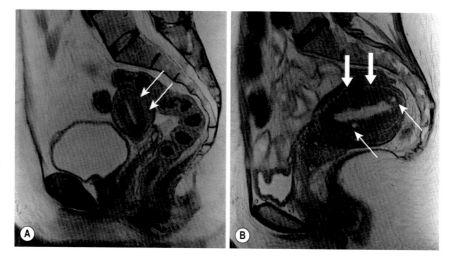

FIGURE 18-21 ■ **MRI of adenomyosis.** (A) Sagittal T2-weighted MRI showing marked thickening of the JZ (arrows). (B) In this case on the sagittal T2-weighted MRI the retroverted uterus has marked thickening of the JZ (block arrows) and small rounded foci of high signal indicating cystic dilatation of glands (thin arrows).

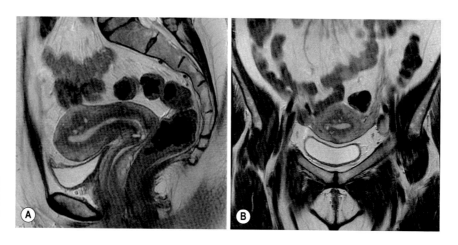

FIGURE 18-22 ■ **Focal adenomyosis.** (A) Sagittal and (B) axial T2-weighted MRI with focal thickening of the JZ and foci of high signal extending into the myometrium.

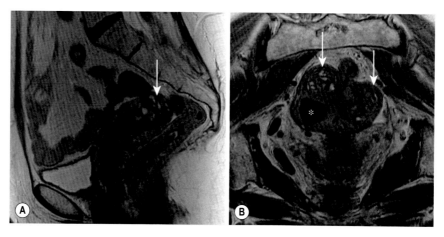

FIGURE 18-23 ■ **Adenomyoma on MRI.** (A) Sagittal and (B) axial T2-weighted MRI with focal adenomyomata (arrows). There is also a fibroid in the posterior myometrium (*).

US is considered the primary imaging technique in the evaluation of pelvic pain, while MRI is reserved as a problem-solving tool.[19]

Endometriosis

Endometrial tissue outside the uterine cavity is termed endometriosis. It usually affects women of reproductive age, and is the most prevalent cause of chronic pelvic pain, also causing dysfunctional uterine bleeding and infertility.[20] Common locations of endometrial tissue include the ovaries, uterine ligaments, fallopian tubes, rectovaginal septum, pouch of Douglas, bladder wall and umbilicus. Although a definitive diagnosis of endometriosis requires a laparoscopy and histological confirmation, transvaginal ultrasound and MRI are commonly

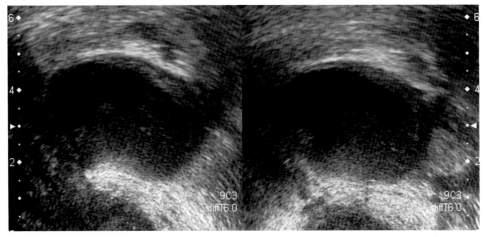

FIGURE 18-24 ■ **Ultrasound of endometrioma.** The cystic mass shows blood products layering posteriorly, seen as fine particulate debris.

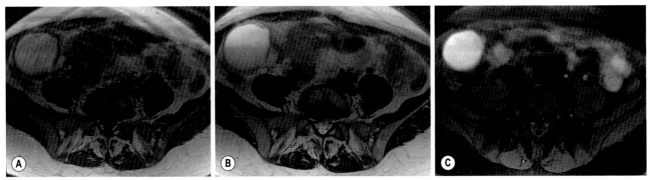

FIGURE 18-25 ■ **Classic MRI appearance of an endometrioma.** (A) T1-, (B) T2- and (C) T1-weighted fat suppression axial images. Note the endometrioma is hyperintense on the T1-weighted image, and of variable signal on the T2-weighted image with the shading sign of old blood products. The fat suppression sequence has increased its conspicuity.

used for initial investigation, and monitoring response to treatment.

Ultrasound

Transvaginal ultrasound is the initial investigation for suspected endometriosis. Endometriomas appear as cystic masses with diffuse uniform low-level echoes. Fluid–fluid levels or fluid–debris levels represent blood products (Fig. 18-24). After repeated episodes of bleeding and re-bleeding, irregular walls and echogenic mural nodules may develop, causing diagnostic difficulty in differentiation from a malignant ovarian mass. Lesions in deeply infiltrating endometriosis are hypoechoic compared to the myometrium, and can appear as mural thickening or focal nodules, sometimes with multiple small cystic areas.

Magnetic Resonance Imaging

MRI is the best imaging investigation for the depiction of endometriosis, due to its ability to detect old haemorrhage, deep pelvic lesions and fibrosis. Endometriomas often appear hyperintense on T1-weighted images and low or variable signal on T2-weighted images. Fat suppression sequences increase their conspicuity[21] and the shading sign on T2-weighted images representing old blood products may help in differentiating from haemorrhagic corpus luteum cysts (Fig. 18-25). Deep endometrial implants can be detected on MRI, where they appear as irregular or indistinct masses, sometimes with cystic and haemorrhagic areas with low signal on T2-weighted images, and intermediate signal on T1-weighted images, and minimal post-IV enhancement. Involvement of the vaginal or rectal wall and uterosacral ligaments should be suspected when they are hypointense, thickened or nodular in appearance (Fig. 18-26).[22] The detection of adhesions can be suggested by the appearances of angulated bowel loops, posterior displacement of the uterus and 'kissing' ovaries (Fig. 18-27). Hydro- or haematosalpinx is often seen.[2]

Pelvic Inflammatory Disease

Pelvic inflammatory disease (PID) is common, and due to infection of the endometrium, fallopian tubes and/or contiguous structures. It is a significant complication of

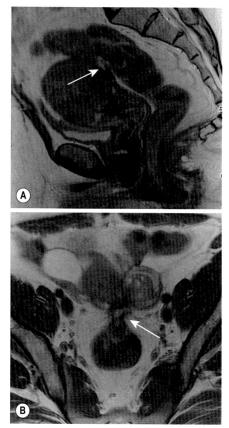

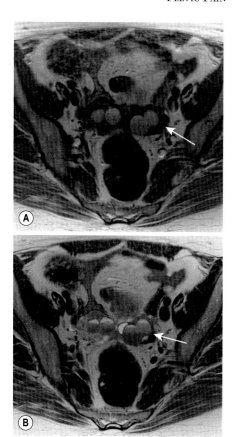

FIGURE 18-26 ■ **Advanced endometriosis.** (A) Sagittal and (B) axial T2-weighted MRI with a deposit of endometriosis between the rectum and uterus (arrows). There is tethering of the rectum to the serosal surface of the uterus. High signal in the centre of the deposit indicates active disease with haemorrhage. Note also bilateral ovarian endometriosis.

FIGURE 18-27 ■ **Endometriosis 'kissing ovaries'.** (A) Axial T1- and (B) T2-weighted sequences of the pelvis which shows the ovaries tethered by adhesions in the mid-line ('kissing ovaries'). There are bilateral endometriotic cysts with classic layering of haemorrhagic debris (arrows).

sexually transmitted diseases, usually caused by *Chlamydia trachomatis* and *Neisseria gonorrhoeae*, and is also associated with the use of intrauterine contraceptive devices (IUCDs).

Early diagnosis is important to prevent chronic inflammation, which leads to pelvic pain, adhesions and infertility.

Radiology has an important role in identifying subtle changes associated with early PID as well as the investigation and management of more obvious findings in complicated PID.

Ultrasound

Transabdominal ultrasound is useful for getting an overview of the pelvis, identifying free fluid and excluding other abnormalities (e.g. ovarian cysts). It can identify complicated pelvic inflammatory disease and tubo-ovarian abscess. Transvaginal ultrasound demonstrates various stages of tubo-ovarian inflammation which cannot be seen by transabdominal ultrasound alone. Findings will depend on the extent and duration of the disease.[23] The uterus may be normal in the early stages or may be slightly enlarged, with ill-defined margins ('indefinite uterus') due to the presence of pelvic exudate. The endometrium may be thickened, measuring more than

14 mm, with variable echogenicity, a poorly defined endometrial/myometrial interface and fluid present within the endometrial cavity.

The myometrium can be hypoechoic, with poorly defined areas of decreased echogenicity due to oedema and inflammation.

Normal fallopian tubes are not usually seen on transvaginal ultrasound but, as the disease progresses, exudate accumulates within the lumen of the tube and the ultrasound may show a thickened tubular structure in the adnexal region, extending from the cornual region.

The inflammation may eventually occlude the ostium and the tube dilates with an elongated convoluted or club-shaped configuration. Internal echoes may be seen within the distended fluid-filled tube, as fluid debris, or layered pus inferring a *pyosalpinx* (Fig. 18-28).

As active infection subsides, the pus undergoes proteolysis, becoming thin serous fluid (anechoic compared to the echogenic purulent fluid in pyosalpinx) and a hydrosalpinx is formed.

A hydrosalpinx has four distinct features (Figs. 18-29 and 18-30):
• Tubular shape;
• Folded configuration;
• Well-defined echogenic wall; and
• Short linear echoes protruding into the lumen.

The linear intraluminal echoes have been described as possibly due to the wrinkled nature of the tubal epithelium. The fluid of hydrosalpinx is anechoic in comparison with the purulent and debris component on the pyosalpinx. Colour Doppler distinguishes a hydrosalpinx from dilated pelvic veins.

If the ovaries are involved (oophoritis), they can be enlarged and globular with multiple cysts (polycystic-like ovaries). In late PID a tubo-ovarian mass may form. Tubo-ovarian abscesses can have a variable and complex appearance on ultrasound. Typically they are unilocular or multilocular complex cystic masses with irregular borders, thickened walls and echogenic fluid, sometimes with debris levels (Fig. 18-31). These ultrasound findings are not specific and the differential diagnosis includes endometriosis, abscesses of non-gynaecological origin related to diverticulitis or appendicitis, and malignancy.

Computed Tomography

CT is helpful for evaluating the extent of the inflammatory process and identifying associated complications, particularly in patients who may need surgical or percutaneous drainage.[24]

CT findings are subtle in early PID. Mild pelvic oedema results in thickening of the uterosacral ligaments and haziness of the pelvic fat, with obscuration of the pelvic fascial planes (Fig. 18-32). The uterus may be bulky. Abnormal endometrial enhancement and fluid within the endometrial cavity indicates endometritis (Fig. 18-33A).

Salpingitis is seen as thickening of the fallopian tubes, and oophoritis as enlarged and abnormally enhancing ovaries that may demonstrate a polycystic appearance, as seen with ultrasound.

If the fallopian tubes exhibit a degree of wall thickening and enhancement and are distended with complex fluid, these findings usually indicate pyosalpinx (Fig. 18-33A). Tubo-ovarian and pelvic abscesses are indicated by the presence of thick-walled, complex fluid collections that may contain internal septa and fluid–debris level (Fig. 18-33B). Gas in PID abscesses is relatively uncommon.

CT findings are, however, not specific, and the clinical picture has to be considered.

In patients with poor response to antibiotic therapy, percutaneous drainage of the collections may be guided by ultrasound or CT.

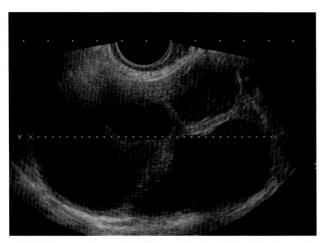

FIGURE 18-28 ■ **US of a pyosalpinx.** The fallopian tube is dilated with an elongated convoluted configuration. Internal echoes are seen within the distended fluid-filled tube. Careful scanning will distinguish a dilated tube from a multi-septated ovarian cyst, and demonstration of the ovary as a separate structure is also useful.

Magnetic Resonance Imaging

MRI shows a variety of findings in PID cases, including tubo-ovarian abscesses, slightly to massively dilated fluid-filled fallopian tubes and polycystic-like ovaries with free

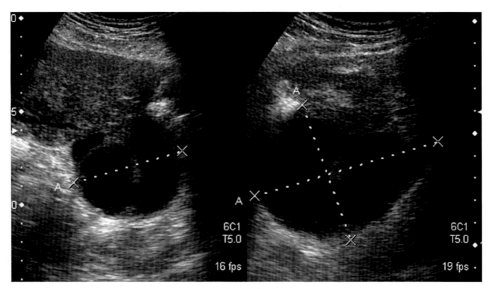

FIGURE 18-29 ■ **US of hydrosalpinx.** Axial and sagittal transvaginal US of a hydrosalpinx, easily recognised by its convoluted tubular shape.

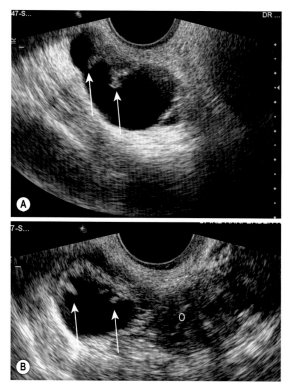

FIGURE 18-30 ■ **US of hydrosalpinx.** These (A) sagittal and (B) axial transvaginal US images demonstrate the typical features of a hydrosalpinx of a well-defined echogenic wall and short linear echoes protruding into the lumen, thought to be due to wrinkling of the tubal epithelium (arrows). Note adjacent ovary (O).

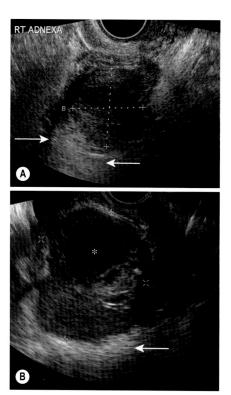

FIGURE 18-31 ■ **Transvaginal US of tubo-ovarian abscess.** (A, B) There is a right adnexal complex mass. The ovary cannot be discerned as a separate structure. Posterior acoustic enhancement (arrows) indicates the mass contains echogenic fluid contents. Note hypoechoic loculation in centre of mass (*), which usually represents pus.

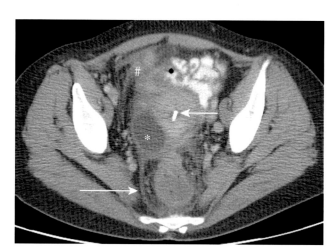

FIGURE 18-32 ■ **CT of pelvic Inflammatory disease.** This CT shows some of the typical features of PID on CT. The presence of an IUCD (small arrow), inflammatory changes (#), thickening of the uterosacral ligaments (large arrow) and right adnexal cystic mass (*) are all suggestive of PID.

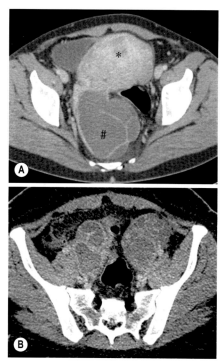

FIGURE 18-33 ■ **CT findings in late pelvic inflammatory disease.** (A) Axial enhanced CT in late PID. Note bulky enhancing uterus with some fluid in the cavity (*). The convoluted tubular structure containing slightly turbid fluid is a pyosalpinx (#). (B) Bilateral thick-walled, complex fluid collections containing enhancing internal septae due to tubo-ovarian abscesses.

Pelvic Varices

Pelvic varices are dilated veins in the broad ligament and ovarian plexus. When symptomatic, the condition is called 'pelvic congestion syndrome', a common cause of chronic pelvic pain. Varices are most often found in multiparous women of reproductive age and are associated with varicose veins in the vulva, buttocks and legs.

The criteria for diagnosis include venous structures greater than 4 mm in diameter, slower than 3 cm s^{-1} velocity flow and connecting arcuate veins within the myometrium.

BENIGN OVARIAN CONDITIONS

Functional Ovarian Cysts

Functional ovarian cysts include follicular, corpus luteum and theca lutein cysts. They are common, frequently asymptomatic and often resolve spontaneously, but may cause pain and dysfunctional uterine bleeding.[26] Simple unilocular cysts without solid components are very unlikely to be malignant; more complex cysts require a serum CA125 and repeat US or MRI.

Follicular cysts represent failure of reabsorbtion of an incompletely developed follicle. They vary in size from 3 to 8 cm in diameter. On US they are thin-walled, hypoechoic and unilocular, and on MRI demonstrate low signal on T1-weighted images and high signal on T2. No treatment is required in the majority of cases as the cysts are often asymptomatic and usually regress spontaneously in 2 months (Fig. 18-35). Simple thin-walled follicular cysts are commonly seen in postmenopausal women and if less than 3 cm can be safely disregarded (Fig. 18-35).

Corpus luteum cysts are functional cysts which occur following ovulation, and may demonstrate internal haemorrhage, giving rise to a complex appearance on US. A persistent corpus luteum cyst may cause local pain and tenderness and either amenorrhoea or delayed menstruation, simulating the clinical picture associated with ectopic pregnancy. A variable echogenic pattern on US depends on the appearances of altered blood products, with high T1 signal on MRI due to internal haemorrhage. They commonly resolve spontaneously, and a repeat US after 6 weeks to check regression is the usual management.

Theca lutein cysts are less common, and result from excessive BHCG stimulation or hypersensitivity in association with polycystic ovarian disease, hydatidiform mole or clomifene therapy. They are often bilateral and, although usually of small-to-medium size, they can grow larger and cause ovarian torsion or haemorrhage.

Polycystic Ovaries

The diagnostic conundrum of possible polycystic ovarian syndrome (PCOS) is frequently encountered. The joint meeting of the ASRM and ESHRE in Rotterdam in 2003[27] was key to the agreement of a refined definition of PCOS and included a specific description of the

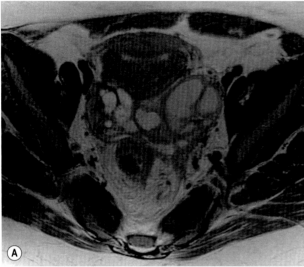

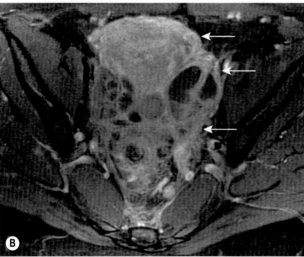

FIGURE 18-34 ■ MRI of pelvic inflammatory disease. (A) Axial T1-weighted image of bilateral tubo-ovarian abscesses. Note hyperintense fluid in the collections due to debris and haemorrhage. (B) Axial T1-weighted fat saturation post-contrast images. Note enhancement shown by the arrows compared to the T1-weighted image.

pelvic fluid.[25] An abscess is seen as a thick-walled, fluid-filled mass in an adnexal location. The abscess wall and adjacent soft-tissue inflammation enhance intensely on T1-weighted post-contrast images (Fig. 18-34). The contents of a pyosalpinx or abscess are slightly **hypointense** on T2-weighted images and slightly **hyperintense** on T1-weighted images relative to urine because of the presence of haemorrhage or debris.

The MRI differential diagnosis of tubo-ovarian abscess includes endometrioma, ovarian tumor, infected cyst and abscesses from other sources, such as Crohn's disease or appendicitis.

MRI is usually used as a problem-solving investigation where there is uncertainty about the cause of a complex adnexal mass, since transvaginal ultrasound is far more cost-effective.

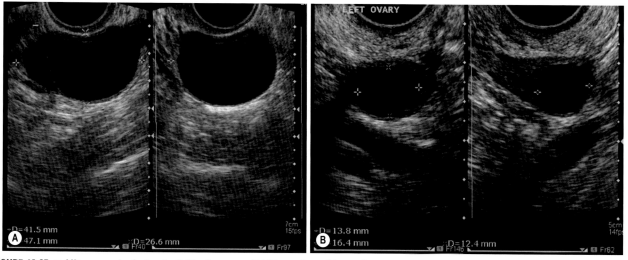

FIGURE 18-35 ▪ **Ultrasound of simple follicular cyst.** (A) There is a thin-walled, hypoechoic and unilocular cyst measuring 4.7 cm maximum diameter. (B) Same patient 5 weeks later. The cyst has resolved.

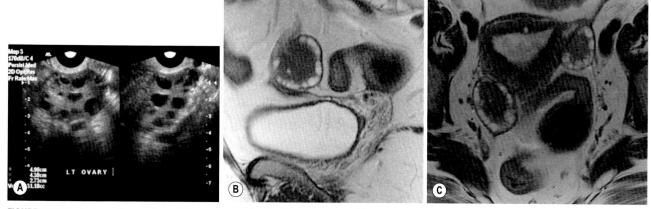

FIGURE 18-36 ▪ **Polycystic ovaries.** (A) Transvaginal US, (B) sagittal and (C) axial T2-weighted MRI demonstrating the classic appearances of polycystic ovaries with 12 or more follicles of 2–9 mm in diameter, and increased ovarian volume.

ultrasound morphology, requiring two out of three of the following criteria:

1. Oligo- and/or anovulation;
2. Hyperandrogenism (clinical and/or biochemical); and
3. Polycystic ovaries.

Despite this, many sonographers and radiologists remain unaware of the revised definitions and continue to make assessments of the ovaries without mention of size, volume, number or size of follicles or reference to the phase of the cycle in the report. This has led to many women being incorrectly labelled as having polycystic ovaries.

Polycystic ovaries (PCO) are often found incidentally in women undergoing ultrasound for unrelated gynaecological symptoms. Approximately 20% of young women have ovaries which appear polycystic and of these, about 40–70% have symptoms of infertility, menstrual irregularity or hirsutism, consistent with the diagnosis of PCOS.[28]

Transvaginal ultrasound is a sensitive method for identification of polycystic ovaries because of the better spatial resolution afforded by high-frequency transvaginal probes. The ovaries, particularly in obese patients, can appear homogeneous on Transabdominal images.[29] The transvaginal route is omitted in patients who are virgo intacta or who decline transvaginal ultrasound.

The ultrasound findings should be interpreted in relation to the cycle. The presence of a follicle >10 mm diameter or a corpus luteum will result in an increased ovarian volume and, therefore, ultrasound should be repeated during the early days of the next cycle. In oligo-amenorrhoeic women, ultrasound can be performed at random.

Assessment of the size and number of follicles, and volume are key to making the ultrasound diagnosis of PCO. There should be 12 or more follicles of 2–9 mm in diameter; the distribution of the follicles is unimportant[27,29] (Fig. 18-36A).

Increased stromal echogenicity of the ovary is no longer considered to be an important diagnostic feature. Ovarian volume correlates well with the increase in stroma, and therefore this measurement is crucial. The volume for diagnosis should be greater than 10 cm³; normal ovaries never have a volume of greater than 8.0 cm³. Just one ovary fulfilling the criteria is sufficient to define PCOS.[27,29]

Magnetic Resonance Imaging

MRI is expensive, and rarely provides more information in PCOS than transvaginal ultrasound. It may have a limited role where transvaginal ultrasound is not practical or diagnostic (for example, in very obese patients or those who are virgo intacta). T2-weighted sequences elegantly demonstrate ovarian morphology (Fig. 18-36B, C).[30]

Benign Tumours of the Ovary

Ninety per cent of all ovarian tumours are benign, although this varies with age. Transvaginal ultrasound is the first-line investigation for a suspected ovarian mass. In most cases of non-complex masses, malignancy can be confidently excluded, but in 20% of cases the ovarian mass remains indeterminate. The strength of MRI is its ability to further characterise adnexal lesions (Fig. 18-37).

The MRI appearance of benign ovarian neoplasms is variable, depending on the combination of cystic, solid and haemorrhagic components. Whilst the likelihood of malignancy may increase with the proportion of solid component, the overlap between benign and malignant lesions is wide but dynamic contrast-enhanced MRI and diffusion-weighted imaging have been shown to be effective in differentiating benign from malignant masses.[31,32]

Epithelial Tumours

Benign epithelial tumours arise from the ovarian surface epithelium. They demonstrate smaller, less numerous

papillary projections than borderline or malignant varieties.[33]

Serous cystadenomas are the commonest and are bilateral in 20% of patients; they are usually unilocular with low signal on T1-weighted images and high signal on T2-weighted images (Fig. 18-38). They can become very large, and can have a fibrous component, when they are known as cystadenofibromas.

Mucinous cystadenomas account for 15–25% of all ovarian tumours. They contain thick mucinous material, are often multiloculated with thin septa and can grow to

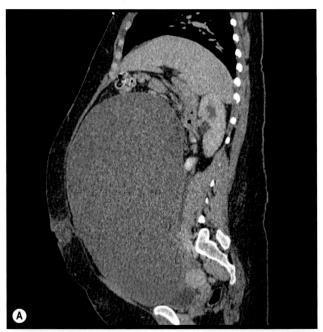

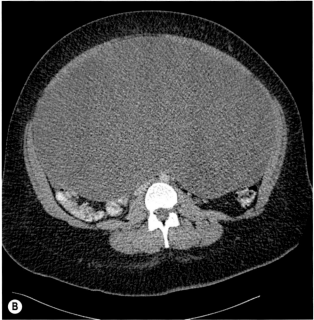

FIGURE 18-38 ■ **CT of a serous cystadenoma.** A 25-year-old complained of abdominal distension. There is a huge unilocular cyst arising from the pelvis with no discernible papillary projections or mural nodules. (A) Axial image. (B) Sagittal reconstruction.

	T1W	T2W	FST1W	CET1W
Simple cyst				
Haemorrhagic cyst				
Endometrioma				
Dermoid				
Fibroma/ Brenner				
Cystic epithelial neoplasm				
Solid malignant neoplasm				

FIGURE 18-37 ■ **Diagram of enhancement patterns of adnexal lesions.** (Image kindly supplied by Dr John Spencer, Consultant Radiologist, Leeds, UK.)

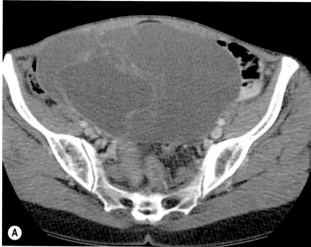

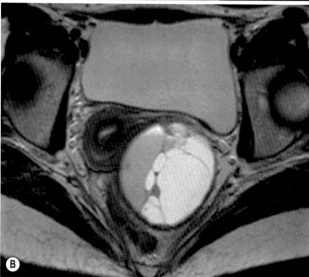

FIGURE 18-39 ■ **Mucinous cystadenoma.** (A) CT of mucinous cystadenoma of the pelvis. Note subtle changes in attenuation between the cyst locules. (B) T2-weighted axial MRI of the pelvis elegantly demonstrates variable signal of the locules due to differing amounts of proteinaceous and mucinous material within.

a large size. The locules can demonstrate variable signal on MRI, depending on the combination of proteinaceous, mucinous and haemorrhagic content (Fig. 18-39).

Transitional cell or Brenner tumours are rare epithelial tumours. They are usually small, unilateral and solid and require surgical removal.

Germ Cell Tumours

Germ cell tumours are among the most common ovarian tumours seen in women less than 30 years of age. Overall, only 2–3% of germ cell tumours are malignant.

Mature cystic teratomas, or dermoid cysts, are derived from one or more of the three germ cell layers. The three most common appearances on ultrasound are: (a) a cystic mass with an echogenic nodule projecting into the lumen;

(b) a predominantly echogenic mass with posterior sound attenuation owing to the presence of sebaceous material and hair; and (c) a cystic mass with fine internal echogenic lines also representing hair (Figs. 18-40A, B). A fluid–fluid level which represents sebaceous material floating on fluid may be seen. The presence of fat and calcification also aids in diagnosis on CT (Fig. 18-40C). MRI is sensitive and specific in the diagnosis of dermoid cysts. The demonstration of fat with fat saturation techniques, fat–water chemical shift artefact, fat–fluid and/or fluid–fluid levels, layering debris, low signal intensity calcifications (e.g. teeth) and soft-tissue protuberances (Rokitansky nodules or dermoid plugs) attached to the cyst wall are all features that can be detected on MRI (Figs. 18-37 and 18-41).

Stromal Cell Tumours

Fibromas are uncommon tumours which are usually asymptomatic, but may be rarely associated with Meigs syndrome (ascites and a right-side pleural effusion) and Gorlin's syndrome (basal cell carcinoma, jaw keratocysts and dural calcification). They can be mistaken for malignant tumours due to their solid nature, and are best characterised on MRI, where they demonstrate characteristic isointense to low signal compared to myometrium on T2- as well at T1-weighted images, enhancing less than myometrium. They can be confused with pedunculated leiomyomas, which also demonstrate low T2 signal, but the absence of a normal ipsilateral ovary and the presence of small follicular cysts help to determine their ovarian origin[33] (Figs. 18-37 and 18-42).

Thecomas are another type of stromal cell tumour, often unilateral, solid and most commonly seen in postmenopausal women. They can produce oestrogen in sufficient quantity to produce systemic effects, including endometrial hyperplasia and malignancy.

Other benign conditions which may be encountered during imaging of the female pelvis include para-ovarian cysts, peritoneal inclusion cysts, lymphoceles and haematomas, which can mimic ovarian cystic lesions on imaging. The identification of normal ovaries separate to the cystic mass is key to the diagnosis.[34] Para-ovarian cysts are usually simple unilocular cysts which are in close proximity to but separate from the ovary. Peritoneal inclusion cysts occur secondary to peritoneal damage from infection, inflammation or surgery and usually conform to the shape of the peritoneum. Lymphoceles occur at pelvic node dissection sites, lateral to the pelvic vessels.

Ovarian Torsion

Torsion of the ovaries and fallopian tubes results from partial or complete rotation of the ovary on its vascular pedicle. It is commonest in women in their reproductive years, and is often associated with a cyst or benign tumour, the commonest being a mature cystic teratoma. Early diagnosis is important for preventing irreversible ovarian damage, and US is often used as the first-line investigation. The most constant finding is ovarian enlargement (>7 cm), without which the diagnosis is unlikely to be

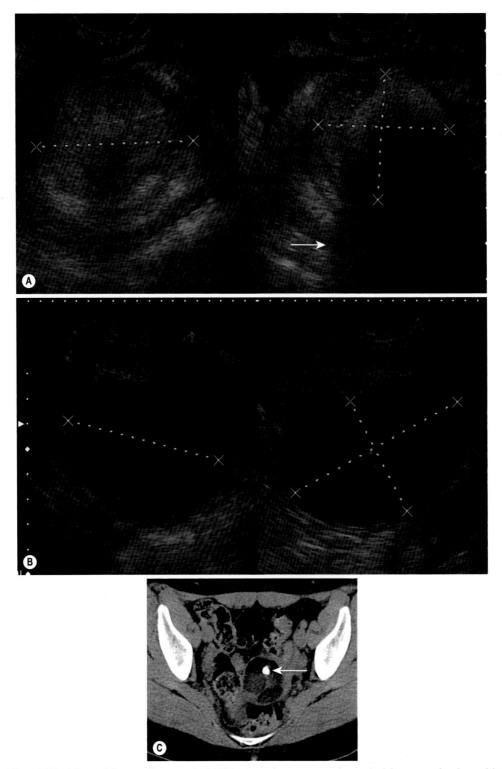

FIGURE 18-40 ■ **US and CT of dermoid cysts.** Transvaginal US images demonstrate the typical features of a dermoid. (A) A predominantly echogenic mass with posterior sound attenuation owing to the presence of sebaceous material and hair (arrow). (B) A cystic mass with echogenic mass projecting into the cyst. (C) CT of a dermoid cyst with a characteristic fat–fluid level, and tooth (small arrow).

torsion.[35] Pelvic free fluid, a complex adnexal mass and multiple small peripheral cysts representing displaced follicles may also be seen. Lack of Doppler signal or a twisted vascular pedicle sign on colour Doppler are also suggestive of ovarian torsion, with the presence of flow suggesting the ovary may be viable. CT is not routinely used for diagnosis of ovarian torsion, and findings are relatively non-specific, including a large adnexal mass, deviation of the uterus to the affected side and ascites.

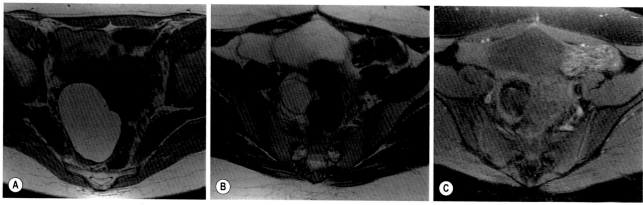

FIGURE 18-41 ■ **MRI of a dermoid cyst.** (A) T1-, (B) T2- and (C) T1-weighted fat saturation axial images which demonstrate the typical findings of a dermoid cyst on MRI. There is a right adnexal mass with areas of high and intermediate signal on the T1-weighted image, intermediate signal on the T2-weighted image and suppression of the high signal from fat on the T1-weighted fat saturation sequence.

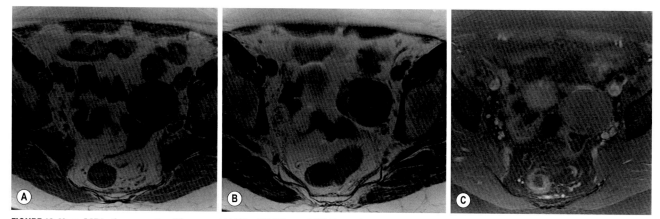

FIGURE 18-42 ■ **MRI of an ovarian fibroma.** (A) T1-, (B) T2- and (C) T1-weighted post-contrast fat saturation axial images showing the typical findings of a fibroma on MRI, with low signal on T1- and T2-weighted images and little enhancement.

VAGINAL CYSTS

Vaginal cysts are often asymptomatic and discovered as incidental findings on imaging. Gartner duct cysts are usually found above the pubic symphysis in the anterolateral wall of the upper vagina, whereas Bartholin gland cysts are found below the pubic symphysis in the posterolateral vaginal introitus. They are usually well-defined lesions, isointense to fluid on MRI unless they contain proteinaceous fluid when they will demonstrate high signal on T1-weighted imaging. They can be differentiated from periurethral cysts (Skene gland cysts) and cervical cysts (Nabothian cysts) based on their anatomical location.[36]

REFERENCES

1. Thurmond AS. Fallopian tube catheterization. Semin Intervent Radiol 2008;25(4):425–431.
2. Imaoka I, Wada A, Matsuo M, et al. MR imaging of disorders associated with female infertility: use in diagnosis, treatment, and management. Radiographics 2003;23(6):1401–21.
3. The American Fertility Society. Classification of adnexal adhesions, distal tubal obstruction, tubal occlusion secondary to tubal ligation, tubal pregnancies, müllerian anomalies and intrauterine adhesions. Fertil Steril 1998;49:661–79.
4. Edmonds DK. Rokitansky syndrome and other Müllerian anomalies. In: Balen AH, Creighton SM, Davies MC, et al, editors. Paediatric and Adolescent Gynaecology. Cambridge, UK: Cambridge University Press; 2004. pp. 267–74.
5. Troiano RN, McCarthy SM. Müllerian duct anomalies: imaging and clinical issues. Radiology 2004;233(1):19–34.
6. Carrington BM, Hricak H, Nuruddin RN, et al. Müllerian duct anomalies: MR imaging evaluation. Radiology 1990;176:715–20.
7. Chavhan GB, Parra DA, Oudjhane K, et al. Imaging of ambiguous genitalia: classification and diagnostic approach. Radiographics 2008;28(7):1891–904.
8. Bajekal N, Li TC. Fibroids, infertility and pregnancy wastage. Hum Reprod Update 2000;6(6):614–20.
9. Kim HS, Baik JH, Pham LD, Jacobs MA. MR-guided high-intensity focused ultrasound treatment for symptomatic uterine leiomyomata: long term outcomes. Acad Radiol 2011;18(8):970–6.
10. Murase E, Siegelman ES, Outwater EK, et al. Uterine leiomyomas: histopathologic features, MR imaging findings, differential diagnosis and treatment. Radiographics 1999;19:1179–97.

11. Ascher SM, Jha RC, Reinhold C. Benign myometrial conditions: leiomyomas and adenomyosis. Top Magn Reson Imaging 2003; 14:281–304.

12. Ueda H, Togashi K, Konishi I, et al. Unusual appearances of uterine leiomyomas: MR imaging findings and their histopathologic backgrounds. Radiographics 1999;19:S131–45.

13. Grasel RP, Outwater EK, Siegelman ES, et al. Endometrial polyps: MR imaging features and distinction from endometrial carcinoma. Radiology 2000;214(1):47–52.

14. Fleischer AC. Transvaginal sonography of endometrial disorders: an overview. Radiographics 1998;18(4):923–30.

15. Ascher SM, Imakoa I, Lage J. Tamoxifen-induced uterine abnormalities: the role of imaging. Radiology 2000;214:29–38.

16. Nalaboff KM, Pellerito JS, Ben-Levi E. Imaging the endometrium: disease and normal variants. Radiographics 2001;21(6):1409–24.

17. Tamai K, Togashi K, Ito T, et al. MR imaging findings of adenomyosis: correlation with histopathologic features and diagnostic pitfalls. Radiographics 2005;25:21–40.

18. Reinhold C, Tafazoli F, Mehio A, et al. Uterine adenomyosis: endovaginal US and MR imaging features with histopathologic correlation. Radiographics 1999;19:S147–60.

19. Kuligowska E, Deeds L 3rd, Lu K 3rd. Pelvic pain: overlooked and underdiagnosed gynecologic conditions. Radiographics 2005;25: 3–20.

20. Steinkeler JA, Woodfield CA, Lazarus E, Hillstrom MM. Female infertility: a systematic approach to radiologic imaging and diagnosis. Radiographics 2009;29(5):1353–70.

21. Woodward PJ, Sohaey R, Mezzetti TP Jr. Endometriosis: radiologic–pathologic correlation. Radiographics 2001;21:193–216; questionnaire 288–94.

22. Coutinho A Jr, Bittencourt LK, Pires CE, et al. MR imaging in deep pelvic endometriosis: a pictorial essay. Radiographics 2011;31(2):549–67.

23. Horrow MM, Rodgers SK, Naqvi S. Ultrasound of pelvic inflammatory disease. Ultrasound Clin 2007;2(2):297–309.

24. Sam JW, Jacobs JE, Birnbaum BA. Spectrum of CT findings in acute pyogenic pelvic inflammatory disease. Radiographics 2002; 22:1327 34.

25. Tukeva TA, Aronen HJ, Karjalainen PT, et al. MR imaging in pelvic inflammatory disease: comparison with laparoscopy and US. Radiology 1999;210(1):209–16.

26. Stany MP, Hamilton CA. Benign disorders of the ovary. Obstet Gynecol Clin N Am 2008;35(2):271–84.

27. The Rotterdam ESHRE/ASRM-Sponsored PCOS consensus workshop group. Revised 2003 consensus on diagnostic criteria and long-term health risks related to polycystic ovary syndrome (PCOS). Hum Reprod 2004;19:41–7.

28. Clayton RN, Ogden V, Hodgkinson J, et al. How common are polycystic ovaries in normal women and what is their significance for the fertility of the population? Clin Endocrinol 1992;37: 127–34.

29. Balen AH, Laven JS, Tan S, et al. Ultrasound assessment of the polycystic ovary: international consensus definitions. Hum Reprod Update 2003;9(6):505–14.

30. Kimura I, Togashi K, Kawakami S, et al. Polycystic ovaries: implications of diagnosis with MR imaging. Radiology 1996;201: 549–52.

31. Bernardin L, Dilks P, Liyanage S, et al. Effectiveness of semiquantitative multiphase dynamic contrast-enhanced MRI as a predictor of malignancy in complex adnexal masses: radiological and pathological correlation. Eur Radiol 2012;22(4):880–90.

32. Thomassin-Naggara I, Toussaint I, Perrot N, et al. Characterization of complex adnexal masses: value of adding perfusion- and diffusion-weighted MR imaging to conventional MR imaging. Radiology 2011;258(3):793–803.

33. Jeong YY, Outwater EK, Kang HK. Imaging evaluation of ovarian masses. Radiographics 2000;20(5):1445–70.

34. Moyle PL, Kataoka MY, Nakai A, et al. Nonovarian cystic lesions of the pelvis. Radiographics 2010;30(4):921–38.

35. Chang HC, Bhatt S, Dogra VS. Pearls and pitfalls in diagnosis of ovarian torsion. Radiographics 2008;28(5):1355–68.

36. Walker DK, Salibian RA, Salibian AD, et al. Overlooked diseases of the vagina: a directed anatomic-pathologic approach for imaging assessment. Radiographics 2011;31(6):1583–98.

CHAPTER 19

GENITOURINARY TRACT TRAUMA

Lisa A. Miller • Stuart E. Mirvis

INTRODUCTION

There has been a steady advance in the imaging, management and treatment of genitourinary (GU) system trauma. Multidetector CT (MDCT) has become the primary diagnostic tool for the rapid and accurate assessment of acute injuries of the kidneys, ureters and bladder. Advances in computer speed and use of thinner MDCT slices now allow for rapid reconstruction of axial images and faster generation of 3D multiplanar, maximal intensity projections and volumetric imaging. Use of these non-axial images can enhance visualisation and comprehension of selected urinary system injuries.

This chapter describes imaging findings seen with injury to the urinary system and male genitalia from both blunt and penetrating force. The emphasis of the chapter is on the MDCT findings of acute traumatic injury, but also considers complications arising from injuries to these structures. In selected situations, other techniques—including intravenous and retrograde urography, ultrasound and renal nuclear scintigraphy—are required. However, in the acute phase of post-traumatic imaging, MDCT is the most efficient and information-intensive study to assess the injured GU system.

Interventional radiology has increasingly been used to manage vascular renal injury and complications of urinary tract injury, such as infected urinoma or partial ureteral tear, thus avoiding the need for surgical exploration. The manner in which diagnostic findings and interventional techniques are integrated with clinical observations and therapeutic decisions will also be described in this chapter.

RENAL INJURY

Clinical Aspects

Renal injury is common, occurring in 8–10% of cases of blunt and penetrating trauma.[1] About 90% of renal injuries result from blunt force and 10% from penetrating trauma.[2] Gunshot or stab wounds are the most common cause of penetrating injury, although iatrogenic injuries sustained during renal biopsy or laparotomy for non-genitourinary disease also unfortunately occur. Patients with an acquired or congenital renal anomaly such as renal transplant, horseshoe kidney, ectopic kidney, renal cyst, renal neoplasm or hydronephrosis are more vulnerable to traumatic renal injury.[3] An underlying renal lesion should be suspected if a patient presents with CT findings of renal injury out of proportion to the mechanism of injury (Fig. 19-1).[4]

The clinical indications for imaging evaluation of the GU system depend on several factors, including the overall haemodynamic status of the patient, other injuries sustained, the site of blunt or penetrating trauma and the presence or absence of gross haematuria. Patients who are haemodynamically unstable and cannot be rapidly resuscitated are usually taken directly to surgery. Although no longer commonly used, a rapid intravenous urogram (IVU) can be performed in the admission area, but is probably best obtained in the operating room, once haemodynamic stability is achieved. This single radiograph will allow visualisation of both kidneys, if functional, and detect the majority of major renal parenchymal injuries.[5] IVU is approximately 68% accurate for staging penetrating trauma;[6] it may not detect minor renal parenchymal lacerations and contusions, but these are unlikely to have major clinical ramifications.

Although ultrasound is often used in the diagnosis of medical renal disease and for rapid assessment of the peritoneal cavity for free fluid, it cannot assess renal function and is relatively insensitive for detection of renal lacerations and contusions, extravasation of blood or urine, collecting system disruption and parenchymal haematoma. Because of these limitations, a negative ultrasound examination cannot exclude a renal injury and is not commonly used in the assessment of acute renal injury.[7]

The significance of haematuria as an indicator of significant renal injury has been the subject of debate, but a

TABLE 19-1   Indications for Renal Imaging in Acute Trauma

Indication	Imaging Study
Penetrating flank and back trauma	Chest, abdominal-pelvic CT with IV and oral contrast medium
Gross haematuria	Abdominal-pelvic CT with oral and IV contrast medium if haemodynamically stable or resuscitated
Haemodynamically unstable requiring emergency surgery	Intraoperative IVU when stabilised
Haemodynamically stable with microscopic haematuria, but no other indication for abdominal-pelvic CT	Observation until resolution of haematuria
Haemodynamically stable with microscopic haematuria, but other indications for abdominal-pelvic CT (+ abdominal examination, decreasing haematocrit, indeterminate result of peritoneal lavage or abdominal ultrasound, unreliable physical examination)	Abdominal-pelvic CT with oral and IV contrast medium
Haemodynamically stable with or without microscopic haematuria with evidence of major flank impact (e.g. lower posterior rib or lumbar transverse process fracture, major contusion of flank soft tissues)	Abdominal-pelvic CT with oral and IV contrast medium

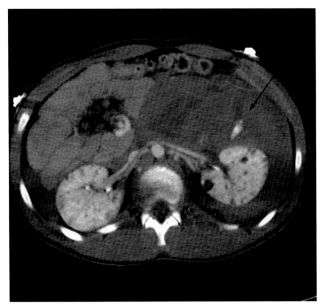

FIGURE 19-1 ■ A 17-year-old man involved in a sledding accident. Note innumerable renal angiomyolipomas in this patient with tuberous sclerosis. Large perinephric haematoma surrounds the left kidney with site of active bleeding (arrow). This is a significant renal injury for a low-velocity injury.

consensus appears to be developing. Hardeman et al. found that 21 of 25 patients (84%) presenting with gross haematuria following blunt trauma had documented renal injury.[8] As a rule, all patients with penetrating flank and back trauma should have a CT examination. Microscopic haematuria without hypotension is very unlikely to be associated with major renal injury. Miller and McAninch reviewed 1588 blunt trauma patients without haematuria or shock on admission.[9] Only three had significant renal injuries, all of which were diagnosed at laparotomy performed for other indications. A combination of four series comprising 2873 blunt trauma patients with microscopic haematuria, but without shock on admission, reported only 10 with significant renal injuries, most of which were also detected at laparotomy performed for other indications. These authors also reported that 78 of 422 patients admitted with gross

haematuria or microscopic haematuria with shock had grade II–V renal injuries, of whom 34 required repair. Haematuria may be absent in patients with severe renal injury, particularly those with vascular pedicle injury, ureteral tear, ureteropelvic disruption and penetrating urinary system injury.[10] One series reported a normal urinalysis in 24% of patients with major renal artery occlusion.[8]

However, in the paediatric population, Stein et al. have shown that microscopic haematuria without hypotension can be associated with significant renal injury, and recommend CT imaging for both gross and microscopic haematuria.[11] Several other clinical factors should also be considered and are reflected in the imaging guidelines utilised at the Maryland Shock Trauma Center, as listed in Table 19-1.

CT Technique for Renal Injury

In general, the kidneys and proximal collecting systems are evaluated as part of the abdominal-pelvic CT study without special protocols. In our centre, the abdomen and pelvis are examined using 40- or 64-channel MDCT with non-ionic IV contrast material as part of a whole-body trauma CT study. An intravenous bolus of 100 mL iodinated contrast agent (350 mg/mL) is given at 6 mL/s for 60 mL and then 4 mL/s for 40 mL by power injector. CT data acquisition is triggered to begin when a threshold density of 100 HU is reached in the ascending aorta. Axial images at 3–5 mm are fused for review and storage on a PACS workstation. The original images are used for all 2D or 3D reformatted imaging and are also saved to a proprietary reconstruction workstation for reference, if required. Since MDCT covers the abdomen and pelvis very quickly, there is no opportunity for opacification of the renal pelvis and ureters, resulting in failure to diagnose potential proximal collecting system injury.[12] Currently, at our centre, if there is radiological suspicion for collecting system injury on the initial CT image set, additional 3- to 20-min delayed images may be obtained as necessary to evaluate for extravasation of intravenous contrast material from the collecting system or ureters. Reduced radiation dose is adequate for additional delayed images since these images are used primarily for detection of high-density contrast material rather than parenchymal injury.[13] Delayed CT has been shown to detect as many as 8.6% of collecting system injuries in patients with blunt renal trauma.[12]

The arterial phase images are most useful in demonstrating presence and symmetry of IV contrast by the kidneys and potential active bleeding or traumatic pseudoaneurysm, while the portal venous images provide more information about the extent of parenchymal damage and help differentiate active bleeding from traumatic pseudoaneurysm.

Grading of Renal Injury and Implications for Management

Management of renal trauma depends to a large degree on extent of the injury and clinical status of the patient. In 1989, the American Association for the Surgery of Trauma (AAST) created a renal organ injury grading system, which was based on surgical observations. This grading system was found to be valid in that increasing renal injury grade was directly correlated with the need for renorrhaphy or nephrectomy,[14] the need for haemodialysis and inpatient mortality after blunt renal injury, the need for nephrectomy after penetrating trauma[15,16] and decreased renal function after major renal injury.[17]

In 2011, a review of 3580 renal injuries by Buckley and McAninch[18] led to the revision of the original AAST renal grading system (Table 19-2). The 2011 revision is not solely based on surgical findings but takes into account radiological findings. The revised grading system includes renal injuries not described in the original grading scale (segmental vascular injuries, ureteral pelvic injuries) and reclassifies grade IV and grade V injuries. In the revised grading system, grades I–III remain the same as the original 1989 renal injury staging. Surgical literature was inconsistent in the definition of a grade IV or V injury and no clear management and outcome data could be obtained for these severe injuries. Grades IV and V were thus reclassified in the revised system with more precise language to optimise management, standardise clinical research and improve outcomes.

Generally, patients with grades I–III renal injuries are managed non-operatively. With the gradual shift in trauma care to a more conservative approach, most revised AAST grade IV injuries will likely be managed with interventional angiography and active surveillance, with the exception of a complete ureteral pelvic junction avulsion, which requires surgery, while most grade V injuries will likely have a higher exploration rate and lower renal salvage rate. Our institution uses a CT-based grading scale similar to the revised AAST renal injury grading system (Table 19-3).

CT of Grade I–III Renal Injury

Most renal injuries are minor (75–98%), represented by grades I–III, and will heal spontaneously without

TABLE 19-2 Revised AAST Renal Injury Grading System

Grade	Injury Location	Definition
I	Parenchyma	Subcapsular haematoma and/or contusion
	Collecting system	No injury
II	Parenchyma	Laceration <1 cm in depth and into cortex, small haematoma contained within Gerota's fascia
	Collecting system	No injury
III	Parenchyma	Laceration >1 cm in depth and into medulla, haematoma contained within Gerota's fascia
	Collecting system	No injury
IV	Parenchyma	Laceration through the parenchyma into the urinary collecting system
		Vascular segmental vein or artery injury
	Collecting system	Laceration, one or more into the collecting system with urinary extravasation
		Renal pelvis laceration and/or complete ureteral pelvic disruption
V	Vascular	Main renal artery or vein laceration, avulsion or thrombosis

A renal unit can sustain more than one grade of injury and should be classified by the higher grade of renal injury.

TABLE 19-3 Contrast-Enhanced Spiral CT Grading of Blunt Renal Injury

Injury Grade	Description or CT Finding
I	Superficial laceration(s) involving cortex
	Renal contusion(s)
	<1 cm subcapsular haematoma
	Perinephric haematoma not filling Gerota's space and no active bleeding
	Segmental renal infarction
II	Deeper renal laceration extending to medulla, with intact collecting system
	>1 cm subcapsular haematoma with intact renal function
	Perinephric haematoma limited to and not distending the perinephric space; no active bleeding
III	Laceration extending into collecting system with urine extravasation limited to retroperitoneum
	Perinephric haematoma distending perinephric space or extending into pararenal spaces; no active bleeding
IV	Fragmentation (three or more segments) of the kidney (usually partially devitalised with large perinephric haematoma)
	Devascularisation >50% of parenchyma
	Main renal pedicle injury
	Active bleeding by CT
	Extravasation of urine into peritoneal cavity or extensive extravasation
	Subcapsular haematoma compromising renal perfusion

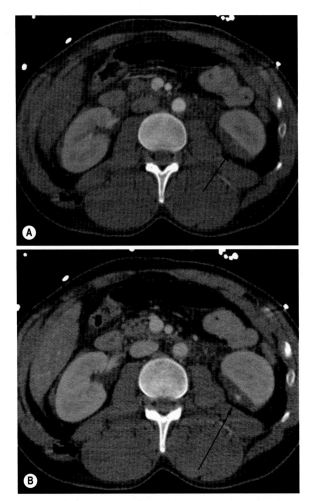

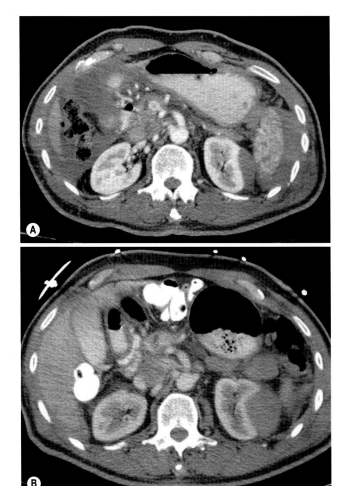

FIGURE 19-2 ■ Arterial phase image of contrast-enhanced MDCT of patient who fell demonstrates subcapsular haematoma flattening the posteromedial aspect of left kidney (A). There is a small focus of hyperdensity within the subcapsular haematoma (arrow). Portal venous phase image (B) shows increase in size of focus of hyperdensity (arrow), indicating active bleeding. Note small amount of right perinephric haemorrhage.

FIGURE 19-3 ■ Contrast-enhanced MDCT of a patient who fell demonstrates a small subcapsular haematoma indenting the lateral aspect of the left kidney (A). A follow-up MDCT obtained three days later for increasing pain (B) demonstrates interval increase in size of subcapsular haematoma with a more pronounced biconvex shape and increased mass effect on underlying renal parenchyma.

intervention. Contusions are visualised as ill-defined low-attenuation areas with irregular margins. They may appear as regions with a striated nephrogram pattern due to differential blood flow through the contused parenchyma. These lesions do not usually require follow-up imaging. Subcapsular renal haematomas are uncommon as the renal capsule is not easily separated from the cortex. A subcapsular haematoma appears as an unenhanced, typically convex fluid collection indenting the underlying parenchyma (Fig. 19-2). Small subcapsular haematomas may become biconvex as they enlarge (Fig. 19-3). Some delay in renal perfusion may be seen with these injuries, secondary to increased resistance to arterial perfusion. In most cases the injury will resolve without specific treatment, although acute or delayed onset of hypertension from renal parenchymal compression (Page kidney) should be sought. Large subcapsular haematomas could theoretically compress the kidney to near systolic level pressures, preventing

perfusion and requiring surgical release of renal tamponade.

Minor renal lacerations can be either superficial, involving the cortex only, or deep, extending to the renal medulla. Lacerations appear as non-enhancing linear defects on a background of otherwise normally enhancing renal parenchyma (Fig. 19-4). As a rule, a minor renal laceration will spare the collecting system. These are usually self-limited injuries, typically accompanied by small amounts of perinephric haemorrhage. Perinephric haemorrhage will appear as a poorly marginated, hyperdense fluid confined by Gerota's fascia. Thickening of the lateral conal fascia may also be seen (Fig. 19-5). Even if the perinephric haematoma is large, it will usually not indent the renal contour as seen with a subcapsular haematoma.

Segmental renal infarctions are also considered minor renal injuries and are relatively common in blunt renal trauma. These result from stretching and subsequent

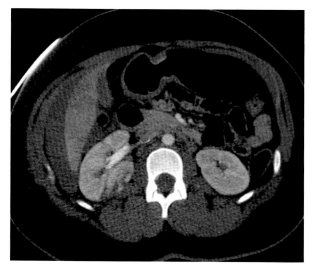

FIGURE 19-4 ■ **A 42-year-old woman involved in motor vehicle collision.** Contrast-enhanced MDCT demonstrates several linear low-density lacerations in the posterior right kidney, characterised as a grade II renal injury using the revised AAST renal injury grading scale.

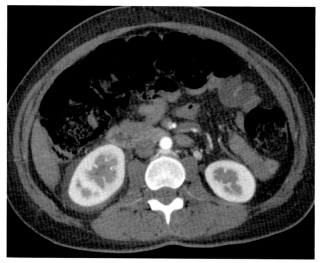

FIGURE 19-5 ■ **Contrast-enhanced MDCT of female patient involved in motor vehicle collision.** There is a small right perinephric haematoma. Note associated thickening of right lateral conal fascia secondary to extension of retroperitoneal blood.

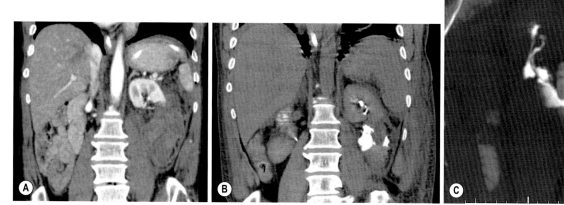

FIGURE 19-6 ■ Coronal reformatted arterial phase image of contrast-enhanced MDCT of 24-year-old male victim of gunshot injury to left flank (A) shows destruction of lower pole of left kidney and large left perinephric haematoma. Because of high likelihood of collecting system injury, additional 13-min delayed images were obtained (B) and show extravasation of high-density IV contrast-enhanced urine from the left collecting system. Maximum intensity projection coronal reformatted image (C) better demonstrates site of collecting system injury.

occlusion of an accessory renal artery, extrarenal or intra-renal branches of the renal artery or a capsular artery.[19] Segmental infarctions appear as sharply demarcated, wedge-shaped areas of very low attenuation with the base of the wedge at the renal capsule and the apex at the renal hilum. Segmental infarctions typically involve the renal pole(s).

CT of Grade IV Renal Injury

More significant renal trauma may require intervention by angiography or surgery. AAST grade IV injuries include deep renal lacerations that extend into the renal collecting system with or without urinary extravasation,

segmental vascular injury within the kidney and renal pelvis laceration or ureteropelvic junction disruption.

Lacerations of the collecting system are identified on CT by extravasation of urine into the perirenal space (Fig. 19-6). A collecting system injury can be missed if the CT images are obtained before intravenous contrast has reached the collecting system. Visualisation of any fluid around the kidney on the admission CT may require additional, delayed CT imaging when appropriate. Delayed images will show the collection of high-density, contrast-enhanced urine adjacent to the site of injury. If the injury is not diagnosed on CT, the development of sepsis, decreasing renal function or unexplained increasing serum creatinine and blood urea nitrogen (BUN)

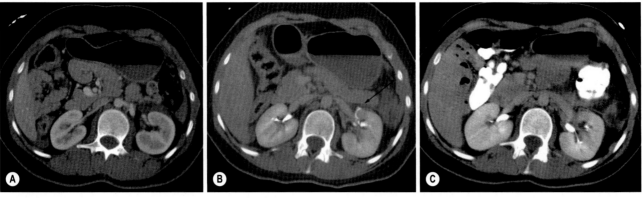

FIGURE 19-7 ■ Axial portal venous MDCT image of patient involved in motor vehicle collision (A) shows small amount of very-low-density fluid along anteromedial aspect of left kidney. Because of high suspicion for collecting system injury, 10-min delayed images were obtained (B) and demonstrate small leak of high-density iodinated contrast-enhanced urine from collecting system (arrow). This patient was managed with observation. Contrast-enhanced MDCT obtained one week later (C) shows resolution of leak, indicating interval healing of collecting system injury.

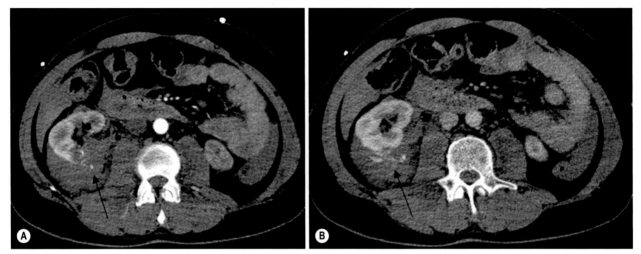

FIGURE 19-8 ■ Arterial phase MDCT image of patient involved in motorcycle collision (A) demonstrates extensive injury to mid-right kidney with moderate amount of perinephric haemorrhage and several small foci of high density (arrow). Portal venous image (B) shows interval increase in size of foci of high density (arrow), consistent with active bleeding. This patient underwent successful angiographic embolisation for treatment of the active bleeding.

should raise concern for urine leak. Urine leaks from collecting system injury spontaneously resolve in 87% of cases and can often be managed with observation alone (Fig. 19-7). Resolution is particularly likely if there is unimpeded antegrade urine flow. Urinomas can become infected due to urine stasis or bacterial contamination from penetrating injury, and are managed by percutaneous drainage. Persistent collecting system leaks may be treated with nephrostomy or a double-J ureteral catheter. Surgical repair may be required if non-surgical interventions do not resolve the leak. This is more likely in cases where the urine leak communicates with a low-pressure space like the pleural or peritoneal cavity.

Segmental vascular injuries include active bleeding and traumatic pseudoaneurysm formation. Active bleeding into the kidney or surrounding tissue appears as patchy or linear dense contrast material surrounded by

less dense haematoma on arterial phase images. On portal venous imaging, the area of extravasated contrast material will increase (Fig. 19-8) and remain high in density. Haemorrhage is apparent because arterial extravasation appears before opacification of the renal collecting system. Typically, the density of extravasated arterial contrast medium is greater than 80 HU and is within 15 HU of an adjacent artery (Fig. 19-9).[20] A traumatic renal pseudoaneurysm will appear as a rounded or oval area of high density on arterial phase imaging that becomes isodense on portal venous images (Fig. 19-10). In stable patients, sites of active bleeding and traumatic pseudoaneurysms can be confirmed by selective renal angiography and treated by angioembolisation with Gelfoam pledgets followed by coils.

Injury to the renal pelvis most likely results from hyperextension with overstretching of the pelvis.[21] The

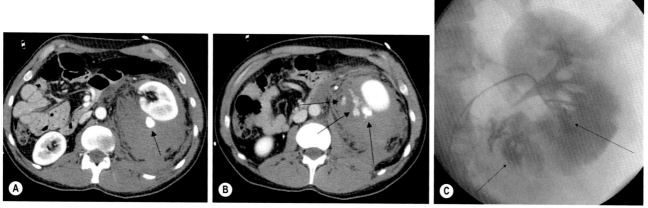

FIGURE 19-9 ■ **A 22-year-old male victim of motor vehicle collision.** Arterial phase MDCT image (A) demonstrates a large left peri-nephric haemorrhage with an oval focus of high density adjacent to the posterior aspect of the mid-kidney (arrow). Portal venous phase image at the level of the lower pole (B) shows the focus has remained dense and increased in size (arrows), diagnostic of active bleeding. Selective left renal angiogram (C) confirms presence of active bleeding (arrows). Treatment of the active bleeding with angiographic embolisation was subsequently performed.

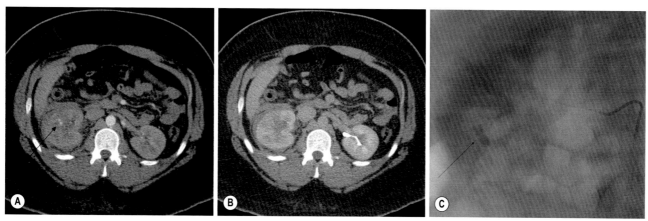

FIGURE 19-10 ■ Arterial phase image of contrast-enhanced MDCT (A) of patient with right renal injury due to gunshot wound shows two foci of high density (arrow) which fade on portal venous imaging (B), consistent with traumatic pseudoaneurysm. Note small amount of right perinephric haemorrhage. Selective right renal angiography (C) confirms presence of bilobed pseudoaneurysm (arrow). This patient was successfully treated with coil angioembolisation.

injury manifests as gross contrast/urine extravasation near the ureteropelvic junction (UPJ). The involved kidney is typically intact with limited or no parenchymal dysfunction. Mulligan et al. described five adult patients with UPJ disruption, of whom three had false-negative diagnoses as a result of CT being performed in the pre-excretory phase, resulting in absent or subtle contrast extravasation.[22] As with intrarenal collecting system injuries, a renal pelvis injury can be missed if the images are obtained before intravenous contrast has reached the renal pelvis. This emphasises the need for suspicion of injury when fluid is seen near the UPJ and performance of delayed CT. Extravasation of contrast-enhanced urine into the right anterior pararenal space could mimic duodenal rupture with leakage of oral contrast. Renal pelvic injury with visualisation of the distal ureter indicates only partial disruption exists. Partial disruption can be managed with transureteral catheter stenting, whereas large or complete disruptions require operative repair. A

dilated renal pelvis resulting from congenital or acquired urinary outflow obstruction is at increased risk for rupture from a traumatic impact (Fig. 19-11).[23]

CT of Grade V Injury

AAST grade V injuries include laceration, avulsion or thrombosis of the main renal artery or vein. Main renal artery injury following blunt trauma is rare, with an estimated incidence of only 0.05%.[24] Main renal artery thrombosis is thought to be due to lateral displacement of the kidneys. This motion stretches the intima beyond its elastic limit, leading to dissection. Clot then begins to form on and around the disrupted intima, leading to partial or complete artery occlusion.[25] The artery usually occludes between its proximal and middle third. It is common for the non-perfused kidney to otherwise appear intact. Using contrast-enhanced MDCT, the absence of perfusion is obvious from the lack of renal opacification,

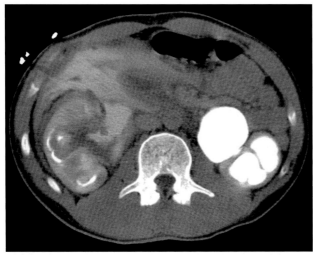

FIGURE 19-11 ■ **A 24-year-old man with bilateral UPJ obstruction involved in motor vehicle collision.** A 10-min delayed image of contrast-enhanced MDCT demonstrates extensive iodinated urine extravasation from injured right collecting system. The left collecting system shows UPJ obstruction without injury.

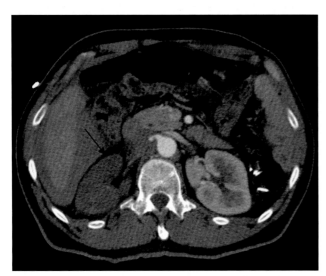

FIGURE 19-12 ■ **Arterial phase MDCT image of patient involved in motor vehicle collision demonstrates characteristic findings of main renal artery injury.** There is abrupt cut-off of the proximal right renal artery with small amount of surrounding haemorrhage, small renal size and lack of perfusion to most of the kidney. Note minimal peripheral renal enhancement (arrow) due to intact collateral capsular vessels (rim sign).

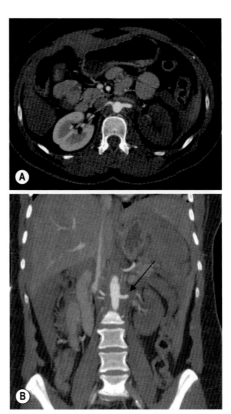

FIGURE 19-13 ■ **A 53-year-old female bicyclist hit by motor vehicle.** Arterial phase MDCT (A) shows abrupt cut-off of left main renal artery, lack of renal perfusion and small renal size indicating left renal arterial injury. Coronal reformatted image (B) better demonstrates the abrupt termination of the injured proximal left renal artery (arrow).

diminished kidney size and, occasionally, preserved peripheral enhancement (rim sign) from intact collateral flow (Fig. 19-12). The precise site of occlusion can often be seen, especially using multiplanar reformatted (MPR) images (Fig. 19-13).

Optimal management of main renal artery occlusion remains controversial. Treatment options include immediate nephrectomy, non-operative management or endovascular or surgical revascularisation. Currently, non-operative management is usually chosen. Surgical revascularisation results are dismal, with long-term preservation of renal function in fewer than 25%.[26] There

are only case reports of treatment of main renal artery occlusion with endovascular stent placement[24,27] (Fig. 19-14) that seldom report long-term results. Lopera et al. recently described eight patients with main renal artery occlusion after blunt abdominal trauma.[28] Renal artery recanalisation with stent placement was successful in six patients (75%), with a mean time from injury to recanalisation of 5 hours. Although endovascular stent placement can be technically possible in some patients, long-term results appear mixed.

Clinically, significant renal vein disruption is also rare. It can produce extensive perinephric bleeding, but as the venous pressure is low this is usually limited to the retroperitoneum. CT findings include an enlarged renal vein containing thrombus, increased renal size, a delayed and progressively dense nephrogram due to high venous outflow resistance and delayed excretion of IV contrast medium into the collecting system.

Severe fragmentation of the renal parenchyma is also considered a major renal injury and typically results in nephrectomy. However, in selected cases, non-operative management, supplemented by renal angiography and percutaneous drainage, if needed, can be attempted— even in cases of major renal parenchymal disruption. On occasion the authors have seen considerable restoration of renal anatomy and function after non-operative treatment after renal fragmentation.

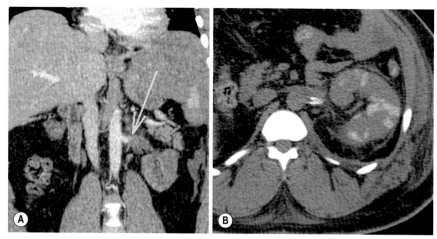

FIGURE 19-14 ■ Coronal reformatted MDCT image of bicyclist struck by automobile (A) shows abrupt cut-off of proximal left renal artery (arrow), small amount of perivascular haemorrhage and decreased perfusion to left kidney. Selective angiography of the left renal artery with stent placement was performed and follow-up CT (B) shows satisfactory placement of stent with patchy perfusion of the kidney.

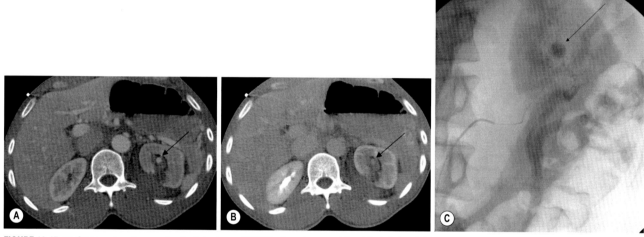

FIGURE 19-15 ■ Contrast-enhanced arterial phase MDCT of patient stabbed in left back (A) demonstrates a posterior left renal laceration, small amount of perinephric haemorrhage and round focus of high density in the central kidney (arrow) that slightly fades in density on portal venous imaging (B) (arrow), consistent with traumatic pseudoaneurysm. Selective left renal angiography (C) confirms the presence of the pseudoaneurysm (arrow). This patient was successfully treated with angiographic coil embolisation.

Penetrating Renal Trauma

Significant renal injuries are seen in about 10% of cases of penetrating trauma to the flank and back (Fig. 19-15).[29] Although gross haematuria is typically present, major injuries can be seen in 15–25% of such patients who present with only microscopic haematuria. A normal urinalysis does not exclude a major renal or ureteral injury. Kansas et al. reported that haematuria was absent in 54–58% of patients with renal injury from gunshot and stab wounds.[30]

Historically, patients with penetrating flank and back trauma were explored surgically to determine the extent of injury. More recently, contrast-enhanced MDCT (CE-MDCT) has been used in stable patients to assess

the extent of injury and potentially permit conservative management. Federle et al. performed CT in 22 patients with penetrating flank and back wounds and were able to manage 20 patients successfully without surgery.[29] Because additional associated injuries can be seen in up to 80% of patients with renal injury from penetrating trauma, these patients are more likely than blunt injury patients to be surgically explored. The typical non-sterile condition of penetrating injury is associated with increased risk of infection, which may require management with interventional radiology or surgical debridement.

A study of 143 patients with penetrating renal stab wounds by Armenakas et al. was performed using the AAST grade classification.[6] The majority of injuries were minor but all grades were seen. Trauma to other organs occurred in 61% of these patients, typically involving the liver, spleen, diaphragm and pleural space. Conservative treatment was instituted in 54% of cases and only 3 patients required delayed surgical intervention for bleeding.

In the authors' institution CE-MDCT is routinely used to ascertain extent of injury for patients with penetrating back and flank wounds and has shown excellent accuracy. Contrast medium is administered (oral and rectal) to opacify the bowel and identify colonic and intraperitoneal wound extension. Increased use of CE-MDCT for stable patients with penetrating torso injury should decrease surgical exploration by accurately defining the trajectory of penetrating objects and site(s) and extent of injuries, including the presence or absence or peritoneal space violation.[31]

Renal artery aneurysms are more common in penetrating than blunt renal trauma. These injuries may present several days after injury with haematuria or rupture, or may remain asymptomatic for years and present with delayed rupture.[32]

Intervention in Renal Injury

If surgical exploration of a renal injury is performed, there is a 64% chance of nephrectomy, regardless of operative intent.[15] Surgery is currently required in less than 10% of renal injuries and its use will likely continue to decrease. Interventional radiology procedures have become increasingly valuable in permitting non-operative management of major renal injuries. Percutaneously placed catheters can assist in draining persistent urinomas or perinephric abscesses. Nephrostomy can divert urine flow and lower pressure on injuries to the renal collecting system.

Management of renal injuries with angioembolisation (AE) has become increasingly common.[33] Currently, there is no consensus on exactly what CT findings can predict or exclude the need for AE. CT criteria that have been evaluated include the AAST grade of renal injury, the complexity of the laceration, the site of laceration, discontinuity of Gerota's fascia, presence of active bleeding and size of perirenal haematoma. Several authors have shown that the presence of active bleeding on CT predicts the need for AE.[34,35] Fu et al. demonstrated that discontinuity of Gerota's fascia had a positive predictive value (PPV) of 92% and negative predictive value (NPV) of 78% in predicting need for AE.[36]

Recently, Charbit et al. looked at all of the aforementioned CT criteria to predict need for AE in 53 patients with high-grade renal injuries, defined as AAST grade III or higher, treated by conservative management.[37] Results showed that no one CT finding could exclude the need for AE. AAST grade, complexity of laceration and laceration site were found to have no relationship with need for AE. The presence of active bleeding was found to have a PPV of 78% for AE. In those patients without active bleeding the size of the perirenal haematoma was used to guide further management. These authors proposed, in the absence of active bleeding, angiography should be considered if perirenal haematoma size was

>25 mm, but not for haematoma size <25 mm. AE was recommended for patients with active renal bleeding.

URETERAL INJURY

Ureteral injures from blunt trauma are very rare. In a review of 22,706 genitourinary injuries, Siram et al. found only 224 cases (<1% incidence) from blunt trauma.[38] The ureters are protected by the vertebral column, psoas muscles and bony pelvis and significant blunt force is needed to cause injury. Injuries to other organs are almost always present and the diagnosis of ureteral injury may be delayed due to management of associated injuries.

Ureteral injury associated with blunt trauma typically occurs at the UPJ although injury to the mid-ureter has also been described. Hyperextension causing ureteral stretching or ureter compression against lumbar transverse processes is a likely mechanism. Ureteral injury may involve contusion, partial tear or complete disruption. In cases of blunt trauma, CT findings on arterial and portal venous phase imaging may be very subtle. Mild fat stranding or a small amount of low-density fluid around the kidney, renal pelvis or ureter may be the only abnormalities identified. The most common associated injury is pelvic fracture.[38] Lack of precise clinical findings adds difficulty in detecting ureteral injury.[39] Haematuria may be absent in up to one-third of patients with ureteral injury.

Delayed, excretory phase images are usually needed to make the diagnosis. Delayed images will show contrast material accumulating in the periureteral soft tissues. The integrity of the ureter can be determined by demonstration of contrast below the level of injury and dictates management. Retrograde urography can be used to document the site and extent of disruption, especially when IVP or CT is inconclusive. Radionuclide scintigraphy can also be used to detect urine extravasation. Penetrating injury to the ureter is twice as common as blunt injury. Penetrating injury, typically from gunshot injury or stab wound, involves the upper portion of the ureter in 70% and distal portion in 22% of cases.[39] Gunshot wounds to the abdomen result in ureteral injury in 2 to 5% of cases[40] (Fig. 19-16). Gunshot injuries can damage the ureter directly or by blast effect. Blast effect may disrupt the intramural blood supply of the ureter, resulting in ureteral necrosis. Penetrating injuries are usually focal, involving only a short ureteral segment. Bowel and vascular injuries, usually iliac vein or artery, are the most commonly associated.[38]

Iatrogenic ureteral injury occurs in 0.4–2.5% of patients undergoing gynaecological surgery for non-malignant conditions.[41] Conditions that increase the likelihood of iatrogenic ureteral injury include haemorrhage, endometriosis, uterine enlargement, cancer and adhesions. When the injury is recognised at the time of surgery, immediate repair can be performed. In many cases, the injury remains unrecognised, and patients present with fever, loin pain, fistula formation or signs of infection or obstruction. Once the diagnosis is suspected, it is best confirmed by retrograde urography.

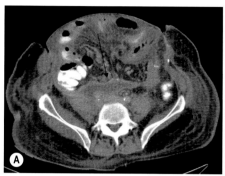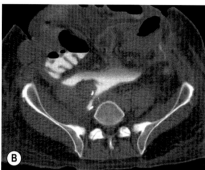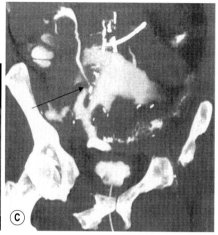

FIGURE 19-16 ■ **A 54-year-old man who sustained an abdominal gunshot injury was found to have multiple organ injuries at laparotomy.** The fluid from an abdominal surgical drain had a high creatinine level. (A) shows a rim-enhancing hypodense fluid collection (arrow) in the mesenteric root. One-hour delayed MDCT image (B) shows extravasation of iodinated urine into the collection. Coronal maximum intensity projection image (C) better demonstrates the injured mid-right ureter draining into the urinoma (arrow).

BLADDER INJURY

Diagnostic Technique

Between 60 and 90% of patients with traumatic bladder rupture have also sustained concurrent fractures of the pelvis and 2–11% of patients with pelvic fractures have a ruptured bladder.[42] The severity of the pelvic injury roughly correlates with the likelihood of bladder and urethral injury.[43] Haematuria, typically gross, almost always accompanies significant bladder injury.[44] Additional signs and symptoms of bladder injury include suprapubic pain or tenderness, difficulty or inability to void, distension, guarding, or rebound tenderness, ileus and ascites. Abnormal electrolytes and elevation of the serum creatinine and BUN can also appear if diagnosis is delayed.

Cystography, by either radiography or CT, must be performed in all patients with gross haematuria associated with pelvic fractures. Cystography is performed after urethral injury has been excluded and retrograde bladder catheterisation is deemed safe. To reliably diagnose bladder injury sufficient bladder distension must be obtained to initiate detrusor muscle contraction. Instillation of less than 250 mL of iodinated contrast material can produce a falsely negative cystogram due to inadequate distension. At the authors' trauma centre at least 300 mL of 30% contrast medium is instilled. Scout, full bladder and postvoid frontal pelvic radiographs are obtained. If it is highly likely that a bladder injury exists, based on the extent and type of pelvic fracture, initial instillation of 100 mL of contrast medium followed by AP pelvic radiography is performed to avoid extensive extravasation which might obscure potential sites of pelvic bleeding if selective pelvic angiography and embolisation is required. If no injury is seen, the remaining contrast material is instilled and full and postvoid radiographs obtained. If a question of minimal extravasation exists, a bladder washout with normal saline can be

performed to localise any contrast remaining after voiding. If pelvic angiography is contemplated for ongoing haemorrhage, cystography should await completion of that procedure. An 'on-table' cystogram can be conveniently performed in the angiographic suite upon completion of the arteriogram.

MDCT cystography is rapidly becoming the preferred study for suspected bladder trauma.[45] A drip bladder infusion of up to 400 mL of 4% contrast material, from a reservoir at a maximum height of 100 cm, is instilled unless limited by detrusor contraction. After installation, the pelvis is examined at 5-mm sections with a full bladder and after voiding or catheter drainage. A cystogram should be performed when there are pelvic fractures (excluding isolated acetabular fractures), gross haematuria or free pelvic fluid, or pelvic haematoma of unknown source (Fig. 19-17). The absence of shock and microscopic haematuria are strong negative predictors for bladder injury.[43]

While bladder injuries may be seen on standard CT with intravenous contrast medium and a clamped bladder catheter, this antegrade approach to bladder distension cannot reliably exclude bladder injury.[43] MDCT cystography has proven to be as accurate as conventional cystography, with 95% sensitivity and 99% specificity in detecting bladder rupture.[46]

Classification

Intraperitoneal bladder rupture (IBR) usually occurs at the anatomically weak bladder dome and results from blunt impact to a full bladder or transmission of hydraulic pressure waves in a partially full bladder.[43] Blunt trauma may lead to a rapid rise in intraperitoneal pressure and cause bursting of the bladder dome. IBR accounts for 10–20% of all bladder ruptures in adults and requires surgical repair to avoid urinary peritonitis. Standard cystography or CT cystography show free intraperitoneal contrast medium outlining the peritoneal recesses and

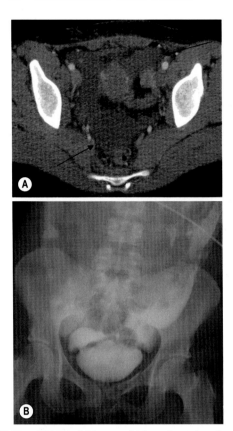

FIGURE 19-17 ▪ MDCT of 31-year-old female patient involved in motor vehicle collision (A) shows moderate amount of low-density pelvic free fluid (arrows). A cystogram (B) shows large amount of extravasated contrast material surrounding bowel loops and layering in the colonic gutters, findings diagnostic of intraperitoneal bladder rupture.

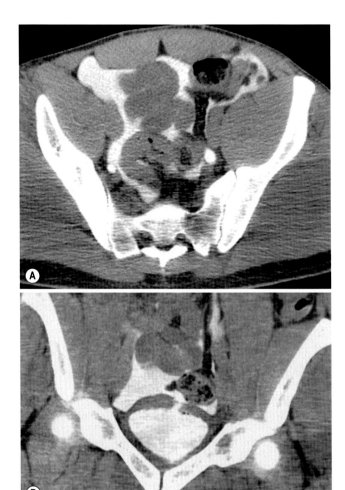

FIGURE 19-18 ▪ CT cystogram of patient with intraperitoneal bladder injury (A) demonstrates high-density fluid surrounding bowel loops. (B) Coronal reformatted MDCT image shows the precise site of bladder injury at the bladder dome.

bowel loops (Fig. 19-18). Leak of opacified urine into the vagina (posterior fornix) can mimic IBR into the pelvis. On CT, spillage of iodinated contrast into the peritoneal cavity can mimic bowel rupture with leakage of oral contrast medium or even haemorrhage into the peritoneal cavity. In many cases a clear demarcation in CT density is seen between urine extravasated before and after contrast enhancement. In addition, dense urinary contrast medium can obscure intraperitoneal blood or intestinal contents, diminishing overall diagnostic accuracy of abdominal-pelvic CT.

Cystography can be falsely negative for intraperitoneal bladder rupture when contrast media is blocked from leaking by detrusor contraction, a small tear, a blood clot or a Foley catheter. IRBs are believed to occur more frequently in small children in motor vehicle accidents than in adults as the seat belt fits over the anterior lower abdomen rather than the superior iliac spines and the bladder is positioned in the lower abdomen rather than deep in the pelvis.[42]

Extraperitoneal bladder rupture (EBR) is caused by perforation of the bladder by bone spicules or by pulling of fascial connections between the bladder and pelvis during pelvic deformation. Most injuries occur in the anterolateral bladder wall near the base (Fig. 19-19).[42] The pattern of iodinated urine extravasation into the surrounding extraperitoneal tissues creates a streaky or flame-shaped appearance. Contrast material often dissects through fascial planes into the anterior prevesical space of Retzius, the anterior abdominal wall, the inguinal regions(s) and upper thigh(s), the lateral paravesical space and the presacral space (Fig. 19-20). In EBR there is often concurrent disruption of the urogenital diaphragm (posterior urethra) and bladder base with contrast media seen extending into the perineum and scrotum. Rarely, extravesical contrast material can extend retroperitoneally to the level of the kidneys, suggesting a renal source of contrast extravasation. Careful review of sequential CT images should avoid this pitfall. CT can often directly demonstrate the exact site of bladder wall disruption. Most cases of EBR are treated with transurethral or suprapubic bladder drainage. In 90% of extraperitoneal injuries, the bladder is healed within 10 days.[47] However, surgical repair of extraperitoneal injuries may be considered, especially in patients with pelvic fractures requiring orthopaedic surgery. Approximately 5–10% of cases of bladder rupture are combined intraperitoneal and extraperitoneal ruptures. Cystography will demonstrate features typical of both injuries.

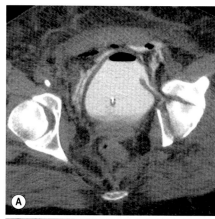
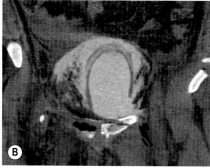

FIGURE 19-19 ■ CT cystogram of victim of motor vehicle collision (A) shows streaky extravasated contrast material around urinary bladder consistent with extraperitoneal bladder injury. (B) Coronal reformatted image better demonstrates the site of injury at the left bladder base. Note adjacent left superior ramus fracture.

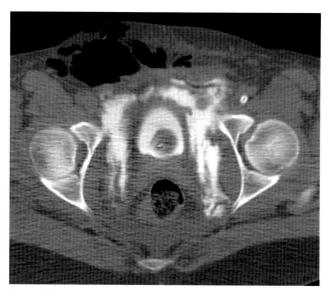

FIGURE 19-20 ■ CT cystogram of trauma patient with extraperitoneal bladder rupture shows extensive streaky extravasation of contrast into the fascial planes of the pelvis.

Rarely, the bladder can be entrapped in a displaced pelvic fracture requiring open reduction and repair.[48] On cystography, the bladder has a distorted shape and is in close proximity to an adjacent displaced fracture. Cystography can reveal the presence of pelvic haematomas

displacing the bladder, but CT provides this information with greater accuracy, indicating the site and extent of other pelvic injuries and in many cases, the location of pelvic arterial injury. Mucosal lacerations and bladder wall contusions may produce haematuria or haematomas.

Intravesical blood clots may result from trauma to the urinary tract. Clots arising from the ureteral orifices are most likely to be due to renal or ureteral rather than direct bladder injury. Rarely, intravesical clots can mask a full-thickness bladder injury by temporarily blocking urine leakage.

Complications of missed bladder injury include urinary tract infection, abdominal distension, pelvic abscess and bladder neck fistula or constriction and incontinence.[42]

Penetrating injuries of the bladder, usually from pelvic gunshot or stab wounds, account for 15–40% of bladder ruptures. Stab wounds and low-velocity missile wounds without evidence of urine extravasation can probably be managed conservatively with good outcomes. High-velocity missile wounds producing evidence of bladder or ureteral injury should be surgically explored.[49]

URETHRAL INJURY

Urethral injuries occur in about 10% of major pelvic fractures and typically involve the proximal (posterior) portion. The overwhelming majority of urethral injuries occur in young men sustaining high-velocity blunt trauma, but these injuries can rarely occur in women. The different configuration of the female pelvic floor and shorter urethral length reduce the risk of urethral injuries in women with pelvic ring fractures.[50] In women with pelvic fractures, the presence of vaginal bleeding, labial oedema, voiding difficulty, blood at the meatus, haematuria or urine leak through the rectum should raise suspicion for urethral injury. In men, urethral injury is associated with blood at the urethral meatus, inability to void, elevation of the prostate on digital rectal examination and perineal swelling or haematoma.[43] Urethral injury should be suspected in men with unstable pelvic ring disruption or lateral compression injury of the pelvis. Lückhoff et al.[51] reviewed 27 patients with urethral trauma. He found the presence of pubic symphysis disruption on AP pelvic radiography had 100% sensitivity for urethral injury. Imaging assessment of the urethra should precede cystography and should be delayed until after pelvic arteriography if the latter is indicated. A retrograde urethrogram is performed using 30 mL of 60% contrast medium via a Foley balloon catheter positioned in the distal urethra and inflated with 2 mL of saline. Ideally, the study should be conducted using fluoroscopy, but is often performed using oblique radiographs obtained with the shaft of the penis perpendicular to the femur to visualise the full extent of the urethra. Urethrography results can be used to classify the injury using the Goldman system[52] (Table 19-4), permitting effective treatment planning.

Anterior urethral injury is caused more commonly by iatrogenic or penetrating rather than blunt trauma. The bulbous urethra may be injured when crushed between

TABLE 19-4 Classification of Urethral Injuries

Grade	Colapinto & McCallum	Goldman & Sandler
I	Posterior urethra stretched, but intact (OldFig 43-23)	Posterior urethra stretched but intact
II	Posterior urethral tear above intact urogenital diaphragm (UGD)	Partial or complete posterior urethral tear above intact UGD
III	Posterior urethral tear with extravasation through torn UGD (OldFig 43-24)	Partial or complete tear of combined anterior and posterior urethra with torn UGD
IV	—	Bladder neck injury with extension to the urethra (OldFig 43-25)
IVa	—	Injury to bladder base with extravasation simulating type IV (pseudo-grade IV)
V	—	Isolated anterior urethral injury

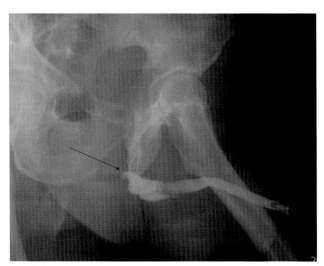

FIGURE 19-21 ■ Retrograde urethrogram of 71-year-old man who suffered straddle injury after falling while walking on a beam demonstrates abrupt cut-off of contrast material due to transection at junction of penile and bulbous urethra (arrow).

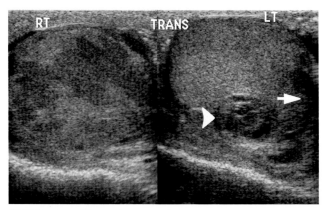

FIGURE 19-22 ■ The patient sustained a kick to the scrotum. The right testicle shows areas of lower echogenicity in an irregular pattern, suggesting contused parenchyma. The left testicle shows a linear fracture (arrow) and a rounded focus of mixed echo texture indicating haematoma (arrowhead).

the impacting object and the inferior surface of the symphysis pubis (Fig. 19-21). The leak from the anterior urethral injury may be limited to the corporal bodies if Buck's fascia remains intact or may spread extensively throughout the scrotum, perineum and anterior abdominal wall if Buck's fascia is disrupted. Posterior urethral injuries are usually diagnosed by retrograde urethrography, but are occasionally seen on pelvic CT. Although non-specific, other CT findings associated with urethral injury include haematoma of the ischiocavernous or obturator internus muscles, distortion or obscuration of the urogenital diaphragm fat plane and distortion or obscuration of the prostatic contour.[53] The use of CT retrograde urethrography to diagnose urethral injuries has recently been described and provides an alternative radiological modality for diagnosing these injuries.[54] Chronic complications of missed urethral injuries include urethral stricture, impotence and incontinence.[51]

SCROTAL INJURY

Injury to the testis may occur from penetrating wounds, direct impact of high-velocity objects against the testis or

compression of the testis against the pubic arch and impacting object. Sporting injuries account for 50% of these injuries. Clinical assessment of the extent and type of scrotal injury is difficult, particularly concerning distinction between testicular haematoma, rupture and torsion.[43] The distinction is essential because a ruptured testis can be salvaged in 90% of patients if repaired within 72 h, but decreases to 55% after this period.[55]

Ultrasound is the imaging technique of choice in acute scrotal trauma and is performed with 5- or 7.5-MHz transducer. Both gray scale and colour Doppler are used.

Intratesticular haematomas are common after trauma (Fig. 19-22). The ultrasound appearance depends on the time between occurrence of trauma and ultrasound evaluation. Acute haematomas are typically isoechoic to the normal testicular parenchyma and can be difficult to identify. If ultrasound findings are equivocal, a repeat study is performed within 12–24 hours to exclude haematoma. Although a testicular haematoma is usually managed conservatively, follow-up to resolution is recommended because of the high incidence of infection and necrosis, which may necessitate orchiectomy.[56]

Testicular rupture implies tearing of the tunica albuginea with extrusion of testicular parenchyma into the scrotal sac. The margins of the testis are poorly defined and the echogenicity of the testis is heterogeneous. The use of colour Doppler is essential as rupture of the tunica

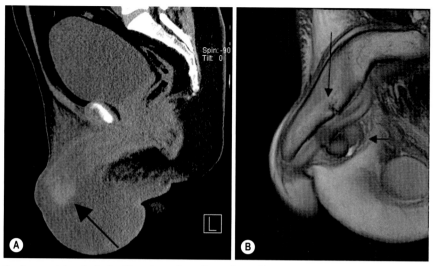

FIGURE 19-23 ■ The patient complained of significant penile pain and swelling after sexual intercourse. Sagittal reformatted image of contrast-enhanced MDCT (A) shows significant scrotal swelling and round focus of haematoma adjacent to penis (arrow). (B) Sagittal T2 fat-saturated MRI demonstrates rupture (long arrow) of the mid left posterior tunica albuginea surrounding the corpora cavernosum. A portion of the haematoma is visible (short arrow).

albuginea will almost always be associated with a loss of vascularity to a portion of or the entire testis.[57] The amount of viable testicular tissue will help determine the appropriate method of surgical management. Guichard et al. found ultrasound to have a sensitivity of 100% and specificity of 65% in detecting testicular rupture in a study of 33 patients.[58] Testicular rupture is usually associated with laceration, fragmentation, intratesticular haematoma and infarction.

Trauma to the testis can also result in dislocation or torsion. Dislocation most commonly results from impact of the scrotum against the fuel tank in motorcycle accidents. Testicular dislocation, typically into the inguinal canal, may be detected by CT or ultrasound. Delayed diagnosis of dislocation may lead to cellular changes in the testis and predispose it to malignant degeneration.[59] Testicular torsion is preceded by trauma in 5–8% of cases.[60]

PENILE INJURIES

Penile fractures typically result from vigorous sexual intercourse or masturbation. The corpus cavernosum is typically fractured with disruption of the tunica albuginea, often accompanied by a cracking sound of the erect penis, pain and detumesence.[61] Thinning of the tunica albuginea in the erect penis increases vulnerability to rupture with sudden bending. Injury to the corpora spongiosum and urethra occurs in 10–20% of cases.[61] Corporal laceration can result from direct trauma to flaccid penis such as a direct kick or penetrating injury. Physical examination is often limited due to painful swelling. Ultrasound can identify the exact site of tear with interruption of the thin echogenic line of tunica albuginea and adjacent haematoma. Colour Doppler may show blood flush through the tunica defect with squeezing of

the penile shaft.[61] MRI reveals discontinuity of the hypointense tunica albuginea, with or without adjacent haematoma (Fig. 19-23). MRI has been reported to demonstrate disruption of the tunica spongiosum and associated anterior urethral tear.[62]

REFERENCES

1. Bower P, Paul J, Brosman SA. Urinary tract abnormality presenting as a result of blunt abdominal trauma. J Trauma 1978;18:719–22.
2. Margenthaler JA, Weber TR, Keller MS. Blunt renal trauma in children: experience with conservative management at a pediatric trauma center. J Trauma 2002;52:928–32.
3. Tezval H, Tezval M, von Klot C, et al. Urinary tract injuries in patients with multiple trauma. World J Urol 2007;25:177–84.
4. Suson KD, Gupta AD, Wang MH. Bloody urine after minor trauma in a child: isolated renal injury versus congenital anomaly? J Pediatr 2011;159:870.
5. Roberts RA, Belitsky P, Lannon SG, et al. Conservative management of renal lacerations in blunt trauma. Can J Surg 1987;30:253–5.
6. Armenakas NA, Duckett CP, McAninch JW. Indications for non-operative management of renal stab wounds. J Urol 1999;161:768–71.
7. McGahan JP, Richards JR. Blunt abdominal trauma: the role of emergent sonography and a review of the literature. Am J Roentgenol 1999;172(4):897–903.
8. Hardeman SW, Husmann DA, Chinn HKW, Peters PC. Blunt urinary tract trauma: identifying those patients who require radiologic diagnostic studies. J Urol 1987;138:99–101.
9. Miller KS, McAninch JW. Radiographic assessment of renal trauma: our 15-year experience. J Urol 1995;154:352–5.
10. Kawashima A, Sandler CM, Corl FM. Imaging evaluation of post-traumatic renal injuries. Abdom Imaging 2002;27:199–213.
11. Stein JP, Kaji DM, Eastjam J, et al. Blunt renal trauma in the pediatric population: indications for radiologic diagnosis. Urology 1994;44:406–10.
12. Brown SL, Hoffman DM, Spirnak JP. Limitations of routine spiral computerized tomography in the evaluation of blunt renal trauma. J Urol 1998;160:1979–81.
13. Stuhlfaut JW, Lucey BC, Varghese JC, Soto JA. Blunt abdominal trauma: utility of 5-minute delayed CT with a reduced radiation dose. Radiology 2006;238(2):473–9.

14. Santucci RA, McAninch JW, Safir M, et al. Validation of the American Association for the Surgery of Trauma organ injury severity scale for the kidney. J Trauma 2001;50:195–200.

15. Kuan JK, Wright JL, Nathens AB, et al. American Association for the Surgery of Trauma Organ Injury Scale for kidney injuries predicts nephrectomy, dialysis, and death in patients with blunt injury and nephrectomy for penetrating injuries. J Trauma 2006; 60:351–6.

16. Wright JL, Nathens AB, Rivara FP, Wessells H. Renal and extra-renal predictors of nephrectomy from the national trauma data bank. J Urol 2006;175:970–5.

17. Tasian GE, Aaronson DS, McAninch JW. Evaluation of renal function after major renal injury: Correlation with the American Association for the Surgery of Trauma Injury Scale. J Urol 2010; 183:196–200.

18. Buckley JC, McAninch JW. Revision of current American Association for the Surgery of Trauma renal injury grading system. J Trauma 2011;70:35–7.

19. Lewis DR, Mirvis SE, Shanmuganathan K. Segmental renal artery infarction following blunt abdominal trauma. Clinical significance and appropriate management. Emerg Radiol 1996;3: 236–40.

20. Cerva DS, Mirvis SE, Shanmuganathan K, et al. Detection of bleeding in patients with major pelvic fractures: value of contrast-enhanced CT. Am J Roentgenol 1996;166:131–6.

21. Mirvis SE, Dunham CM. Abdominal-pelvic trauma. In: Mirvis SE, Young JWR, editors. Imaging in Trauma and Critical Care. Baltimore: Williams & Wilkins; 1992. pp. 145–242.

22. Mulligan JM, Cagiannos I, Collins JP, Millward SF. Ureteropelvic junction disruption secondary to blunt trauma: excretory phase imaging (delayed films) should help prevent a missed diagnosis. J Urol 1998;159:67–70.

23. Yaofeng H, Zhihui Z. Massive hydronephrosis associated with traumatic rupture. Injury 1997;28:505–6.

24. Sangthong B, Demetriades D, Martin M, et al. Management and hospital outcomes of blunt renal artery injuries: analysis of 517 patients from the National Trauma Data Bank. J Am Coll Surg 2006;203:612–17.

25. Santucci RA, McAninch JW. Diagnosis and management of renal trauma: past, present, and future. J Am Coll Surg 2000;191: 443–51.

26. Elliott SP, Olwenhy EO, McAninch JW. Renal arterial injuries: a single center analysis of management strategies and outcomes. J Urol 2007;178:2451–5.

27. Chabrot P, Cassagnes L, Alfidja A, et al. Revascularization of traumatic renal artery dissection by endoluminal stenting: three cases. Acta Radiol 2010;51:21–6.

28. Lopera JE, Suri R, Kroma G, et al. Traumatic occlusion and dissection of the main renal artery: endovascular treatment. J Vasc Interv Radiol 2011;22:1570–4.

29. Federle MP, Brown TR, McAninch JW. Penetrating renal trauma: CT evaluation. J Comput Assist Tomogr 1987;11:1026–30.

30. Kansas BT, Eddy MJ, Mydlo JH, Ozzo RG. Incidence and management of penetrating renal trauma in patients with multiorgan injury: extended experience at an inner city trauma center. J Urol 2004;172:1355–60.

31. Shanmuganathan K, Mirvis SE, Chiu WC, et al. Penetrating torso trauma: triple-contrast helical CT in peritoneal violation and organ injury—a prospective study in 200 patients. Radiology 2004;231: 775–84.

32. Mizobata Y, Junichiro Y, Fujimura I, Sakashita K. Successful evaluation of pseudoaneurysm formation after blunt renal injury and dual-phase contrast enhanced helical CT. Am J Roentgenol 2001; 177:136–8.

33. Breyer BN, McAninch JW, Elliott SP, Master VA. Minimally invasive endovascular techniques to treat acute renal hemorrhage. J Urol 2008;179:2248–52.

34. Dugi DD III, Morey AF, Gupta A, et al. American Association for the Surgery of Trauma grade 4 renal injury substratification into grades 4A (low risk) and 4B (high risk). J Urol 2010;183: 592–7.

35. Nuss GR, Morey AF, Jenkins AC, et al. Radiographic predictors of need for angiographic embolization after traumatic renal injury. J Trauma 2009;67:578–82.

36. Fu CY, Wu SC, Chen RJ, et al. Evaluation of need for angioembolization in blunt renal injury: discontinuity of Gerota's fascia has an increased probability of requiring angioembolizaiton. Am J Surg 2010;199:154–9.

37. Charbit J, Manzanera J, Millet I, et al. What are the specific computed tomography scan criteria that can predict or exclude the need for renal angioembolizaiton after high-grade renal trauma in a conservative management strategy? J Trauma 2011;70(5): 1219–27.

38. Siram SM, Gerald SZ, Greene WR, et al. Ureteral trauma: patterns and mechanisms of injury of an uncommon condition. Am J Surg 2010;199:566–70.

39. Elliott SP, McAninch JW. Ureteral injuries from external violence: the 25-year experience at San Francisco General Hospital. J Urol 2003;170:1213–16.

40. Franco I, Eshghi M, Schutte H, et al. Value of proximal diversion and ureteral stenting in management of penetrating ureteral trauma. Urology 1988;1998(32):99–102.

41. Drake MJ, Noble JG. Ureteric trauma in gynecologic surgery. Int Urogynecol J Pelvic Floor Dysfunct 1998;9:108–17.

42. Gomez RG, Ceballos L, Coburn M, et al. Consensus statement on bladder injuries. BJU Int 2004;94:27–32.

43. Mirvis SE. Trauma. Radiol Clin North Am 1996;34:1225–56.

44. Lis LE, Cohen AJ. CT cystography in the evaluation of bladder trauma. J Comput Assist Tomogr 1990;14:386–9.

45. Ishak C, Kanth N. Bladder trauma: multidetector computed tomography cystography. Emerg Radiol 2011;18:321–7.

46. Chan DP, Abujudeh HH, Cushing GL Jr, Novelline RA. CT cystography with multiplanar reformation for suspected bladder rupture: experience in 234 cases. Am J Roentgenol 2006;187(5): 1296–302.

47. Tezval H, Tezval M, von Klot C, et al. Urinary tract injuries in patients with multiple trauma. World J Urol 2007;25:177–84.

48. Wright DG, Taitsman L, Laughlin RT. Pelvic and bladder trauma: a case report and subject review. J Orthop Trauma 1996;10: 351–4.

49. Baniel J, Schein M. The management of penetrating trauma to the urinary tract. J Am Coll Surg 1994;178:417–25.

50. Mundy AR, Andrich DE. Urethral trauma part II: types of injury and their management. BJU Int 2011;108:630–50.

51. Lückhoff C, Mitra B, Cameron PA, et al. The diagnosis of acute urethral trauma. Injury 2011;42:913–16.

52. Goldman SM, Sandler CM, Corriere JN Jr, McGuire EJ. Blunt urethral trauma: a unified, anatomic mechanical classification. J Urol 1997;157:85–9.

53. Ingram MD, Watson SG, Skippage PL, Patel U. Urethral injuries after pelvic trauma: evaluation with urethrography. Radiographics 2008;28:1631–43.

54. Moore FO, Petersen SR, Norwood SH. Diagnosis of blunt urethral injuries with computed tomogram retrograde urethrography. J Trauma 2010;68:1264.

55. Krone KD, Carroll BA. Scrotal ultrasound. Radiol Clin North Am 1985;23:121–39.

56. Dogra V, Bhatt S. Acute painful scrotum. Radiol Clin North Am 2004;42:349–63.

57. Deurdulian C, Mittelstaedt CA, Chong WK, Fielding JR. US of acute scrotal trauma: optimal technique, imaging findings and management. Radiographics 2007;27:357–69.

58. Guichard G, El Ammari J, Del Coro C, et al. Accuracy of ultrasonography in diagnosis of testicular rupture after blunt scrotal trauma. Urology 2008;71:52–6.

59. Bromberg W, Wong C, Kurek S, Salim A. Traumatic bilateral testicular dislocation. J Trauma 2003;54:1009–11.

60. Lrhorfi H, Manunta A, Rodriguez A, Lobel B. Trauma induced testicular torsion. J Urol 2002;168:2548.

61. Eke N. Fracture of the penis. Br J Surg 2002;89:555–65.

62. Pretorius ES, Siegelman ES, Ramchandan P, Banner MP. MR Imaging of the penis. Radiographics 2001;21:S283–98.

CHAPTER 20

ADRENAL IMAGING

Anju Sahdev • Rodney H. Reznek

CHAPTER OUTLINE

THE ADRENAL GLANDS

With the increasing use of cross-sectional imaging, adrenal lesions are frequently identified in routine practice and are seen in up to 5% of abdominal CTs.[1] Pathognomonic imaging features have been established for many of these lesions, including myelolipomas, adenomas, haematomas and cysts. Most adrenal lesions are benign. However as the adrenal gland is also a frequent site for metastastic disease, distinguishing between benign and malignant masses on imaging in patients with primary cancers elsewhere is essential. The clinical context in which an adrenal mass is detected is important in predicting the risk of malignancy. Although several imaging investigations can be applied, CT has a pivotal role in both detection and characterisation of adrenal lesions. In functioning adrenal disease, clinical and biochemical findings should direct the radiologist to the correct interpretation and diagnosis. This chapter looks at adrenal anatomy, physiology, the characteristic imaging features of common adrenal lesions, the application of modern imaging techniques in evaluating an incidental adrenal mass and functioning and non-functioning adrenal disease.

ANATOMY AND PHYSIOLOGY

Anatomy

The adrenal gland is a composite gland made up of two neuroendocrine organs, the adrenal cortex of mesodermal orgin and adrenal medulla of neuroectodermal origin. Modern imaging techniques cannot distinguish between cortex and medulla as separate zones.

Each gland is found in the suprarenal fossa, the left gland is crescentic and right gland is pyramidal in adults. Although variable, the approximate size of each gland is $5 \times 3 \times 1$ cm and weighs between 4 and 6 g each. Prolonged stress, however, can induce hypertrophy and hyperplasia, increasing both size and weight. The adrenal arterial supply comes from the adrenal arteries arising directly from the abdominal aorta or from the inferior phrenic and renal arteries. The shorter right adrenal vein drains directly to the inferior vena cava whilst the longer left adrenal vein may drain to the renal vein or IVC. Lymphatic channels are only present in the capsule and not within the glands.

The ideal imaging parameters for imaging the adrenal glands on CT and MRI are summarised in Tables 20-1 and 20-2. On cross-sectional imaging, both adrenal glands can be divided into a body, medial and lateral limbs. The right adrenal body should not exceed 8 mm and the left adrenal body should not exceed 10 mm in maximum dimension. The maximum normal adrenal limb thickness is 5 mm. The normal adrenal demonstrates uniform contrast enhancement on arterial and venous phase CT and the cortex cannot be distinguished from the medulla (Fig. 20-1). On MRI, both glands have a uniform intermediate T1 and a low-to-intermediate T2 signal intensity and are better demonstrated on T1 fat-saturated images as nulling the signal from surrounding retroperitoneal fat augments the adrenal signal (Fig. 20-2).

Physiology

The adrenal cortex synthesises and secretes corticosteroids which include mineralocorticoids, glucocorticoids and sex hormones, all derived from cholesterol (Fig. 20-3).

The outer zona glomerulosa produces aldosterone and other mineralocorticoids and is chiefly under the control of angiotensin II.

The central broad zona fasciculata and zona reticularis are influenced primarily by ACTH and produce glucocorticoids and some androgens and oestrogens, respectively. The main glucocorticoid is cortisol and it has an

TABLE 20-1	CT Parameters for Imaging the Adrenals	
	Slice Thickness (mm)	Plane
Unenhanced	3–5	Axial
60 s post-contrast	1–3	Axial and coronal
15 min post-contrast	1–3	Axial and coronal

TABLE 20-2	MRI Parameters for Imaging the Adrenal Glands	
Weighting	Plane	Slice Thickness (mm)/Gap (mm)
Standard Sequences		
T1	Axial	3–5/3
T2	Axial and coronal	3–5/3
CSI (in- and out-phase)	Axial	3–5
T1 fat sat	Axial	5–7/3
Optional Sequences		
T1 fat sat with gadolinium	Axial and coronal	5–7/3
DWI (b = 0, 250, 500, 1000, 1200)	Axial	3–5

important role in carbohydrate, fat and protein metabolism.

The adrenal medulla contains the chromaffin cells producing catecholamines (noradrenaline and adrenaline) and is the major source of noradrenaline (in addition to the organ of Zuckerkandl located at the aortic bifurcation). The medulla synthesises and secretes the catecholamines in response to signals from preganglionic nerve fibres in the sympathetic nervous system.

INCIDENTALLY DETECTED ADRENAL MASS

Incidentally detected adrenal masses in patients with no known malignancy occur in 5% of all abdominal CT examinations.[1–3] These masses are usually benign, but when detected they often present a diagnostic dilemma and require clinical evaluation to exclude endocrine disease, primary adrenal cancer and metastases from other malignancies. The important questions to answer before a suitable management plan can be made are to determine if the lesion is functioning or non-functioning and if it is benign or malignant. Function is clinically and biochemically established, whilst benign adrenal masses such as lipid-rich adenomas, myelolipomas, adrenal cysts and adrenal haemorrhage have pathognomonic cross-sectional imaging appearances, as discussed below.

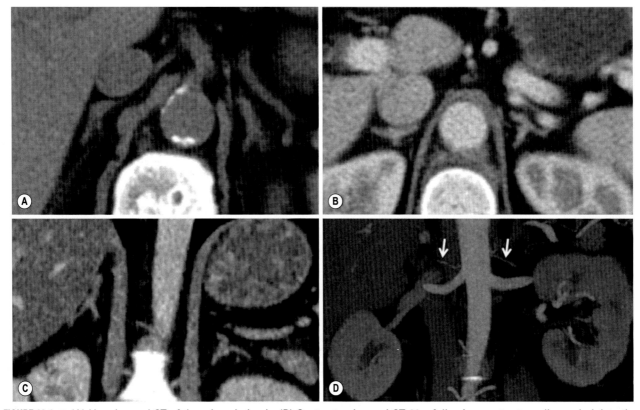

FIGURE 20-1 ■ (A) Unenhanced CT of the adrenal glands. (B) Contrast-enhanced CT 60 s following contrast medium administration. (C) Coronal reconstruction of the enhanced CT. Normal adrenal glands on CT with homogeneous appearances pre- and post-contrast administration. The adrenal body of each gland is demonstrated by the arrows and medial and lateral limbs by the dashed arrows. (D) Contrast-enhanced CT 30 s following injection, demonstrating the adrenal arteries (arrows).

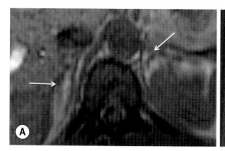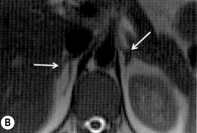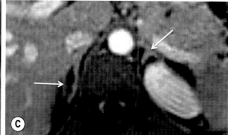

FIGURE 20-2 ■ (A) Axial T1-, (B) axial T2- and (C) axial T1-weighted image with fat saturation of normal adrenal glands, which have homogeneous intermediate T1 signal, low T2 signal and high T1 signal following fat saturation. The fat saturation sequences enhance the visibility of the normal adrenal glands by nulling the surrounding fat signal.

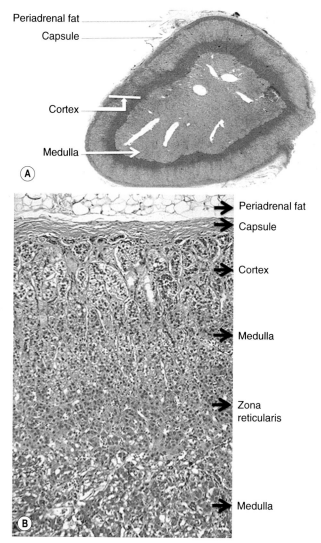

FIGURE 20-3 ■ (A) Gross morphological cross-sectional anatomy of the adrenal gland demonstrating the outer cortex and inner medulla. The thin adrenal capsule is surrounded by retroperitoneal fat. (B) Histology of the normal adrenal gland. The adrenal cortex is composed of the zona glomerulosa, zona fasciculata and zona reticularis. The zona glomerulosa produces aldosterone and other mineralocorticoids and is chiefly under the control of angiotensin II. The zona fasciculata and zona reticularis are influenced primarily by ACTH and produce glucocorticoids and androgens. The adrenal medulla contains the chromaffin cells producing catecholamines and is the major source of noradrenaline (in addition to the organ of Zuckerkandl located at the aortic bifurcation).

Adrenal adenomas are more common in some inherited diseases, including multiple endocrine neoplasia type I, Beckwith–Weidmann syndrome and the Carney complex. The likelihood of developing an adenoma increases with age. Based on pathological studies, about 6% of the population over 60 years of age harbour an adrenal adenoma.[4] Of these, 80% are benign non-functioning adenomas. Adrenal masses are also frequently discovered during imaging performed for staging of patients with cancer. The prevalence of adrenal masses increases to 9–13% in patients with a known underlying malignancy.[1,2] The adrenal gland is a relatively frequent site for metastatic disease but even in patients with a known carcinoma, only 26–36% of adrenal masses are metastatic.[5] This incidence of metastatic adrenal lesions increases to 71% if the adrenal mass is larger than 4 cm and demonstrates an increase in size on follow-up imaging within 1 year.[6]

The nature of incidentally detected adrenal masses can be determined with a high degree of accuracy using computed tomography (CT) or magnetic resonance imaging (MRI) alone. Positron emission tomography (PET) is also increasingly used in clinical practice to characterise adrenal lesions in patients being staged for cancer.

A small minority of adrenal masses elude precise characterisation on cross-sectional imaging and remain indeterminate. These are usually some lipid-poor adenomas, adrenal metastases, adrenal carcinomas and phaeochromocytomas. It is clearly important to make the distinction between these lesions in patients undergoing staging for a known carcinoma, as the presence of metastases contraindicates radical curative surgery or radiotherapy. On occasion the distinction can be difficult as there remains an overlap between imaging features of some benign and malignant lesions. CT and MRI techniques are optimised to maximise specificity for benign adrenal adenomas whilst still maintaining an acceptable sensitivity. Conversely, PET techniques are optimised for detection of malignant disease.

A variety of combinations of imaging techniques are used for characterisation of adrenal masses and these are discussed in the following section.

Computed Tomography (CT)

Lesion Size and Contour

On unenhanced CT, imaging findings that suggest a higher likelihood of malignancy include a large lesion size, irregular contour, heterogeneous appearance and a temporal increase in size. Lesions greater than 4 cm in diameter have a higher likelihood to be either metastases or primary adrenal carcinomas.[6,7] However, size alone is a poor discriminator between adenomas and non-adenomas. In a study by Lee et al., using 3.0 cm as the maximum size cut-off, the sensitivity and specificity for adenomas was only 79 and 84%, respectively (Figs. 20-4 and 20-5).[7] Although it has been suggested that adenomas have a smooth contour, whilst malignant lesions have an irregular shape, this as a single feature is insufficient in discriminaing.

Rapid change in size does raise the suspicion of malignancy as adenomas are slow-growing lesions.

Guidelines published by the American College of Radiology suggest that for lesions >4 cm in size, adrenal resection without any other additional imaging work-up should be considered once biochemical evaluation to exclude phaeochromocytomas has been performed if

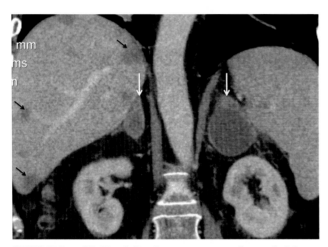

FIGURE 20-4 ■ **CT 60 s following contrast medium administration.** Coronal reconstruction. Bilateral heterogeneous adrenal masses with necrotic centres are seen. In addition there are several liver metastases.

typical imaging features such as those seen in benign lesions such as myelolipomas, adenomas, cysts are not present.[8] The same guidelines also controversially suggest that in patients with no history of prior malignancy who present with a <4 cm adrenal mass with benign imaging features such as smooth external contour and homogeneous appearance, a follow-up in 6–12 months is adequate and no additional imaging with contrast enhancement or chemical shift imaging (CSI) MRI is required. In the authors' experience, other confirmative features of a benign lesion are needed before this guideline can be safely applied.

Intracellular Lipid Content of the Adrenal Mass

The majority (>70%) of adenomas have a high intracellular lipid content which lowers their non-contrast CT density and hence their attenuation value. If an adrenal mass measures 0 HU or less, the specificity of the mass being a benign lipid-rich adenoma is 100% but the sensitivity is only an unacceptable 47%. Boland et al. performed a meta-analysis of 10 studies demonstrating that if a threshold attenuation value of 10 HU was adopted, specificity was 98% and sensitivity increased to a clinically acceptable 71%.[9] Therefore, 10 HU is the most widely used threshold value for the diagnosis of a lipid-rich adrenal adenoma. In another study by Song et al.,[3] in 973 consecutive patients with 1049 incidental adrenal masses, adenomas accounted for 75% of incidental masses, of which 78% were lipid-rich adenomas, with a non-contrast CT attenuation value of less than 10 HU. By using a threshold of 10 HU, the sensitivity and specificity for the detection of an adenoma at unenhanced CT is 89% and 100%, respectively.[10] Therefore most lesions can be fully characterised by CT alone and require no further confirmatory imaging (Fig. 20-6). Lesions on unenhanced CT with an attenuation greater than 10 HU require further evaluation with either contrast-enhanced washout CT, MRI or scintigraphy.

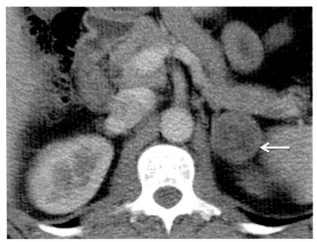

FIGURE 20-5 ■ **Contrast-enhanced CT of the adrenal glands.** A 3-cm enhancing heterogeneous mass is seen in the left adrenal, which had washout criteria consistent with an adenoma.

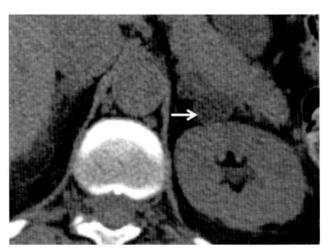

FIGURE 20-6 ■ **Unenhanced CT of the adrenal glands demonstrating a left-sided adenoma.** The non-contrast-enhanced CT attenuation value of the mass is –13 HU, consistent with a lipid-rich adenoma. If the adenoma demonstrates no biochemical function, no further imaging or follow-up would be necessary.

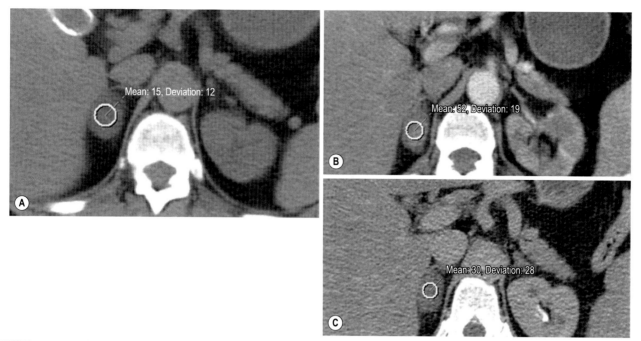

FIGURE 20-7 ▪ A left adrenal mass as seen on CT with the attenuation values shown on the images. (A) Unenhanced CT. (B) Sixty seconds following contrast medium administration. (C) Fifteen minutes following contrast medium administration. The region of interest should include at least 50% of the mass but without contamination from the surrounding fat. On the unenhanced CT, the attenuation of 15 HU indicates an indeterminate mass. The attenuation values above provide an absolute contrast washout value of 60%, in keeping with a benign adenoma.

Contrast Enhancement and Contrast Washout Characteristics

On unenhanced CT, up to 12–30% of benign adenomas have an attenuation value of greater than 10 HU and are considered lipid poor.[9–13] Malignant lesions and phaeochromocytomas are also lipid poor. Characterisation of adrenal masses using contrast-enhanced CT relies on the unique physiological perfusion patterns of adenomas. Adenomas enhance rapidly after contrast medium administration and also demonstrate a rapid washout of contrast medium—a phenomenon termed contrast medium washout. Malignant lesions and phaeochromocytomas enhance rapidly but demonstrate a slower washout of contrast medium.

The difference in contrast enhancement washout characteristics between adenomas and malignant lesions has been shown to be a consistent and reliable technique. The percentage of contrast enhancement washout between enhanced images acquired 60 s after contrast medium administration and the delayed images acquired 15 min after contrast medium administration can be used to differentiate adenomas from malignant lesions.[14–16] Measurements of the attenuation values of the mass before injection of contrast medium, at 60 s following injection of contrast medium and then again at 15 min, are made using an electronic cursor that encompasses at least two-thirds of the mass. These contrast medium enhancement washout values are only applicable to relatively homogeneous masses without large areas of necrosis or haemorrhage. Both lipid-rich and -poor adenomas behave similarly, as this property of adenomas is independent of their lipid content (Fig. 20-7). The

percentage of absolute contrast enhancement washout (ACEW) can be calculated thus:

$$\% \text{ ACEW} = \frac{\text{CE CT attenuaton at 60 s} - \text{delayed CT attenuation}}{\text{CT attenuation at 60 s} - \text{unenhanced CT attenuation}} \times 100$$

The contrast-enhanced CT (CE CT) value is the attenuation value of the mass, in Hounsfield units, 60 seconds after commencement of intravenous contrast medium administration. The delayed attenuation value is the attenuation value of the mass, in Hounsfield units 15 min after commencement of contrast medium administration. Unenhanced CT attenuation is the attenuation value of the mass before administration of contrast media.

If a 15-min delayed protocol is used, an absolute contrast enhancement washout of 60% or higher has a sensitivity of 86–88% and a specificity of 92–96% for the diagnosis of an adenoma.[16]

However, the measurement of this absolute contrast medium enhancement washout requires a non-contrast image. Frequently, in clinical practice, only post-contrast are available (Fig. 20-8). In these patients, by performing a delayed 15-min CT the percentage relative contrast enhancement washout can be calculated thus:

$$\% \text{ RCEW} = \frac{\text{CE CT attenuaton at 60 s} - \text{delayed CT attenuation}}{\text{CT attenuation at 60 s}} \times 100$$

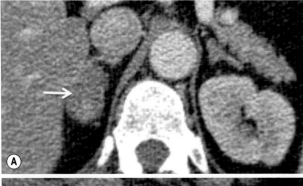

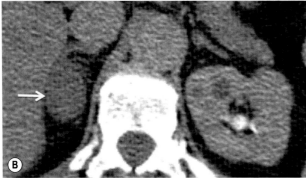

FIGURE 20-8 ■ (A) Sixty seconds following intravenous contrast medium administration. A right adrenal mass is incidentally detected with an attenuation value of 100 HU. (B) Delayed images 15 min following enhancement show the mass has an attenuation value of 32 HU. The relative washout is therefore 68% consistent with an adenoma.

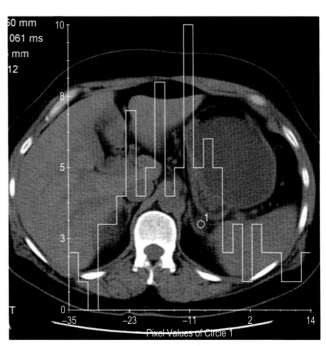

FIGURE 20-9 ■ **Histogram analysis of adenoma.** A small left-sided adrenal lesion is seen on the unenhanced CT. The attenuation value is 14 HU and therefore indeterminate on unenhanced CT alone. On histogram analysis, obtained by drawing a region of interest over the mass, there are pixels ranging between −35 HU and +14 HU (x-axis). The presence of more than 5% negative pixels indicates an adenoma. This was confirmed on washout criteria.

The enhanced and delayed attenuation values are measured as described previously. After 15 min, if a relative enhancement washout of 40% or higher is achieved, this has a sensitivity of 96% and a specificity of 100% for the diagnosis of an adenoma.[11]

Phaeochromocytomas may cause confusion as they may be of sufficiently low attenuation (1.8–42 HU) on non-contrast-enhanced CT to be mistaken for adenomas and show contrast washout profiles similar to adenomas (absolute washout 40–89% and relative washout 16–83%). Phaeochromocytomas, although rare, may present as incidental masses and on CT mimic both adenomas and malignant masses.[12] Therefore, if there is doubt, a phaeochromocytoma should be excluded by clinical and biochemical evaluation.

Histogram Analysis Method

Although contrast enhancement washout criteria have a high sensitivity and specificity for adenomas, the technique is somewhat cumbersome, requiring contrast medium administration and delayed images up to 15 min after contrast enhancement. Unenhanced CT alone, when using a threshold of 10 HU or less, has a 100% specificity but a low sensitivity for adenomas. CT histogram analysis is a technique that has been applied to both non-contrast-enhanced and contrast-enhanced images.[17–21] A region of interest (ROI) cursor is drawn covering at least two-thirds of the adrenal mass,

excluding areas of necrosis. The individual attenuation values of all the pixels in the ROI are plotted against their frequency and the amount of lipid in the mass is proportional to the number of negative pixels (less than 0 HU). The original studies demonstrated 97% of adenomas contain negative pixels. Eighty-five per cent have more than 5% negative pixels and 83% have more than 10% negative pixels. No metastases had negative pixels.[18] The performance of histogram analysis is variable in the literature and subsequent studies have reported negative pixels in non-adenomas including metastases, phaeochromocytomas, and carcinomas.[19,20]

CT histogram analysis on unenhanced images may be a useful adjunct to the CT attenuation values, as the combination of CT attenuation value <10 HU or > 10% negative pixel content would correctly identify 91% of adenomas compared with 66% using CT attenuation values alone (Fig. 20-9).[10,20,21] On enhanced CT, the low sensitivity of histogram analysis precludes clinical usefulness.[20]

Magnetic Resonance Imaging

Conventional Spin-Echo Imaging

On conventional T1 and T2 images, considerable overlap exists between the signal intensities of adenomas and metastases and up to a third of lesions remain indeterminate.[22–24]

Gadolinium-Enhanced Magnetic Resonance Imaging

The accuracy of MRI in differentiating benign from malignant masses can be improved by using intravenous gadolinium injection and T1-weighted sequences. After gadolinium enhancement, 90% of adenomas demonstrate homogeneous or ring enhancement while 60% of malignant masses have heterogeneous enhancement. Adenomas again show early peak enhancement, and the time to reach peak enhancement is the strongest discriminator between adenomas and malignant adrenal masses. The value of peak enhancement has no statistical difference between adenomas and metastases.[25] However, as with signal characteristics alone, there is considerable overlap in enhancement characteristics of benign and malignant masses, limiting its clinical application in distinguishing adenomas from malignant masses.

Chemical Shift Imaging

Chemical shift imaging (CSI) relies on the fact that, within a magnetic field, protons in water molecules oscillate or precess at a slightly different frequency than the protons in lipid molecules. As a result, water and fat protons cycle in and out of phase with respect to one another. By selecting appropriate sequencing parameters, separate images can be acquired with the water and fat protons oscillating in-phase and out-of-phase to each other. The signal intensity of a pixel on in-phase images is derived from the signal of water plus fat protons when water and fat are present in the same pixel. On out-of-phase sequences, the signal intensity is derived from the difference of the signal intensities of water and fat protons. Therefore, adenomas which contain intracellular lipid lose signal intensity on out-of-phase images compared to in-phase images, whereas malignant lesions and phaeochromocytomas, which lack intracellular lipid, remain unchanged.

Simple visual assessment of relative signal intensity loss is accurate in most cases, but quantitative methods may be useful in equivocal cases (Fig. 20-10).

There are several quantitative ways of assessing the degree of loss of signal intensity. Quantitative analysis can be made using adrenal-splenic ratio (ASR) and signal intensity index (SII). MR signal intensity units are arbitrary units and therefore comparison of signal intensity of the adrenal mass to an internal reference provides a more accurate analysis than evaluation of two values from the same organ. A variety of ratios comparing the loss of signal intensity in the adrenal mass with that of the liver, paraspinal muscle or spleen on in-phase and out-of-phase images have been used. Fatty infiltration of the liver (particularly in oncology patients receiving chemotherapy) and iron overload make the liver an unreliable internal standard. Fatty infiltration in mainly elderly patients or due to disuse may also affect skeletal muscle to a lesser extent. To calculate adrenal-lesion-to-spleen ratio (ASR), regions of interest (ROIs) are used to acquire the signal intensity (SI) within the adrenal mass and the spleen from in-phase and out-of-phase images. The ASR reflects the percentage signal drop-off within the adrenal lesion compared with the spleen and it can be calculated thus:

$$ASR = \frac{\text{SI adrenal lesion out-of-phase/}\ \text{SI spleen out-of-phase}}{\text{SI adrenal lesion in-phase/}\ \text{SI spleen in-phase}} \times 100$$

An ASR ratio of 70 or less has been shown to be 100% specific for adenomas but only 78% sensitive (Fig. 20-11).[26]

Signal intensity index uses the same characteristics of the adrenal mass on both in- and out-of-phase imaging and can be calculated thus:

$$SII = \frac{\text{In-phase lesion SI} - \text{Out-of-phase lesion SI}}{\text{In-phase lesion SI}} \times 100$$

Signal intensity indices have been shown to discriminate between adenomas and metastases with an accuracy of 100%.[27] Adenomas characteristically have signal intensity indices greater than 5%, whilst metastases have indices lower than 5% (Fig. 20-12). However subsequent studies have used thresholds of between 1 and 30% in identifying adenomas.[28] This variability can be partly explained by the difference in imaging parameters like T1 weighting, repetition time, and flip angles which affect the quantification of lipid.[29] Individual centres need to determine which threshold to use depending on the imaging parameters employed.

The combination of spin-echo signal characteristics, gadolinium enhancement and chemical shift imaging is currently 85–90% accurate in distinguishing between adenomas and non-adenomas. There are few direct comparisons between CT and MRI. As both unenhanced CT and chemical shift imaging rely upon the same property of adenomas, namely their lipid content, the performance of the techniques correlate. Recent studies indicate that CSI is more sensitive in the detection of intracellular lipid than CT. Whereas on unenhanced CT, up to 30% of adenomas are lipid poor, only 8% demonstrate no loss of signal intensity on CSI. In addition, more lipid-poor adenomas can be distinguished from non-adenomas using signal intensity indices without the use of intravenous contrast media. When CSI was applied to lipid-poor adenomas with non-contrast CT attenuation values between 10 and 30 HU, CSI detected adenomas with a sensitivity of 89%. Therefore in this group of adrenal masses, CSI detects more adenomas than non-contrast-enhanced CT.[30,31]

Further modification of CSI to subtraction CSI entails post processing of the CSI data whereby the out-of-phase images are subtracted from the in-phase images. The subtracted images can be evaluated either quantitatively or qualitatively. Qualitative assessment is visual, with adenomas demonstrating higher signal intensities than metastases on subtracted images. Quantitatively, the mean signal intensity from a region of interest in the subtracted image is obtained. If the cutoff values of the subtracted signal intensities selected are above 106 for adenomas and below 36 for metastases, the reported

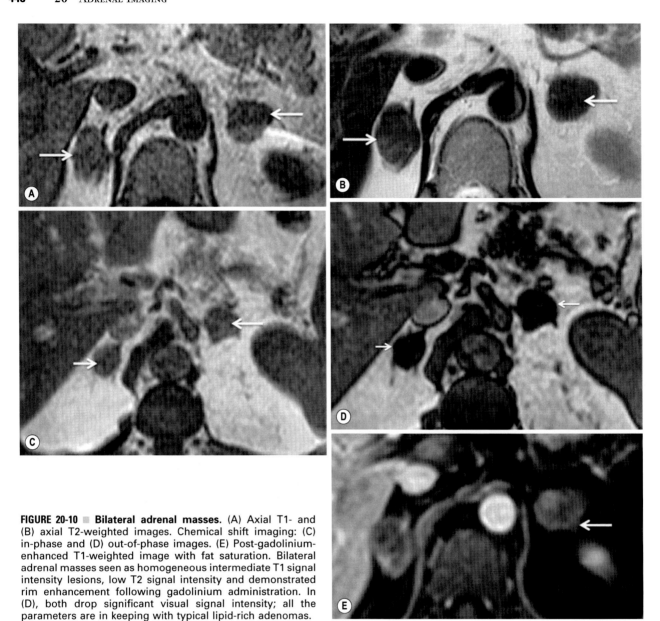

FIGURE 20-10 ■ **Bilateral adrenal masses.** (A) Axial T1- and (B) axial T2-weighted images. Chemical shift imaging: (C) in-phase and (D) out-of-phase images. (E) Post-gadolinium-enhanced T1-weighted image with fat saturation. Bilateral adrenal masses seen as homogeneous intermediate T1 signal intensity lesions, low T2 signal intensity and demonstrated rim enhancement following gadolinium administration. In (D), both drop significant visual signal intensity; all the parameters are in keeping with typical lipid-rich adenomas.

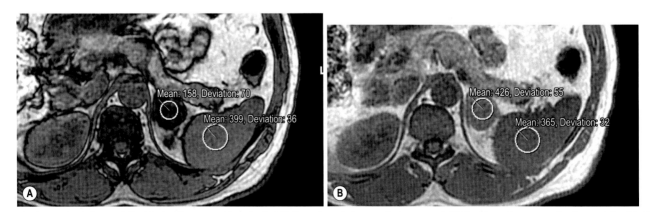

FIGURE 20-11 ■ **A large left-sided adenoma.** Chemical shift imaging: (A) out-of-phase and (B) in-phase images of a large left-sided adenoma seen with visual signal dropout on the out-of-phase images. The signal intensities of the mass and the spleen are obtained using a region of interest. The adrenosplenic ratio of the mass is 33%, confirming an adenoma. The signal intensity index is greater than 50%, in keeping with an adenoma.

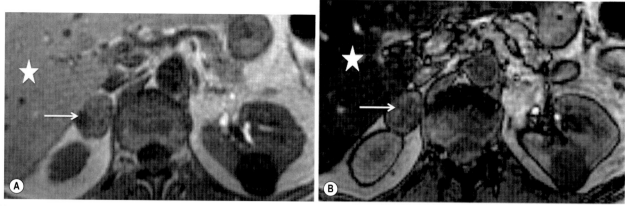

FIGURE 20-12 ■ **Right adrenal mass.** (A) In-phase and (B) out-of-phase images of a right adrenal mass. The imaging was performed in a patient clinically suspected of a phaeochromocytoma. On visual inspection no significant signal dropout is seen in the mass. The signal intensity index was 3%, consistent with a phaeochromocytoma, which was later surgically confirmed.

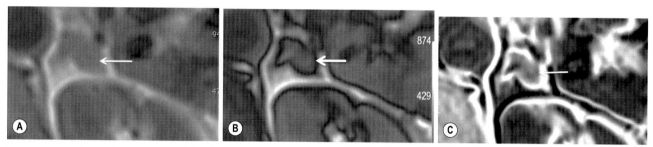

FIGURE 20-13 ■ **Left adrenal mass.** (A) In-phase and (B) out-of-phase images of a left adrenal mass. (C) Subtraction image (in-phase minus out-of-phase). A small left adrenal mass, which does not demonstrate visual drop of signal intensity on the out-of-phase images, is noted. Subtraction of the CSI images shows an increase in high signal in the mass consistent with an adenoma.

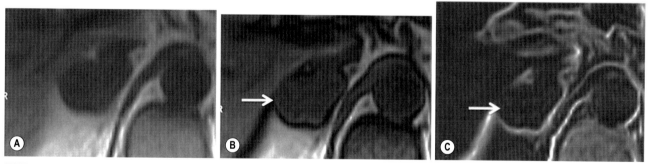

FIGURE 20-14 ■ **Right adrenal mass.** (A) In-phase and (B) out-of-phase images of a right adrenal mass. (C) Subtraction image (in-phase minus out-of-phase). A large right adrenal mass, which does not demonstrate visual drop of signal intensity on the out-of-phase images, is noted. Subtraction of the CSI images shows no increase in signal after subtraction, indicating no signal dropout. Hence, the lesion is a non-adenoma or a lipid-poor adenoma. In this patient the mass was an adrenal metastasis from small cell lung cancer.

accuracy of distinguishing between the two lesions is 100%. One advantage of subtraction MRI is that the technique uses no calculation of ratios or formulas. This technique can be used in equivocal cases to further improve diagnostic CSI accuracy in distinguishing adenomas from non-adenomas (Figs. 20-13 and 20-14).[32]

Positron Emission Tomography

Whole-body positron emission tomography (PET) with [18F]-fluorodeoxyglucose (18F-FDG) improves the characterisation of malignant adrenal lesions. In early studies,

in relation to lung cancer, 18F-FDG PET was shown to be highly accurate in differentiating adrenal benign non-inflammatory lesions from malignant disease. Larger, more recent studies confirm the high sensitivity of PET-CT in detecting malignant lesions but the specificity is lower, ranging between 87 and 97%. This loss of specificity is attributable to a small number of adenomas and other benign lesions that mimic the high metabolic activity of malignant lesions.[33,34]

To distinguish between adenomas and non-adenomas, qualitative visual assessment alone of FDG activity in benign adrenal adenomas is variable, ranging from mild,

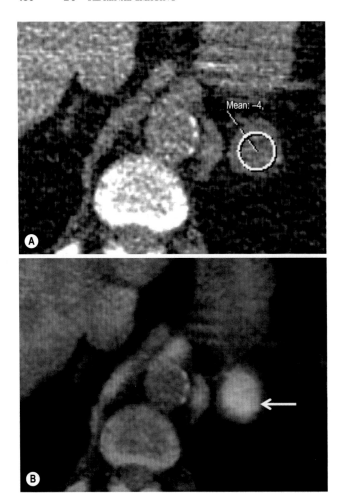

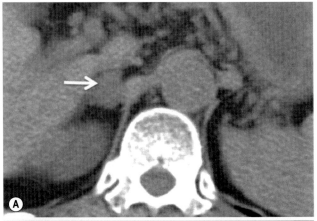

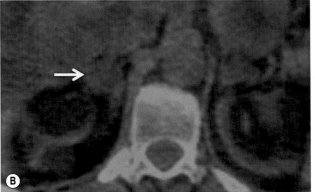

FIGURE 20-16 ■ (A) Unenhanced CT component and (B) fused image from PET-CT component of ¹⁸F-FDG PET-CT. A 2.4-cm right-sided adrenal mass with an attenuation value of 8 HU in keeping with a lipid-rich adenoma. The adenoma typically has FDG uptake less than the liver.

FIGURE 20-15 ■ (A) Unenhanced CT component and (B) fused image from PET-CT component of ¹⁸F-FDG PET-CT. A 2-cm left adrenal mass with a CT attenuation value of –4HU consistent with a lipid-rich adenoma is present. The adenoma demonstrates significant FDG uptake, greater than the background uptake in the liver. The adenoma remained stable over a follow-up period of 3 years.

moderate to high FDG uptake while malignant masses have moderate to high uptake. When compared to FDG uptake in the liver, benign adenomas have been shown to have FDG uptake less than, equal to, or more than the liver in 51, 38 and 10%, respectively. No non-adenomas had activity less than the liver and FDG uptake equal to, or more than the liver in 25 and 75%, respectively. However, as 48% of adenomas demonstrate moderate and high FDG, they mimic malignant masses, thereby limiting the role of ¹⁸F-FDG PET in clinical practice (Figs. 20-15 and 20-16).[35,36]

Quantitative evaluation using standardised uptake values (SUVs) using a cutoff value of 2.68–3.0 separates malignant from benign adrenal masses with a high sensitivity (99%), specificity (92%), positive predictive value (89%), and negative predictive values (99%). When combined FDG PET and CT data, including contrast washout characteristics, are analysed, the sensitivity, specificity, positive predictive value and negative predictive value for malignant adrenal masses improve to 100, 98, 97 and 100%, respectively.[35–37] False-positive lesions

for malignancy encountered at integrated PET-CT include adrenal adenomas, phaeochromocytomas, adrenal endothelial cysts, inflammatory and infectious lesions. False negatives for malignancy have been reported in adrenal metastases with haemorrhage or necrosis, small (5–10 mm) metastatic nodules, and metastases from pulmonary bronchioloalveolar carcinoma or carcinoid tumours (Fig. 20-17).

Although the maximum SUV uptake values for adenomas are lower than metastases, as for qualitative evaluation considerable overlap remains. More sophisticated quantification methods have been proposed looking at the ratio of SUV of the adrenal mass and the liver. Lesions that demonstrate visual uptake and SUV less than the liver have now been confirmed on several studies to be benign lesions with a specificity of 100%. A negative PET may predict a benign tumour that would potentially prevent the need for biopsy or surgery in lesions with inconclusive CT or MR imaging. However, lesions with visual and SUV uptake equal to or greater than the liver still remain problematic as the specificity for malignant disease is between 88 and 94%.[35]

The specificity of PET can be improved with the use of [¹¹C]metomidate (MTO), a marker of 11β-hydroxylase, as a tracer for adrenocortical tissue. With this tracer, phaeochromocytomas, metastases to the adrenal gland, and non-adrenal cortical masses are all

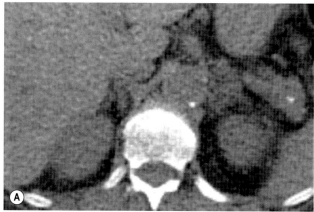

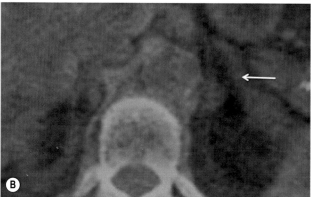

FIGURE 20-17 ■ (A) Unenhanced CT from a PET-CT study obtained as a staging investigation for a 78-year-old woman with biopsy-proven bronchioalveolar carcinoma. A 3-cm left adrenal mass measuring 23 HU is seen. (B) Fused PET-CT image demonstrating low-level uptake only in the left adrenal mass. Following chemotherapy, the pulmonary and adrenal mass reduced significantly in size, thereby proving the adrenal mass was a metastasis.

MTO-uptake negative. However, the tracer has an increased uptake in both adenomas and adrenocortical carcinomas, hence being unable to distinguish between these lesions.[38]

Percutaneous Adrenal Biopsy

The indications for adrenal biopsy have devolved with the availability of new imaging techniques which can characterise adrenal adenomas with high specificity. With improved imaging, only a small percentage of adrenal masses cannot be characterised. The main indication currently is when the mass retains imaging features suggestive of a solitary adrenal metastasis in patients with extra-adrenal primary malignancy, prior to deeming them unresectable. These patients should have a percutaneous biopsy for confirmatory diagnosis. However, prior to percutaneous biopsy the possibility of a phaeochromocytoma must be excluded due to the risk of an adrenal crisis induced by the biopsy. Percutaneous CT-guided adrenal biopsy is a relatively safe procedure in patients with a known extra-adrenal malignancy. Minor complications of adrenal biopsy include abdominal pain, haematuria, nausea and small pneumothoraces. Major complications, generally regarded as those requiring treatment, occur in

2.8–3.6% of cases and include pneumothoraces requiring intervention and haemorrhage, with isolated reports of adrenal abscesses, pancreatitis and seeding of metastases along the needle track.[39]

Adrenal Scintigraphy

Adrenal scintigraphy allows functional characterisation based on uptake and accumulation of radiotracers. Tracers such as iodocholesterol-labelled analogues (^{131}I-6-β-iodomethyl-19-norcholesterol [NP-59] and ^{75}Se-6-β-selenomethyl cholesterol) are markers of adrenal cortical tissue. Tumours of adrenocortical origin including functioning and non-functioning adenomas and adrenocortical carcinomas will show radiocholesterol uptake.

Adrenal medullary scintigraphy requires radioiodinated guanethidine analogues, ^{131}I-MIBG and ^{123}I-MIGB. ^{123}I-MIGB scintigraphy localises phaeochromocytoma as focal increased adrenal uptake. Detailed discussion of the performance of MIBG is under medullary hyperfunction.

INCIDENTALLY DETECTED NON-FUNCTIONING ADRENAL MASSES

Although adrenal adenomas are the most frequently detected non-functioning adrenal mass, other lesions include adrenal cysts, myelolipomas and nodular hyperplasia. Adrenal metastases are rarely detected incidentally but, as discussed previously, form part of a differential diagnosis of an adrenal mass in patients with a known malignancy.

Adrenal Cysts

Benign adrenal cysts are rare, with a range of histological types indistinguishable from each other on imaging. Autopsy series report an incidence of 0.06% and most adrenal cysts are detected incidentally, but, when large, patients may present with flank pain. These cysts can be categorised into 5 subtypes, summarised in Table 20-3.

The lesions demonstrate the expected imaging characteristics of cysts, with fluid attenuation on CT, no enhancement following contrast medium administration, anechois on ultrasound and low T1 and high T2 signal characteristics on MRI (Fig. 20-18). The presence of solid components, thickened walls and septae increase the likelihood of a necrotic mass or infective cyst rather than a benign cyst.

If an incidentally discovered adrenal lesion meets all the radiologic criteria for an uncomplicated benign cyst, a conservative approach is recommended. Large symptomatic adrenal cysts should be surgically excised, but small, asymptomatic, non-functional cysts with benign characteristics may be treated conservatively with regular follow-up by ultrasound or CT and biochemical evaluation. Aspiration of the cysts to confirm benignancy has also been proposed and this has the added benefit of also being therapeutic.[40] Where there is diagnostic uncertainty and the lesion is >4 cm, following ACR guidelines, these lesions should be excised.

TABLE 20-3 **Types of Adrenal Cysts**

Endothelial (Vascular) Cyst with Endothelial Lining	Haemorrhagic Cyst (Pseudocyst)	Parasitic Cyst	Epithelial-Lined (True) Cyst	Lymphangioma
45% of adrenal cysts	39% of adrenal cysts	Usually echinococcal, asymptomatic but serology positive in up to 90%	Rare	Rare (0.06% incidence)
2/3 in females	Usually middle-aged women	Has 2 layers: • The inner, germinal layer is composed of the parasite, which is one-cell thick, produces the laminar membrane and scoleces and secretes the cystic fluid	Mesothelial origin	Thin-walled cyst with smooth lining and flattened endothelial cells
8% bilateral	May be associated with Beckwith–Wiedemann syndrome.	• The outer layer allows the passage of nutrients	Qretention cysts, embryonal cysts or arising within adenomas	
May have residual adrenocortical tissue in wall	Originally an endothelial or lymphangioendothelial cyst with haemorrhage, fibrosis and hemosiderin deposition	Ultrasound classification: • Type 1 are simple cysts with no internal architecture • Type 2 cysts have the 'water lily sign' with seperation of the membrane layers • Type 3 have complex internal septa and floating debris • Types 4 and 5 have increasing solid walls and calcification		
	Enlargement due to haemorrhage and fluid accumulation			

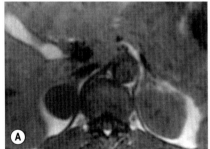 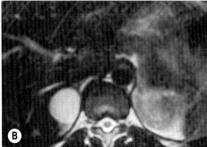 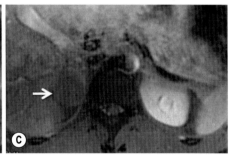

FIGURE 20-18 ■ (A) T1-, (B) T2- and (C) T1-weighted image with fat saturation and gadolinium enhancement of a right-sided simple adrenal cyst demonstrated with uniform low T1 and high T2 signal intensity. No internal architecture or wall thickening is seen. Following gadolinium enhancement, no internal soft tissue or wall enhancement is present. The lesion was asymptomatic and incidental and therefore followed up for 3 years with no progression.

Myelolipoma

Although described as rare (0.1–0.2% of cases), these benign lesions are increasingly detected incidentally on imaging and their true incidence is likely to be higher. Usually the tumour is small (<5 cm), solitary and is composed of haematopoietic precursor cells and mature adipose tissue in varying proportions. Most are hormonally inactive.

The tumour may have areas of fibromyxoid degeneration, haemorrhage, necrosis and calcification.

The appearance of myelolipomas on CT depends on their histologic composition, with some tumours showing only small regions of fatty tissue in a predominantly soft-tissue mass, whilst others are almost completely composed of fat (Figs. 20-19 and 20-20). The masses often have a recognisable capsule and may contain calcification. The soft-tissue component usually enhances after administration of intravenous contrast. If there is haemorrhage within the tumour, high attenuation fluid may be present. The key to CT diagnosis is a focal area of fat in the adrenal mass. In nearly all myelolipomas, some regions with attenuation values less than –30 HU can be identified. This is done most reliably using unenhanced CT. Although an adrenal adenoma may have low-attenuation values due to a large amount of intracellular lipid, this is usually not less than –20 HU.[41]

Similarly, on MRI, the diagnosis is based on the demonstration of fat in the lesion. Fat has high signal intensity on both T1- and T2-weighted images. Hematopoietic

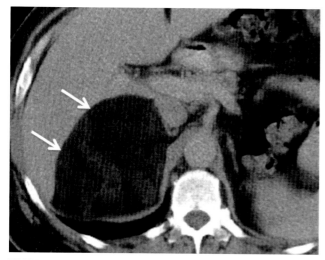

FIGURE 20-19 ■ **Post-contrast-enhanced CT, 90 s following contrast medium administration.** A large predominantly fatty mass is seen in the right adrenal gland. The mass has an attenuation value between –30 and –50 HU, similar to the retroperitoneal fat. The appearances are typical of a fat-rich myelolipoma.

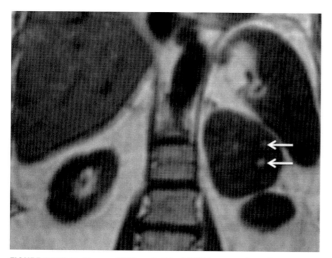

FIGURE 20-20 ■ **Coronal T1-weighted MR image showing a large solid left adrenal mass.** Although predominantly solid, there are small foci of high T1 signal consistent with fat. Surgical resection of the mass confirmed a myelolipomatous mass in association with an adrenocortical carcinoma.

marrow elements have low signal intensity on T1-weighted images and intermediate signal intensity on T2-weighted images. The signal intensity of haemorrhage varies depending on the age of blood. The presence of fat in myelolipomas can be proven on MR sequences that suppresses signal from fat. The most frequently applied sequence is T1-weighted gradient-echo sequence with fat suppression. Areas of fat with high T1 signal intensity lose signal on the fat-saturated sequence (Fig. 20-21). Chemical shift imaging also may demonstrate loss of signal intensity on the opposed phase images in areas of mixed adipose and myeloid tissue. Other sequences including STIR and T2 fat saturation will also show loss of signal within the fat of the tumour.

Myelolipomas are asymptomatic in most cases, although, especially, the large ones can present with abdominal pain or retroperitoneal bleeding. Adrenocortical dysfunction occurs in 10% and may present as Addison's disease, Cushing's disease, hyperandrogenism or hypertension due to catecholamine or aldosterone secretion.

Other adrenal masses containing fat (e.g. lipomas, teratomas and liposarcomas) are extremely rare.

The treatment for myelolipomas, if small and asymptomatic, is conservative and surgical in large and symptomatic lesions.

IMAGING FUNCTIONAL DISORDERS OF THE ADRENAL GLAND

Diseases of adrenal dysfunction are detected clinically and biochemically. The purpose of imaging is to identify the site of the lesion, determine whether lesions are unilateral or bilateral, plan surgical or medical management and to characterise the lesions. There are three major types of adrenal dysfunction;
1. Hyperfunction of the adrenal cortex, including:
   a. Cushing's syndrome
   b. Conn's syndrome
   c. Adrenogenital syndrome
2. Adrenal medullary hyperfunction, including: adrenal medullary hyperplasia and phaeochromocytomas

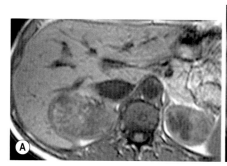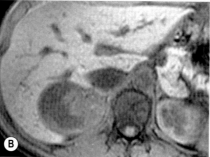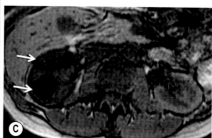

FIGURE 20-21 ■ (A) Axial T1- and (B) axial T1-weighted with fat saturation images, and (C) axial out-of-phase chemical shift image of a large right-sided adrenal mass with multiple foci of high T1 signal intensity present within the mass (arrows). These areas of high T1 signal lose signal on fat saturation sequences, and on out-of-phase chemical shift sequences, confirming the fatty tissue. The lesion was surgically confirmed as a myelolipoma with several pockets of fat.

3. Adrenal hypofunction, including:
   a. Addison's disease due to autoimmune disease, granulomatous diseases (TB, sarcoidosis and histoplasmosis), amyloid, metastases, haemorrhagic necrosis
   b. Secondary adrenocortcal insufficiency due to decreased ACTH levels.

Hyperfunctioning Adrenal Cortical Disorders

Cushing's Syndrome

Cushing's syndrome is made up of symptoms and signs that result from long-term inappropriate elevation of free circulating glucocorticoid levels: the incidence is about 30 per 1,000,000 per annum. Although the outlook of the condition has improved greatly over the years, it remains a physically and psychologically disabling condition, even though the disease is suspected and investigated much earlier now in those who present with diabetes, hypertension, osteoporosis, psychiatric and gynaecological disorders. Imaging has come to play a key and central role in the early diagnosis of these patients.

In 80–85% of cases, Cushing's syndrome is ACTH-dependent usually secondary to a pituitary ACTH secreting tumour (Cushing's disease). Less frequently ACTH secretion is from a non-pituitary source or ectopic secretion (10%). In the remaining 15–20% of patients the syndrome is ACTH-independent due to primary adrenal disease. The treatment of Cushing's syndrome depends on distinguishing between ACTH-dependent and ACTH-independent disease. In ACTH-independent disease, the role of imaging is to identify, localise and characterise adrenal masses. In ACTH-dependent Cushing's disease imaging is important to identify an anterior pituitary adenoma or to identify a source of ectopic ACTH.

ACTH-Independent Cushing's Syndrome. Eighty per cent of ACTH-independent disease is in women. ACTH-independent Cushing's syndrome is always due to autonomous primary adrenal disease producing cortisol. Adrenal adenomas and carcinomas account for 95% of the cases. Rarely primary pigmented nodular adrenal dysplasia (PPNAD) and ACTH-independent macronodular hyperplasia (AIMAH) are responsible. In children carcinomas are more frequent than adenomas, whilst adults have a similar frequency of adenomas and carcinomas.

Biochemically the cortisol levels are high and the ACTH levels are low. There is no suppression of ACTH with high- or low-dose dexamethasone suppression testing.

Adrenal Adenomas. Hyperfunctioning ACTH-secreting adenomas, which account for most of the cases, have similar imaging features to other benign adrenal adenomas. They are usually between 2 and 7 cm in size and 95% of these hyperfunctioning adenomas are lipid-rich. The contralateral adrenal gland is either normal or atrophic due to low circulating ACTH levels (Fig. 20-22).

Rarely, cortisol-producing adenomas may be bilateral or occur simultaneously with PPNAD.[42,43] Heterotopic

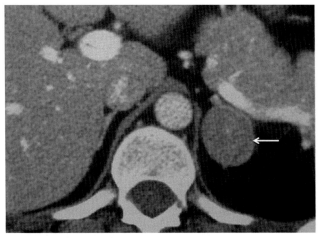

FIGURE 20-22 ■ **Post-contrast-enhanced CT, 60 s following contrast medium administration.** A large left histologically confirmed adrenal adenoma is seen in a patient presenting with ACTH-independent Cushing's syndrome. The contralateral adrenal is small due to the low circulating ACTH levels.

adrenal tissue can be found anywhere along the embryological migration path of the adrenal glands. The adrenal cortex is already prominent in the suprarenal ridges by 7 weeks' gestation. At this time the medullary chromaffin cells migrate to invaginate the adrenal cortex, dividing it into its three layers and central medulla. As the medullary elements migrate into the cortex, multiple primordia or secondary separated fragments of the parent gland may split of, forming accessory adrenal nests. Usually such nests remain close to the original gland but may be dragged along with the genital structures into the pelvis and scrotum. Although in the majority this is normal accessory adrenal tissue, secretory adenomas causing Cushing's syndrome have been reported.[44]

Adrenal Carcinoma. Adrenal carcinomas are rare, with an incidence of approximately 0.6–1.67 cases per 1,000,000 per year. The female-to-male ratio is approximately 2.5–3:1. Male patients tend to be older and have a worse overall prognosis than female patients. Adrenal carcinomas are associated with Li–Fraumeni syndrome, Beckwith–Wiedemann syndrome and congenital adrenal hyperplasia. Fifty per cent are functional and associated with Cushing's syndrome and virilisation. Adrenal carcinoma occurs in two major peaks: in the first decade of life and again in the fourth to fifth decades. Approximately 75% of children with adrenal carcinoma are younger than 5 years. Adrenocortical carcinomas are staged according to the TNM system summarised in Table 20-4. Functioning tumours are more common in women and children with resultant Cushing's syndrome or virilisation, while non-functional tumours are more common in adults. In adults, 30–40% of adrenal carcinomas are hyperfunctioning. Hypercortisolism and virilisation is the most common endocrine manifestation, although trace amounts of other hormones may be produced. Carcinomas account for 27% of ACTH-independent Cushing's syndrome, ranging in size between 6 and 10 cm. These carcinomas are highly necrotic tumours and may cause fever simulating an infectious

TABLE 20-4 **Adrenocortical Carcinoma TNM Staging System from AJCC, 7th Edition**

Primary Tumour (T)	Regional Lymph Nodes (N)	Distant Metastasis (M)
TX: Primary tumour cannot be assessed T0: No evidence of primary tumour T1: Tumour 5 cm or less in greatest dimension, no extra-adrenal invasion T2: Tumour greater than 5 cm, no extra-adrenal invasion T3: Tumour of any size with local invasion, but not invading adjacent organs* T4: Tumour of any size with invasion of adjacent organs*	Note: regional lymph nodes are aortic (para- and peri-aortic) and retroperitoneal NOS NX: Regional lymph nodes cannot be assessed N0: No regional lymph node metastasis N1: Metastasis in regional lymph node(s)	M0: No distant metastasis M1: Distant metastasis

*Adjacent organs are kidney, diaphragm, great vessels, pancreas, spleen and liver.

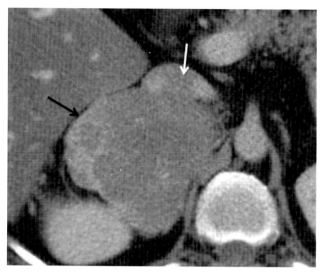

FIGURE 20-23 ■ **Post contrast-enhanced CT, 60 s following contrast medium administration.** A large right heterogeneous, irregular adrenocortical carcinoma with variable enhancement is seen. The carcinoma invades the inferior vena cava and the thrombus can be clearly seen within the lumen of the IVC.

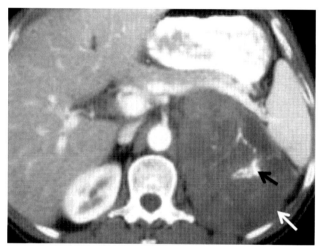

FIGURE 20-24 ■ **Post contrast-enhanced CT, 60 s following contrast medium administration.** A left-sided adrenocortical carcinoma is present, demonstrating the irregular margins anteriorly, speckled calcification, heterogeneous enhancement and large size, characteristic of a carcinoma.

process clinically. Adrenal vein, vena cava, adjacent kidney, retroperitoneal invasion is frequently present at the time of presentation (Fig. 20-23). However, increasingly, these carcinomas are detected early and venous invasion may not be present. The commonest sites of metastatic disease are the liver (60%), regional lymph nodes (40%), lungs (40%) and rarely peritoneal and pleural surfaces, bone and skin (anaplastic tumours).[45]

Large adenomas can be indistinguishable from carcinomas on imaging. CT typically shows a unilateral mass, usually > 6 cm in size with necrosis, haemorrhage, fibrosis and calcification (Fig. 20-24). However, recent studies combining unenhanced, delayed enhancement CT attenuation and percentage of contrast enhancement washout attenuation values at 10 min for adrenal carcinomas were all in the range for non-adenomas. Using these criteria, adenomas were distinguished from adrenal carcinomas and phaeochromocytomas with a sensitivity and specificity of 100%.[46,47] Multiplanar imaging using MDCT and MRI allows better assessment of invasion into adjacent

structures, important for surgical planning. A large mass, high suspicion of malignancy and surrounding invasion preclude laproscopic adrenalectomy, which may be suitable for benign adenomas. Currently the only true definitive criteria for diagnosing malignancy are the presence of distant metastasis or local invasion on imaging or surgical specimen.

Primary Pigmented Nodular Adrenocortical Disease (PPNAD). This is a rare cause of Cushing's syndrome in infants, children and young adults. The disease may be familial and frequently associated with the Carney complex (spotty skin pigmentation, endocrine hyperfunction, testicular tumours and cardiac myxomas). Sporadic and non-familial patients are usually infants or young adults <30 years of age.

On imaging, adrenal glands in PPNAD may be normal or minimally hyperplastic with multiple, benign cortical nodules. Secondary to pigmentation, the nodules demonstrate lower T1 and T2 signal intensity on MRI compared to surrounding atrophic cortical tissue. The nodules do not normally exceed 5 mm but in older patients may be 1–3 cm[48] (Fig. 20-25). Histologically, there are

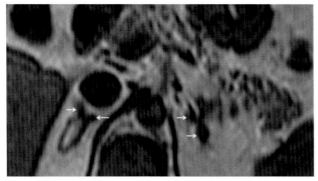

FIGURE 20-25 ■ **A 20-year-old female patient with Cushing's syndrome.** Axial T1-weighted image of the adrenals demonstrating multiple small bilateral low T1 signal intensity nodules shown by the arrows ('black adenomas'). These are also of low signal intensity on T2-weighted images and pigmented on histology.

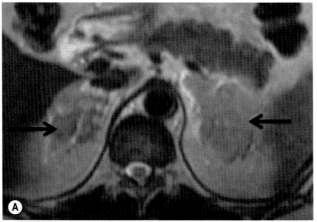

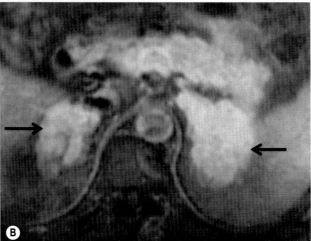

FIGURE 20-26 ■ **A 27-year-old woman presented with new ACTH-independent Cushing's syndrome.** (A) Axial T2- and (B) axial T1-weighted image with fat saturation and gadolinium enhancement of both adrenal glands which demonstrate massive enlargement with numerous nodules. The appearances of the adrenal glands in the context of ACTH independence are consistent with adult idiopathic massive adrenal hyperplasia.

multiple brown-black pigmented cortical nodules in both adrenal glands and atrophy of the intervening cortex due to low circulating ACTH levels. In the absence of gradients on petrosal venous sampling and normal cross-sectional imaging, a presumptive diagnosis of PPNAD may be confirmed by bilateral uptake of ^{131}I-cholesterol scintigraphy. The adrenal uptake of ^{131}I-cholesterol analogues confirms an adrenal source of cortisol excess as opposed to ectopic adrenal rests.[49] Occasionally in older patients where nodules are 1–2 cm in size, atrophy of intervening cortex helps distinguish this from ACTH-dependent hyperplasia.

ACTH-Independent Macronodular Adrenal Hyperplasia (AIMAH). ACTH-independent macronodular adrenal hyperplasia is a very rare cause of Cushing's syndrome. There is a bimodal age distribution, with the first peak in newborns (associated with McCune–Albright syndrome) and the second peak in adults >40 years. Clinically the patients, usually male, present about 10 years older than the mean age of presentation for Cushing's syndrome and the clinical manifestations of the syndrome tend to be mild. The pathophysiology of AIMAH remains obscure. The imaging appearances of the adrenal glands are striking. They show massive bilateral adrenal enlargement, nodularity and distortion of adrenal contour. Nodules vary in size from 1 to 5.5 cm and on CT are of low attenuation in keeping with their high lipid content. Coronal imaging, either with MDCT reconstruction or MR imaging, best demonstrate the craniocaudal extent of the adrenal glands, which frequently extend from the diaphragm to below the renal hila (Fig. 20-26).[50] On MRI, nodules are hypointense relative to the liver on T1-weighted images and hyperintense or isointense to liver on T2-weighted images. In ACTH-dependent Cushing's syndrome, nodules are isointense to liver on T2 images, while in PPNAD nodules are hypointense on both T1- and T2-weighted images. On chemical shift imaging, nodules, due to their high lipid content, lose signal intensity on out-of-phase images.

ACTH-Dependent Cushing's Syndrome. ACTH-dependent Cushing's syndrome is secondary to increased ACTH production either by a pituitary adenoma (Cushing's disease) or an ectopic source. Having confirmed a biochemical diagnosis, it is imperative to locate the source of ACTH production. Clinically and biochemically it may be difficult to distinguish between a pituitary or occult (covert) ectopic ACTH-secreting tumour. Chronic hyperstimulation of the adrenal glands can result in bilateral enlargement. Adrenals usually exhibit nodular or diffuse hyperplasia affecting the entire adrenal cortex. The largest glands, usually lobular and nodular, result from an ectopic rather than pituitary source. Two types of hyperplasia are seen pathologically and on imaging: smooth (diffuse) or nodular. Smooth hyperplasia, on histology, is more common and in 30% of cases the adrenal glands appear normal on imaging (Fig. 20-27). A normal MRI or CT therefore does not exclude the diagnosis. Nodular hyperplasia can be micro- or macronodular. In macronodular hyperplasia there is bilateral enlargement of adrenal glands with one or more nodules. The presence of a dominant unilateral nodule, reaching up to 4 cm, may be misinterpreted as a hyperfunctioning

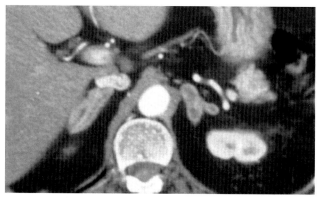

FIGURE 20-27 ■ **Post-contrast-enhanced CT, 60 s following contrast medium administration.** A 19-year-old woman with a known Cushing's disease secondary to a small pituitary adenoma. Both adrenal glands demonstrate smooth enlargement due to the excess ACTH levels. Note the adrenal glands are not as large as when stimulated by ectopic ACTH production.

adenoma, conflicting with biochemical evidence of ACTH dependence.[51,52] The remainder of the glands are enlarged and nodular, aiding the imaging diagnosis of bilateral ACTH-dependent hyperplasia rather than a functional adrenal adenoma (Fig. 20-28).

Rarely, Cushing's syndrome may be due to ectopic production of ACTH from a malignant tumour. In such cases, hypercortisolism is associated with increased levels of ACTH-like peptide; however, no pituitary lesions are found. Ectopic ACTH-like substances may be secreted by small cell carcinomas of the lung and thymus, medullary carcinoma of the thyroid, pancreatic neuroendocrine neoplasms, phaeochromocytomas and some benign ovarian tumours. In children phaeochromocytomas, neuroblastoma, thymic or pancreatic endocrine neoplasms are usually the cause of ectopic ACTH secretion.

The lungs are the commonest organs harbouring an ectopic ACTH source (48%), with the majority of cases being bronchial carcinoid tumours (30%) followed by small cell lung cancer (SCLC) (18%) (Fig. 20-28). In approximately 12–20% of patients, despite repeated biochemical and radiological investigations, the source of the ectopic ACTH production may not be identified.[53]

Contrast-enhanced CT of the chest, abdomen and pelvis is the most sensitive investigation for the identification of the ectopic source, detecting liver and nodal metastases. Bronchial carcinoids are small, typically between 3 and 15 mm in size, and may be difficult to distinguish from granulomas and hamartomas. ACTH-producing SCLC and neuroendocrine tumours of the pancreas and colon have radiological features similar to non-ACTH-producing tumours. Thus in patients suspected of ectopic ACTH production, all small intrapulmonary lesions should be viewed with suspicion. In the abdomen, MRI may identify small islet cell tumours of the pancreas not seen on CT.[54] Overall, two large studies have found ^{111}In-octreotide scintigraphy and whole-body venous sampling generally unhelpful in localising the source of ectopic ACTH. [^{18}F]-fluorodeoxyglucose positron emission tomography (FDG PET) has been recently evaluated and shown to be inferior to CT and MRI in

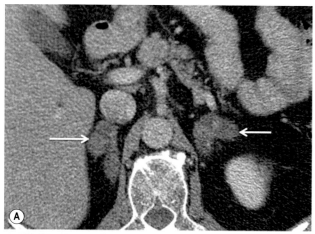
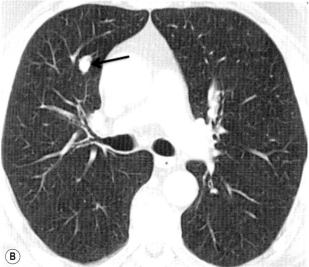

FIGURE 20-28 ■ (A) Post-contrast-enhanced CT, 60 s following contrast medium administration. (B) CT of the chest with lung reconstruction. There is large bilateral macronodular enlargement of the adrenal glands in a patient presenting with ACTH-dependent Cushing's syndrome. The marked enlargement raises the suspicion on imaging of ectopic ACTH production. In this patient a small right-sided pulmonary nodule is seen. Resection of the nodule confirmed an ACTH-secreting small cell carcinoma of the lung.

the detection of ectopic ACTH sources. The hyperstimulated, hyperplastic adrenal glands also obscure the detection of any ACTH-secreting adrenal lesion.[55,56]

Primary Hyperaldosteronism (Conn's Syndrome)

Primary hyperaldosteronism is due to excess production of aldosterone either by a unilateral adrenocortical adenoma (aldosteronoma) or bilateral adrenal cortical hyperplasia (BAH). Rarely an adrenocortical carcinoma may cause mixed secretion of glucocorticoids and mineralocorticoids resulting in both Cushing's and Conn's syndrome. Patients with Conn's syndrome present with early and severe hypertension and biochemical alkalosis, hypokalemia and hypernatraemia. The distinction between an aldosteronoma and bilateral adrenal hyperplasia is crucial as the management of the two causes

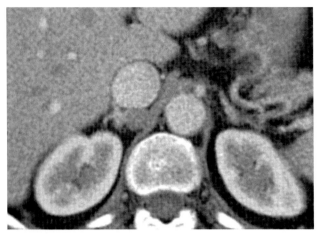

FIGURE 20-29 ■ Post-contrast-enhanced CT 60 s after contrast medium administration in a patient presenting with biochemical Conn's disease. A typical small right aldosteronoma is present with the remainder of the ipsilateral adrenal cortex showing normal appearances.

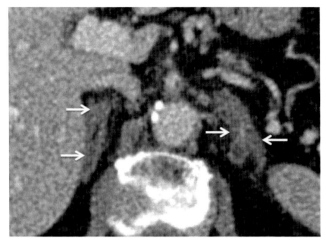

FIGURE 20-30 ■ Post-contrast-enhanced CT 60 s after contrast medium administration. Both adrenal glands are enlarged and the limb thickness bilaterally measures greater than 5 mm.

differs entirely. Surgical resection is the primary treatment for aldosteronoma and carcinomas, but medical treatment with spironolactone and antihypertensives is the treatment of choice for adrenal hyperplasia. CT and MRI are used to differentiate between the two causes after clinical and biochemical confirmation of Conn's syndrome. Aldosterone-producing adenomas (APAs) are of low attenuation on CT, less than 10 HU, usually small, rarely calcify and demonstrate no significant contrast enhancement. The mean size of aldosteronomas is 1.6–2.2 cm, median size of 2 cm and range between 1 and 5 cm.[57] The small size of aldosteronomas makes their detection challenging. Several studies have examined the performance of thin-section CT (3 mm) in the detection of APAs, with sensitivities and specificities varying between 88 and 100% and 33 and 100%, respectively.[57–59] In favour of BAH is enlargement of the adrenal limbs compared to patients with APA or healthy control subjects. On CT if the adrenal limb width is 3 mm or greater, sensitivity for diagnosing BAH is 100% but the specificity is only 54%. The specificity is improved to 100% if the limb width is 5 mm or greater (Figs. 20-29 and 20-30).[59]

In the detection of APA, MRI has a sensitivity, specificity and accuracy of 70, 100 and 85%, respectively. As much as 86% of adenomas and 89% of glands with BAH have intracellular lipid, thereby demonstrating loss of signal intensity on CSI.[57] CT and MRI have a comparative performance in the detection of APAs, with a sensitivity and specificity of 87–93% and 82–85% for CT and 83 and 92% for MRI, respectively.[58] There are several reasons for the poor specificity in the detection of APA, including concomitant contralateral non-functioning nodules masking the small functional adenoma, the presence of unilateral dominant nodules in BAH simulating an APA and the increasing bilateral nodularity with age and hypertension. The sensitivity is limited by the small size of APAs, although this should improve with the increasing use of thinner adrenal sections (1–2 mm)

acquired by multidetector CT. In the overall management of Conn's syndrome a high specificity for the detection of APAs is desirable to avert unsuccessful surgery in patients with BAH.

Adrenal venous sampling (AVS) for aldosterone levels is very accurate in preoperative assessment of Conn's syndrome. It is the most accurate method for distinguishing between unilateral and bilateral aldosterone production. Although now generally safe, it is technically difficult and even with modern techniques and per-procedural ACTH stimulation, bilateral adrenal vein catherisation may only be successful in 44–50% of patients.[60] Catherisation of the right adrenal vein, in particular, remains elusive. The accuracy of AVS in lateralising an APA exceeds 95% when the procedure is technically successful.[61] As AVS is not without risks, it is used selectively and reserved for patients with:

• normal or equivocal adrenal glands on CT;
• presence of bilateral adrenal nodules, which may be either macronodules of adrenal hyperplasia or multiple adenomas; and
• there is disagreement between CT and MRI findings or between imaging and biochemical findings.

AVS is essential in the above patients to avoid unnecessary and inappropriate adrenalectomy.

Virilisation

Virilisation is the development of exaggerated masculine characteristics, usually in women, which may be as a result of the adrenal cortex overproducing androgens. The most common adrenal cause is congenital adrenal hyperplasia (CAH) in both male and female children, adrenal androgen-producing adenomas and adrenocortical carcinomas in adults. In boys, virilisation may signal precocious puberty as part of CAH.

The role of imaging lies in detection of surgically resectable sources of androgen excess in the adrenals, ovaries or testes. In young patients MRI or ultrasound avoid ionising radiation from CT. Adrenal and pelvic

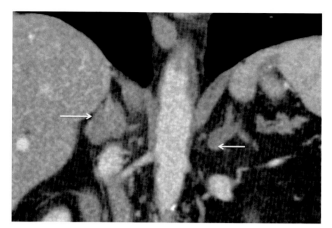

FIGURE 20-31 ■ Post-contrast-enhanced CT 60 s after contrast enhancement, coronal reconstruction. Both adrenal glands are markedly enlarged in CAH with preservation of adreniform shape.

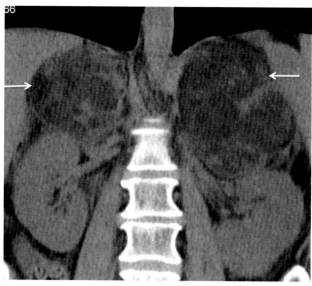

FIGURE 20-32 ■ Post-contrast-enhanced CT 60 s after contrast enhancement, coronal reconstruction. A patient with known CAH and long-term steroid replacement. Both adrenal glands are hugely enlarged and demonstrate lipomatous replacement, a described change in this group of patients.

venous catherisation is reserved for patients in whom uncertainty remains to the presence of small ovarian tumours which cannot be excluded biochemically or on transvaginal ultrasound.[62]

Congenital Adrenal Hyperplasia (CAH). Congenital adrenal hyperplasia refers to several autosomal recessive diseases resulting from defects in steroidogenesis of cortisol from cholesterol by the adrenal cortex. Most of these conditions result in excessive or deficient production of sex steroids, altering the development of primary or secondary sexual characteristics in affected infants, children, and adults. 21-Hydroxylase deficiency accounts for about 95% of CAH. Severe 21-hydroxylase deficiency causes salt-wasting CAH and is life-threatening in the first weeks of life. It is also the most common cause of ambiguous genitalia due to prenatal virilisation of genetically female infants. Moderate 21-hydroxylase deficiency is referred to as simple virilising CAH and typically causes virilisation of prepubertal children. Still milder forms of 21-hydroxylase deficiency are referred to as non-classical CAH and can cause androgen effects and infertility in adolescent and adult women.[63]

In CAH there is a combination of precocious puberty and an androgen excess due to an increase in circulating ACTH with chronic adrenal hyperstimulation. This results in gross enlargement of the adrenal glands seen on CT and MRI as diffuse or nodular adenomatoid enlargement of both adrenal glands with preservation of normal adreniform configuration (Fig. 20-31).[64] Adrenocortical adenomas have been reported in children with long-standing untreated or undertreated CAH.[65] These adenomas are thought to be ACTH-dependent and most regress after adequate steroid replacement. However, not all such adenomas regress and they may even increase in size with lipomatous replacement despite adequate treatment (Fig. 20-32).

Adrenal Virilising Tumours. These are most commonly carcinomas and rarely adenomas. In children 80% of carcinomas present with virilisation. In contrast, only

20–30% of adults with adrenal carcinoma present with virilisation.[66] They usually exceed 2 cm in diameter and have the same imaging characteristics for adenomas and carcinomas.

Hyperfunctioning Adrenal Medullary Disorders

Medullary tumours can be broadly classified into sympathetic system tumours (neuroblastoma, ganglioneuroblastoma, ganglioneuroma) or adult neuroendocrine tumours (phaeochromocytoma).

Phaeochromocytomas

Phaeochromocytomas, the commonest tumours of the adrenal medulla, are paragangliomas arising from neural crest cells. Adrenal phaeochromocytomas constitute 90% of all paragangliomas. Ten per cent of adrenal phaeochromocytomas are multiple, 10% are malignant with the incidence increasing in tumours larger than 6 cm, 10% are associated with neuroectodermal syndromes (neurofibromatosis, tuberosclerosis, von Hippel–Lindau disease, multiple neuroendocrine neoplasia types 11a and 11b) and 10% are non-functioning tumours. Functioning phaeochromocytomas mainly secrete catecholamines—adrenaline and nor-adrenaline. The tumours may also secrete dopamine, parathyroid hormones, calcitonin, gastrin, serotonin and ACTH with or without the catecholamines. Symptomatic patients present with paroxysmal hypertension, headaches, visual blurring, sweating and vasomotor changes caused by the transient elevation in catecholamines. The diagnosis of a phaeochromocytoma is made clinically and biochemically by detection of elevated plasma and urinary levels of catecholamines or

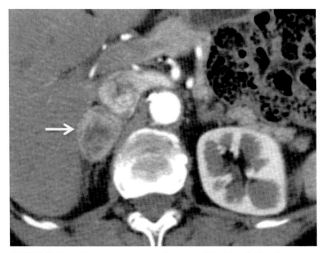

FIGURE 20-33 ■ **Post-contrast-enhanced CT, 60 s following contrast medium administration.** A typical sporadic right-sided phaeochromocytoma is present. This is >3 cm in size, demonstrating heterogeneous avid enhancement with central areas of necrosis.

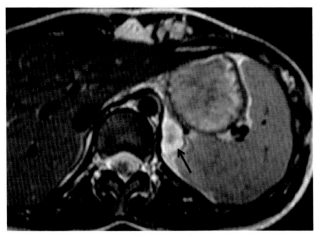

FIGURE 20-34 ■ **Axial T2-weighted image of a 25-year-old male patient, known to have succinate dehydrogenase deficiency (SDHD).** A small homogeneous high T2 signal left adrenal mass is detected on a screening MRI (arrow). The very high T2 signal intensity is consistent with a phaeochromocytoma in association with SDHD.

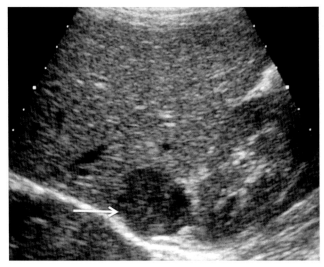

FIGURE 20-35 ■ **Longitudinal ultrasound image of the right suprarenal area in a 14-year-old female presenting with virilisation.** A smooth hypoechoeic mass is present in the adrenal bed separate from the upper pole of the right kidney. The mass is homogeneous and has smooth contours. The mass was resected and confirmed as a functional adenoma secreting androgens.

their metabolites, vanillylmandelic acid (VMA) and metanephrine.

Once a clinical and biochemical diagnosis of phaeochromocytoma has been made, imaging studies are performed to localise the tumour and to aid surgical planning for resection. Sporadic adrenal phaeochromocytomas are usually large at time of diagnosis (90% larger than 2 cm) and readily detected on imaging. Phaeochromocytomas occuring in association with neuroectodermal syndromes (MEN, VHL, neurofibromatosis) are smaller at the time of detection, as these patients are actively screened, usually by MRI (Figs. 20-33 and 20-34).

On ultrasound, phaeochromocytomas are well-defined, ovoid or round suprarenal masses (Fig. 20-35). They frequently have an inhomogeneous internal architecture due to haemorrhage and necrosis. Ultrasound has a lower sensitivity for the detection of phaeochromocytomas than CT or MR imaging as smaller lesions particularly on the left may be obscured by bowel gas.

On unenhanced CT, the tumours have a soft-tissue density and speckled calcification is present in up to 12% of tumours.[67] Phaeochromocytomas characteristically demonstrate intense contrast enhancement (Fig. 20-33). The internal architecture of the tumours is variable, depending on the degree of central necrosis. In tumours with a large amount of central necrosis, the tumour may appear cystic. Even in these tumours a peripheral rim of intensely enhancing soft tissue can still be demonstrated (Fig. 20-36). To perform contrast-enhanced CT, non-ionic contrast has been shown to be safe for patients with phaeochromocytomas without the use of α-adrenergic blockade.[68] Contrast-enhanced CT is highly accurate in the detection of adrenal phaeochromocytomas, with the reported sensitivities between 93 and 100% and a positive predictive value exceeding 90%.[69]

On MR imaging, most phaeochromocytomas are iso- or hypointense to the liver on spin-echo (SE) T1-weighted imaging. High T1-weighted signal intensity corresponding to areas of haemorrhage has been reported in up to 20% of phaeochromocytomas. On spin-echo T2-weighted images the typical phaeochromocytoma has a very high signal intensity. Larger tumours tend to be inhomogeneous, containing cystic central necrosis, calcification or haemorrhage. These typical appearances are not demonstrated by up to 35% of adrenal phaeochromocytomas,[70] which demonstrate only moderately high T2 signal intensity (Fig. 20-37). On chemical shift imaging typical phaeochromocytomas do not show signal intensity loss on opposed-phase images. The typical appearances of phaeochromocytomas overlap with necrotic adrenal metastasis. Intravenous gadolinium is rarely useful as both phaeochromocytomas and adrenal metastasis enhance markedly after injection.

Meta-iodobenzylguanidine (MIBG) is a noradrenaline analogue taken up by the chromaffin cells in paragangliomas including phaeochromocytomas. MIBG is most commonly labelled with iodine-123 (for diagnosis) or I-131 (for treatment) for whole-body scintigraphy in the detection and localisation of primary and metastatic paragangliomas. The sensitivity of MIBG is reported between 87 and 90%, lower than that for both CT and MRI, as the detection of lesions depends on ability of the tumour to take up the tracer. However, the strength of MIBG is its high specificity, which exceeds 90%.[71]

Patients with a phaeochromocytoma may have more than one tumour in the adrenal glands or in an ectopic location. The commonest sites of extra-adrenal paragangliomas are the para-aortic region at the level of the renal hila (46%), at the organ of Zuckerkandl (29%), thoracic paraspinal region (10%), bladder (10%) and head and neck (2–4%). In the head and neck 80% are carotid body or glomus vagale tumours. Owing to the superior MR tissue contrast and tissue characterisation, the sensitivity of MR imaging has been shown to be equivalent or better than CT in the demonstration of extra-adrenal paragangliomas. In addition to tissue characterisation, MR is useful in problem areas such as spinal cord, bladder wall, intracardiac tumours and those adjacent to the IVC, internal jugular vein and carotid arteries. MR shows excellent natural contrast on T2-weighted images between the hyperintense paraganglioma and the hypointense flowing blood (Fig. 20-38).[72]

The choice of initial imaging in a patient suspected of having a phaeochromocytoma depends on the institutional availability of CT, MR imaging and MIBG. Unlike CT and MR imaging, MIBG examines the whole body with the advantage of simultaneously detecting extra-adrenal locations of tracer uptake in metastasis or extra-adrenal paragangliomas. CT and MR imaging have similar sensitivity and specificity. They have the advantage of concurrently detecting associated tumours (pancreatic tumours, renal cell carcinoma, neurofibromata, thyroid carcinoma, extra-adrenal paragangliomas) in patients with neuroendocrine syndromes. The multiplanar ability or MRI and MDCT imaging are very useful in the surgical planning for resection of phaeochromocytomas and extra-adrenal paragangliomas.

PET CT has also been evaluated in localising phaeochromocytomas, when cross-sectional imaging and MIBG are negative but a phaeochromocytoma is biochemically suspected. Different PET tracers have been used, including [11C]-hydroxyephedrine, [11C]-epinephrine, 6-[18F]-fluorodopamine or [18F]-fluorodihydroxyphenylalanine. The most reliable has been shown to be 6-[18F]-fluorodopamine, which can localise adrenal and extra-adrenal lesions, including metastatic lesions. FDG PET displays a relatively low sensitivity (70%) and therefore is not recommended for the initial diagnostic evaluation. Nonetheless, it can be useful for a metastatic lesion.

Despite encouraging data, the cost and availability of PET, particularly 6-[18F]-fluorodopamine, limits its application to specialised centres only.

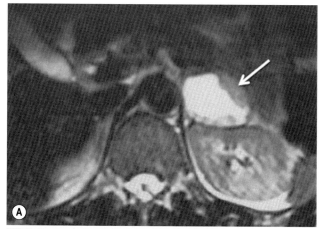
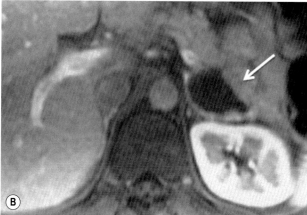

FIGURE 20-36 ■ A 38-year-old male presented with uncontrolled hypertension and palpitations and biochemical profile suggesting a phaeochromocytoma. MRI of the abdomen demonstrated a cystic mass in the left adrenal gland. (A) Axial T2- and (B) axial T1-weighted image with fat saturation and gadolinium enhancement. The mass has a thick enhancing wall (arrows), thereby excluding a simple cyst. In view of the high suspicion of a phaeochromocytoma, the mass was resected and histologically confirmed as a necrotic phaeochromocytoma.

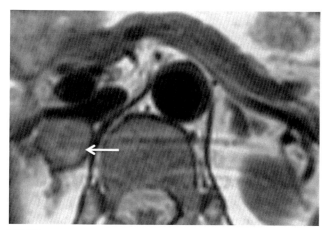

FIGURE 20-37 ■ Axial T2-weighted image of a proven right phaeochromocytoma. In the newer MRI imaging and with the increasing use of gradient T2-weighted images, the T2 signal intensity of the phaeochromocytoma may not appear as high as on turbo spin-echo images. However, the signal is as high as the CSF T2 signal intensity.

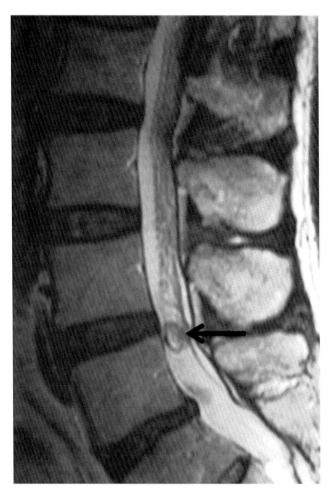

FIGURE 20-38 ■ **Sagittal T2-weighted image of the lumbar spine.** A 35-year-old woman presented with biochemical evidence of a phaeochromocytoma but with no detected lesion on CT of the chest, abdomen and pelvis. ^{123}I-MIBG was also negative. As the patient had vague symptoms of back pain, an MRI of the lumbar spine was performed. This revealed a small hypervascular lesion, confirmed as an extra-adrenal phaeochromocytoma.

Adrenal Medullary Hyperplasia (AMH)

The normal adrenal gland weighs approximately 5 g, with the medulla accounting for 1 g of its weight. The adrenal medulla is only found in the body of the gland. The diagnosis of medullary hyperplasia is made pathologically when the medulla extends into the adrenal limbs and there is an increase in the medullary/cortical ratio within the body. The adrenal medulla shows a two-to-three-fold increase in medullary volume and weight compared to age- and sex-matched controls.[73] It is associated with cystic fibrosis, non-familial Beckwith–Wiedemann syndrome, MEN 2a or 2b and familial medullary thyroid carcinoma. Adrenal medullary hyperplasia is a rare cause of clinical and biochemical findings, mimicking phaeochromocytomas. On MR imaging, adrenal glands may be normal and demonstrate unilateral or bilateral involvement with diffuse or nodular disease. The bodies of the adrenal glands are most frequently enlarged, with relative preservation of the limbs (Fig. 20-39). In patients with clinical and biochemical evidence of raised catecholamines, absence of a focal mass on imaging and increased adrenal MIBG uptake should raise the suspicion of adrenal medullary hyperplasia, especially in the setting of an associated syndrome. The management of AMH is surgical. In unilateral disease, adrenalectomy is performed. In patients with bilateral disease or asynchronous recurrence of AMH in the contralateral adrenal, cortical-sparing surgery or resection of the largest gland has been proposed to preserve adrenal cortical function. Long-term follow-up indicates patients thus treated retain normal clinical and biochemical function for up to 20 years.[74,75]

Neuroblastoma and Ganglioneuroblastoma

Neuroblastomas and ganglioneuroblastomas are primitive tumours derived from neuroblastic and mature ganglion cells distributed along the sympathetic nervous

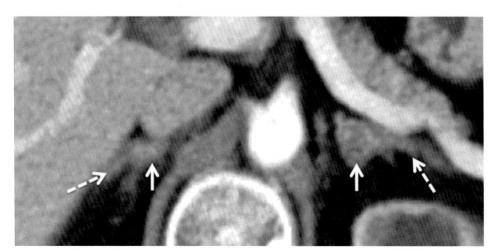

FIGURE 20-39 ■ **Post-contrast-enhanced CT, 60 s following contrast medium administration.** Bilateral adrenal medullary hyperplasia with enlargement of both adrenal bodies (arrows). The adrenal limbs are relatively spared (dashed arrows), as there is little or no medullary tissue in the normal adrenal limbs.

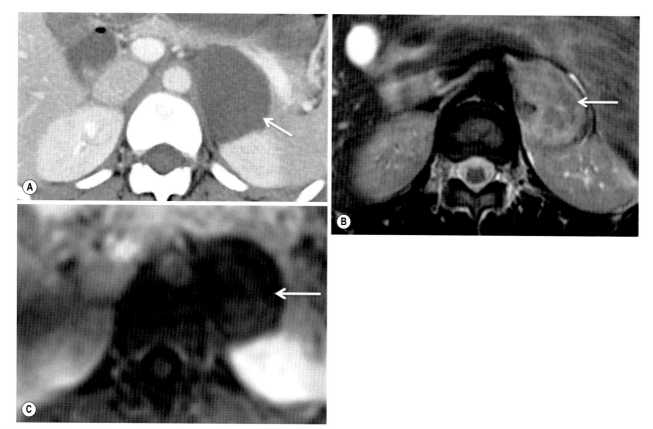

FIGURE 20-40 ■ **A 17-year-old female patient was investigated for vague abdominal pain and a left adrenal mass was noted.** (A) Contrast-enhanced CT 60 s after contrast medium administration, (B) axial T2-weighted and (C) axial T1-weighted image with fat saturation and gadolinium enhancement. The mass measured 18 HU post-contrast and therefore was originally thought to be an adrenal cyst. An MRI was performed and T2 and post-gadolinium images demonstrate a complex solid internal architecture and low-level enhancement of the soft tissues. The well-defined nature of the solid mass raises the probability of a benign neurogenic tumour and histology confirmed a benign ganglioneuroma of the adrenal gland.

system. There is a continuum of aggressive tumours from neuroblastoma (most immature and aggressive) to ganglioneuroblastoma to ganglioneuroma (most mature and low malignant potential) (Fig. 20-40). Both neuroblastomas and ganglioneuroblastomas produce abnormally high catecholamine precursors that are detected by measurement of urinary catecholamine metabolites, vanillylmandelic acid (VMA) and homovanillic acid (HVA). Whereas phaeochromocytomas secrete adrenaline, neuroblastomas and ganglioneuroblastomas secrete noradrenaline and gastrointestinal hormones, particularly, vasoactive intestinal peptide (VIP). Neuroblastoma and ganglioneuroblastoma occur most frequently in infants and children. It is the most common extracranial, solid malignant tumour of childhood, accounting for 8% of childhood malignancies, with 50–80% arising in adrenal glands; 60% of patients have metastases in cortical bone, bone marrow, lymph nodes, liver and rarely to lung or brain. On gross examination, ganglioneuroblastomas have variable amounts of calcification and their appearance depends upon degree of differentiation and primitive elements. Neuroblastomas are aggressive tumours; the majority are irregularly shaped, lobulated and unencapsulated. They invade adjacent organs or encase adjacent vessels, and tend to be inhomogeneous owing to tumour necrosis and haemorrhage. They

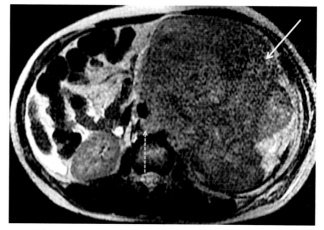

FIGURE 20-41 ■ **Axial T2-weighted image.** A very large mass is present in the left adrenal gland, filling the entire retroperitoneum. The mass extends posterior to and lifts the aorta and IVC anteriorly. This is a characteristic feature of neuroblastomas.

contain coarse, amorphous, mottled peripheral calcification in approximately 85% of cases (Fig. 20-41).

Assessment of disease status requires multiple imaging investigations. Plain radiography can identify lytic lesions. Ultrasound usually detects the characteristically large suprarenal mass and liver involvement.[76] MRI and CT features of neuroblastoma are a large mass, with calcification, often extending across the midline to engulf and displace the aorta anteriorly. Heterogeneous contrast enhancement is usual. Imaging is useful for defining morphological features, precisely assessing tumour extent for planning biopsies and surgical resection and helps determine tumour extension to retroperitoneal lymph nodes and liver, around central vessels, and into the vertebral canal. Liver metastases may take one of two forms: diffuse infiltration, or focal hypoenhancing masses. MRI has become the investigation of choice for staging due to its multiplanar capabilities, lack of ionising radiation and good contrast between the very high signal tumour and surrounding tissues on T2-weighted images. MRI is the preferred investigation for assessing intraspinal extension of primary tumour (the so-called dumbbell tumours, seen in 10% of abdominal, 28% of thoracic and occasionally in cervical neuroblastomas) and for detection of diffuse hepatic metastases; these metastases manifest as areas of high signal intensity on T2-weighted images. Recent studies show MRI has the highest staging sensitivity (86%), MIBG the highest specificity (85%) and combined integrated imaging improves both sensitivity (99%) and specificity (95%).[76,77]

Adrenal Hypofunction (Addison's Disease)

Primary Adrenal Hypofunction

Adrenal hypofunction affects about 1 in 100,000 people. This can result either from primary adrenal insufficiency or may be secondary to hypothalamic–pituitary ACTH deficiency. In primary adrenal hypofunction there is a reduction in aldosterone, whilst in ACTH deficiency this remains unaffected as aldosterone production is controlled by the renin–angiotensin pathway rather than ACTH. The acquired causes of primary adrenal hypofunction include autoimmune disease, infection (tuberculosis (TB), AIDS, cytomegalovirus, histoplasmosis), drugs, adrenal haemorrhage, Waterhouse–Friderichsen syndrome, metastatic disease, sarcoidosis, amyloidosis and haemochromatosis. The prevalence of primary adrenal insufficiency has increased threefold in the general population since the 1970s.[78] Autoimmune disease is the most common cause in the Western countries, accounting for 68–94% of primary adrenocortical failure. Worldwide, TB of the adrenal glands remains the commonest cause of adrenal insufficiency. Congenital or hereditary causes of primary adrenal insufficiency include congenital adrenal hyperplasia, X-linked adrenoleukodystrophy, congenital familial glucocorticoid deficiency and triple A syndrome. X-linked adrenoleukodystrophy is the most frequent genetic cause of primary adrenal insufficiency, accounting for up to 20% of male cases.[79] The causes of adrenal hypofunction are summarised in Table 20-5.

The clinical symptoms and signs of Addison's disease manifest when more than 90% of the adrenal cortex is destroyed. Addison's disease may be acute, subacute or chronic. Acute disease is rare and usually results from acute bilateral adrenal haemorrhage. Chronic Addison's

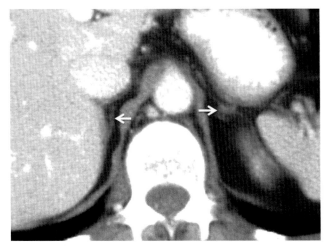

FIGURE 20-42 ■ **Contrast-enhanced CT 60 s after contrast medium administration.** Both adrenal glands are very small, irregular and difficult to detect. The appearances are typical for autoimmune adrenal atrophy.

disease is most commonly due to autoimmune adrenal atrophy. On imaging, autoimmune adrenal disease results in often barely discernible atrophic non-calcified adrenal glands (Fig. 20-42).

Bilateral adrenal haemorrhage may result from anticoagulant use or other bleeding diathesis and in the context of septicaemia in Waterhouse–Friderichsen syndrome. The commonest pathogens in Waterhouse–Friderichsen syndrome are meningococcus, *Haemophilus influenzae*, *Pseudomonas aeruginosa*, *Escherichia coli* and *Streptococcus pneumoniae*. Non-traumatic acute adrenal haematomas characteristically appear as well-defined round or oval areas within the adrenal glands. On MRI, in the acute stage (less than 7 days), haematomas typically appear as iso- or hypointense masses on T1-weighted images and markedly hypointense on T2-weighted images. Subacute haematomas (7 days–7 weeks) are hyperintense on both T1- and T2-weighted imaging. Chronic haematomas (>7 weeks) have a hypointense rim on T1- and T2-weighted imaging (Fig. 20-43). Over time, adrenal haematomas decrease in size, and may calcify or organise, appearing as adrenal cysts which may contain areas of calcification.

In patients without discernible risk factors with unilateral or bilateral non-traumatic adrenal haemorrhage, careful imaging is essential for excluding an underlying adrenal mass. Underlying mass lesions including phaeochromocytomas, lymphoma and metastases from bronchogenic carcinoma and melanoma may cause bilateral adrenal haemorrhage and an acute Addisonian crisis. Contrast-enhanced MRI is of value in distinguishing between an uncomplicated haemorrhage where non-enhancing blood products are the sole component and haemorrhage within an underlying mass lesion which demonstrates contrast enhancement.[80]

Adrenal hypofunction present for less than 2 years is defined as subacute Addison's disease and is usually a result of adrenalitis. Imaging plays an important role in evaluating these cases. Typically in untreated adrenalitis

TABLE 20-5 **Causes of Adrenal Hypofunction**

	Causes	Clinical	Imaging Appearances
Primary insufficiency Addison's disease	a. Rapid withdrawal of exogenous steroids or failure to increase steroids with acute stress		a. Normal or small adrenals
Often insidious in onset, patients may present in shock due to acute stress No symptoms until 90% of cortex is compromised	b. Hypotension/shock that causes mild or massive corticomedullary haemorrhagic necrosis, including Waterhouse–Friderichsen syndrome	b. More common in children <2 years. Usually bilateral, more commonly in right adrenal. Usually due to bacteraemia, *Neisseria, Pseudomonas,* pneumococci, staphylococcus. Less common causes are burns, cardiac failure, hypothermia, birth trauma	b. Adrenals are enlarged and haemorrhagic with extensive necrosis
	c. Infections that destroy substantial adrenal cortical tissue. No symptoms until almost complete cortical destruction has occurred	c. HIV and HIV-related infections, e.g. CMV, cryptococcus, histoplasmosis, herpes simplex/varicella zoster, TB and *Mycobacterium avium-intracellulare*	c. Enlarged glands with necrosis and granulomatous inflammatory enhancement. Chronic disease may show small calcified glands
	d. Amyloidosis e. Drugs, radiation f. Autoimmune disorders: also called idiopathic primary adrenal insufficiency (autoimmune adrenalitis or polyglandular autoimmune syndromes)	e. Metapyrone, Mitotane f. 70–90% of adrenal insufficiency, usually white women ages 20–50, sporadic or familial. Up to 75% have autoantibodies against adrenal cortical zones; antibodies appear months to years before onset of adrenal insufficiency	f. Irregular very small glands, may be hard to find
Secondary insufficiency	Caused by any disorder of pituitary gland which decreases ACTH production and causes adrenal cortical atrophy		Small or normal glands
Tertiary insufficiency	Caused by any disorder of the hypothalamus, respectively, which decreases ACTH production and causes adrenal cortical atrophy		Small or normal glands

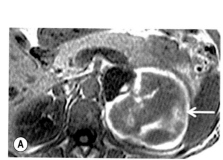 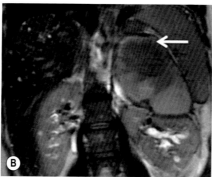 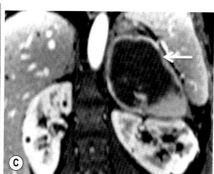

FIGURE 20-43 ■ (A) Axial T1-, (B) coronal T2- and (C) coronal T1-weighted image with fat saturation and gadolinium enhancement of a sporadic large left adrenal haemorrhage in a 43-year-old man. There is a high T1 signal intensity rim, low T2 signal intensity foci within the lesion, and no internal contrast enhancement. The lack of internal architecture and enhancement excludes an underlying lesion.

the adrenal glands are enlarged and may demonstrate central necrosis and rim enhancement. These features are not typical of any one pathogen and adrenal biopsy may be required to distinguish between the causes of adrenalitis which include TB, histoplasmosis and other fungal infections. In acute adrenal TB, bilateral adrenal enlargement is seen in 91% of cases. This can be mass-like and calcification is seen in up to 59%. Peripheral rim enhancement is seen in 47% of patients (Fig. 20-44). After successful treatment, 88% of enlarged glands decrease or return to normal size and configuration. Calcification in atrophic adrenal glands is most often seen in

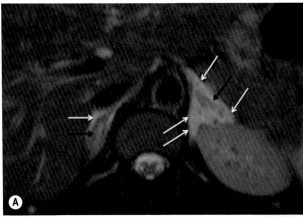

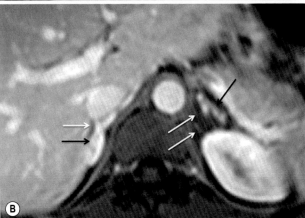

FIGURE 20-44 ■ **A patient presents with abnormal adrenal glands and with acute pulmonary cytomegalovirus infection in the context of HIV.** (A) Axial T2-weighted image with fat saturation and (B) axial T1-weighted image with fat saturation and gadolinium enhancement. There is marked oedema, seen as high T2 signal intensity (white arrows) surrounding the adrenal parenchyma (black arrows). Following contrast medium administration the adrenal parenchyma enhances but no enhancement of the surrounding oedema is seen. A presumptive diagnosis of CMV adrenalitis was made and the patient treated accordingly. Following 6 weeks of treatment, the adrenal glands returned to normal (not shown).

granulomatous diseases (TB, histoplasmosis and sarcoidosis). However, calcification in adrenal glands is not pathognomonic for granulomatous adrenalitis and is indistinguishable from calcification due to previous haemorrhage.[81]

Secondary Adrenal Hypofunction

Secondary adrenal insufficiency is much more common than primary adrenal insufficiency. In secondary adrenal insufficiency, the pituitary gland no longer triggers the adrenals to produce cortisol, and DHEA production also declines. Causes of pituitary hypofunction include tumours or infections of the pituitary, pituitary infarction and radiation or surgery for the treatment of pituitary or hypothalamic tumours. Hypopituitarism due to any cause results in ACTH and cortisol deficiency but not aldosterone deficiency.

Exogenous steroid administration by any route can also result in ACTH deficiency and the patient is at risk

of Addisonian crisis if the steroids are stopped abruptly. Imaging of the hypothalamic–pituitary axis excludes pituitary apoplexy in acute onset of secondary adrenal failure and granulomatous diseases, macroadenomas and metastases in insidious secondary adrenal failure. The low circulating levels of ACTH result in normal or small adrenal glands on MRI.

CONCLUSION

Adrenal imaging has become increasingly important with the emeregence of incidental adrenal masses. Imaging is also an essential adjunct to clinical and biochemical findings in the evaluation and management of adrenal dysfunction. CT remains the mainstay of adrenal imaging but MRI is increasingly used to detect and characterise adrenal masses, especially in patients unable to undergo CT, in children and in patients being screened for adrenal tumours. The majority of adrenal lesions have characteristic imaging features. However, in a small number of masses, there is an overlap in the imaging features of benign and malignant masses. Emerging technologies such as PET-CT add to the radiologists armentarium to distinguishing between benign and malignant masses. Close collaboration is required between the endocrinologists and radiologist to obtain the correct diagnosis and to select the most appropriate imaging strategy.

REFERENCES

1. Glazer HS, Weyman PJ, Sagel SS, et al. Non-functioning adrenal masses: incidental discovery on computed tomography. Am J Roentgenol 1982;139:81–5.
2. Bovio S, Cataldi A, Reimondo G, et al. Prevalence of adrenal incidentaloma in a contemporary computerized tomography series. J Endocrinol Invest 2006;29:298–302.
3. Song JH, Chaudhry FS, Mayo-Smith WW. The incidental adrenal mass on CT: prevalence of adrenal disease in 1,049 consecutive adrenal masses in patients with no known malignancy. Am J Roentgenol 2008;190:1163–8.
4. Libe R, Bertherat J. Molecular genetics of adrenocortical tumours, from familial to sporadic diseases. Eur J Endocrinol 2005;153: 477–87.
5. Oliver TW Jr, Bernardino ME, Miller JI, et al. Isolated adrenal masses in non small-cell bronchogenic carcinoma. Radiology 1984;153:217–18.
6. Frilling A, Tecklenborg K, Weber F, et al. Importance of adrenal incidentaloma in patients with a history of malignancy. Surgery 2004;136:1289–96.
7. Lee MJ, Hahn PF, Papanicolaou N, et al. Benign and malignant adrenal masses: CT distinction with attenuation coefficients, size, and observer analysis. Radiology 1991;179:415–8.
8. Francis IR, Casalino DD, Arellano RS, et al. ACR Appropriateness Criteria. Incidentally Discovered Adrenal Mass. <http://gm.acr.org/SecondaryMainMenuCategories/quality_safety/app_criteria/pdf/ExpertPanelonUrologicImaging/IncidentallyDiscoveredAdrenalMassDoc7.aspx> 2009. Accessed 20 February 2012.
9. Boland GW, Lee MJ, Gazelle GS, et al. Characterization of adrenal masses using unenhanced CT: an analysis of the CT literature. Am J Roentgenol 1998;171:201–4.
10. Korobkin M, Brodeur FJ, Yutzy GG, et al. Differentiation of adrenal adenomas from nonadenomas using CT attenuation values. Am J Roentgenol 1996;166:531–6.
11. Pena CS, Boland GW, Hahn PF, et al. Characterization of indeterminate (lipid-poor) adrenal masses: use of washout characteristics at contrast-enhanced CT. Radiology 2000;217:798–802.
12. Blake MA, Krishnamoorthy SK, Boland GW, et al. Low-density pheochromocytoma on CT: a mimicker of adrenal adenoma. Am J Roentgenol 2003;181(6):1663–8.

13. Szolar DH, Kammerhuber FH. Adrenal adenomas and nonadenomas: assessment of washout at delayed contrast-enhanced CT. Radiology 1998;207:369–75.

14. Blake MA, Kalra MK, Sweeney AT, et al. Distinguishing benign from malignant adrenal masses: multi-detector row CT protocol with 10-minute delay. Radiology 2006;238:578–85.

15. Caoili EM, Korobkin M, Francis IR, et al. Adrenal masses: characterization with combined unenhanced and delayed enhanced CT. Radiology 2002;222:629–33.

16. Korobkin M, Brodeur FJ, Francis IR, et al. CT time-attenuation washout curves of adrenal adenomas and nonadenomas. Am J Roentgenol 1998;170(3):747–52.

17. Bae KT, Fuangtharnthip P, Prasad SR, et al. Adrenal masses: CT characterization with histogram analysis method. Radiology 2003;228:735–42.

18. Remer EM, Motta-Ramirez GA, Shepardson LB, et al. CT histogram analysis in pathologically proven adrenal masses. Am J Roentgenol 2006;187:191–6.

19. Jhaveri KS, Wong F, Ghai S, Haider MA. Comparison of CT histogram analysis and chemical shift MRI in the characterization of indeterminate adrenal nodules. Am J Roentgenol 2006;187:1303–8.

20. Halefoglu AM, Bas N, Yasar A, Basak M. Differentiation of adrenal adenomas from nonadenomas using CT histogram analysis method: A prospective study. Eur J Radiol 2010;73(3):643–51.

21. Ho LM, Paulson EK, Brady MJ, et al. Lipid-poor adenomas on unenhanced CT: does histogram analysis increase sensitivity compared with a mean attenuation threshold? Am J Roentgenol 2008;191:234–8.

22. Reinig JW, Doppman JL, Dwyer AJ, et al. Adrenal masses differentiated by MR. Radiology 1986;158:81–4.

23. Chang A, Glazer HS, Lee JK, et al. Adrenal gland: MR imaging. Radiology 1987;163:123–8.

24. Glazer GM, Woolsey EJ, Borrello J, et al. Adrenal tissue characterization using MR imaging. Radiology 1986;158:73–9.

25. Inan N, Arslan A, Akansel G, et al. Dynamic contrast enhanced MRI in the differential diagnosis of adrenal adenomas and malignant adrenal masses. Eur J Radiol 2008;65:154–62.

26. Mayo-Smith WW, Lee MJ, McNicholas MM, et al. Characterization of adrenal masses by use of chemical shift MR imaging: observer performance versus quantitative measures. Am J Roentgenol 1995;165:91–5.

27. Tsushima Y, Ishizaka H, Matsumoto M. Adrenal masses: differentiation with chemical shift, fast low-angle shot MR imaging. Radiology 1993;186:705.

28. Korobkin M, Giordano TJ, Brodeur FJ, et al. Adrenal adenomas: relationship between histologic lipid and CT and MR findings. Radiology 1996;200:743–7.

29. Al-Hawary MM, Francis IR, Korobkin M. Non-invasive evaluation of the incidentally detected indeterminate adrenal mass. Best Pract Res Clin Endocrinol Metab 2005;19:277–92.

30. Israel GM, Korobkin M, Wang C, et al. Comparison of unenhanced CT and chemical shift MRI in evaluating lipid-rich adrenal adenomas. Am J Roentgenol 2004;183:215–19.

31. Haider MA, Ghai S, Jhaveri K, Lockwood G. Chemical shift MR imaging of hyperattenuating (410 HU) adrenal masses: does it still have a role? Radiology 2004;231:711–16.

32. Savci G, Yazici Z, Sahin N, et al. Value of chemical shift subtraction MRI in characterization of adrenal masses. Am J Roentgenol 2006;186:130–5.

33. Erasmus JJ, McAdams HP, Patz EF Jr. Non-small cell lung cancer: FDG-PET imaging. J Thorac Imaging 1999;14:247–56.

34. Boland GW, Blake MA, Holalkere NS, Hahn PF. PET/CT for the characterization of adrenal masses in patients with cancer: qualitative versus quantitative accuracy in 150 consecutive patients. Am J Roentgenol 2009;192:956–62.

35. Caoili EM, Korobkin M, Brown RK, et al. Differentiating adrenal adenomas from nonadenomas using (18)F-FDG PET/CT quantitative and qualitative evaluation. Acad Radiol 2007;14:468–75.

36. Chong S, Lee KS, Kim HY, et al. Integrated PET-CT for the characterization of adrenal gland lesions in cancer patients: diagnostic efficacy and interpretation pitfalls. Radiographics 2006;26:1811–24.

37. Blake MA, Slattery JM, Kalra MK, et al. Adrenal lesions: characterization with fused PET/CT image in patients with proved or suspected malignancy—initial experience. Radiology 2006;238:9707.

38. Hennings J, Lindhe O, Bergstrom M, et al. [11C]metomidate positron emission tomography of adrenocortical tumours in correlation with histopathological findings. J Clin Endocrinol Metab 2006;91:1410–4.

39. Harisinghani MG, Maher MM, Hahn PF, et al. Predictive value of benign percutaneous adrenal biopsies in oncology patients. Clin Radiol 2002;57:898–901.

40. Tung GA, Pfister RL, Papanicolaou N, et al. Adrenal cysts: imaging and percutaneous aspiration. Radiology 1989;173:107–10.

41. Miyake H, Maeda H, Tashimo M, et al. CT of adrenal tumors: frequency and clinical significance of low-attenuation lesions. Am J Roentgenol 1989;152:1005–7.

42. Nomura K, Saito H, Aiba M, et al. Cushing's syndrome due to bilateral adrenocortical adenomas with unique histological features. Endocr J 2003;50(2):155–62.

43. Tung SC, Wang PW, Huang TL, et al. Bilateral adrenocortical adenomas causing ACTH-independent Cushing's syndrome at different periods: a case report and discussion of corticosteroid replacement therapy following bilateral adrenalectomy. J Endocrinol Invest 2004;27(4):375–9.

44. Ayala AR, Basaria S, Udelsman R, et al. Corticotropin-independent Cushing's syndrome caused by an ectopic adrenal adenoma. J Clin Endocrinol Metab 2000;85(8):2903–6.

45. Stojadinovic A, Ghossein RA, Hoos A, et al. Adrenocortical carcinoma: clinical, morphologic and molecular characterization. J Clin Oncol 2002;20:941–50.

46. Szolar DH, Korobkin M, Reittner P, et al. Adrenocortical carcinomas and adrenal pheochromocytomas: mass and enhancement loss evaluation at delayed contrast-enhanced CT. Radiology 2005;234(2):479–85.

47. Slattery JM, Blake MA, Kalra MK, et al. Adrenocortical carcinoma: contrast washout characteristics on CT. Am J Roentgenol 2006;187(1):W21–4.

48. Doppman JL, Travis WD, Nieman L, et al. Cushing syndrome due to primary pigmented nodular adrenocortical disease: findings at CT and MR imaging. Radiology 1989;172(2):415–20.

49. Rockall AG, Babar SA, Sohaib SA, et al. CT and MR imaging of the adrenal glands in ACTH-independent Cushing syndrome. Radiographics 2004;24(2):435–52.

50. Doppman JL, Chrousos GP, Papanicolaou DA, et al. Adrenocorticotropin-independent macronodular adrenal hyperplasia: an uncommon cause of primary adrenal hypercortisolism. Radiology 2000;216(3):797–802.

51. Isidori AM, Kaltsas GA, Pozza C, et al. The ectopic adrenocorticotropin syndrome: clinical features, diagnosis, management, and long-term follow-up. J Clin Endocrinol Metab 2006;91(2):371–7.

52. Sohaib SA, Hanson JA, Newell-Price JD, et al. CT appearance of the adrenal glands in adrenocorticotrophic hormone-dependent Cushing's syndrome. Am J Roentgenol 1999;172(4):997–1002.

53. Ilias I, Torpy DJ, Pacak K, et al. Cushing's syndrome due to ectopic corticotropin secretion: twenty years' experience at the National Institutes of Health. J Clin Endocrinol Metab 2005;90(8):4955–62.

54. Vincent JM, Trainer PJ, Reznek RH, et al. The radiological investigation of occult ectopic ACTH-dependent Cushing's syndrome. Clin Radiol 1993;48(1):11–17.

55. Pacak K, Ilias I, Chen CC, et al. The role of [(18)F]fluorodeoxyglucose positron emission tomography and [(111)In]-diethylenetriaminepentaacetate-D-Phe-pentetreotide scintigraphy in the localization of ectopic adrenocorticotropin-secreting tumors causing Cushing's syndrome. J Clin Endocrinol Metab 2004;89(5):2214–21.

56. Tsagarakis S, Christoforaki M, Giannopoulou H, et al. A reappraisal of the utility of somatostatin receptor scintigraphy in patients with ectopic adrenocorticotropin Cushing's syndrome. J Clin Endocrinol Metab 2003;88:4754–8.

57. Sohaib SA, Peppercorn PD, Allan C, et al. Primary hyperaldosteronism (Conn syndrome): MR imaging findings. Radiology 2000;214:527–31.

58. Lingam RK, Sohaib SA, Rockall AG, et al. Diagnostic performance of CT versus MR in detecting aldosterone-producing adenoma in primary hyperaldosteronism (Conn's syndrome). Eur Radiol 2004;14:1787–92.

59. Geisinger MA, Zelch MG, Bravo EL, et al. Primary hyperaldos-teronism: comparison of CT, adrenal venography, and venous sam-pling. Am J Roentgenol 1983;141:299–302.

60. Lau JH, Sze WC, Reznek RH, et al. A prospective evaluation of postural stimulation testing, computed tomography and adrenal vein sampling in the differential diagnosis of primary aldosteronism. Clin Endocrinol (Oxf) 2012;76(2):182–8.

61. Young WF, Stanson AW, Thompson GB, et al. Role for adrenal venous sampling in primary aldosteronism. Surgery 2004;136:1227–35.

62. Kaltsas GA, Mukherjee JJ, Kola B, et al. Is ovarian and adrenal venous catheterization and sampling helpful in the investigation of hyperandrogenic women? Clin Endocrinol (Oxf) 2003;59(1):34–43.

63. Bonfig W, Bittmann I, Bechtold S, et al. Virilising adrenocortical tumours in children. Eur J Pediatr 2003;162(9):623–8.

64. Harinarayana CV, Renu G, Ammini AC, et al. Computed tomog-raphy in untreated congenital adrenal hyperplasia. Pediatr Radiol 1991;21(2):103–5.

65. Bhatia V, Shukla R, Mishra SK, Gupta RK. Adrenal tumor com-plicating untreated 21-hydroxylase deficiency in a 5 1/2-year-old boy. Am J Dis Child 1993;147(12):1321–3.

66. Allolio B, Fassnacht M. Clinical review: Adrenocortical carcinoma: clinical update. J Clin Endocrinol Metab 2006;91(6):2027–37.

67. Dunnick NR, Korobkin M, Francis I. Adrenal radiology: distin-guishing benign from malignant adrenal masses. Am J Roentgenol 1996;1667:861–7.

68. Muckerjee JJ, Peppercorn PD, Reznek RH, et al. Phaeochromocy-toma: effect of non-ionic contrast media in CT on circulating catecholamine levels. Radiology 1997;202:227–31.

69. Quint LE, Gazer GM, Francis IR, et al. Phaeochromocytomas and paraganglioma: comparison of MR imaging with CT and 131-I MIBG scintigraphy. Radiology 1987;165:89–93.

70. Jacques AET, Sahdev A, Sandrasagara M, et al. Adrenal phaeochro-mocytoma: correlation of MRI appearances with histology and function. Eur Radiol 2008;18:2885–92.

71. Bhatia KS, Ismail MM, Sahdev A, et al. ^{123}I-metaiodobenzylguanidine (MIBG) scintigraphy for the detection of adrenal and extra-adrenal phaeochromocytomas: CT and MRI correlation. Clin Endocrinol 2008;69:181–8.

72. Sahdev A, Sohaib A, Monson JP, et al. CT and MR imaging of unusual locations of extra-adrenal paragangliomas. Eur Radiol 2005;15:85–92.

73. Lack EE. Tumours of the Adrenal Gland and Extra-adrenal Para-ganglia. Third series edn. Washington, DC: Armed Forces Insti-tute of Pathology; 1997.

74. Yung BC, Loke TK, Tse TW, et al. Sporadic bilateral adrenal medullary hyperplasia: apparent false positive MIBG scan and expected MRI findings. Eur J Radiol 2000;36(1):28–31.

75. Jansson S, Khorram-Manesh A, Nilsson O, et al. Treatment of bilateral pheochromocytoma and adrenal medullary hyperplasia. Ann N Y Acad Sci 2006;1073:429–35.

76. Kushner BH. Neuroblastoma: a disease requiring a multitude of imaging studies. J Nucl Med 2004;45(7):1172–88.

77. Pfluger T, Schmied C, Porn U, et al. Integrated imaging using MRI and ^{123}I metaiodobenzylguanidine scintigraphy to improve sensitiv-ity and specificity in the diagnosis of pediatric neuroblastoma. Am J Roentgenol 2003;181(4):1115–24.

78. Lovas K, Husebye ES. High prevalence and increasing incidence of Addison's disease in western Norway. Clin Endocrinol (Oxf) 2002;56(6):787–91.

79. Falorni A, Laureti S, De Bellis A, et al. SIE Addison Study Group. Italian addison network study: update of diagnostic criteria for the etiological classification of primary adrenal insufficiency. J Clin Endocrinol Metab 2004;89(4):1598–604.

80. Kawashima A, Sandler CM, Ernst RD, et al. Imaging of nontrau-matic hemorrhage of the adrenal gland. Radiographics 1999;19(4):949–63.

81. Yang ZG, Guo YK, Li Y, et al. Differentiation between tuberculosis and primary tumors in the adrenal gland: evaluation with contrast-enhanced CT. Eur Radiol 2006;16(9):2031–6.

SUBJECT INDEX

Page numbers followed by 'f' indicate figures, 't' indicate tables, and 'b' indicate boxes.

Notes

To simplify the index, the main terms of imaging techniques (e.g. computed tomography, magnetic resonance imaging etc.) are concerned only with the technology and general applications. Users are advised to look for specific anatomical features and diseases/disorders for individual imaging techniques used.

vs. indicates a comparison or differential diagnosis.

To save space in the index, the following abbreviations have been used:

CHD—congenital heart disease
CMR—cardiac magnetic resonance
CT—computed tomography
CXR—chest X-ray
DECT—dual-energy computed tomography
DWI-MRI—diffusion weighted imaging-magnetic resonance imaging
ERCP—endoscopic retrograde cholangiopancreatography
EUS—endoscopic ultrasound
FDG-PET—fluorodeoxyglucose positron emission tomography
HRCT—high-resolution computed tomography
MDCT—multidetector computed tomography
MRA—magnetic resonance angiography
MRCP—magnetic resonance cholangiopancreatography
MRI—magnetic resonance imaging
MRS—magnetic resonance spectroscopy
PET—positron emission tomography
PTC—percutaneous transhepatic cholangiography
SPECT—single photon emission computed tomography
US—ultrasound

A

AAST (American Association for the Surgery of Trauma), 427, 427*t*
Abdomen imaging, plain radiograph *see* Plain abdominal radiograph
Abdominal bowel wall pattern *see* Gastrointestinal system
Abdominal imaging
  CT
    radiation concerns, 15–16
Abnormal gas distribution *see* Gastrointestinal system
Abscesses
  kidney/renal *see* Renal abscesses
  liver, 151–152, 151*f*–152*f*

perirenal *see* Perirenal abscesses
peritoneum, 122
prostate gland, 276, 277*f*
Acalculous cholecystitis *see* Cholecystitis
Accessory spleen, 181, 182*f*
Accessory unilateral renal arteries, 282
Achalasia, 32–33, 33*f*
ACKD (acquired cystic kidney disease), 260
Acquired cystic kidney disease (ACKD), 260
ACTH *see* Adrenalocorticotropic hormone (ACTH)
ACTH-dependent Cushing's syndrome *see* Cushing's syndrome
ACTH-independent Cushing's syndrome *see* Cushing's syndrome
ACTH-independent macronodular adrenal hyperplasia (AIMAH), 454
  Cushing's syndrome, 456, 456*f*
Actinomycosis
  small intestine, 82
Acute acalculous cholecystitis, 201
Acute appendicitis, 12, 13*t*
Acute bacterial cholangitis, 211
Acute bacterial prostatitis, 276, 277*f*
Acute calculous cholecystitis *see* Cholecystitis
Acute cholecystitis, 15
Acute diverticulitis, 15
Acute epididymitis, 377*f*, 380, 380*f*–381*f*
Acute focal pyelonephritis, 309
Acute fulminant colitis, 109–110, 110*f*
Acute mesenteric ischaemia (AMI), 84–85
  MDCT, 84
Acute necrotic collections (ANC), acute pancreatitis, 227–228
  drainage, 247–249, 248*f*
Acute pancreatitis, 123, 124*f*, 224–231
  acute necrotic collections *see* Acute necrotic collections (ANC), acute pancreatitis
  causes, 224, 224*f*
  CT, 225–226
    contrast-enhanced CT, 224–225
    severity index, 225, 225*t*
  diagnosis, 224–225
  gastrointestinal involvement, 230–231
  imaging, 225–226
    see also specific imaging methods
  interstitial oedematous pancreatitis, 226–227, 226*f*–227*f*
  MRCP, 226, 226*f*
  necrotizing pancreatitis *see* Necrotizing pancreatitis
  pancreatic collections, 227–228
  peripancreatic collections, 227–228
  pseudocysts, 228, 229*f*–230*f*
  US, 225
  vascular complications, 229–230, 230*f*
  walled-off necrosis *see* Walled off necrosis (WON), acute pancreatitis
Acute Pancreatitis Classification Group, 224–225

Acute peripancreatic fluid collections (APFC), 227–228
Acute pyelonephritis (APN), 261–266
  CT, 258*f*, 262–263, 263*f*–264*f*
  Doppler US, 262
  haematogenous seeding, 261–262
  intravenous urography, 262
  MRI, 263–264, 265*f*
  paediatric, 261–262
  renal scintigraphy, 264–266
  US, 262
  vesicoureteric reflux, 261
Acute rejection
  renal transplantation, 321
Acute tubular necrosis (ATN)
  paediatric, 261–262
  renal transplantation, 319, 321
Adaptive statistical iterative reconstruction (ASIR), CT, 301
Addison's disease (adrenal hypofunction), 464–466, 464*f*, 466*f*
  causes, 465*t*
    acquired causes, 464
    autoimmune disease, 464
  contrast-enhanced MRI, 464
  primary adrenal hypofunction, 464–466
  secondary, 466
Adenitis, mesenteric, 80–81
Adenocarcinoma
  bladder cancer, 350–351, 352*f*
  Helicobacter pylori infection, 41
  oesophagus, 28
  small intestine, 76–78, 78*f*
Adenoma
  adrenal glands, 443
  gallbladder cholesterol polyps *vs.*, 202–203, 203*f*
  large intestine, 93
  liver *see* Hepatic adenoma
  malignancy, 93–94
  nephrogenic, 353
  periampullary, duodenum, 66, 67*f*
Adenomatous polyps, 48
  small intestine, 80
Adenomyomatous hyperplasia, gallbladder, 202, 203*f*
Adenomyosis, 411–412
  MRI, 412, 413*f*
  US, 412, 412*f*
ADPKD *see* Autosomal dominant polycystic kidney disease (ADPKD)
ADPKD (adult polycystic kidney disease), 308
Adrenal gland(s), 441–468
  adenoma, 443
  CT, 441, 442*t*
  functional disorders, 453–466
    adrenal medullary hyperplasia, 462, 462*f*
    ganglioneuroblastoma, 462–464, 463*f*
    hyperfunctioning disorders, 459–464

Pseudomonas aeruginosa infection
acute epididymitis, 380
Pseudomyxoma peritonei, 129
Pseudo-obstruction, large-bowel
obstruction, 9
Psoas muscle hypertrophy, 287
PTC *see* Percutaneous transhepatic
cholangiography (PTC)
PTLD (post-transplantation
lymphoproliferative disorder),
325
PUNLMP (papillary urothelial neoplasms
of low malignant potential),
337
PUV *see* Posterior urethral valves (PUV)
Pyelography, retrograde *see* Retrograde
pyelography
Pyelonephritis
acute *see* Acute pyelonephritis (APN)
acute focal, 309
emphysematous *see* Emphysematous
pyelonephritis
Pyelonephrosis, 270
chronic, 270–271, 271f–272f
CT, 270, 270f
MRI, 270, 271f
Pyloroplasty, 59
Pylorus, stomach, 36
Pyosalpinx, 415–416, 416f

Q

Quality control, CT urography, 333

R

Radiation dose issues
CT, 15–16
urinary tract CT, 301
urinary tract IVU, 300–301
urinary tract radiography, 300
Radiation dose optimisation, CT urography,
333
Radiation enteritis, chronic, 82, 82f
Radical nephroureterectomy, open, 331
Radical prostatectomy (RP), 367
Radical radiotherapy, oesophageal cancer
treatment, 27, 29f
Radiofrequency ablation (RFA)
oesophageal endoscopy, 21–22
Radiography
plain abdominal *see* Plain abdominal
radiograph
Radionuclide scintigraphy, 434
Radiotherapy
brachytherapy *see* Brachytherapy
prostate cancer recurrence, 367
RAS *see* Renal artery stenosis (RAS)
RCC *see* Renal cell carcinoma (RCC)
RECIST (response evaluation criteria in
solid tumours), 349, 350f
Rectal cancer, 99–100
endorectal US, 93f, 100
MRI, 100
nodal staging, 100
PET-CT, 100
resection, 99–100
transanal endoscopic microsurgery, 100
Rectorectal lesions, 113, 113f, 113t
Rectovaginal septum, 90–91
Rectum, 90–91
anatomy, 90
lymphatic vessels, 90
mesorectal fascia, 90–91, 91f
Recurrent pyogenic cholangitis (RPC),
211–212, 212f

Reflux oesophagitis, gastro-oesophageal
reflux disease, 31, 31f
Regional lymphadenectomy, 331–332
Regions of interest (ROI), adrenal mass
MRI, 447
Rejection, acute *see* Acute rejection
Renal abscesses, 266, 309, 309f
CT, 266
DWI-MRI, 266, 267f–268f
US, 266, 266f
Renal agnesis, 283
Renal artery
occlusion, 432f
stenosis *see* Renal artery stenosis (RAS)
Renal artery stenosis (RAS), 431–432, 432f
renal transplantation, 324–325, 324f
Renal calculi
renal transplantation, 323f, 324
Renal calyces, 282
Renal cancer *see* Renal masses
Renal cell carcinoma (RCC), 311–313
angiography, 313
chromophobe tumours, 312, 314f
clear cell carcinoma, 311, 312f
CT, 255f, 314f
staging, 314, 315f
MRI, 299, 299f, 313
papillary tumours, 312, 313f
radiography, 293
staging, 313–315
Renal cyst(s), 306–308
adult polycystic kidney disease, 308
complicated cysts, 307–308, 307f
hydatid cysts, 308
localised cystic disease, 308
multicystic renal dysplasia, 308
parapelvic cysts, 308
peripelvic cysts, 308
serous cysts, 306–307
Renal dysplasia, multicystic, 308
Renal ectopia
crossed fused ectopic *see* Cross fused renal
ectopia
Renal failure, 259–261
acquired cystic kidney disease, 260
autosomal dominant polycystic kidney
disease, 260
chronic *see* Chronic renal failure
contrast medium-induced nephrotoxicity,
261
CT, 259–260
MRI, 259–260
nephrogenic systemic fibrosis, 261
non-focal biopsy, 260
obstruction, 259–260
renal size, 260
renovascular disease, 260–261
tuberous sclerosis, 260
US, 259
Renal masses, 305–318
arteriography, 306
CT, 305, 306f
cysts *see* Renal cyst(s)
intravenous urography, 305
malignant neoplasms, 311–317
non-parenchymal, 316–317
parenchymal, 311–316
see also specific diseases/disorders
MRI, 305–306
multislice CT, 305
needle aspiration and biopsy, 306
neoplastic, 311–317
benign, 311
non-neoplastic, 306
parenchymal malignant, 311–316
parenchymal tumour, 297, 297f

pathological, 306–311
angiomyolipomas *see* Angiomyolipoma
focal hydronephrosis, 311
inflammatory masses, 309
non-renal masses, 311
renal sinus lipomatosis, 311
vascular masses, 309–310
see also specific types
plain abdominal radiography, 305
radionuclide imaging, 305
US, 305
see also Renal cell carcinoma (RCC)
Renal parenchyma fragmentation, 432
Renal parenchymal tumour, 297, 297f
Renal pelvic dilatation (RPD) *see*
Hydronephrosis
Renal pelvis
congenital abnormalities, 286–288
trauma, 430–431, 432f
Renal sinus lipomatosis, 282, 311
Renal stones, 253, 253f–254f
haematuria *see* Haematuria
Renal tract calcification, haematuria,
252–253
Renal transplantation, 319–329
biopsy, 328, 328f–329f
donor kidney evaluation, 328–329
CT, 328
DMSA scan, 328
dynamic MRI, 329
US, 328
historical aspects, 319
imaging techniques, 319–320
colour flow US, 320
CT, 320
cystogram, 320, 320f
Doppler US, 319
MRA, 320
MRI, 320
steady-state free precision MRA, 320
time-of-flight MRI, 320
US, 319, 320f
isotope scans, 326–328
MAG3 renography, 327
nonvascular complications, 321–324
false aneurysm, 325f
fluid collection, 321f–322f
hydronephrosis, 323
lymphocoele, 322f–323f, 323
MRI, 322f
postoperative haematoma, 322f
renal calculi, 323f, 324
ureteric strictures, 323, 323f
urinoma, 322–323, 322f
rejection *vs.* acute tubular necrosis, 319
surgical techniques, 319
vascular complications, 321, 324–326
acute rejection, 321
acute tubular necrosis, 321
cancer, 325, 325f–327f
chronic rejection, 325, 326f
infarction, 321, 324f
infection, 326, 327f
renal artery stenosis, 324–325, 324f
Renal trauma, 425–434
active bleeding, 430, 430f–431f
clinical aspects, 425–426
collecting system injury, 429–430, 430f
congenital anomalies, 425
CT, 425–427, 426f
grade I, 427–429
grade II, 427–429
grade III, 427–429
grade IV, 429–431, 429f
grade V injury, 431–432, 432f
grading, 427, 427t

Printed in the United States
By Bookmasters